The Brain Adapting with Pain

Contribution of Neuroimaging Technology to Pain Mechanisms

The Brain Adapting with Pain

Contribution of Neuroimaging Technology to Pain Mechanisms

The Brain Adapting with Pain

Contribution of Neuroimaging Technology to Pain Mechanisms

Editor

A. Vania Apkarian, PhD

Professor, Department of Physiology
Northwestern University
Feinberg School of Medicine
Chicago, Illinois

Wolters Kluwer

Philadelphia • Baltimore • New York • London
Buenos Aires • Hong Kong • Sydney • Tokyo

International Association for the Study of Pain
IASP®
Working together for pain relief

Acquisitions Editor: Keith Donnellan
Product Development Editor: Nicole Dernoski
Editorial Assistant: Kathryn Leyendecker
Production Project Manager: Marian Bellus
Design Coordinator: Joan Wendt
Manufacturing Coordinator: Beth Welsh
Marketing Manager: Dan Dressler
Prepress Vendor: S4Carlisle Publishing Services

9 8 7 6 5 4 3 2 1

Printed in China

Library of Congress Cataloging-in-Publication Data

The brain adapting with pain : contribution of neuroimaging technology to pain mechanisms / [edited by] A. Vania Apkarian. — First edition.
p. ; cm.
Includes bibliographical references.
ISBN 978-1-4963-1749-0
I. Apkarian, A. V., editor.
[DNLM: 1. Pain—physiopathology. 2. Brain—physiopathology. 3. Functional Neuroimaging—trends. WL 704]
RC368
616'.0472—dc23

2015000734

LWW.com

CCS0615

CONTRIBUTORS

A. Vania Apkarian, PhD
Professor
Department of Physiology
Northwestern University
Feinberg School of Medicine
Chicago, Illinois

Qasim Aziz, MD, PhD
Professor
Centre for Digestive Diseases
Blizard Institute
Wingate Institute for Neurogastroenterology
Barts and the London School of Medicine and Dentistry
Queen Mary University of London
London, United Kingdom

Marwan N. Baliki, PhD
Research Scientist
Department of Physiology
Northwestern University School of Medicine
Chicago, Illinois

Alexis T. Baria, PhD
Post-Doctoral Fellow
National Institute of Neurological Disorders and Stroke
National Institutes of Health
Bethesda, Maryland

Ulf Baumgärtner, MD, PhD
Chair of Neurophysiology
University of Heidelberg
Department of Neurophysiology
Center for Biomedicine and Medical Technology Mannheim
Heidelberg University
Mannheim, Germany

Lino Becerra, PhD
Professor
Center for Pain and the Brain
Boston Children's Hospital
Pain Medicine Division
Boston, Massachusetts

Ulrike Bingel, MD
Professor
Department of Neurology
University Hospital Essen
University Duisberg-Essen
Essen, Germany

David Borsook, MD, PhD
Professor
Anesthesia, Perioperative & Pain Medicine
Boston Children's at Waltham
Center for Pain and the Brain
Boston Children's Hospital
Pain Medicine Division
Waltham, Massachusetts

Christian Büchel, MD
Professor
Department of Systems Neuroscience
University Medical Center Hamburg-Eppendorf
Hamburg, Germany

Rami Burstein, PhD
Professor
P.A.I.N. Group, Boston Children's Hospital
Massachusetts General Hospital and McLean Hospital
Harvard Medical School and Department of Anesthesia, Critical Care, and Pain Medicine
Boston Children's Hospital
Boston, Massachusetts

Kenneth L. Casey, MD
Professor Emeritus/A of Neurology
Professor Emeritus of Molecular and Integrative Physiology
University of Michigan
Ann Arbor, Michigan

Franco Cauda, PhD
Professor
CCS fMRI, Koelliker Hospital and Department of Psychology
Functional Neuroimaging and Complex Systems Group
Department of Psychology
University of Turin
Turin, Italy

Guillermo Cecchi, PhD
Research Staff Member
Biometaphorical Computing
IBM Thomas J. Watson Research Center
Yorktown Heights, New York

Li Min Chen, MD, PhD
Assistant Professor of Radiology and Radiological Sciences
Vanderbilt University
School of Medicine
Nashville, Tennessee

J. J. Cheng, MD
Assistant Resident
Department of Neurosurgery
Johns Hopkins Hospital
Baltimore, Maryland

J. H. Chien, MS, PhD
Research Study Coordinator and Post-Doctoral Fellow
Department of Neurosurgery
Johns Hopkins Hospital
Baltimore, Maryland

Robert C. Coghill, PhD
Senior Scientist and Director of Research
Department of Anesthesiology
Cincinnati Children's Hospital
Cincinnati, Ohio

Camilo Diaz Cruz, MD
Pre-Doctoral Fellow
Spaulding Center of Neuromodulation
Spaulding Rehabilitation Hospital
Harvard Medical School
Boston, Massachusetts

Karen D. Davis, PhD
Professor
Department of Brain, Imaging and Behaviour
Toronto Western Research Institute
University Health Network
Institute of Medical Science and Department of Surgery
University of Toronto
Toronto, Canada

Flavia Di Pietro, PhD
Pre-Doctoral Fellow
Neuroscience Research Australia
Sydney, Australia
University of New South Wales
New South Wales, Australia

Melissa A. Farmer, PhD
Research Scientist
Department of Physiology
Feinberg School of Medicine
Northwestern University
Chicago, Illinois

Herta Flor, MD, PhD
Professor
Department of Cognitive and Clinical Neuroscience
Central Institute of Mental Health
Medical Faculty Mannheim
Heidelberg University
Mannheim, Germany

Felipe Fregni, MD, PhD, MPH
Director
Spaulding Center of Neuromodulation
Spaulding Rehabilitation Hospital
Associate Professor of Neurology and Physical Medicine and Rehabilitation
Harvard Medical School
Boston, Massachusetts

Randy L. Gollub, MD, PhD
Associate Director
Psychiatric Neuroimaging
Psychiatric Research Program
Associate Professor,
Department of Psychiatry
Massachusetts General Hospital
Harvard Medical School
Charlestown, Massachusetts

J. D. Greenspan, PhD
Professor and Chair
Department of Neural and Pain Sciences
University of Maryland School of Dentistry
Professor and Chair of the Department of Neural and Pain Sciences
Baltimore, Maryland

Arpana Gupta, PhD
Post-Doctoral Researcher, Ingestive Behavior and Obesity Program
Oppenheimer Center for Neurobiology of Stress
Departments of Medicine, Physiology, and Psychiatry
UCLA, CURE Digestive Diseases Research Center
UCLA Division of Digestive Diseases
Los Angeles, California

Biyu J. He, PhD
Independent Investigator
National Institutes of Neurological Disorders and Stroke
National Institutes of Health
Bethesda, Maryland

Catherine S. Hubbard, PhD
Post-Doctoral Research Fellow
Department of Neural and Pain Sciences
University of Maryland School of Medicine
Baltimore, Maryland

G. D. Iannetti, MD, PhD
Professor
Department of Neuroscience, Physiology and Pharmacology
University College London
London, United Kingdom

J. H. Kim, MD, PhD
Professor
Department of Neurosurgery
Johns Hopkins Hospital
Baltimore, Maryland

Jian Kong, MB, MS, MPh
Associate Professor
Psychiatric Neuroimaging
Psychiatric Research Program
Department of Psychiatry
Massachusetts General Hospital
Harvard Medical School
Charlestown, Massachusetts

Jean-Pascal Lefaucheur, MD, PhD
Faculty of Medicine
Universite Paris Est Creteil
Service de Physiologie
Explorations Fonctionnelles
Henri Mondor Hospital
Assistance Publique
Hopitaux de Paris
Creitel, France

F. A. Lenz, MD, PhD
Professor
Department of Neurosurgery
Johns Hopkins Hospital
Baltimore, Maryland

C. C. Liu, PhD
Assistant Professor
Department of Neurosurgery
Johns Hopkins Hospital
Baltimore, Maryland

Martin Lotze, MD
Professor
Functional Imaging
Center for Diagnostic Radiology and Neuroradiology
University of Greifswald
Greifswald, Germany

Radi Masri, DDS, MS, PhD
Associate Professor
Department of Endodontics Prosthodontics and Operative Dentistry
University of Maryland School of Dentistry
Department of Anatomy and Neurobiology and Program in Neuroscience
University of Maryland School of Medicine
Baltimore, Maryland

Arne May, MD
Assistant Professor
Institute for Systems Neuroscience
Hamburg University
Hamburg, Germany

Emeran A. Mayer, MD, PhD
Director
Oppenheimer Center for Neurobiology of Stress
Professor, Department of Medicine, Physiology, and Psychiatry
UCLA, CURE Digestive Diseases Research Center
UCLA Division of Digestive Diseases
Los Angeles, California

Melvin Mezue, BSc
Pre-Doctoral Fellow
Oxford Centre for Functional Magnetic Resonance Imaging of the Brain
Nuffield Division of Anaesthetics
Nuffield Department of Clinical Neurosciences
University of Oxford
England, United Kingdom

Massieh Moayedi, PhD, BSc
Post-Doctoral Fellow
Department of Brain, Imaging and Behaviour
Toronto Western Research Institute
University Health Network
Institute of Medical Science
University of Toronto
Toronto, Canada
Department of Neuroscience, Physiology and Pharmacology
Division of Biosciences
University College London
London, United Kingdom

Jeffrey S. Mogil, PhD
EP Taylor Professor of Pain Studies Canada Research Chair in the Genetics of Pain (Tier I)
Department of Psychology and Alan Edwards Centre for the Study of Pain
McGill University
Montreal, Quebec, Canada

A. Mouraux, MD, PhD
Professor
Institute of Neurosciences (IoNS)
Catholic University of Louvain
Brussels, Belgium

Vitaly Napadow, PhD LicAc
Associate Professor
Martinos Center for Biomedical Imaging
Massachusetts General Hospital
Harvard Medical School
Charlestown, Massachusetts

Yasser Al Omran, BSc (Hons)
Pre-Doctoral Fellow
Centre for Digestive Diseases
Blizard Institute
Wingate Institute for Neurogastroenterology
Barts and the London School of Medicine and Dentistry
Queen Mary University of London
London, United Kingdom

Todd Parrish, PhD
Professor of Radiology
Northwestern University
Feinberg School of Medicine
Chicago, Illinois

Markus Ploner, PhD
Research Group Leader and Consultant Neurologist
Department of Neurology
Department of Neurology and TUM-Neuroimaging Center
Technical University of Munich
Munich, Germany

Tobias Schmidt-Wilcke, PhD
Professor
Department of Neurology
Berufsgenossenschaftliches Universitatsklinikum Bergmannsheil
Ruhr University Bochum
Bochum, Germany

David A. Seminowicz, PhD
Assistant Professor
Department of Neural and Pain Sciences
University of Maryland School of Medicine
Baltimore, Maryland

Christian Sprenger, MD
Professor
Department of Systems Neuroscience
University Medical Center Hamburg-Eppendorf
Hamburg, Germany

Diana M. Torta, PhD
Pre-Doctoral Fellow
CCS fMRI, Koelliker Hospital and Department of Psychology, Functional Neuroimaging and Complex Systems Group
Department of Psychology
University of Turin
Turin, Italy
Institute of Neuroscience (IoNS)
Universite Catholique de Louvain
Brussels, Belgium

Irene Tracey, PhD
Professor
Oxford Centre for Functional Magnetic Resonance Imaging of the Brain
Nuffield Division of Anaesthetics
Nuffield Department of Clinical Neurosciences
University of Oxford
England, United Kingdom

Rolf-Detlef Treede, PhD
Chair of Neurophysiology
Medicine Faculty at Mannheim
Department of Neurophysiology
Center for Biomedicine and Medical Technology Mannheim
Heidelberg University
Mannheim, Germany

Jaymin Upadhyay, PhD
Post-Doctoral Fellow
Center for Pain and the Brain
Boston Children's Hospital
Pain Medicine Division
Waltham, Massachusetts

Tor D. Wager, PhD
Associate Professor
Department of Psychology and Neuroscience
University of Colorado, Boulder
Boulder, Colorado

PREFACE

This book is a collection of chapters written by leading scientists in the field who volunteered to create this body of knowledge. It is an effort to convey the latest ideas percolating in the field of pain and brain imaging, with the dual intention of covering the state of our understanding as well as raising critical questions that remain to be addressed. Many of the chapters are coauthored by scientists that I thought held diverging views on the specific subject. This perhaps delayed completion of the project. However, I also hope it made the chapters more critical, with serious attempts of either highlighting or reconciling differences of opinion.

Based on the simplistic metric of the number of papers published in the topic, brain imaging in relation to pain has had a huge impact. As of May 2014, a PubMed search for "pain" AND "neuroimaging" yields more than 31,000 papers. On the other hand, performing the same PubMed search for the years 2006–2010 or for 2010–2014 yields almost exactly the same number of papers. Thus, the field also seems to have reached a mature steady state. Note that the field did not even exist prior to 1990. With this scale of explosion of science, one wonders what can be covered within the bounds of a book. Given the existence of many very high-quality reviews in the specific subjects tackled here, each chapter in this book attempts to convey briefly where the field stands and where it is going. The chapters are intended to include minimal jargon and yet be substantive, hoping to appeal to the next-generation scientists as well as to clinicians who feel the urge to follow and interpret the brain imaging knowledge to themselves and to their patients. After all, despite repeated pronouncements of disclaimers by many authors throughout this book, objective brain markers of acute and chronic pain are at least on the horizon if not here already, and we must seriously contemplate the use of this information in bettering pain treatment/management.

The research endeavour addressed here has dramatically changed our notions in both the fields of pain and the brain. There is little doubt that our ability to peer within the human brain, and scrutinize the human brain for myriads of clinical pain conditions, has and will continue to hone our concepts regarding mechanisms of pain. At the same time, the painful brain has provided intriguing new information about the adaptability of the brain that can be identified and tracked at the gross macroscopic level. Along these lines, the title of this book is intended to suggest the fundamental novel achievement of the field, namely, that pain and the brain dynamically interact with each other and shape, carve, and predict each other. Over the last 10 years, this notion has been firmly established, yet its details and specifics remain to be understood in future studies, especially from cellular and molecular mechanistic viewpoints. The book makes a concerted effort both to cover the historical past and to contemplate the possible future directions, given what has been achieved in the last 20 years. I characterize the first 10 years of MRI-based brain imaging as an effort to establish the existence of pain-related signals in the human brain, the second decade as pursuing ways to differentiate between pain conditions and establishing the modulatory properties of cognitive states on brain responses to pain; all of it embedded strongly within the Cartesian notion of the brain as real estate dedicated to solving specific problems. I envision that the current, third, decade in the topic is moving in very exciting new directions where the dynamics of information processing is being pursued, based on notions of the brain as a highly interconnected, inter-related, network. These notions are built upon both theoretical and technological foundations that this book attempts to cover extensively. The book also attempts to present the brain MRI-based technology together with the electrical and magnetic methodologies, at least implicitly emphasizing the complementarity of these approaches, with the continued hope that the approaches would become fully mature only when they smoothly merge with each other. Perhaps my prejudice emerges most blatantly by the clear separation that I have imposed between topics in relation to acute in contrast to chronic pain. Additionally, the limited number of chapters dedicated to animal neuroimaging highlights the fact that this direction of research remains in its infancy, and far more development will be necessary to reach its potential influence on the science of pain.

Unravelling scientific rules behind perception remains the Holy Grail of all of neuroscience, and current concepts regarding perception across all sensory modalities remain as mysterious today as it did in the days of Plato and Aristotle. Yet I remain confident and hopeful that the field of brain imaging of pain will play a critical role in this endeavour, if we are ever to crack this nut.

As with any communal project, the sum total is far more exciting than the individual parts. Given that a large number of leading scientists in the field participated in creating this book, I am forever indebted to them all. There are missing topics, and I would have loved for us to pursue additional relevant subjects, but limits of time and space that dog academic life constrained the project. Still, I take full responsibility for what is amiss or inadequate, and wholeheartedly thank participant authors.

If there is a single overarching idea that I hope this book would impart to the reader, it can be summarized by one of my favourite lines by the philosopher Jerry Fodor: "There is plenty of tunnel at the end of the light."

A. Vania Apkarian

ACKNOWLEDGEMENT

I would like to thank the members of my laboratory for their reading of many of the chapters of this book and their suggestions regarding editing many of those chapters. Special thanks go to Melissa A. Farmer, Don Davis, and Charents Apkarian for their editorial help. It is important to emphasize that the book is a compilation of work by many scientists researching the topic in different directions, and their participation is highly appreciated. Moreover, the book is a reflection of brain imaging studies that require the participation of many volunteers, healthy or otherwise, who have given time and often suffered painful stimuli applied to diverse body parts, with the conviction that this effort will advance science and decrease future suffering from pain. Thus, I also want to specifically thank all the volunteers who took part in the studies reviewed in the book, and hope that the book can be a testimonial of their aspirations regarding advancing the science of pain.

CONTENTS

SECTION THREE Technology: Animal Neuroimaging

SECTION FOUR Acute Pain

SECTION FIVE Neuroplasticity and Chronic Pain

SECTION SIX The Brain Adapting with Chronic Pain

SECTION 1

Historical Overview

CHAPTER 1

Brain Imaging and Pain: A Historical Perspective

Kenneth L. Casey

Anatomical and functional brain imaging has had a profound and indelible effect on the conceptual models of pain mechanisms that guide experiments, diagnosis, and treatment. These conceptual models are seldom articulated explicitly, but there is little doubt that they influence research and clinical practice. A background theme of this historical perspective is that technology, in this case making the living brain visible, drives the theory behind conceptual models. In physics, it seems that theory most often drives technology. For example, we have the Large Hadron Collider to test the theory that predicted the Higgs boson. We do not have a similar example in the neurosciences where the reverse order of influence seems to apply more often.

Each stage in the development of modern brain imaging was not accompanied by an explicit annunciation of some new theory of pain mechanisms. Rather, as documented recently by Moayedi and Davis [81] and by Perl [86], theories and ideas about pain evolve gradually as new information becomes available. Here, I suggest how advancements in brain imaging laid the foundation for changes in the conceptual models of pain that are evolving among clinicians and researchers today.

THE LIVING BRAIN WAS INVISIBLE

Consequences for Theory

The invisibility of the living brain persisted through the 1970s and influenced the range of thinking about brain function, including concepts of pain mechanisms. Most of the information we had about human pain mechanisms was derived from descriptions of the clinical presentation of patients and, if available, the examination of biopsy or postmortem specimens of peripheral or central nervous system tissue. From these clinical reports, it was clear that thalamocortical structures receiving direct or transsynaptic input from the spinothalamic tract were critical for pain; however, the reports typically lacked critical anatomical and neurological examination details [51, 74, 104]. Even after it became clear that somatic and visceral tissues are innervated by specialized nociceptors that encode impending or actual tissue damage [9, 19, 26], the lack of information about how this input was processed at the spinal and supraspinal levels allowed us only to speculate about the central mechanisms mediating the pain experience. A major debate has been about the degree to which the physiological specificity of nociceptors is preserved as sensory afferent information is transmitted to those central neurons mediating pain. One form of this debate has been referred to as "pattern versus specificity." The term "labelled line" has been used to represent the view that pain results only from the activation of central pathways and brain structures with responses that closely mimic the physiological properties of peripheral nociceptors [34]. Pattern theories, as described before the characterization of physiologically specific nociceptors [112, 119], have been largely replaced by hypotheses emphasizing the integration of nociceptive and nonnociceptive information among central neurons mediating various components of pain [77, 96, 98], defined by the International Association for the Study of Pain (IASP) as: "An unpleasant sensory and emotional experience associated with actual or potential tissue damage, or described in terms of such damage" [78]. In essence, the discussion centres around the degree to which the concept of distributed parallel processing applies to pain [30, 43, 79, 80, 101]. This brief review will show that the results of anatomical and functional brain imaging have eclipsed the old "pattern versus specificity" debate.

Another major concept left in the shadow of the invisible brain was the modulation of pain by various brain functions, including hedonic* and cognitive processes long considered "psychological" and therefore somehow removed from neurophysiology. The prevailing concepts of pain mechanisms began to change when the living brain became visible.

Consequences for Practice

The invisibility of the living brain had consequences for the practice of medicine. Physicians in training before the 1980s would be taught how to superimpose two images of a skull X-ray acquired in 3-D mode, thus allowing one to view a beautiful stereoscopic rendering of an empty skull. If a calcified pineal gland was present, one could determine whether the brain was displaced from the midline. Depending on the clinical presentation, the patient might be moved to the angiography suite, where a large-bore needle was inserted into the carotid artery for the injection of liquid contrast material, thus allowing X-ray visualization of the intracranial vasculature. Alternatively, a pneumoencephalogram could be performed by forcefully injecting about 50 cc of air into the spinal intrathecal space and thence into the brain ventricular system and subarachnoid space. Of course, the detection of abnormalities of internal brain structure was out of the question. Except as observed through a small skull opening in the neurosurgery suite, the living brain was invisible, leading to the execution of the very risky, highly unpleasant procedures described above. The reported successes of spinothalamic tractotomy reinforced the "labelled line" concept and led to the practice of conducting several types of central ablative procedures for the relief of pain [69, 120]; most of these had very limited success and sometimes substantial risks and long-term complications.

THE LIVING BRAIN BECOMES VISIBLE

Shortly before the structure of the living brain became visible, radioactive tracer and labelling methods were developed to detect intracranial vascular changes that accompanied normal brain activity or focal pathological conditions. In 1890, Roy and Sherrington [103] demonstrated that a product of brain metabolism increased regional cerebral blood volume

* From definition 1b of *Webster's third new international dictionary (unabridged)*, Springfield, MA; 1971: "Involving the psychological range of feelings from pleasant to unpleasant."

in the dog or rabbit. The subsequent development of clinical and experimental evidence linking regional cerebral blood flow (rCBF) to local synaptic activity has been reviewed recently [69, 99]. On the basis of the evidence then available, Ingvar and Risberg [57], using ^{133}Xenon and the intracarotid injection method developed by Lassen et al. [66], were able to detect hemispheric grey matter (cortical) rCBF increases of 5–8% in the suprasylvian area of human volunteers and patients as they performed a reverse digit span task. This result contrasted with the earlier negative study of Sokoloff et al. [113], who used the nitrous oxide inhalation method for estimating global CBF changes during mental arithmetic. The study by Ingvar and Risberg thus represents a major advance in the localization of cognitive brain function, although the location of the rCBF changes had to be plotted on bony landmarks of skull X-rays because the living brain was still invisible.

The Development of Computerized Tomography

In 1961, William H. Oldendorf, a neurologist at the UCLA-affiliated West Los Angeles VA Medical Center, first demonstrated the feasibility of radiologically detecting structures behind the skull barrier by constructing a home-made apparatus using ^{131}I as a gamma ray source (Fig. 1-1). Oldendorf obtained patent protection for this device, but was unable to secure the interest of the radiological industry because, according to Oldendorf's [84] review of this history, the manufacture of such a device "... would result in nothing but a

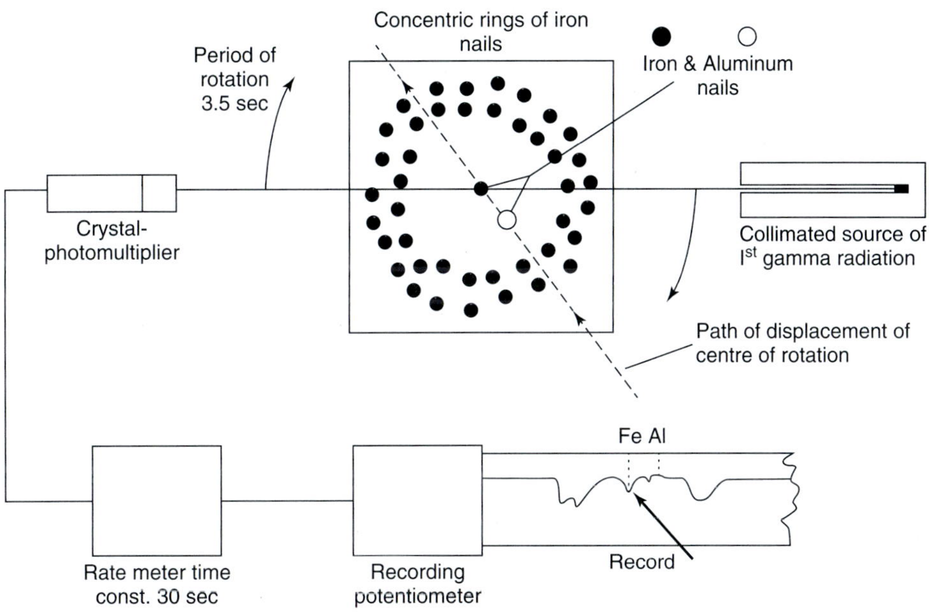

FIGURE 1-1 Diagram of Oldendorf's apparatus for demonstrating a radiological method for detecting structures of different radiodensities behind a barrier. An iron and an aluminium nail were placed inside a circular barrier of iron nails, and the whole assembly was rotated on a phonograph turntable while being pulled along a toy railroad track by an alarm clock motor. The combined motion along the path of displacement (labelled) allowed only the inner two nails to remain equidistant from the radiation source during the experiment. Radioactive counts were picked up by the crystal photomultiplier and fed to the integrating rate meter with the output displayed on a recorder. The diagrammed recording shows the deflections caused by the barrier ("skull") nails on each side of the two deflections caused by the inner iron (Fe) and aluminium (Al) nails, which have different radiodensities (*bold arrow* added). (From Oldendorf [84].)

radiographic cross-section of brain." Given the technology of the time, it was not possible to pursue this concept further.

It remained for Godfrey Hounsfield, a computer engineer at EMI Ltd., and Allan Cormack, a radiation biophysicist, to develop the mathematical foundation for, and practical development of, the computerized tomographic (CT) scanner and share the 1979 Nobel Prize in Medicine and Physiology [33, 52, 53]. In his Nobel lecture, Hounsfield cites the pioneering work of Oldendorf; indeed, the description of Hounsfield's early experiments shows Oldendorf's influence. Oldendorf was not included in the Nobel Prize award.

With the development of the CT scanner, the living brain became visible. Clinicians and researchers could then begin to identify brain locations associated with estimates of brain function, including pain, from living individuals and groups. It soon became clear that brain lesions affecting pain also impaired other neurological functions, including somesthesis. Bogousslavsky and colleagues [13] were among the first to use CT in an investigation of 40 patients with focal (lacunar) thalamic infarctions, 18 involving the ventrolateral thalamus with associated hemisensory loss. The sensory loss included tactile, vibratory, and kinesthetic functions in addition to pain and temperature. The observation that these small thalamic infarctions, unlike spinothalamic infarctions (e.g., Wallenberg syndrome) or surgical spinothalamic tractotomies, did not result in a selective loss of pain and temperature sensation, confirmed earlier clinical reports of autopsied cases [38] and could be considered as early evidence for the distribution of thermal and nociceptive information among brain structures with functions that were not limited to the mediation of pain. In addition, central poststroke pain developed in a significant minority of these patients, again confirming earlier autopsy-based reports [36–38, 51] and suggesting the interruption of an endogenous sensory control mechanism. Schmahmann and Leifer [109] used CT to study six patients with central pain and sensory loss following stroke or trauma involving the parietal lobe ("pseudothalamic" pain). All but one of these patients had impaired somesthetic discriminative function in addition to hypalgesia and hypothermesthesia. The common lesion was not in the cortex but in the white matter deep to the posterior insula and the rostral posterior parietal cortex, including secondary somatosensory cortex (S2), and the cortex of the inferior parietal lobule. The authors suggested that the central pain in their patients might be attributed to a thalamocortical disconnection syndrome. Cohen and colleagues [32] conducted a CT and neuropsychological pre- and postoperative study of patients with bilateral stereotactic focal cingulotomy for chronic, intractable pain. They observed that 66% of their patients gave postoperative pain ratings that were moderately but significantly lower and reported a robust reduction of the negative hedonic or affective component of their pain.

The Development of Magnetic Resonance Imaging

CT did not monopolize brain imaging for long because magnetic resonance imaging (MRI) of the brain soon developed [62] and has since dominated the combination of anatomical brain imaging and clinical correlation. Bassetti and colleagues used both CT and MRI to characterize the clinical presentation of 20 patients with parietal lobe strokes. Ten of their patients had "pseudothalamic syndrome" with tactile, pinprick, and thermal sensory impairment; none had central pain. Similar to the observations of Schmahmann and Leifer, the common lesion affected the white matter underlying the parietal operculum (including S2 cortex), posterior insula, and inferior parietal lobule; however, the cortex of these areas was also involved. Greenspan and colleagues [48] used MRI anatomical analysis and psychophysical testing in a study of six patients with lesions involving the parasylvian cortex. Three patients with destruction of the posterior insula and posterior parietal operculum had impaired innocuous tactile and thermal sensation in addition to elevated mechanical and thermal pain thresholds. The three patients with sparing of these areas did not show these deficits, although one with involvement limited to the posterior insula had a markedly increased cold pain tolerance. Cereda and colleagues [25] conducted an MRI and clinical examination study of four patients with infarctions confined to the insular cortex. One patient with a lesion confined to the posterior insula had no clinically detectable sensory deficit. The remaining three patients all had impaired tactile, thermal, and painful pinprick sensations; some patients had gustatory, vestibular, and language disturbances also. Other MRI-based anatomical–clinical correlations confirmed earlier reports [7, 39, 56] that surgical cingulotomy provides relief from chronic pain in a majority of selected patients [50, 93, 122, 123]; however, the effects of cingulotomy included attenuated affective and attentional aspects of pain, consistent with the findings of Cohen and colleagues (see above). Ploner and colleagues [94] had the unusual opportunity to provide evidence that an unpleasant affective experience is an integral part of pain and not simply a secondary feature that follows some hedonically neutral nociceptive detection. A patient with an infarction confined, on MRI analysis, to the S1 and S2 hand area of the postcentral gyrus had contralaterally impaired tactile, kinesthetic, and absent thermal sensations. Noxious infrared laser stimulation of the involved hand at over twice the pain threshold of the normal hand failed to evoke any sensation except for a "... 'clearly unpleasant' intensity dependent feeling ... (that the subject) ... wanted to avoid [94, p. 213] arising from somewhere in the arm." In a related magnetoencephalographic study of normal subjects, these investigators demonstrated that the contralateral S1 and S2 cortices are activated simultaneously by noxious laser stimulation [95].

The above sample of anatomical–clinical correlation studies began to modify significantly a simple phrenological model of pain mechanisms by showing that nociceptive information is distributed to brain areas that participate in sensory and neurological functions other than pain, and that some act in parallel to mediate both the discriminative and affective components of acute pain. In addition, the combined psychophysical and MRI study of 73 patients with central poststroke pain by Bowsher et al. [15] confirmed earlier reports [24] that the critical lesion for central pain also impaired pain perception and could be located anywhere along the neuraxis; this again provided evidence for an endogenous pain-activated control mechanism.

The Contribution of Electrophysiology and Optical Imaging

Throughout the period preceding and during the development of imaging technology, pain mechanisms were investigated by comparing the electrical responses of single or small groups of neurons to innocuous and noxious stimuli in anesthetized and, occasionally, awake animals. The number and diversity of these electrophysiological studies is far too great to include in this historical perspective. However, two major findings are relevant here: (1) central neurons responsive to noxious stimuli do so either exclusively (NS or nociceptive specific responses) or differentially, with a greater response to noxious than to innocuous stimuli (WDR or wide dynamic range responses); and (2) central neurons with either or both of these nociresponsive properties are found among a wide variety of brainstem and brain structures, including, but not limited to, those discussed above.

For example, nociresponsive cells are found in the dorsal, medial, and ventral grey matter of the spinal cord, the reticular formation and periaqueductal grey matter, basal ganglia, amygdala, medial and lateral thalamic nuclei, hypothalamus, hippocampus, cingulate gyrus, insula, and the primary and secondary somatosensory cortices. The divergence and convergence revealed by the results of these electrophysiological studies are consistent with the distribution of nociceptive information among brain structures mediating different aspects of pain. However, the recording of individual cellular responses fails to capture encoding features that may be present within larger clusters of neurons.

The primary somatosensory cortex (S1) has long been known to encode features of somesthesis that include the detection of location, timing, and stimulus intensity. Nociresponsive neurons with these encoding properties have been recorded from areas 3b and 1 of S1 cortex, although in relatively sparse numbers compared with the number of neurons responding to innocuous tactile stimuli [60, 61]. The development of optical imaging of the exposed cortex permitted the investigation of the biophysical and neurovascular responses of clusters of cortical neurons within the confines of cytoarchitecturally defined areas [45, 49]. Tommerdahl and colleagues [116] used the new optical imaging technology to identify, within S1 cortical area 3a, a population of neurons that are responsive exclusively to noxious thermal stimuli in an intensity-dependent manner and have a reciprocally inhibitory interaction with tactile and nociresponsive cells in the adjacent areas 3b and 1. The area 3a nociresponsive neurons reflect the slow, prolonged responses of unmyelinated (C-fibre-innervated) nociceptors in contrast to the rapid, brief responses of area 3b cells to noxious heat pulses, which are characteristic of finely myelinated nociceptive afferents (Aδ fibres) [121]. These observations suggest that this population of S1 neurons provides spatial, temporal, and intensity-dependent information necessary for normal pain perception mediated through unmyelinated C fibres. It is notable that these uniquely nociresponsive neurons are located within the cytoarchitectural boundaries of an area (3a) that responds also to tactile and kinesthetic stimuli and has robust anatomical connections with cortical and thalamic components of motor mechanisms [54]. Together, these observations show that highly specific nociceptive information is distributed within and among functionally diverse brain regions.

THE FUNCTIONAL ACTIVITY OF THE LIVING BRAIN BECOMES VISIBLE

PET Activation Studies

The studies cited above investigated pain mechanisms by focusing on one or very few brain areas or regions at a time. However, with the development of methods for radioisotope scanning of the whole brain [63] and of radiolabelled (^{14}C) deoxyglucose [59] for estimating the metabolic activity of the synaptic neuropil [75, 110], the path was open for investigating the neuronal activity of the whole brain (Fig. 1-2).

Mapping metabolic responses of the human brain to sensory stimulation soon followed the development of positron emission tomography (PET) and the use of intravenous ^{18}F deoxyglucose (FDG) as the radiolabelled agent [92, 102]. In the seminal report by Phelps et al. [92], it was shown that the metabolic response of the visual cortex to a complex stimulus (outdoor park scene) was much greater than that to simpler stimuli, the association cortex response being even more active than the primary visual cortex.

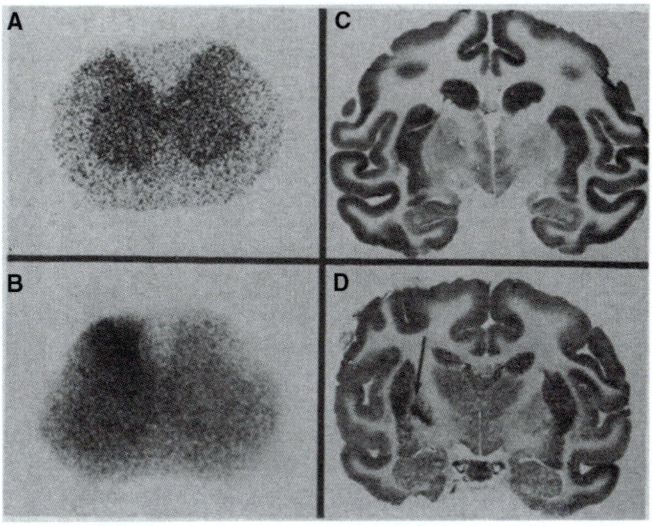

FIGURE 1-2 Autoradiographs of the uptake of ^{14}C deoxyglucose into rat spinal cord at rest **(A)**, rat spinal cord following unilateral (reader's left) electrical stimulation of the sciatic nerve **(B)**, rhesus monkey brain at rest **(C)**, and following unilateral (reader's left) application of penicillin on the motor cortex, resulting in increased activity in the putamen and globus pallidus (*arrow*) **(D)**. (From Kennedy et al. [59].)

The use of intravenous 99m'Tc-exametazime (previously 99m'Tc-HMPAO) as a tracer for single photon emission tomographic (SPECT) studies added further flexibility to the design and conduct of human and animal investigations of activity-related changes in rCBF [67, 68]. The rapid compartmentalization and minimal delayed redistribution of this tracer made it ideal for certain types of human and animal investigations [29]. Apkarian et al. [4] used SPECT to demonstrate a contralateral inhibition of rCBF in S1 cortex during 3 minutes of noxious heat stimulation. Cesaro and colleagues [27] used isopropyliodoamphetamine (IMP) as an rCBF tracer to show thalamic hyperresponsiveness in two patients with hyperpathia following a stroke. Thus, the ability to compare anatomically and functionally distinct brain responses simultaneously now focused attention towards the analysis of structural groups, rather than individual sites, in the mediation of neurological functions.

The time required for the incorporation and retention of FDG (30–50 minutes for each stimulation period) made this method unsuitable for the study of acute, stimulus-evoked pain in awake humans. But the development of the $H_2{}^{15}O$ method for estimating relatively rapid changes in rCBF (or perfusion) [42] with a greater spatial resolution than SPECT enabled the study of responses to a series of brief noxious stimuli. Talbot et al. [115] and Jones and colleagues [58] were the first to use the $H_2{}^{15}O$ PET method to reveal multiple cortical responses to noxious contact heat. Both studies showed activation of the anterior cingulate cortex; the Talbot study revealed responses in the S1 and S2 cortices, and the Jones investigation demonstrated thalamic and lenticular nucleus activation. To determine whether these results were related specifically to pain and not simply to the detection of differences in thermal intensity, Casey et al. [21] performed a similar experiment, but added a control condition with comparable stimulus temperature increases below the noxious range; pain-specific activations were again observed in multiple cortical locations (S1, S2, anterior cingulate, and insula) as well as in the thalamus, medial midbrain (periaqueductal grey region), and cerebellar vermis (Fig. 1-3). These early $H_2{}^{15}O$ PET

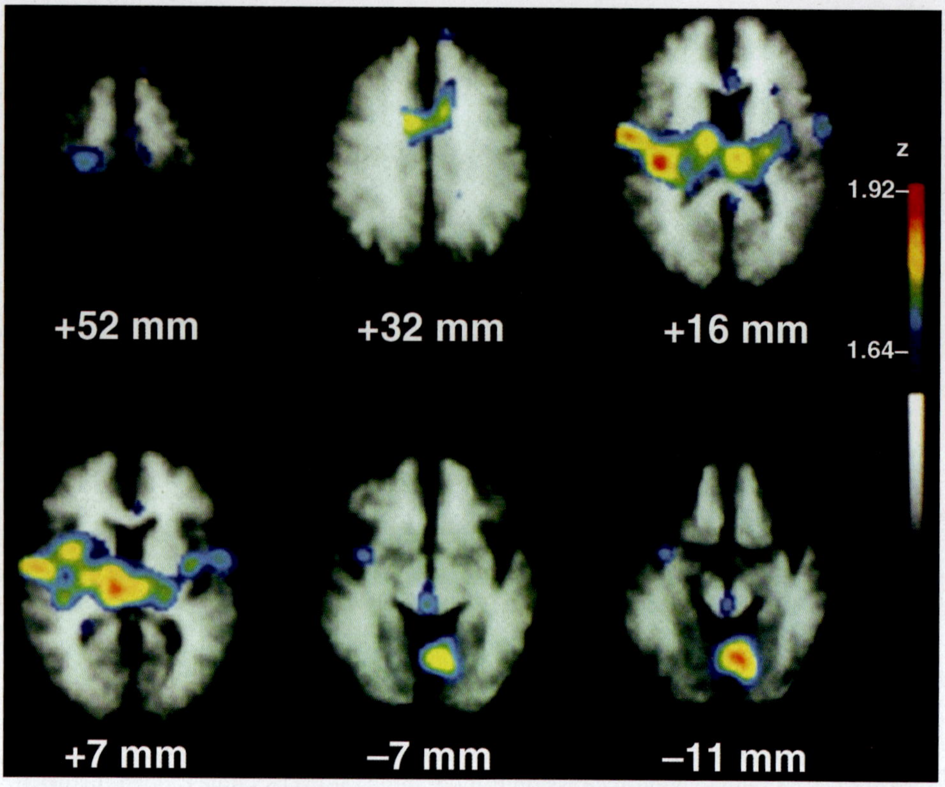

FIGURE 1-3 Early $H_2^{15}O$ PET subtraction study showing heat pain (50°–40°C contrast) activation of: S1 cortex **(upper left)**; bilateral anterior cingulate cortex **(upper middle)**; contralateral insula, S2 cortex, lenticular nucleus, and ipsilateral thalamus **(upper right)**; bilateral S2 cortex and insula, contralateral thalamus **(lower left)**; dorsomedial midbrain (region of PAG) and cerebellar vermis **(lower middle and right)**. Innocuous heat stimulation (42°–32°C contrast) did not activate these structures. Numbers below images indicate millimetres above (+) or below (–) the intercommissural plane. Colour bar numbers indicate *Z*-score deviation from mean CBF change (pooled variance; $P < 0.05$ uncorrected). (From Casey et al. [21].)

studies were quickly followed by a series of pain imaging investigations using the same or similar methods and exploring different types and aspects of pain and pain modulation (for review of this period through 2005, see [2, 91]). For example, Coghill et al. [31] showed that: (1) compared with vibrotactile stimulation, pain-related activation is more widely distributed among anatomically and functionally distinct cortical and subcortical brain areas, and (2) perceived painful stimulus intensity is positively related to the intensity of rCBF changes in a diverse group of brain sites including the bilateral cerebellum, putamen, thalamus, insula, anterior cingulate, and S2 cortex and the contralateral S1 cortex and supplementary motor area [30]. The parallel processing of affective and sensory-discriminative components of pain was revealed by Rainville and colleagues [101], who used hypnotic suggestion to uncouple these experiences during noxious stimulation and demonstrate a specific affect-related activation in the cingulate gyrus but not in the somatosensory cortex. $H_2^{15}O$ PET studies also revealed the temporal dynamics of heat pain [22] and the increased excitability of heat-responsive structures in patients with central sensory loss and central pain [20]. Thus, the simultaneous recording, by $H_2^{15}O$ PET, of multiple localized brain responses in communicating humans further focused attention on the activation of spatially distributed, temporally dynamic networks of brain regions mediating experimental and pathological pain.

Defining the "Default (Resting) Brain"

A common observation during PET studies is that medial prefrontal, posterior cingulate, and precuneate cortical areas are deactivated (reduced blood perfusion) during tasks of any type. In a series of seminal investigations, Raichle and colleagues [100] used PET measures of blood flow and oxygen extraction to show that these brain regions are active in the waking brain at rest (eyes closed). This result established a default (task-free) mode of brain function as a basis for the interpretation of brain activations and deactivations during task performance, including the experience of pain.

A BOLD Contribution to the Functional Imaging of Pain: The Morphology of Chronic Pain

While some of the above studies were being conducted, Ogawa et al. [82, 83] and Kwong et al. [64] reported that changes in tissue magnetic susceptibility, caused by changes in the concentration of blood deoxy- and oxyhemoglobin, could be used to detect increases in tissue oxygenation and thus serve as indicators of neuronal activity. Characterization of this blood oxygenation-level-dependent (BOLD) response led directly to the application of functional magnetic resonance imaging (fMRI) studies of pain. Among the first of these investigations was that of Davis et al. [35], showing that painful electrical stimulation resulted in the conjoint activation of cingulate and S1 cortices, whereas only S1 responded during painless stimulation.

An important advantage of the hemodynamic (BOLD) response is that its amplitude and time course can be measured and correlated with neuronal activity in response to individual stimuli, thus extending and facilitating the design of functional imaging experiments [17, 71, 72]. Furthermore, spontaneous fluctuations in the BOLD signal can be found in the resting, task-free brain, as reported initially by Biswal and colleagues [12], who noted that these spontaneous fluctuations were correlated within and among functionally and anatomically related brain regions. Fox et al. [40, 41] used these fluctuating BOLD signals to reveal distinct, widely distributed networks comprised of autocorrelated BOLD fluctuations in the resting brain. Using the BOLD fluctuations in a priori "seed" voxels, these investigators identified one network comprised of structures activated during a cognitively demanding task and a separate anticorrelated network that is correspondingly deactivated. These and related investigations led to the application of similar methods to examine BOLD responses to transient or sustained fluctuations of ongoing pain in patients with chronic back pain [6]. Activation of the medial prefrontal and rostral cingulate cortex appeared during high-level sustained pain, while rapid increases in pain activated the somatosensory and insular cortices. The authors interpret these results as evidence of a neurophysiologically unique brain response during chronic pain, a predominant emotional and cognitive component of this condition being suggested by the activation of the medial prefrontal and rostral cingulate cortices. An earlier study used the recently developed method of voxel-based morphometry (VBM) [5] to demonstrate a loss of thalamic and dorsolateral prefrontal grey matter in chronic back pain patients [3], suggesting that a loss of inhibition by the dorsolateral prefrontal area could produce an exaggerated medial prefrontal response to noxious input. The histopathological significance and persistence of VBM changes in chronic pain remains to be determined, but the continued use of this technology is beginning to provide information about the longer-term consequences of prolonged or recurrent pain [76] and its degree of dependence on continuing nociceptive input as in some cases of peripheral neuropathic pain [47].

Attention to Connectivity and Networks

As it became obvious that pain was mediated by the activation of a network of brain structures, attention focused on an analysis of the correlation of activity among network components [107]. The correlation of activation intensities among activated voxels could be used to determine connectivity and thus define the emergence of activation networks for specified conditions. Connectivity can be defined as "functional" (temporal correlations among a set of activated sites) or "effective," as the influence of one set of activations on another [16, 44]. In an early example of applying connectivity concepts in pain imaging, Lorenz and colleagues [73] used multiple regression, correlation, and principal components analysis to show, in an experimental model of heat allodynia, a decrease in pain during high levels of allodynia-evoked activity in the dorsolateral prefrontal cortex (DLPFC), which in turn correlated inversely with functional connectivity between the medial thalamus and the dorsomedial midbrain. Shortly thereafter, Apkarian et al. [3] reported their VBM study (cited above) of patients with chronic back pain and atrophy within the DLPFC and thalamic grey matter. These results and those of Baliki [6] (cited above) emphasize the participation of the prefrontal cortex as part of a network modulating the affective component of chronic pain. In another analysis of network connectivity and interaction, Seminowicz and Davis [111] used independent components analysis to demonstrate that both pain and cognitive demand enhance the connectivity of an attention-specific frontoparietal-insular network, suggesting a mechanism for pain interference with cognitively demanding tasks. The emerging emphasis on connectivity and network analysis in pain imaging is reflected in the recent interest in this approach in brain neuroscience generally [8, 18].

PAIN MODULATION BECOMES VISIBLE IN THE LIVING BRAIN

Opioid Receptors and Analgesia Mechanisms

The discovery of opiate receptors [87] and endogenous opioids [55] in the nervous system and later specifically in the limbic structures of the primate brain [65, 105, 106] opened the way for human behavioural [70] and imaging studies of the mechanisms of opioid-based analgesia. Early PET studies revealed a sensory- and site-specific attenuation of pain-related activations by exogenous [1, 23] or endogenous [125] μ-opioid receptor agonists, and suggested the participation of the rostral anterior cingulate cortex and related subcortical systems in analgesic mechanisms. These studies were soon followed by an elucidation of the mechanisms of the placebo effect in healthy persons [117] and patients [97] and the role of opioids in mediating placebo analgesia [118, 124]. In a study using functional and effective

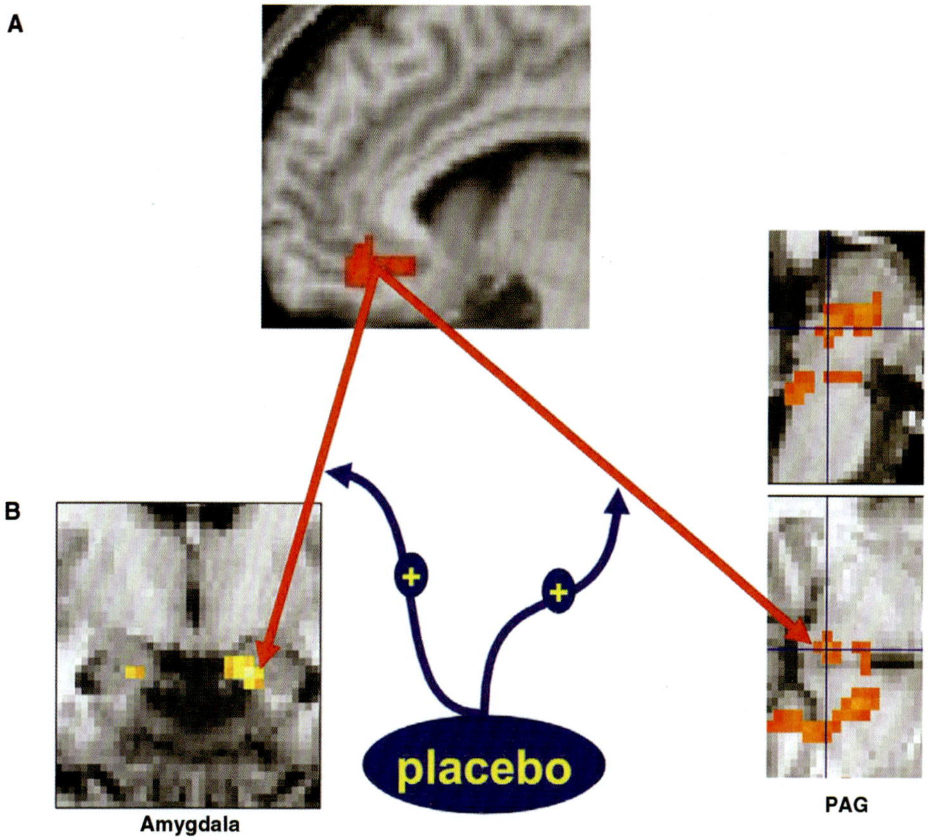

FIGURE 1-4 During placebo analgesia, BOLD responses to noxious laser stimulation were enhanced in the rostral (perigenual) anterior cingulate cortex (rACC, **top image**). BOLD responses in brainstem opioid-related endogenous analgesia circuits (periaqueductal grey, amygdala) covaried with those in the rACC **(lower images)**. Activation related to the rACC is also seen in the rostral dorsal pons, suggesting participation by the noradrenergic locus coeruleus. (From Bingel et al. [10].)

connectivity, for example, Bingel et al. [10] combined psychophysical and physiological measurements to reveal enhanced BOLD responses to noxious laser stimulation in the rostral anterior cingulate cortex (rACC) during the placebo condition; BOLD activity in brainstem opioid endogenous analgesia sites (periaqueductal grey and amygdala) covaried with these placebo-enhanced rACC responses (Fig. 1-4). Although not discussed by the authors, this study also revealed rACC-related activation in the dorsal rostral pons, at a location suggesting participation by noradrenergic neurons in the locus coeruleus, a structure known to participate in nociceptive modulation [88].

Additional Mechanisms of Endogenous Analgesia

Although imaging studies represented by the few examples cited earlier revealed much about opioid-mediated analgesic mechanisms, additional investigations showed that other neuronal systems with diverse neuropharmacology [85, 88] also contribute to endogenous analgesia or other forms of pain modulation. As referenced above, Pertovaara [88] has reviewed the extensive evidence for the participation of central noradrenergic neurons in the modulation of pain and nociception. Both PET and fMRI studies have provided information about the mechanisms of pain modulation during central electrical stimulation [46], cognition [89, 90], expectation [108], acupuncture, and other counterirritative methods [11, 28, 114] (see also [11] for a review of this topic). Indeed, ongoing pain itself attenuates the pain of a superimposed noxious stimulus, as demonstrated by a recent study using connectivity analysis to reveal a partially opioid-dependent activation of a subcortical analgesia network by the anterior cingulate cortex [114].

CONCLUSION

The progress made towards understanding the neurophysiological foundation of pain would have been beyond imagination 50+ years ago when the living human brain was invisible. Simply making the living brain visible opened the way for anatomical analyses of clinical cases with abnormalities of pain perception. These anatomical–clinical correlations showed that lesions in widely different brain regions could affect different aspects of the pain experience and revealed that lesions affecting pain also simultaneously affected other sensory, hedonic, and cognitive functions. These findings were in accord with the finding that cellular responses encoding pain, either exclusively or differentially, were widely distributed in the central nervous system. Moreover, imaging studies of patients with central pain syndromes suggested the distributed anatomy of a pain-activated endogenous control mechanism.

The functional brain imaging of pain confirmed and extended the findings of anatomical–clinical correlations by revealing that pain is marked by the near-simultaneous activation of multiple anatomically and functionally distinct brain regions that are spatially distributed and connected to form interacting networks. Contemporary analyses show that changes in pain perception, whether induced by drugs, suggestion, or other means, are attributable to variations in the intensity and connectivity of activation within specific networks.

We have moved well beyond the old “pattern versus specificity” debate. Flesh and detail has been added to a conceptual skeleton constructed over 40 years ago when the living brain was invisible [77]. Today, there is no doubt about the existence of a diverse set of nociceptors that respond uniquely or differentially to potentially damaging stimuli or that are active only in damaged tissue. There is also no doubt that the brain develops unique and highly specific pain experiences from this nociceptive information and pathological versions of it. Moreover, it is now clear that this specific nociceptive information is not hidden in a neuronal maze; rather, it is widely distributed among identifiable central structures, where it undergoes analysis and modification at all levels of the neuraxis to mediate the complex experience of pain. We can now conceive of pain in terms of identifiable, dynamic, interacting networks with specific functions. These networks are being recognized as specific physiological and anatomical identities. Moreover, the ongoing development of magnetic resonance spectroscopy promises to add biochemical signatures to circuits that participate in developing, maintaining, and controlling chronic pain [14]. The conceptual model of pain mechanisms that is emerging from imaging the working brain should lead to increasingly sophisticated methods that engage physiological mechanisms for more effective pain control.

REFERENCES

1. Adler LJ, Gyulai FE, Diehl DJ, Mintun MA, Winter PM, Firestone LL. Regional brain activity changes associated with fentanyl analgesia elucidated by positron emission tomography. Anesth Analg 1997;84(1):120–6.
2. Apkarian AV, Bushnell MC, Treede RD, Zubieta JK. Human brain mechanisms of pain perception and regulation in health and disease. Eur J Pain 2005;9(4):463–4.
3. Apkarian AV, Sosa Y, Sonty S, Levy RM, Harden RN, Parrish TB, Gitelman DR. Chronic back pain is associated with decreased prefrontal and thalamic gray matter density. J Neurosci 2004;24(46):10410–5.
4. Apkarian AV, Stea RA, Manglos SH, Szeverenyi NM, King RB, Thomas FD. Persistent pain inhibits contralateral somatosensory cortical activity in humans. Neurosci Lett 1992;140:141–7.
5. Ashburner J, Friston KJ. Voxel-based morphometry—the methods. Neuroimage 2000;11(6):805–21.
6. Baliki MN, Chialvo DR, Geha PY, Levy RM, Harden RN, Parrish TB, Apkarian AV. Chronic pain and the emotional brain: specific brain activity associated with spontaneous fluctuations of intensity of chronic back pain. J Neurosci 2006;26(47):12165–73.
7. Ballantine HT Jr, Cassidy WL, Flanagan NB. Stereotaxic anterior cingulotomy for neuropsychiatric illness and intractable pain. J Neurosurg 1967;26:488–95.
8. Behrens TE, Sporns O. Human connectomics. Curr Opin Neurobiol 2012;22(1):144–53.
9. Bessou P, Perl ER. Response of cutaneous sensory units with unmyelinated fibers to noxious stimuli. J Neurophysiol 1969;32:1025–43.
10. Bingel U, Lorenz J, Schoell E, Weiller C, Buchel C. Mechanisms of placebo analgesia: rACC recruitment of a subcortical antinociceptive network. Pain 2006;120(1–2):8–15.
11. Bingel U, Tracey I. Imaging CNS modulation of pain in humans. Physiology 2008;23(6):371–80.
12. Biswal B, Yetkin FZ, Haughton VM, Hyde JS. Functional connectivity in the motor cortex of resting human brain using echo-planar MRI. Magn Reson Med 1995;34(4):537–41.
13. Bogousslavsky J, Regli F, Uske A. Thalamic infarcts: clinical syndromes, etiology, and prognosis. Neurology 1988;38:837–48.
14. Borsook D, Moulton EA, Schmidt K, Becerra L. Neuroimaging revolutionizes therapeutic approaches to chronic pain. Mol Pain 2007;3(1):25.
15. Bowsher D. Pathophysiology of central pain. Pain Forum 1998;7:15–7.
16. Büchel C, Friston KJ. Modulation of connectivity in visual pathways by attention: cortical interactions evaluated with structural equation modelling and fMRI. Cereb Cortex 1997;7(8):768.
17. Buckner RL. The hemodynamic inverse problem: making inferences about neural activity from measured MRI signals. Proc Natl Acad Sci USA 2003;100(5):2177–9.
18. Bullmore E, Sporns O. The economy of brain network organization. Nat Rev Neurosci 2012;13(5):336–49.
19. Burgess PR, Perl ER. Myelinated afferent fibers responding specifically to noxious stimulation of the skin. J Physiol 1967;190:541–62.
20. Casey KL, Geisser ME, Lorenz J, Morrow TJ, Paulson P, Minoshima S. Psychophysical and cerebral responses to heat stimulation in patients with central pain, painless central sensory loss, and in healthy persons. Pain 2012;153(2):331–41.
21. Casey KL, Minoshima S, Berger KL, Koeppe RA, Morrow TJ, Frey KA. Positron emission tomographic analysis of cerebral structures activated specifically by repetitive noxious heat stimuli. J Neurophysiol 1994;71:802–7.
22. Casey KL, Morrow TJ, Lorenz J, Minoshima S. Temporal and spatial dynamics of human forebrain activity during heat pain: analysis by positron emission tomography. J Neurophysiol 2001;85(2):951–9.
23. Casey KL, Svensson P, Morrow TJ, Raz J, Jone C, Minoshima S. Selective opiate modulation of nociceptive processing in the human brain. J Neurophysiol 2000;84:525–33.
24. Cassinari V, Pagni CA. Central Pain: A Neurosurgical Survey. Cambridge, MA: Harvard University Press; 1969.
25. Cereda C, Ghika J, Maeder P, Bogousslavsky J. Strokes restricted to the insular cortex. Neurology 2002;59(12):1950–5.
26. Cervero F, Sharkey KA. An electrophysiological and anatomical study of intestinal afferent fibres in the rat. J Physiol 1988;401:381–98.
27. Cesaro P, Mann MW, Moretti JL, Defer G, Roualdes B, Nguyen JP, Degos JD. Central pain and thalamic hyperactivity: a single photon emission computerized tomographic study. Pain 1991;47:329–36.
28. Chae Y, Chang DS, Lee SH, Jung WM, Lee IS, Jackson S, Kong J, Lee H, Park HJ, Lee H, et al. Inserting needles into the body: a meta-analysis of brain activity associated with acupuncture needle stimulation. J Pain 2013;14(3):215–22.

29. Coghill RC, Morrow TJ. Functional imaging of animal models of pain: high-resolution insights into nociceptive processing. In: Casey KL, Bushnell MC, editors. Pain imaging, Vol. 18. Seattle, WA: IASP Press; 2000. pp. 211–39.
30. Coghill RC, Sang CN, Maisog JH, Iadarola MJ. Pain intensity processing within the human brain: a bilateral, distributed mechanism. J Neurophysiol 1999;82(4):1934–43.
31. Coghill RC, Talbot JD, Evans AC, Meyer E, Gjedde A, Bushnell MC, Duncan GH. Distributed processing of pain and vibration by the human brain. J Neurosci 1994;14(7):4095–108.
32. Cohen RA, Kaplan RF, Moser DJ, Jenkins MA, Wilkinson H. Impairments of attention after cingulotomy. Neurology 1999;53(4):819–24.
33. Cormack AM. Early two-dimensional reconstruction (CT scanning) and recent topics stemming from it. Nobel lecture, December 8, 1979. J Comput Assist Tomogr 1980;4(5):658–64.
34. Craig AD. Pain mechanisms: labeled lines versus convergence in central processing. Annu Rev Neurosci 2003;26:1–30.
35. Davis KD, Wood ML, Crawley AP, Mikulis DJ. fMRI of human somatosensory and cingulate cortex during painful electrical nerve stimulation. Neuroreport 1995;7(1):321–5.
36. Davison C, Schick W. Spontaneous pain and other subjective sensory disturbances: a clinicopathological study. In: Patten C, Frantz A, Hare C, editors. Proceedings of Association for Research in Nervous and Mental Disease. Baltimore, MD: Willams & Wilkins; 1935. pp. 457–96.
37. Dejerine J, Roussy G. La syndrome thalamique. Rev Neurol 1906;12:521–32.
38. Fisher CM. Lacunar strokes and infarcts: a review. Neurology 1982;32:871–6.
39. Foltz EL, White LE. Pain "relief" by frontal cingulumotomy. J Neurosurg 1962;19:89–100.
40. Fox MD, Raichle ME. Spontaneous fluctuations in brain activity observed with functional magnetic resonance imaging. Nat Rev Neurosci 2007;8(9):700–11.
41. Fox MD, Snyder AZ, Vincent JL, Corbetta M, Van Essen DC, Raichle ME. The human brain is intrinsically organized into dynamic, anticorrelated functional networks. Proc Natl Acad Sci USA 2005;102(27):9673–8.
42. Fox PT, Mintun MA, Raichle ME, Herscovitch P. A noninvasive approach to quantitative functional brain mapping with $H_2{}^{15}O$ and positron emission tomography. J Cereb Blood Flow Metab 1984;4(3):329–33.
43. Friedman DP, Murray EA. Thalamic connectivity of the second somatosensory area and neighboring somatosensory fields of the lateral sulcus of the macaque. J Comp Neurol 1986;252:348–73.
44. Friston KJ, Frith CD, Liddle PF, Frackowiak RS. Functional connectivity: the principal-component analysis of large (PET) data sets. J Cereb Blood Flow Metab 1993;13(1):5–14.
45. Frostig RD, Lieke EE, Ts'o DY, Grinvald A. Cortical functional architecture and local coupling between neuronal activity and the microcirculation revealed by in vivo high-resolution optical imaging of intrinsic signals. Proc Natl Acad Sci USA 1990;87(16):6082–6.
46. Garcia-Larrea L, Peyron R, Mertens P, Gregoire MC, Lavenne F, Bonnefoi, Mauguiere F, Laurent B, Sindou M. Positron emission tomography during motor cortex stimulation for pain control. Stereotact Funct Neurosurg 1997;68(1–4, Pt 1):141–8.
47. Gracely RH, Lynch SA, Bennett GJ. Painful neuropathy: altered central processing maintained dynamically by peripheral input. Pain 1992;51(2):175–94.
48. Greenspan JD, Lee RR, Lenz FA. Pain sensitivity alterations as a function of lesion location in the parasylvian cortex. Pain 1999;81(3):273–82.
49. Grinvald A, Frostig RD, Lieke E, Hildesheim R. Optical imaging of neuronal activity. Physiol Rev 1988;68(4):1285–366.
50. Hassenbusch SJ, Pillay PK, Barnett GH. Radiofrequency cingulotomy for intractable cancer pain using stereotaxis guided by magnetic resonance imaging. Neurosurgery 1990;27:220–3.
51. Head H, Holmes G. Sensory disturbances from cerebral lesions. Brain 1911;34:102–254.
52. Hounsfield GN. Computerized transverse axial scanning (tomography), 1: description of system. Br J Radiol 1973;46(552):1016–22.
53. Hounsfield GN. Computed medical imaging. Nobel lecture, December 8, 1979. J Comput Assist Tomogr 1980;4(5):665–74.
54. Huffman KJ, Krubitzer L. Thalamo-cortical connections of areas 3a and M1 in marmoset monkeys. J Comp Neurol 2001;435(3):291–310.
55. Hughes J. Isolation of an endogenous compound from the brain with pharmacological properties similar to morphine. Brain Res 1975;88:295–308.
56. Hurt RW, Ballantine HT. Stereotactic anterior cingulate lesions for persistent pain: a report on 68 cases. Clin Neurosurg 1974;21:334–51.
57. Ingvar DH, Risberg J. Increase of regional cerebral blood flow during mental effort in normals and in patients with focal brain disorders. Exp Brain Res 1967;3(3):195–211.

58. Jones AK, Brown WD, Friston KJ, Qi LY, Frackowiak RS. Cortical and subcortical localization of response to pain in man using positron emission tomography. Proc Roy Soc Lond B Biol Sci 1991;244:39–44.
59. Kennedy C, Des Rosiers MH, Jehle JW, Reivich M, Sharpe F, Sokoloff L. Mapping of functional neural pathways by autoradiographic survey of local metabolic rate with (^{14}C) deoxyglucose. Science 1975;187:850–3.
60. Kenshalo DR, Iwata K, Sholas M, Thomas DA. Response properties and organization of nociceptive neurons in area 1 of monkey primary somatosensory cortex. J Neurophysiol 2000;84(2):719–79.
61. Kenshalo DR Jr, Isensee O. Responses of primate S1 cortical neurons to noxious stimuli. J Neurophysiol 1983;50:1479–96.
62. Kramer DM, Schneider JS, Rudin AM, Lauterbur PC. True three-dimensional nuclear magnetic resonance zeugmatographic images of a human brain. Neuroradiology 1981;21(5):239–44.
63. Kuhl DE, Edwards RQ. Cylindrical and section radioisotope scanning of the liver and brain. Radiology 1964;83:926–36.
64. Kwong KK, Belliveau JW, Chesler DA, Goldberg IE, Weisskoff RM, Poncelet BP, Kennedy DN, Hoppel BE, Cohen MS, Turner R. Dynamic magnetic resonance imaging of human brain activity during primary sensory stimulation. Proc Natl Acad Sci USA 1992;89(12):5675–9.
65. LaMotte CC, Snowman A, Pert CB, Snyder SH. Opiate receptor binding in rhesus monkey brain: association with limbic structures. Brain Res 1978;155:374–9.
66. Lassen NA, Hoedt-Rasussen K, Sorensen SC, Skinhoj E, Cronquist S, Bodforss B, Ingvar DH. Regional cerebral blood flow in man determined by krypton. Neurology 1963;13:719–27.
67. Lear JL. Initial cerebral HM-PAO distribution compared to LCBF: use of a model which considers cerebral HM-PAO trapping kinetics. J Cereb Blood Flow Metab 1988;8(6):S31–7.
68. Lear JL. Quantitative local cerebral blood flow measurements with technetium-99m HM-PAO: evaluation using multiple radionuclide digital quantitative autoradiography. J Nucl Med 1988;29(8):1387–92.
69. Lenz FA, Casey KL, Jones EG, Willis WD. The human pain system: experimental and clinical perspectives. Cambridge, MA: Cambridge University Press; 2010.
70. Levine JD, Gordon NC, Fields HL. The mechanism of placebo analgesia. Lancet 1978;2(8091):654–7.
71. Logothetis NK, Pauls J, Augath M, Trinath T, Oeltermann, A. Neurophysiological investigation of the basis of the fMRI signal. Nature 2001;412(6843):150–7.
72. Logothetis NK, Pfeuffer J. On the nature of the BOLD fMRI contrast mechanism. Magn Reson Imaging 2004;22(10):1517–31.
73. Lorenz J, Minoshima S, Casey KL. Keeping pain out of mind: the role of the dorsolateral prefrontal cortex in pain modulation. Brain 2003;126(Pt 5):1079–91.
74. Marshall J. Sensory disturbances in cortical wounds with special reference to pain. J Neurol Neurosurg Psychiatr 1951;14:187–204.
75. Mata M, Fink DJ, Gainer H, Smith CB, Davidsen L, Savaki H, Schwartz WJ, Sokoloff L. Activity-dependent energy metabolism in rat posterior pituitary primarily reflects sodium pump activity. J Neurochem 1980;34(1):213–5.
76. May A. Chronic pain may change the structure of the brain. Pain 2008;137(1):7–15.
77. Melzack R, Casey KL. Sensory, motivational, and central control determinants of pain. In: Kenshalo DR, editor. The skin senses. Springfield, IL: C. C. Thomas, 1968. pp. 423–39.
78. Merskey H, Bogduk N. Classification of chronic pain: descriptions of chronic pain syndromes and definitions of pain terms, Vol. 2. Seattle, WA: IASP Press; 1994.
79. Mesulam MM. From sensation to cognition. Brain 1998;121:1013–52.
80. Mesulam MM, Mufson EJ. Insula of the old world monkey, III: efferent cortical output and comments on function. J Comp Neurol 1982;212(1):38–52.
81. Moayedi M, Davis KD. Theories of pain: from specificity to gate control. J Neurophysiol 2013;109(1):5–12.
82. Ogawa S, Lee TM, Kay AR, Tank D. Brain magnetic resonance imaging with contrast dependent on blood oxygenation. Proc Natl Acad Sci USA 1990;87:9868–72.
83. Ogawa S, Tank DW, Menon R, Ellermann JM, Kim SG, Merkle H, Ugurbil K. Intrinsic signal changes accompanying sensory stimulation: functional brain mapping with magnetic resonance imaging. Proc Natl Acad Sci USA 1992;89(13):5951–5.
84. Oldendorf WH. The quest for an image of brain: a brief historical and technical review of brain imaging techniques. Neurology 1978;28(6):517–33.
85. Ossipov MH, Dussor GO, Porreca F. Central modulation of pain. J Clin Invest 2010;120:3779.
86. Perl ER. Ideas about pain: a historical view. Nat Rev Neurosci 2007;8(1):71–80.
87. Pert CB, Snyder SH. Opiate receptor: demonstration in nervous tissue. Science 1973;179:1011–4.
88. Pertovaara A. Noradrenergic pain modulation. Prog Neurobiol 2006;80(2):53–83.
89. Petrovic P, Ingvar M. Imaging cognitive modulation of pain processing. Pain 2002;95(1–2):1–5.

90. Petrovic P, Petersson KM, Ghatan PH, Stone-Elander S, Ingvar M. Pain-related cerebral activation is altered by a distracting cognitive task. Pain 2000;85(1–2):19–30.
91. Peyron R, Laurent B, Garcia-Larrea L. Functional imaging of brain responses to pain: a review and meta-analysis. Neurophysiol Clin 2000;30(5):263–88.
92. Phelps ME, Kuhl DE, Mazziota JC. Metabolic mapping of the brain's response to visual stimulation: studies in humans. Science 1981;211(4489):1445–8.
93. Pillay PK, Hassenbusch SJ. Bilateral MRI-guided stereotactic cingulotomy for intractable pain. Stereot Funct Neurosurg 1992;59:33–8.
94. Ploner M, Freund HJ, Schnitzler A. Pain affect without pain sensation in a patient with a postcentral lesion. Pain 1999;81(1–2):211–4.
95. Ploner M, Schmitz F, Freund HJ, Schnitzler A. Parallel activation of primary and secondary somatosensory cortices in human pain processing. J Neurophysiol 1999;81(6):3100–4.
96. Price DD. Psychological and neural mechanisms of the affective dimension of pain. Science 2000;288:1769–72.
97. Price DD, Craggs J, Verne GN, Perlstein WM, Robinson ME. Placebo analgesia is accompanied by large reductions in pain-related brain activity in irritable bowel syndrome patients. Pain 2007;127(1–2):63–72.
98. Price DD, Greenspan JD, Dubner R. Neurons involved in the exteroceptive function of pain. Pain 2003; 106(3):215–9.
99. Raichle ME. Behind the scenes of functional brain imaging: a historical and physiological perspective. Proc Natl Acad Sci USA 1998;95(3):765–72.
100. Raichle ME, MacLeod AM, Snyder AZ, Powers WJ, Gusnard, DA, Shulman GL. A default mode of brain function. Proc Natl Acad Sci USA 2001;98(2):676–82.
101. Rainville P, Duncan GH, Price DD, Carrier M, Bushnell MC. Pain affect encoded in human anterior cingulate but not somatosensory cortex. Science 1997;277:968–71.
102. Reivich M, Kuhl D, Wolf A, Greenberg J, Phelps M, Ido T, Casella V, Fowler J, Hoffman E, Alavi A, et al. The [^{18}F]fluorodeoxyglucose method for the measurement of local cerebral glucose utilization in man. Circ Res 1979;44(1):127–37.
103. Roy CS, Sherrington CS. On the regulation of the blood-supply of the brain. J Physiol (Lond) 1890;11:85–108.
104. Russell WR. Transient disturbances following gunshot wounds of the head. Brain 1945;68:79–97.
105. Sadzot B, Franck G. Non-invasive methods to study drug disposition: positron emission tomography: detection and quantification of brain receptors in man. Eur J Drug Metabol Pharmacokinet 1990;15(2):135–42.
106. Sadzot B, Mayberg HS, Frost JJ. Detection and quantification of opiate receptors in man by positron emission tomography: potential applications to the study of pain. Neurophysiol Clin 1990;20(5):323–34.
107. Salinas E, Sejnowski TJ. Correlated neuronal activity and the flow of neural information. Nat Rev Neurosci 2001;2(8):539–50.
108. Sawamoto N, Honda M, Okada T, Hanakawa T, Kanda M, Fukuyama H, Konishi J, Shibasaki H. Expectation of pain enhances responses to nonpainful somatosensory stimulation in the anterior cingulate cortex and parietal operculum/posterior insula: an event-related functional magnetic resonance imaging study. J Neurosci 2000;20(19):7438–45.
109. Schmahmann JD, Leifer D. Parietal pseudothalamic pain syndrome: clinical features and anatomic correlates. Arch Neurol 1992;49:1032–7.
110. Schwartz WJ, Smith CB, Davidsen L, Savaki H, Sokoloff L, Mata M, Fink DJ, Gainer H. Metabolic mapping of functional activity in the hypothalamo-neurohypophysial system of the rat. Science 1979;205(4407):723–5.
111. Seminowicz DA, Davis KD. Pain enhances functional connectivity of a brain network evoked by performance of a cognitive task. J Neurophysiol 2007;97(5):3651–9.
112. Sinclair DC. Cutaneous sensation and the doctrine of specific energy. Brain 1955;78(4):584–614.
113. Sokoloff L, Mangold R, Wechsler RL, Kennedy C, Kety SS. The effect of mental arithmetic on cerebral circulation and metabolism. J Clin Invest 1955;34:1101–8.
114. Sprenger C, Bingel U, Buchel C. Treating pain with pain: supraspinal mechanisms of endogenous analgesia elicited by heterotopic noxious conditioning stimulation. Pain 2011;152(2):428–39.
115. Talbot JD, Marrett S, Evans AC, Meyer E, Bushnell MC, Duncan GH. Multiple representations of pain in human cerebral cortex. Science 1991;251:1355–8.
116. Tommerdahl M, Delemos KA, Vierck CJ Jr, Favorov OV, Whitsel BL. Anterior parietal cortical response to tactile and skin-heating stimuli applied to the same skin site. J Neurophysiol 1996;75:2662–70.
117. Wager TD, Rilling JK, Smith EE, Sokolik A, Casey KL, Davidson RJ, Kosslyn SM, Rose RM, Cohen JD. Placebo-induced changes in fMRI in the anticipation and experience of pain. Science 2004;303:1162–7.
118. Wager TD, Scott DJ, Zubieta JK. Placebo effects on human mu-opioid activity during pain. Proc Natl Acad Sci USA 2007;104(26):11056–61.

119. Weddell G. Somesthesis and the chemical senses. Annu Rev Psychol 1955;6:119–36.
120. White JC, Sweet WH. Pain and the neurosurgeon: a forty-year experience. Springfield, IL: C. C. Thomas; 1969.
121. Whitsel BL, Favorov OV, Li Y, Quibrera M, Tommerdahl M. Area 3a neuron response to skin nociceptor afferent drive. Cereb Cortex 2009;19(2):349–66.
122. Wilkinson HA, Davidson KM, Davidson RI. Bilateral anterior cingulotomy for chronic noncancer pain. Neurosurgery 1999;45(5):1129–34.
123. Yen CP, Kung SS, Su YF, Lin WC, Howng SL, Kwan AL. Stereotactic bilateral anterior cingulotomy for intractable pain. J Clin Neurosci 2005;12(8):886–90.
124. Zubieta JK, Bueller JA, Jackson LR, Scott DJ, Xu Y, Koeppe RA, Nichols TE, Stohler CS. Placebo effects mediated by endogenous opioid activity on mu-opioid receptors. J Neurosci 2005;25(34):7754–62.
125. Zubieta JK, Smith YR, Bueller JA, Xu Y, Kilbourn MR, Jewett DM, Meyer CR, Koeppe RA, Stohler CS. Regional mu opioid receptor regulation of sensory and affective dimensions of pain. Science 2001;293(5528):311–15.

SECTION 2

Technology: Human Neuroimaging

CHAPTER 2

Using Neuroimaging to Understand Pain: Pattern Recognition and the Path from Brain Mapping to Mechanisms

Tor D. Wager

The brain is the proximal generator of pain. Certainly, many kinds of pain start in the body, in the skin, muscles, or bones; but without a brain none of them become experiences. They do not lead to avoidance, inspire fear, or cause any worry or suffering whatsoever.

To understand pain, we need to understand its brain mechanisms—the central brain processes that represent noxious events in the body and the actual or potential harm they imply. In many forms of pathological pain, the brain is functioning normally, responding appropriately to bodily insult. If a peripheral cause can be identified and removed, the problem may be solved. Too often, however, what starts with an initially healthy brain response to peripheral injury can become pathological. Neurons in the spinal cord and brain may sensitize. Central representations of pain may trigger avoidance, disuse, and ultimately isolation and depression. Innocuous events may become reminders of pain, and pain may take on special significance in the central nervous system, dominating attention, memory, and internal thought. We need better models of how these processes work at the brain level.

Researchers have been using neuroimaging techniques—fMRI and PET—to study the brain mechanisms of pain for over 20 years, since the first seminal publications in 1991 [34, 58]. We have moved rapidly from the first groundbreaking, exploratory studies to a mature literature that has yielded reliable procedures and findings on acute and chronic pain, including functional responses to pain [2, 14] and structural changes that accompany chronic pain [42, 55]. We now have the potential to take a "quantum leap" forward, but we have not done so yet. What is that quantum leap? It is the translation from basic findings to having useful brain markers that can help diagnose pain in individuals, determine the *neurophysiological type* of pain, and understand its mechanisms and connections with other brain systems (e.g., those that mediate fear, avoidance, and depression). This chapter is about some of the things we must consider as we prepare to make the jump.

The central thesis of this chapter is that we are now ready to make the transition from brain mapping, the dominant approach for the first 20 years of neuroimaging, to the *brain biomarker* approach, the use of brain patterns as markers for functional outcomes (e.g., pain and performance under pain). I first describe the brain biomarker approach and how it is supported by a new class of algorithms, *machine learning* or *statistical learning*, that are now in widespread use in research and commercial applications across fields [1, 28]. Then, I describe the criteria for developing brain biomarkers that can be applied and used in research and clinical settings, and some of the potential applications. I will argue that the ultimate goal of the biomarker approach is to identify brain representations of pain and other outcomes. Importantly, not all applications of machine learning are equally viable as biomarkers, but building systematically on carefully developed biomarkers could transform the way pain is understood, assessed, and treated.

BRAIN BIOMARKERS

The potential applications and markets for an understanding of how the brain generates and regulates pain are substantial [8, 25]. Both optimists and skeptics are waiting for breakthrough applications of neuroimaging techniques in clinical and commercial use. But, with few exceptions, those applications have not appeared in the first 20 years of neuroimaging. As one recent, authoritative review put it: "Why has it taken so long for biological psychiatry to develop clinical tests and what to do about it?" [37].

One simple answer is that we have not really tried to develop neuroimaging-based clinical tests. The vast majority of the thousands of human neuroimaging studies, including early neuroimaging studies of pain, have not attempted to do anything that could lead to a clinical test based on measures of human brain activity. These studies have focused on *brain mapping*—an endeavour that seeks to identify which brain regions respond to events in a particular psychological or stimulus category (e.g., painful events, remembered items, or attended objects). The outcome of these studies is a statistical map of brain responses, and these maps have taught us much about the brain. For example, the human insula, cingulate, and thalamus respond to multiple kinds of noxious events, and are hyperactivated in at least some forms of hyperalgesia [14]. A characteristic feature of brain maps is that they subject each region or "voxel" to an independent analysis, seeking to explain its activity level over time as a function of psychological and physical states. Another characteristic is that the outcome is a "yes/no" answer at each voxel—a test of whether there is a statistically nonzero response to the psychological event being mapped.

This is a worthy, and even critical, scientific goal. However, a translational approach requires something qualitatively different: the use of measured brain activity across multiple systems to (a) predict both performance and long-term functional outcomes, and (b) test effects of cognitive, behavioural, or pharmacological interventions (Fig. 2-1). This approach is tantamount to first developing *brain biomarkers* of outcomes of clinical or translational interest, and then using those brain biomarkers to provide mechanistic information on how potential treatments work [9, 10].

The brain biomarker approach inverts the traditional analysis. Instead of treating brain activity in a "voxel" as the outcome, the outcome is the function to be explained or predicted (e.g., pain intensity, pain duration, cognitive performance, or other affective symptoms). All brain information available, including measured activity in multiple regions within and across brain areas, is used to predict the outcome. Brain data can be combined across types of imaging (e.g., functional and structural imaging) or with other measures (traditional clinical assessments, blood biomarkers) to refine the predictions; the limits depend on the application, for example, which measures will be available for test cases.

CONTRASTING THE BIOMARKER APPROACH WITH STANDARD BRAIN MAPPING

In brain mapping as practiced over the last 20 years, efforts are not generally made to (a) evaluate how large and meaningful reported effects are using unbiased techniques and (b) perform exact replications. These shortcomings have had major repercussions for the translation of scientific findings into clinical and commercial settings.

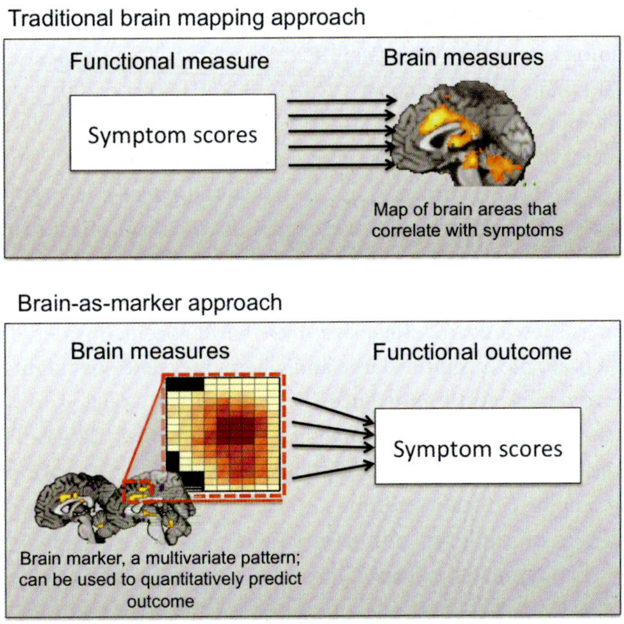

FIGURE 2-1 Traditional and emerging approaches to neuroimaging analysis. Top: A traditional approach with limited potential for translation. Every brain "voxel" or region is treated as a separate outcome, and the goal is to explain brain responses with symptoms and tasks. Bottom: The "brain biomarker" approach, in which machine learning algorithms are used to identify patterns of brain activity that closely predict symptoms or other functional outcomes.

In the area of drug discovery, this has led to failed attempts by pharmaceutical companies to replicate basic research findings and develop them commercially, at great expense to the companies and, ultimately, the public [7, 25, 32]. These failures have caused pharmaceutical companies to dramatically scale back mental health research in some cases. As Dr. Thomas Insel writes, "Despite high prevalence and unmet medical need, major pharmaceutical companies are de-emphasising or exiting psychiatry, thus removing significant capacity from efforts to discover new medicines" [31].

Translational approaches require a very different strategy. Rather than cataloguing statistically significant differences [37], brain markers must be identified that are *strongly predictive* of diagnostic categories or functional outcomes. The diagnostic value of these markers must be assessed across individuals, samples, settings, and research groups. Markers must be *optimized* so that they are maximally diagnostic and robust, including markers that integrate multiple brain measures and systems.

Brain Markers and Effect Sizes

Traditional brain mapping approaches focus on hypothesis testing and correction for multiple comparisons, to reduce false-positive brain findings. However, they are not suitable for testing how *large* the effects are. This point was the core of a heated debate about effect sizes in neuroimaging studies several years ago, which received widespread media coverage and debate in journal editorial offices and funding agencies [62]. Essentially, in neuroimaging as in any other domain, if one performs many tests, the ones that pass the threshold for statistical significance and reporting will tend to include error that favours a significant finding—the "winner's curse." In meta-analysis, the same problem is called the "file drawer problem"—if one runs 100 studies on a phenomenon with no effect, on average 5 of them will be "significant" at $P < 0.05$. If the 5 studies are the only ones published and the 95 null findings go in the proverbial file drawer, then it will appear as though the effect is reliable. Brain maps routinely consist of between 50,000 and 200,000 tests, and the significant findings appear to have much larger effect sizes (correlations with symptoms, *t*- or *Z*-values for effects) than they actually have. Correcting for multiple comparisons limits the reporting of false-positive findings, but it makes the effect-size problem *worse*: By raising the bar for statistical significance, the degree to which significant findings capitalize on chance is increased [65].

Why should we care about effect sizes? Traditional scientific findings are based on hypothesis testing, and effect sizes have hardly been considered. But if one cares about which effects are meaningfully large and where interventions might make a difference, effect sizes are of paramount importance. They are directly related to the ability to classify (or diagnose) cases and accurately predict future outcomes. Large effects (not small ones) are likely to be replicable, important, and useful. Of the thousands of potential causes and correlates of complex clinical conditions, those with large effects deserve particular follow-up study and can inform interventions and policy.

The brain biomarker approach circumvents the effect-size estimation obstacle. The primary analysis metric is an effect size: the error in predicting the outcome in new test cases (e.g., new individuals). The important consideration is whether the estimate of the effect size is valid, and what test cases it applies to. Useful predictions about pain will typically be about new individuals: How much pain (or what type of pain) an individual is feeling, based on their brain state. If a model is developed that relates brain activity maps to one type of pain, and then predictions are made about a new type of pain, or a different group of individuals from a different demographic, the effect size may shrink. The goal is to estimate predictive accuracy across different samples and test conditions, to determine the *breakdown point* or the boundary conditions for the predictive test.

Brain Markers and Replicability

There is an increasing recognition of the need for replication of results across laboratories [33, 47]. This is true across multiple fields that deal with complex data, including both neuroimaging [15] and genetics [22], and in other fields as well [54].

In traditional brain mapping analyses, findings are aggregated and replications "counted" at the level of gross anatomical regions. For example, if two studies show that a distraction modulates activity in the rostral dorsal anterior cingulate (rdACC), then the pair will be counted as a replicated effect by many scientists. This is not unreasonable, as this region is usually circumscribed within one functional zone or "parcel," and is treated as a homogenous region [61]. However, the rdACC contains hundreds of voxels, and there is a question about how close is "close enough" for two brain findings to be considered replicates. In addition, there is ample room for studies that activate different sets of voxels to be considered as replications. These findings would not replicate if a predefined set of voxels were used, and this flexibility introduces an additional level of uncertainty. Although it is commonplace to think of activation patterns that are nearby or overlapping, but not identical, as similar, one must remember that activity in the rdACC and other brain regions at this scale is not a pure measure, and reflects potentially hundreds of distinct processes.

In the brain biomarker framework, there is an explicit emphasis on using precisely defined brain patterns in new individuals and samples. Testing a brain marker on a new sample constitutes an exact replication of the marker at the level of the brain pattern. And, indeed, the precise brain pattern—including which voxels (or connections) are "active" and exactly how strongly they activate in relation to the outcome—must be specified in advance in order to test generalization to new individuals and samples. By holding the brain pattern constant, the brain biomarker approach is naturally suited to replications, and to assessing how variation in the sample, procedures, conditions tested, or other factors affects the size of brain–outcome relationships.

MACHINE LEARNING: A KEY TO DEVELOPING USEFUL BIOMARKERS

An important trend in the neuroimaging literature is the use of "statistical learning" or "machine learning" algorithms to identify distributed patterns of fMRI activity within and across regions [30, 45]. Machine learning is a broad class of algorithms designed to predict outcomes from multivariate datasets. Techniques encompass "supervised learning" techniques designed to predict outcomes of interest, including regression (for predicting continuous outcomes) and classification (for categorical outcomes), and "unsupervised learning" techniques for identifying clusters and dimensional components in datasets. They also include nonlinear and adaptive techniques such as reinforcement learning. Applied to brain data, the machine learning approach is closely aligned with "multi-voxel pattern analysis" (MVPA), the practice of identifying activity *patterns* across voxels and using them to classify or "decode" stimulus conditions [29].

MVPA techniques do not necessarily involve machine learning, but machine learning provides the most powerful ways of identifying patterns of brain activity that have specific profiles of psychological responsivity. Not all machine learning analyses are suitable for the brain biomarker approach: Machine learning is a class of algorithms, and models estimated using machine learning techniques and their outputs can be more or less interpretable, and thus more or less useful for neuroscientific discovery and measurement. However, machine learning algorithms share several features that make them particularly suited for the brain biomarker approach.

Quantitative Diagnostic Assessment

Although the family of machine learning techniques is broad, several specific principles are particularly germane to the brain biomarker approach. First is the notion of quantitative diagnostic testing—evaluating the diagnostic properties of a defined brain marker. This can be captured fairly well by the sensitivity and specificity of the marker in predicting the outcome, from which can be derived the positive and negative predictive values of the brain pattern when applied as a test of the outcome. The positive predictive value is the probability of an outcome (e.g., pain above a specified threshold) when the brain pattern is present (e.g., expression of the brain pattern above a specified threshold). These values are easily interpretable and meaningful in clinical applications. They are not unique to machine learning, and are routinely applied to all kinds of diagnostic tests, but they are of particular interest in machine learning analyses because of the emphasis on prediction; in machine learning, sensitivity and negative predictive value are called "recall" and "precision," and "precision–recall curves" are typically reported. Neither the brain activity nor the outcome need be treated as a categorical measure, however, and continuous measures of prediction error can also be quantified.

Generalization and Application to Individual Persons

Second is the idea of cross-validation [23], a procedure in which a model is developed ("training") on a subset of the data, and tested on a "holdout" dataset. The assignment of training and test data is done multiple times, often so that each observation (e.g., each individual participant) is part of the test set exactly once. These training–test splits are called "folds," and the model is reestimated on the training data for each fold and applied to the test data from that fold. Performed correctly, cross-validation can provide reasonably unbiased estimates of the accuracy in generalization to the test data.

However, cross-validation can yield optimistically biased estimates if (a) the observations are not truly independent, creating dependence between the errors in training and testing datasets, or (b) cross-validated analyses are repeated on the same dataset many times, with different combinations of data processing or algorithmic choices. The first problem can occur in the presence of any unmeasured confound, for example, slow changes in the sample, scanner, or experimenters with the passage of time. The second can occur whenever researchers seek to optimize accuracy and pick the best among a series of models. For this reason, it is often advantageous to (a) stratify the training–testing assignment on potential confounds and (b) reserve a final holdout set for testing only after all analyses are completed and the "final" model is selected.

Hyper-Resolution

Another powerful idea is that patterns derived from machine learning can circumvent some of the limitations in spatial resolution of fMRI, because patterns can be sensitive to the local structure of functional columns and differential functional organization across microvascular beds [17, 38]. Pattern information about functional topography is often preserved at a mesoscopic level, and is detectable even when the voxels sampled are larger than the columns themselves [17, 35, 36, 57]. In addition, mesoscopic organization is often preserved across individuals, permitting accurate inferences about individuals based on normative group-level data [48, 51, 52, 64]. This means that distributed local patterns of activity can be sensitive to the differential distribution of different types of neurons across a brain region. Thus, whereas any one voxel in a region such as the anterior cingulate may not be highly diagnostic of pain [60, 66], a particular local pattern across voxels within the anterior cingulate may be diagnostic [64].

USING MACHINE LEARNING TO SUPPORT THE BRAIN BIOMARKER APPROACH: CHARACTERISTICS OF A USEFUL BRAIN-BASED BIOMARKER

Machine learning, MVPA, and the brain biomarker approach are all conceptually distinct, and the vast majority of machine learning and MVPA fMRI studies are not suitable for use as biomarkers. Rather, neuroimaging-based biomarkers should conform to a particular set of standards [10]. What is at stake is whether a particular brain marker robustly and specifically reflects the core features that cause an outcome (e.g., that cause pain), or reflects noise or superfluous brain processes. The stronger the evidence for these characteristics, the more useful and trustworthy the marker:

1. **Prospectively defined pattern:** The pattern of activity, connectivity, etc. must be *precisely* defined a priori. A priori definition of regions or networks of interest is common in the literature, but their definition is flexible depending on which prior studies or atlases are used. Activation in brain maps is yet more flexible; two studies may activate a region (e.g., the amygdala or dorsal posterior insula) and yet activate nonoverlapping voxels and uncorrelated patterns across voxels. The most useful markers will specify precisely which voxels (or connections) are used within and across brain regions, and the *specific relative activity levels* across voxels. The dangerous potential for capitalizing on chance by testing multiple algorithms, brain features or patterns, and samples and picking the best ones can hardly be overstated.
2. **Diagnostic for individual people (sensitive and specific):** The stronger a pattern separates patient/control groups or predicts other continuous outcomes like pain, the more likely it is to be useful as a diagnostic or prognostic aid. In addition, strongly diagnostic markers are more likely to represent core brain features linked to outcomes. Diagnosticity can be captured by (at a minimum) two values: sensitivity and specificity. In a pain context, sensitivity relates to the effect size of brain responses to pain or, in probabilistic terms, the probability of observing a response in the brain marker above threshold given pain, $P(\text{brain marker} \mid \text{pain})$. Specificity relates to the probability of observing a response given conditions other than pain, $1 - P(\text{brain marker} \mid \text{no pain})$. Specificity must be evaluated relative to specific alternatives to pain (warmth, negative emotion, other salient cues, or events), and very few studies have attempted to address specificity [64]. Specificity is particularly important because current thinking about brain networks emphasizes the generality of brain responses in the "pain matrix" or pain-processing regions [20, 46, 66], though it is likely that machine learning-derived patterns can be much more specific to pain than regional activation [64].
3. **Interpretable:** Brain markers that reflect core brain features of outcomes are likely to be interpretable, in the sense that they (a) can be evaluated by human scientists and (b) conform to predictions based on other sources of data, including studies in nonhuman animals, lesion studies, human and nonhuman electrophysiology, and other neuroscience methods. For example, an interpretable acute pain biomarker should include activity in dorsal posterior insula and SII, stimulation of which evokes pain in humans [43], as well as other regions known to be important from the vast literature on pain across species. Some machine-learning-based markers that have fared well in prediction—even winning competitions for predictive accuracy—are not interpretable, and appear to capture activity in the ventricles or other brain structures not known to be related to the phenomena they are predicting [24, 56]. In some cases, they appear to be related to confounding variables—for example, a recent competition-winning pattern that "diagnosed" attention-deficit hyperactivity disorder versus control subjects appeared to track head motion, rather than psychological elements of the disorder [24].
4. **Transfer across laboratories, scanners, and populations:** Useful brain markers must be demonstrably diagnostic across multiple laboratories, populations, and scanners. Markers that appear to be diagnostic in one sample from one geographical location may not be diagnostic in other samples. Markers that are robust and

that represent core features of the outcome being measured should transfer across laboratories and populations. In addition, they must be able to be shared and applied prospectively and still yield good results. The imperative of testing on datasets independent from those used to identify the marker has, in part, led to multisite efforts to prospectively share neuroimaging data (e.g., http://fcon_1000.projects.nitrc.org/indi/IndiPro.html). Of course, like any assay, a particular brain marker may not perform well in some populations and with some scanning and data processing procedures. These variations must be quantified, so that markers are applied under conditions where good sensitivity and specificity can be expected.

5. **Transfer across conditions:** The sensitivity and specificity of a brain marker must be evaluated relative to the conditions under which it is tested. For a brain marker to be specific to acute pain, it must be sensitive to multiple types of acute pain (e.g., pain evoked by pressure, heat, cold, chemical signals, and inflammation). Of course, if no single brain system tracks all these kinds of pain, there may not be any single marker that tracks pain across these conditions. There may not be any common representation of "pain" across all types, but there may be multiple representations of acute pain, inflammatory pain, chronic neuropathic pain, etc. Alternatively, the systems that represent heat pain and mechanical pain may be different, implying that there is no single representation of "acute pain." Thus, the pattern of conditions a marker transfers versus does not transfer to can help inform us about how the brain is organized and what the neurophysiological types of pain are.

Thus, the brain biomarker approach is a *specific use* of MVPA and machine learning techniques, and putative markers must be evaluated in terms of these (and related) functional characteristics. The process of demonstrating and testing markers across samples, scanners, populations, and task/condition variants (e.g., types of pain) requires substantially more effort than single studies that simply establish an effect or phenomenon [10, 50].

Seen in this light, most examples of machine-learning-based studies in the literature are not suitable for person-level prediction at all. In particular, "searchlight" MVPA approaches [39]—involving search for multivariate predictors of an outcome across many local patterns—are not suitable. They do provide measures of accuracy, but these measures are biased for the same reasons that whole-brain effect-size maps are biased: They capitalize on chance by searching across many variables and picking the "winners." To be used as markers, predictive regions from a searchlight analysis must be tested on a *completely new set of individuals*, with *no additional model selection or retraining*. Searchlight analyses are useful for identifying and studying what information is represented in different brain regions, but not for use as markers unless searchlights are combined into a single, predictive model and then validated for that purpose.

STATE OF THE FIELD: APPLICATIONS OF MACHINE LEARNING TO DEVELOPING BRAIN MARKERS FOR CLINICALLY RELEVANT OUTCOMES

As neuroimaging is increasingly used in clinical and translational studies, there is increasing focus on the diagnostic value of brain patterns for clinical conditions [6, 11, 18, 21, 67] and treatment responses [19, 44]. To provide diagnostic value, studies like these are beginning to use the brain biomarker approach, combined with various MVPA and machine learning methods, to develop brain markers useful in measuring endogenous brain responses linked to outcomes of clinical, psychological, and behavioural interest. These efforts are in the early stages, and the criteria above have seldom been systematically applied. However, these studies show great promise for increasingly systematic application and testing across laboratories.

To date, several studies have focused on using machine learning techniques to identify patterns within an individual person that predict the intensity or incidence of acute pain for that person [11, 12, 16, 41]. Other studies have used EEG [49] to make predictions, which is promising because the technology is less expensive and deployable on a large scale. These studies do not use prospectively designed patterns and make predictions about individuals, so they do not meet criteria 1 and 2 above, but they are important stepping stones towards biomarker development.

Additional studies have shown that it is possible to predict acute pain *without training data on an individual person*, based on a normative model [13, 64]. This is variously referred to as "between-person classification/prediction" or "generalization to out-of-sample individuals," and fulfils criterion 1 above. Such models can be applied prospectively to data from individual persons, without knowledge of the "ground truth" about pain for that individual. Such approaches are required if the brain biomarker approach is to be used to augment tests for pain and other psychological phenomena (e.g., emotional responses).

In a recent study, Wager et al. [64] attempted to address the other criteria above systematically, and in so doing identify a biomarker for acute pain. We identified a pattern based on a sample ($N = 20$) that was composed mainly of patterns of activity within pain-responsive regions (Fig. 2-2). Linear machine learning techniques were used to stabilize the pattern and increase interpretability (criterion 3), which is evidenced by the fact that

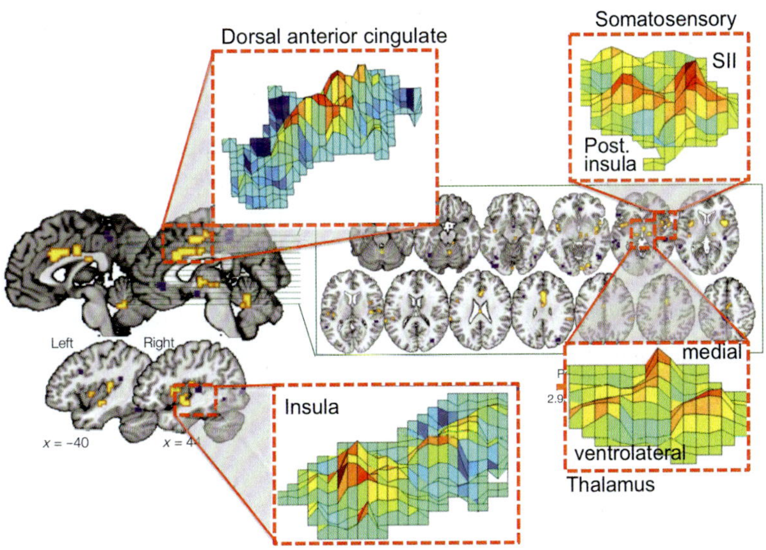

FIGURE 2-2 An example of neuroimaging-based biomarker pattern [64]. This pattern across voxels, including multiple pain-related brain regions, serves as a marker that can be tested in individual persons. The integrated activity across the pattern provides a continuous readout of predicted acute pain intensity. This readout is compared with a threshold to determine whether a condition elicits this pain-related brain pattern or not, and predict which of two conditions is more painful.

increases in predicted pain intensity were driven by increases in activity in multiple "known" pain-related regions. We tested its performance on three additional, independent samples, one from a different scanner (with a different field strength and manufacturer) running different acquisition sequences (criterion 4). In these test samples, we validated that the model has over 90% sensitivity and specificity at the individual person level for discriminating acute pain from nonpainful warmth, pain anticipation, pain judgment, and romantic rejection-related stimuli that otherwise activate very similar brain patterns as acute pain. The rejection condition was negative, arousing, and salient, and activated portions of the dorsal posterior insula and SII that are otherwise quite pain specific [40], providing a strong test case for the pain biomarker.

Applications to clinical samples have, thus far, typically used between-person classification to identify whether a patient has a clinical diagnosis or is a healthy control based on brain activity. For example, functional activity in the nucleus accumbens after pain [5] and brain structural measures related to grey-matter density [59] have been used to classify low back pain patients versus controls. Patient–control separation based on brain measures has also been reported in schizophrenia [21], Alzheimer disease [18], and depression [67]. These studies meet criterion 1, and in some cases are strongly diagnostic of patient versus control status, though their specificity relative to other disorders or confusable controls has not been tested (criterion 2). However, apart from tests in Alzheimer disease—which have benefitted from multisite consortium support and are now used in clinical trials—they have not yet been tested for generalizability across samples, populations, and test conditions (criteria 4 and 5). An additional limitation is that the candidate markers vary in interpretability (criterion 3); and, critically, a marker trained to identify patients versus controls can capitalize on *any* differences between the groups, including those that are irrelevant to the core features of the disorder (e.g., how patients understand task instructions or attend to visual stimuli or move their heads). Therefore, patient versus control classification is a starting point, but not an end point, for biomarker development.

Models that can be applied prospectively are predictive ones that can be used to guess patient status or predict recovery before outcome data become available. These models are particularly promising and important for early identification of risk and intervention. For example, Apkarian's group has used functional connectivity in medial frontal–striatal circuits to predict whether patients will recover from back pain or transition to chronic pain [6, 26]. Machine learning techniques have also been used to predict treatment recovery in depression [53] and social anxiety [19]. This is one of the most promising applications of the brain biomarker approach, as it could be used to (a) identify high-risk individuals who will benefit from intensive treatment; (b) permit early intervention, before disease processes have caused irreparable damage; and (c) predict who will respond best to a particular treatment. Other work has sought to predict who will respond to placebo treatments [27, 63], which could be clinically useful for (a) identifying placebo responders, (b) assessing how placebo and drug responses are related (they may be independent or interact [3, 4]), and (c) screening or controlling for placebo responses in clinical trials.

Machine learning approaches, when used in particular ways, are also particularly suited to *person stratification*—one of the great translational needs described earlier. Approaches such as *collaborative filtering* attempt to identify subgroups of individuals and make predictions specific to that individual's group. These approaches are widely used in commercial "big data" applications, and are just beginning to be applied to neuroimaging data; however, such approaches have not yet been widely applied in clinical settings.

SUMMARY AND POTENTIAL APPLICATIONS

Neuroimaging-based biomarkers for pain can be developed, and they have many uses. They could serve to augment pain measurement as part of multimodal assessments, and could be used in clinical trials for multiple purposes [8]. They could help screen drugs for brain penetrance and pharmacodynamic properties in early-stage (Phase 1) trials, demonstrate efficacy in affecting objective, pain-related outcomes in Phase 2 and 3 trials, and separate drug responses from placebo responses based on physiological outcomes in Phase 3 trials, increasing the efficacy of trials and understanding of the mechanisms of drug action in the brain. They can also be used for early identification of risk factors, and thus cost-effective early treatment. They can potentially be used to identify subgroups of healthy individuals and patients with different neurophysiological "types" (sources) of pain, who may respond to different treatments. And, perhaps most importantly, they can provide an increased understanding of the neurophysiological components, or "ingredients," of pain, and an understanding of how these vary across types of pain, disorders, contexts, and treatments. A biomarker that is predictive of pain or diagnostic of patient status is a first step, an entry point into the assessment of the brain *representations* that constitute the ingredients of pain at the brain level. And understanding pain's representational basis is the key to developing ways of thinking about and treating pain that are beyond our current vision. It is also the key to comparing representations across species and better understanding how mechanisms discovered and studied in animals apply to humans.

However, developing translationally useful biomarkers requires more rigorous evidence than most scientific studies of brain function [10]. Precise markers must be identified and used prospectively, and they must be diagnostic in individual persons. We must characterize what precisely they are diagnostic of (a specific type of pain? Negative affect? Arousal? Salience?), in different populations and relative to multiple potentially confusable alternative states (emotion, apprehension, distress without the *pain*). Obtaining rigorous evidence requires testing of multiple studies across multiple laboratories as well as the establishment of imaging practices and quality controls so that results can be widely used and trusted. If we embrace this goal and work together, then real advances in the understanding, prevention, and treatment of pain in humans and across species are possible.

REFERENCES

1. Anderson JR, Michalski RS, Carbonell JG, Mitchell TM. Machine learning: an artificial intelligence approach, Vol. 2. Los Altos, CA: Morgan Kaufmann; 1986.
2. Apkarian AV, Bushnell MC, Treede RD, Zubieta JK. Human brain mechanisms of pain perception and regulation in health and disease. Eur J Pain 2005;9(4):463–84.
3. Atlas LY, Whittington RA, Lindquist MA, Wielgosz J, Sonty N, Wager TD. Dissociable influences of opiates and expectations on pain. J Neurosci 2012;32(23):8053–64.
4. Atlas LY, Wielgosz J, Whittington RA, Wager TD. Specifying the non-specific factors underlying opioid analgesia: expectancy, attention, and affect. Psychopharmacology 2014;231(5):813–23.
5. Baliki MN, Geha PY, Fields HL, Apkarian AV. Predicting value of pain and analgesia: nucleus accumbens response to noxious stimuli changes in the presence of chronic pain. Neuron 2010;66(1):149–60.
6. Baliki MN, Petre B, Torbey S, Herrmann KM, Huang L, Schnitzer TJ, Fields HL, Apkarian AV. Corticostriatal functional connectivity predicts transition to chronic back pain. Nat Neurosci 2012;15(8):1117–9.
7. Begley CG, Ellis LM. Drug development: raise standards for preclinical cancer research. Nature 2012;483(7391):531–3.
8. Borsook D, Becerra L, Fava M. Use of functional imaging across clinical phases in CNS drug development. Transl Psychiatry 2013;3(7):e282.

9. Borsook D, Becerra L, Hargreaves R. Biomarkers for chronic pain and analgesia, part 1: the need, reality, challenges, and solutions. Discov Med 2011;11(58):197–207.
10. Borsook D, Becerra L, Hargreaves R. Biomarkers for chronic pain and analgesia, part 2: how, where, and what to look for using functional imaging. Discov Med 2011;11(58):209–19.
11. Brodersen KH, Schofield TM, Leff AP, Ong CS, Lomakina EI, Buhmann JM, Stephan KE. Generative embedding for model-based classification of fMRI data. PLoS Comput Biol 2011;7(6):e1002079.
12. Brodersen KH, Wiech K, Lomakina EI, Lin CS, Buhmann JM, Bingel U, Ploner M, Stephan KE, Tracey I. Decoding the perception of pain from fMRI using multivariate pattern analysis. Neuroimage 2012;63(3):1162–70.
13. Brown JE, Chatterjee N, Younger J, Mackey S. Towards a physiology-based measure of pain: patterns of human brain activity distinguish painful from non-painful thermal stimulation. PLoS One 2011;6(9):e24124.
14. Bushnell MC, Čeko M, Low LA. Cognitive and emotional control of pain and its disruption in chronic pain. Nat Rev Neurosci 2013.
15. Button KS, Ioannidis JP, Mokrysz C, Nosek BA, Flint J, Robinson ES, Munafo MR. Power failure: why small sample size undermines the reliability of neuroscience. Nat Rev Neurosci 2013;14(5):365–76.
16. Cecchi GA, Huang L, Hashmi JA, Baliki M, Centeno MaV, Rish I, Apkarian AV. Predictive dynamics of human pain perception. PLoS Compt Bio 2012;8(10):e1002719.
17. Chaimow D, Yacoub E, Ugurbil K, Shmuel A. Modeling and analysis of mechanisms underlying fMRI-based decoding of information conveyed in cortical columns. Neuroimage 2011;56(2):627–42.
18. Cuingnet RM, Gerardin E, Tessieras JRM, Auzias G, Lehricy SP, Habert M-O, Chupin M, Benali H, Colliot O. Automatic classification of patients with Alzheimer's disease from structural MRI: a comparison of ten methods using the ADNI database. Neuroimage 2011;56(2):766–81.
19. Doehrmann O, Ghosh SS, Polli FE, Reynolds GO, Horn F, Keshavan A, Triantafyllou C, Saygin ZM, Whitfield-Gabrieli S, Hofmann SG. Predicting treatment response in social anxiety disorder from functional magnetic resonance imaging treatment prediction in social anxiety disorder. JAMA Psychiatry 2013;70(1):87–97.
20. Downar J, Crawley AP, Mikulis DJ, Davis KD. A cortical network sensitive to stimulus salience in a neutral behavioral context across multiple sensory modalities. J Neurophysiol 2002;87(1):615–20.
21. Du W, Calhoun VD, Li H, Ma S, Eichele T, Kiehl KA, Pearlson GD, Adali Tl. High classification accuracy for schizophrenia with rest and task fMRI data. Front Hum Neurosci 2012;6:145.
22. Duncan LE, Keller MC. A critical review of the first 10 years of candidate gene-by-environment interaction research in psychiatry. Am J Psychiatry 2011;168(10):1041–9.
23. Efron B, Gong G. A leisurely look at the bootstrap, the jackknife, and cross-validation. Am Statist 1983;37(1): 36–48.
24. Eloyan A, Muschelli J, Nebel MB, Liu H, Han F, Zhao T, Barber A, Joel S, Pekar JJ, Mostofsky S. Automated diagnoses of attention deficit hyperactive disorder using magnetic resonance imaging. Front Syst Neurosci 2012;6:61.
25. Hargreaves R, Bullmore E, Becerra LR, Borsook D. Reasons to believe: the potential of imaging in CNS drug development. Imaging CNS Drug Discov Devel 2009;381–6.
26. Hashmi JA, Baliki MN, Huang L, Baria AT, Torbey S, Hermann KM, Schnitzer TJ, Apkarian AV. Shape shifting pain: chronification of back pain shifts brain representation from nociceptive to emotional circuits. Brain 2013;136(9):2751–68.
27. Hashmi JA, Baria AT, Baliki MN, Huang L, Schnitzer TJ, Apkarian AV. Brain networks predicting placebo analgesia in a clinical trial for chronic back pain. Pain 2012;153(12):2393–402.
28. Hastie T, Tibshirani R, Friedman JH. The elements of statistical learning: data mining, inference, and prediction. New York, NY: Springer; 2009.
29. Haxby JV, Gobbini MI, Furey ML, Ishai A, Schouten JL, Pietrini P. Distributed and overlapping representations of faces and objects in ventral temporal cortex. Science 2001;293(5539):2425–30.
30. Horikawa T, Tamaki M, Miyawaki Y, Kamitani Y. Neural decoding of visual imagery during sleep. Science 2013;340(6132):639–42.
31. Insel TR. Next-generation treatments for mental disorders. Sci Transl Med 2012;4(155):155ps119.
32. Ioannidis JP. Contradicted and initially stronger effects in highly cited clinical research. JAMA 2005;294(2):218–28.
33. Ioannidis JP. Why most published research findings are false. PLoS Med 2005;2(8):e124.
34. Jones AK, Brown WD, Friston KJ, Qi LY, Frackowiak RS. Cortical and subcortical localization of response to pain in man using positron emission tomography. Proc Biol Sci 1991;244(1309):39–44.
35. Kamitani Y, Sawahata Y. Spatial smoothing hurts localization but not information: pitfalls for brain mappers. Neuroimage 2010;49(3):1949–52.
36. Kamitani Y, Tong F. Decoding the visual and subjective contents of the human brain. Nat Neurosci 2005;8(5):679–85.

37. Kapur S, Phillips AG, Insel TR. Why has it taken so long for biological psychiatry to develop clinical tests and what to do about it? Mol Psychiatry 2012;17(12):1174–9.
38. Kriegeskorte N, Cusack R, Bandettini P. How does an fMRI voxel sample the neuronal activity pattern: compact-kernel or complex spatiotemporal filter? Neuroimage 2010;49(3):1965–76.
39. Kriegeskorte N, Goebel R, Bandettini P. Information-based functional brain mapping. Proc Natl Acad Sci USA 2006;103(10):3863–8.
40. Kross E, Berman MG, Mischel W, Smith EE, Wager TD. Social rejection shares somatosensory representations with physical pain. Proc Natl Acad Sci USA 2011;108(15):6270–5.
41. Marquand A, Howard M, Brammer M, Chu C, Coen S, Mourao-Miranda J. Quantitative prediction of subjective pain intensity from whole-brain fMRI data using Gaussian processes. Neuroimage 2010;49(3):2178–89.
42. May A. Chronic pain may change the structure of the brain. Pain 2008;137(1):7–15.
43. Mazzola L, Isnard J, Peyron R, Mauguière F. Stimulation of the human cortex and the experience of pain: Wilder Penfield's observations revisited. Brain 2012;135(2):631–40.
44. Miller JM, Schneck N, Siegle GJ, Chen Y, Ogden RT, Kikuchi T, Oquendo MA, Mann JJ, Parsey RV. fMRI response to negative words and SSRI treatment outcome in major depressive disorder: a preliminary study. Psychiatr Res Neuroimaging 2013;214(3):296–305.
45. Mitchell TM, Shinkareva SV, Carlson A, Chang K-M, Malave VL, Mason RA, Just MA. Predicting human brain activity associated with the meanings of nouns. Science 2008;320(5880):1191–5.
46. Mouraux A, Diukova A, Lee MC, Wise RG, Iannetti GD. A multisensory investigation of the functional significance of the "pain matrix". Neuroimage 2011;54(3):2237–49.
47. Pashler H, Wagenmakers EÄ. Editors' introduction to the special section on replicability in psychological science: a crisis of confidence? Perspect Psychol Sci 2012;7(6):528–30.
48. Rissman J, Greely HT, Wagner AD. Detecting individual memories through the neural decoding of memory states and past experience. Proc Natl Acad Sci USA 2010;107(21):9849–54.
49. Schulz E, Zherdin A, Tiemann L, Plant C, Ploner M. Decoding an individual's sensitivity to pain from the multivariate analysis of EEG data. Cereb Cortex 2012;22(5):1118–23.
50. Schwarz AJ, Becerra L, Upadhyay J, Anderson J, Baumgartner R, Coimbra A, Evelhoch J, Hargreaves R, Robertson B, Iyengar S. A procedural framework for good imaging practice in pharmacological fMRI studies applied to drug development# 1: processes and requirements. Drug Discov Today 2011;16(13):583–93.
51. Shinkareva SV, Malave VL, Just MA, Mitchell TM. Exploring commonalities across participants in the neural representation of objects. Hum Brain Mapp 2012;33(6):1375–83.
52. Shinkareva SV, Mason RA, Malave VL, Wang W, Mitchell TM, Just MA. Using fMRI brain activation to identify cognitive states associated with perception of tools and dwellings. PLoS One 2008;3(1):e1394.
53. Siegle G, Carter C, Thase M. Use of fMRI to predict recovery from unipolar depression with cognitive behavior therapy. Am J Psychiatry 2006;163(4):735–8.
54. Simmons JP, Nelson LD, Simonsohn U. False-positive psychology: undisclosed flexibility in data collection and analysis allows presenting anything as significant. Psychol Sci 2011;22(11):1359–66.
55. Smallwood RF, Laird AR, Ramage AE, Parkinson AL, Lewis J, Clauw DJ, Williams DA, Schmidt-Wilcke T, Farrell MJ, Eickhoff SB, et al. Structural brain anomalies and chronic pain: a quantitative meta-analysis of gray matter volume. J Pain 2013;14(7):663–75.
56. Sona D, Olivetti E, Avesani P, Veeramachaneni S. Learning to interpret cognitive states from fMRI Brain images. In: Proceedings of the 2009 Conference on Computational Intelligence and Bioengineering: Essays in Memory of Antonina Starita. Amsterdam, the Netherlands: IOS Press; 2009. pp. 21–35.
57. Swisher JD, Gatenby JC, Gore JC, Wolfe BA, Moon C-H, Kim S-G, Tong F. Multiscale pattern analysis of orientation-selective activity in the primary visual cortex. J Neurosci 2010;30(1):325–30.
58. Talbot JD, Marrett S, Evans AC, Meyer E, Bushnell MC, Duncan GH. Multiple representations of pain in human cerebral cortex. Science 1991;251(4999):1355–8.
59. Ung H, Brown JE, Johnson KA, Younger J, Hush J, Mackey S. Multivariate classification of structural MRI data detects chronic low back pain. Cereb Cortex 2014;24(4):1037–44.
60. van Snellenberg JX, Wager TD. Cognitive and motivational functions of the human prefrontal cortex. In: Christensen A, Goldberg E, Bougakov D, editors. Luria's legacy in the 21st century. Oxford, UK: Oxford University Press; 2009. pp. 30–61.
61. Vogt BA. Pain and emotion interactions in subregions of the cingulate gyrus. Nat Rev Neurosci 2005;6(7):533–44.
62. Vul E, Harris C, Winkielman P, Pashler H. Puzzlingly high correlations in fMRI studies of emotion, personality, and social cognition. Perspect Psychol Sci 2009;4(3):274–90.

63. Wager TD, Atlas LY, Leotti LA, Rilling JK. Predicting individual differences in placebo analgesia: contributions of brain activity during anticipation and pain experience. J Neurosci 2011;31(2):439–52.
64. Wager TD, Atlas LY, Lindquist MA, Roy M, Woo CW, Kross E. An fMRI-based neurologic signature of physical pain. N Engl J Med 2013;368(15):1388–97.
65. Yarkoni T. Big correlations in little studies: inflated fMRI correlations reflect low statistical power-commentary on Vul et al. (2009). Perspect Psychol Sci 2009;4(3):294–8.
66. Yarkoni T, Poldrack RA, Nichols TE, Van Essen DC, Wager TD. Large-scale automated synthesis of human functional neuroimaging data. Nat Methods 2011;8(8):665–70.
67. Zeng L-L, Shen H, Liu L, Wang L, Li B, Fang P, Zhou Z, Li Y, Hu D. Identifying major depression using whole-brain functional connectivity: a multivariate pattern analysis. Brain 2012;135(5):1498–507.

CHAPTER 3

Resting-State Brain Signals and Functional Connectivity Mapping

Biyu J. He

Clinicians commonly localize behavioural deficits to focal lesions in the brain. This principle of "cortical localization of function" is a cornerstone of clinical practice based on two theoretical principles that were articulated in the 1800s. The first is that specific functions are represented in specific parts of the brain [8]. Second, injuries to the brain disrupt localized functions and give rise to corresponding behavioural deficits [7]. Although these localizationist ideas remain the theoretical backbone of clinical neurology, recent advances in neuroscience suggest a much more distributed, parallel, and recursive view of brain function that has deep implications for clinical practice.

It is well accepted that the brain is anatomically organized in widely distributed and highly parallel networks. For example, the visual system is arranged as a hierarchy of cortical areas, each connected bidirectionally with upstream and downstream areas [14]. Moreover, many areas are horizontally connected with other areas at the same level. This anatomical arrangement emphasizes not just a bidirectional flow of information (bottom up from sensory to cognitive to motor areas, and top down from cognitive to sensory levels), but also local and long-range recursive processing through cortico-cortical or cortico-subcortical loops. In other words, perception of a stimulus or performance of a task requires the temporal coordination of multiple regions as the behaviour unfolds.

More generally, execution of any cognitive or behavioural function requires coordination of distributed brain regions. Hence, even in the absence of any localized abnormality, impairment of communication between brain regions could lead to failure in carrying out the corresponding function. Disruption in interregional communication (also called "functional connectivity") could result from damage in the brain regions involved, damage in the white matter pathway connecting them, or imbalance in the larger network(s) that they are embedded in. Traditional clinical practice was primarily concerned with local regional abnormality or the general imbalance of neurotransmitters, whereas modern neuroimaging research emphasizes a network perspective, under which impairment of anatomical or functional connectivity within or across brain networks can contribute significantly to various neurological and psychiatric disorders. In what follows, we will review the methodology for studying interregional connectivity, and highlight some recent progress in using this technique to shed light on brain disorders.

ELECTROPHYSIOLOGICAL APPROACHES FOR STUDYING FUNCTIONAL CONNECTIVITY

The amplitude of brain signals recorded with electroencephalography (EEG), magnetoencephalography (MEG), or invasive EEG (also called electrocorticography, ECoG) directly offers a measure of the degree of local neuronal synchrony [47], because only synchronized activity across a neuronal population can be picked up by these techniques that record brain activity at a relatively coarse spatial scale. To investigate interactions between neuronal groups on a larger spatial scale, that is, interregional connectivity, two approaches are commonly used: coherence [2, 5] and phase synchronization [31, 44]. In essence, both measures assess the maintenance of a constant phase relationship between two signals across time. The difference is that coherence computation derives phase from classical Fourier transformation and thus requires stationarity of the data, whereas phase-synchronization analysis extracts instantaneous phase using wavelet or Hilbert transform. Both methods reveal interactions between spatially discrete brain regions, and have been successfully applied to studying brain functional states in both normal physiology [13, 19, 49, 61] and clinical disorders [59]. Using noninvasive electrophysiological recordings to study brain networks faces the challenges of poor spatial resolution of these techniques and the potential volume conduction effect in scalp-recorded signals. However, recent methodological advances in source modelling have allowed the delineation of resting-state brain networks using MEG that well match those seen with functional magnetic resonance imaging (fMRI) [11, 27].

NEUROIMAGING AND BRAIN STIMULATION APPROACHES FOR STUDYING EFFECTIVE CONNECTIVITY

Over the past two decades, a handful of approaches have been developed for investigating brain networks using fMRI. These approaches can be largely classified into two categories: *effective connectivity*, defined as "the influence that one neural system exerts over another either directly or indirectly" [20], and *functional connectivity*, defined as "temporal correlations between spatially remote neurophysiological events" [21].

Classical approaches to studying effective connectivity include structural equation modelling and dynamic causal modelling. Both methods require an a priori model in which regions and connections of interest are specified; thus, the inferences are restricted to preselected networks and are strongly contingent upon the hypothesis (for detailed reviews, see [42, 56]). These methods are also contingent upon the specific task used, as changes in the system caused by external inputs are an integral part of the model. For examples of its application to patient populations, see [26, 36, 48, 52].

Several model-free approaches for studying effective connectivity have recently been developed. These methods either exploit temporal precedence information or utilize a "perturb-and-measure" approach. The logic behind the former is that cause should happen in advance of consequence. Thus, if activity in region A precedes that in region B, A is likely to exert an influence on B. Temporal precedence can be measured using various analytical methods, including autoregressive modelling ("Granger causality") [23, 45], phase spectrum [57], and asymmetry in lagged covariance function [46]. One major caveat in these analyses, when applied to fMRI data, is that temporal precedence information at the neuronal level may be distorted by heterogeneous hemodynamic delay across brain regions [12]. Nonetheless, because the hemodynamic response of a brain region is stable across different task conditions, one could compare the patterns of causal connectivity across task conditions to get around the hemodynamic confound [6]. We have recently successfully applied this approach to the study of bistable perception [62]. A second caveat is that common influence from a third region might manifest as spurious directed influence; however, this problem can be mitigated by the use of partial-correlation type of analysis, such as partial Granger causality [6].

The "perturb-and-measure" approach to studying effective connectivity uses transcranial magnetic stimulation (TMS) to reversibly perturb neural activity in a selected cortical area, and neuroimaging or electrophysiology to measure the resulting changes in brain activity patterns away from the stimulated area (for a review, see [41]). Interestingly, this effect is contingent not only upon anatomical connections (even including transsynaptic connections), but also on the state of spontaneous neural activity in the system [34, 41]. This approach has been successfully applied to the investigation of multiple altered states of consciousness and yielded impressive results [35].

NEUROIMAGING APPROACHES FOR STUDYING FUNCTIONAL CONNECTIVITY

There are two common approaches for studying functional connectivity in fMRI data: seed-driven correlation analysis and independent component analysis (ICA). Detailed methods for both approaches and their respective pros and cons have been reviewed elsewhere [17]. In brief, the seed-driven approach extracts the fMRI time course from a given brain region ("seed") and examines its temporal correlation with all other brain voxels [4]. This method is simple and intuitive, but does rely on the a priori selection of a seed region. By contrast, ICA decomposes the entire fMRI dataset into separate clusters of voxels that are maximally spatially independent of each other (i.e., "spatial ICA") [10]. Recently, a temporal ICA method has also been developed and applied to fMRI data acquired with fast sampling rate [54]. The temporal ICA method maximizes temporal independence between components but allows them to spatially overlap. In general, the ICA method is data driven and automatically isolates noise components, but it does require user specification of the number of independent components. This choice is often arbitrary and represents a trade-off between richness and robustness. In order to mitigate this arbitrariness, the investigator can perform ICA using different choices of dimensionality (i.e., the number of extracted components) and verify the robustness of the extracted components.

Two methodological issues should receive special attention in fMRI functional connectivity studies. Firstly, it has recently been established that motion artefact in the scanner produces spurious but systematic distortion of resting-state functional connectivity, leading to increased short-range connectivity and decreased long-range connectivity [43, 60]. Because the amount of motion often varies between patient and control populations, or across developmental stages, studies contrasting functional connectivity between these populations must either take great care in matching the amount of motion across groups or control for motion in data analyses [43, 60].

Secondly, the handling of the "global signal" has been a hotly debated issue. In seed-driven correlation analyses, the global signal averaged across all voxels in the brain is often regressed out from each voxel before correlation analyses are performed, in an effort to reduce nonspecific physiological noise in the data [17, 18]. Although this method does help in reducing noise, it produces the unwanted effect of forcing the existence of negative correlations, fuelling a fierce debate about whether anti-correlations [18] are real or artificially introduced by the regression of global signal [39]. Thus far, the observation of anticorrelation has withstood the test of time, being reinforced by the presence of anticorrelation in electrophysiological data [29], as well as fMRI data cleaned up for physiological noise without the use of global signal regression [9]. Nonetheless, caution should be exercised when applying global signal regression, especially in light of the finding that the fMRI global signal correlates with the power of local field potentials (LFPs) in simultaneous LFP–fMRI recordings in macaques, suggesting a potential neural contributor to the global signal [50]. For example, when contrasting functional connectivity between patient and control populations, if properties of the global signal differ between them, applying global signal regression would distort functional connectivity results. In these cases, we recommend repeating the analyses without global signal regression and verifying that the results are robust to this manoeuvre.

RESTING-STATE FUNCTIONAL CONNECTIVITY—APPLICATIONS TO CLINICAL POPULATIONS

Among the various approaches discussed here, the functional connectivity method applied to fMRI data has been most widely adopted for clinical applications because of its robustness (normally seen in single-subject data after 5–15 minute scanning), test–retest reliability [53], reproducibility across healthy subjects, intrinsic nature (i.e., emerging from brain's spontaneous activity, thus no task performance is required of the patient), and persistence under light sedation [24]. Several reviews on this topic already exist [16, 25, 63], covering the applications of resting-state functional connectivity to stroke; Alzheimer disease; presurgical planning; and various psychiatric disorders such as depression, autism, schizophrenia, and attention-deficit hyperactivity disorder (ADHD). Recently, altered functional connectivity has also been characterized in patients with epilepsy [33] and multiple sclerosis (for a review, see [15]). Impressive progress notwithstanding, we are still far from establishing reliable clinical biomarkers for diagnosis on a single-patient basis. Such translational efforts will be well worth making, given the great promises of this approach. In the context of this book, multiple recent studies have begun to explore altered functional connectivity accompanying chronic pain and have yielded promising results [3, 40, 51, 58].

Last but not least, several exciting recent developments in the resting-state fMRI field should be taken full advantage of in future clinical applications. These include the recognition of the importance of interindividual variability [30, 37, 38], the dynamical nature of functional connectivity [1, 11, 28, 32], the genetic contribution to functional connectivity [22], and the higher-quality data with better spatial and temporal resolution allowed by recent improvement of image acquisition methods [55].

ACKNOWLEDGEMENT

This research was supported by the Intramural Research Program of the National Institutes of Health, National Institute of Neurological Disorders and Stroke.

REFERENCES

1. Allen EA, Damaraju E, Plis SM, Erhardt EB, Eichele T, Calhoun VD. Tracking whole-brain connectivity dynamics in the resting state. Cereb Cortex 2014;24(3):663–76.
2. Andrew C, Pfurtscheller G. Event-related coherence as a tool for studying dynamic interaction of brain regions. Electroencephalogr Clin Neurophysiol 1996;98(2):144–8.
3. Baliki MN, Baria AT, Apkarian AV. The cortical rhythms of chronic back pain. J Neurosci 2011;31(39):13981–90.
4. Biswal B, Yetkin FZ, Haughton VM, Hyde JS. Functional connectivity in the motor cortex of resting human brain using echo-planar MRI. Magn Reson Med 1995;34(4):537–41.
5. Bressler SL, Coppola R, Nakamura R. Episodic multiregional cortical coherence at multiple frequencies during visual task performance. Nature 1993;366(6451):153–6.
6. Bressler SL, Seth AK. Wiener–Granger causality: a well established methodology. Neuroimage 2011;58(2):323–9.
7. Broca P. Localisation des fonctions cerebrales. Siege du langage articule. Bullettins del la Societe d'Anthropologie (Paris) 1863;4:200–3.
8. Brodmann K. On the comparative localization of the cortex [originally in German; translated by von Bonin G]. In: Tomas CC, editor. Some papers on the cerebral cortex. Springfield, IL: Charles C. Thomas, 1960. pp. 201–30.
9. Chang C, Glover GH. Effects of model-based physiological noise correction on default mode network anti-correlations and correlations. Neuroimage 2009;47(4):1448–59.
10. Damoiseaux JS, Rombouts SA, Barkhof F, Scheltens P, Stam CJ, Smith SM, Beckmann CF. Consistent resting-state networks across healthy subjects. Proc Natl Acad Sci USA 2006;103(37):13848–53.
11. de Pasquale F, Della Penna S, Snyder AZ, Lewis C, Mantini D, Marzetti L, Belardinelli P, Ciancetta L, Pizzella V, Romani GL, et al. Temporal dynamics of spontaneous MEG activity in brain networks. Proc Natl Acad Sci USA 2010;107(13):6040–5.
12. de Zwart JA, Silva AC, van Gelderen P, Kellman P, Fukunaga M, Chu R, Koretsky AP, Frank JA, Duyn JH. Temporal dynamics of the BOLD fMRI impulse response. Neuroimage 2005;24(3):667–77.
13. Engel AK, Fries P, Singer W. Dynamic predictions: oscillations and synchrony in top-down processing. Nat Rev Neurosci 2001;2(10):704–16.
14. Felleman DJ, Van Essen DC. Distributed hierarchical processing in the primate cerebral cortex. Cereb Cortex 1991;1(1):1–47.
15. Filippi M, Agosta F, Spinelli EG, Rocca MA. Imaging resting state brain function in multiple sclerosis. J Neurol 2013;260(7):1709–13.
16. Fox MD, Greicius M. Clinical applications of resting state functional connectivity. Front Syst Neurosci 2010;4:19.
17. Fox MD, Raichle ME. Spontaneous fluctuations in brain activity observed with functional magnetic resonance imaging. Nat Rev Neurosci 2007;8(9):700–11.
18. Fox MD, Snyder AZ, Vincent JL, Corbetta M, Van Essen DC, Raichle Me. The human brain is intrinsically organized into dynamic, anticorrelated functional networks. Proc Natl Acad Sci USA 2005;102(27):9673–8.
19. Fries P. A mechanism for cognitive dynamics: neuronal communication through neuronal coherence. Trends Cogn Sci 2005;9(10):474–80.
20. Friston KJ, Frith CD, Frackowiak RS. Time-dependent changes in effective connectivity measured with PET. Hum Brain Mapp 1993;1:69–79.
21. Friston KJ, Frith CD, Liddle PF, Frackowiak RS. Functional connectivity: the principal-component analysis of large (PET) data sets. J Cereb Blood Flow Metab 1993;13(1):5–14.
22. Glahn DC, Winkler AM, Kochunov P, Almasy L, Duggirala R, Carless MA, Curran JC, Olvera RL, Laird AR, Smith SM, et al. Genetic control over the resting brain. Proc Natl Acad Sci USA 2010;107(3):1223–8.
23. Goebel R, Roebroeck A, Kim DS, Formisano E. Investigating directed cortical interactions in time-resolved fMRI data using vector autoregressive modeling and Granger causality mapping. Magn Reson Imaging 2003;21(10):1251–61.
24. Greicius MD, Kiviniemi V, Tervonen O, Vainionpaa V, Alahuhta S, Reiss AL, Menon V. Persistent default-mode network connectivity during light sedation. Hum Brain Mapp 2008;29(7):839–47.
25. He BJ, Shulman GL, Snyder AZ, Corbetta M. The role of impaired neuronal communication in neurological disorders. Curr Opin Neurol 2007;20(6):655–60.
26. Hinrichs H, Heinze HJ, Schoenfeld MA. Causal visual interactions as revealed by an information theoretic measure and fMRI. Neuroimage 2006;31(3):1051–60.
27. Hipp JF, Engel AK, Siegel M. Oscillatory synchronization in large-scale cortical networks predicts perception. Neuron 2011;69(2):387–96.

28. Hutchison RM, Womelsdorf T, Allen EA, Bandettini PA, Calhoun VD, Corbetta M, Della Penna S, Duyn JH, Glover GH, Gonzalez-Castillo J, et al. Dynamic functional connectivity: promise, issues, and interpretations. Neuroimage 2013;80:360–78.
29. Keller CJ, Bickel S, Honey CJ, Groppe DM, Entz L, Craddock RC, Lado FA, Kelly C, Milham M, Mehta AD. Neurophysiological investigation of spontaneous correlated and anticorrelated fluctuations of the BOLD signal. J Neurosci 2013;33(15):6333–42.
30. Kelly AM, Uddin LQ, Biswal BB, Castellanos FX, Milham MP. Competition between functional brain networks mediates behavioral variability. Neuroimage 2008;39(1):527–37.
31. Lachaux JP, Rodriguez E, Martinerie J, Varela FJ. Measuring phase synchrony in brain signals. Hum Brain Mapp 1999;8(4):194–208.
32. Liu X, Duyn JH. Time-varying functional network information extracted from brief instances of spontaneous brain activity. Proc Natl Acad Sci USA 2013;110(11):4392–7.
33. Maccotta L, He BJ, Snyder AZ, Eisenman LN, Benzinger TL, Ances BM, Corbetta M, Hogan RE. Impaired and facilitated functional networks in temporal lobe epilepsy. Neuroimage Clin 2013;2:862–72.
34. Massimini M, Ferrarelli F, Huber R, Esser SK, Singh H, Tononi G. Breakdown of cortical effective connectivity during sleep. Science 2005;309(5744):2228–32.
35. Massimini M, Ferrarelli F, Sarasso S, Tononi G. Cortical mechanisms of loss of consciousness: insight from TMS/EEG studies. Archives italiennes de biologie 2012;150(2–3):44–55.
36. Mechelli A, Allen P, Amaro E Jr, Fu CH, Williams SC, Brammer MJ, Johns LC, McGuire PK. Misattribution of speech and impaired connectivity in patients with auditory verbal hallucinations. Hum Brain Mapp 2007;28(11):1213–22.
37. Mennes M, Kelly C, Zuo XN, Di Martino A, Biswal BB, Castellanos FX, Milham MP. Inter-individual differences in resting-state functional connectivity predict task-induced BOLD activity. Neuroimage 2010;50(4):1690–701.
38. Mueller S, Wang D, Fox MD, Yeo BT, Sepulcre J, Sabuncu MR, Shafee R, Lu J, Liu H. Individual variability in functional connectivity architecture of the human brain. Neuron 2013;77(3):586–95.
39. Murphy K, Birn RM, Handwerker DA, Jones TB, Bandettini PA. The impact of global signal regression on resting state correlations: are anti-correlated networks introduced? Neuroimage 2009;44(3):893–905.
40. Otti A, Guendel H, Wohlschlager A, Zimmer C, Noll-Hussong M. Frequency shifts in the anterior default mode network and the salience network in chronic pain disorder. BMC Psychiatry 2013;13:84.
41. Paus T. Inferring causality in brain images: a perturbation approach. Philos Trans R Soc Lond B Biol Sci 2005;360(1457):1109–14.
42. Penny WD, Stephan KE, Mechelli A, Friston KJ. Modelling functional integration: a comparison of structural equation and dynamic causal models. Neuroimage 2004;23(Suppl 1):S264–74.
43. Power JD, Barnes KA, Snyder AZ, Schlaggar BL, Petersen SE. Spurious but systematic correlations in functional connectivity MRI networks arise from subject motion. Neuroimage 2012;59(3):2142–54.
44. Rodriguez E, George N, Lachaux JP, Martinerie J, Renault B, Varela FJ. Perception's shadow: long-distance synchronization of human brain activity. Nature 1999;397(6718):430–3.
45. Roebroeck A, Formisano E, Goebel R. Mapping directed influence over the brain using Granger causality and fMRI. Neuroimage 2005;25(1):230–42.
46. Rykhlevskaia E, Fabiani M, Gratton G. Lagged covariance structure models for studying functional connectivity in the brain. Neuroimage 2006;30(4):1203–18.
47. Scherrer J. Organization of spontaneous electrical activity in the neocortex. Prog Brain Res 1976;45:309–325.
48. Schlosser R, Gesierich T, Kaufmann B, Vucurevic G, Hunsche S, Gawehn J, Stoeter P. Altered effective connectivity during working memory performance in schizophrenia: a study with fMRI and structural equation modeling. Neuroimage 2003;19(3):751–63.
49. Schnitzler A, Gross J. Normal and pathological oscillatory communication in the brain. Nat Rev Neurosci 2005;6(4):285–96.
50. Scholvinck ML, Maier A, Ye FQ, Duyn JH, Leopold DA. Neural basis of global resting-state fMRI activity. Proc Natl Acad Sci USA 2010;107(22):10238–43.
51. Schwedt TJ, Schlaggar BL, Mar S, Nolan T, Coalson RS, Nardos B, Benzinger T, Larson-Prior LJ. Atypical resting-state functional connectivity of affective pain regions in chronic migraine. Headache 2013;53(5):737–51.
52. Seminowicz DA, Mayberg HS, McIntosh AR, Goldapple K, Kennedy S, Segal Z, Rafi-Tari S. Limbic-frontal circuitry in major depression: a path modeling meta-analysis. Neuroimage 2004;22(1):409–18.
53. Shehzad Z, Kelly AM, Reiss PT, Gee DG, Gotimer K, Uddin LQ, Lee SH, Margulies DS, Roy AK, Biswal BB, et al. The resting brain: unconstrained yet reliable. Cereb Cortex 2009;19(10):2209–29.

54. Smith SM, Miller KL, Moeller S, Xu J, Auerbach EJ, Woolrich MW, Beckmann CF, Jenkinson M, Andersson J, Glasser MF, et al. Temporally-independent functional modes of spontaneous brain activity. Proc Natl Acad Sci USA.2012;109(8):3131–6.
55. Smith SM, Vidaurre D, Beckmann CF, Glasser MF, Jenkinson M, Miller KL, Nichols TE, Robinson EC, Salimi-Khorshidi G, Woolrich MW, et al. Functional connectomics from resting-state fMRI. Trends Cogn Sci 2013;17(12):666–82.
56. Stephan KE, Harrison LM, Kiebel SJ, David O, Penny WD, Friston KJ. Dynamic causal models of neural system dynamics: current state and future extensions. J Biosci 2007;32(1):129–44.
57. Sun FT, Miller LM, D'Esposito M. Measuring temporal dynamics of functional networks using phase spectrum of fMRI data. Neuroimage 2005;28(1):227–37.
58. Tagliazucchi E, Balenzuela P, Fraiman D, Chialvo DR. Brain resting state is disrupted in chronic back pain patients. Neurosci Lett 2010;485(1):26–31.
59. Uhlhaas PJ, Singer W. Neural synchrony in brain disorders: relevance for cognitive dysfunctions and pathophysiology. Neuron 2006;52(1):155–68.
60. Van Dijk KR, Sabuncu MR, Buckner RL. The influence of head motion on intrinsic functional connectivity MRI. Neuroimage 2012;59(1):431–8.
61. Varela F, Lachaux JP, Rodriguez E, Martinerie J. The brainweb: phase synchronization and large-scale integration. Nat Rev Neurosci 2001;2(4):229–39.
62. Wang M, Arteaga D, He BJ. Brain mechanisms for simple perception and bistable perception. Proc Natl Acad Sci USA 2013;110(35):E3340–9.
63. Zhang D, Raichle ME. Disease and the brain's dark energy. Nat Rev Neurol 2010;6(1):15–28.

CHAPTER 4

Monitoring Brain Electrical and Magnetic Activity for Assessing Pain: Advantages and Limitations

Rolf-Detlef Treede and Ulf Baumgärtner

Signal processing in the brain involves electrical signalling within neurons and chemical signalling between neurons. Electrical signals can be recorded intracellularly with micropipettes that are inserted into the neuron, and extracellularly with wire electrodes inside the brain or flat electrodes on top of the brain (electrocorticography). Intrinsic optical signals and voltage-sensitive dyes make these signals accessible to microscope imaging as well [8]. There is an ongoing debate over whether some magnetic resonance parameters are sufficiently modulated by electrical potentials to yield a useful signal for MRI.

Since 1929, when the German psychiatrist Hans Berger [3] first described recording electrical signals from the surface of the heads of bald men, EEG has provided a window into the brain. Some of the main applications of ongoing EEG recording are differential diagnosis of epilepsies, sleep staging, and intraoperative monitoring, and standardized guidelines have led to wide clinical use [1, 6, 17, 18, 25]. Signal changes in these applications are pronounced and can be detected by visual inspection of the EEG traces. Effects of cognitive processes in the brain are more subtle and require elaborate digital signal processing. Upon external stimulation, the EEG traces contain evoked potentials, usually of small amplitude, that can be isolated by time-locked averaging [7]. For pain research, investigators have attempted to find correlates of ongoing spontaneous pain in the ongoing EEG, and correlates of evoked pain in evoked potentials [2, 20, 22, 23, 25].

About 40 years after the discovery of the EEG, David Cohen [4] of the MIT (1968) was able to record magnetic fields that reflected the idling activity of the brain called alpha rhythm. Since then, ongoing magnetoencephalography (MEG) activity and evoked magnetic fields have also been studied to shed light on cortical processing of nociceptive inputs [10, 13, 14, 16].

NEUROPHYSIOLOGICAL BASIS OF EEG AND MEG SIGNALS

The grey matter of the neocortex, where cortical neurons are located, consists of six layers, with layer 1 being closest to the surface of the brain and layer 6 adjacent to the white matter, which contains only axons that connect different parts of the brain. In addition to several classes of excitatory and inhibitory interneurons that make connections with only nearby neurons, neocortical grey matter contains pyramidal neurons that send long axons to other

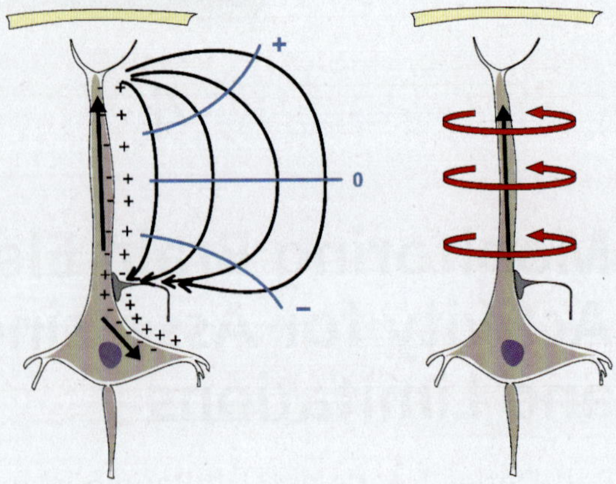

FIGURE 4-1 Schematic drawing of a lamina V cortical pyramidal cell, the intra- and extracellular current flow (*black arrows*) and isopotential lines (*blue*) induced by excitatory synaptic input into lamina IV for EEG signals (**left panel**), and the magnetic fields (*red arrows*) detectable by MEG induced by the intracellular current (**right panel**).

parts of the CNS, where they form glutamatergic excitatory synaptic connections. EEG and MEG signals are thought to be generated by the largest pyramidal neurons that are located in layer 5 and have long dendritic trees extending through most of the cortical layers. These dendrites can be turned into electrical dipoles by synaptic input either in superficial layers (from nonspecific afferents) or in layer 4 (from specific thalamocortical afferents). If layer 5 pyramidal neurons are activated asynchronously, their dipoles cancel each other out, but when they are activated simultaneously, their individual dipoles can add up to a large signal that is detectable from outside the head.

Fig. 4-1 shows evoked potentials (left) and evoked magnetic fields (right) that are induced by synaptic input to layer 4 from specific thalamic nuclei, which is the typical pathway for sensory inputs to the neocortex. While the resting membrane potential is negative at the inside of the neuron, excitatory synapses allow positive current to flow into the neuron via nonselective cation channels. This transmembrane current depolarizes the neuron (excitatory postsynaptic potential [EPSP]), which is now less negative at the site of excitatory synaptic input. This local depolarization is equivalent to a relative positivity compared with other parts of the same neuron, and this electrical potential difference leads to intracellular current flow. While some of the current flows towards the axon hillock where an action potential may be generated to forward a signal to the next neuron, the majority of the intracellular current is directed towards the apical parts of the dendrites that have not been depolarized. This intracellular current is detected by MEG according to the magnetic fields that are present around each electrical current and that are recordable with sensitive instruments (superconducting quantum interference devices [SQUIDs]) even at some distance from the current source.

Since EEG is measured with extracellular electrodes, it cannot detect those intracellular currents. However, the transmembrane current at the excitatory synapse removes positive charges from the outside of the membrane, which therefore becomes relatively negative compared with the outer side of the membrane of the apical nondepolarized parts of the dendrite. This potential difference leads to extracellular current flow, which is detected by EEG. Fig. 4-1 (left) also illustrates that the extracellular current flows through the volume conductor in loops at various distances from the generating neuron, and that there are electrical potential differences along each of these current loops that can be measured by pairs of electrodes even at some distance from the current source.

Thus, both MEG and EEG are generated by electrical dipole sources that lead to current flow perpendicular to the surface of the brain. Since MEG is generated by the intracellular current and EEG by the extracellular current, the direction of the relevant dipole

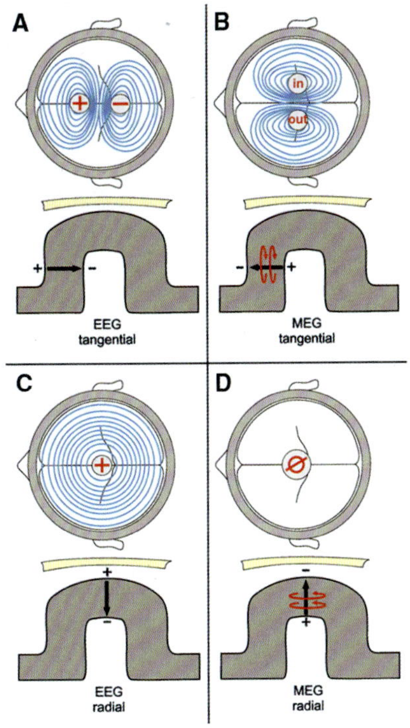

FIGURE 4-2 **A and B:** Scalp topographies of electrical potentials and magnetic fields resulting from source in the anterior wall of a gyrus like in primary somatosensory cortex Brodmann area 3b that generates current flow perpendicular to the surface of area 3b but tangential to the surface of the head. **C and D:** Scalp topographies of electrical potentials and magnetic fields resulting from a source in the crown of a gyrus like the somatosensory cortex Brodmann area 1 that generates current flow perpendicular to the surface, which is radial to the surface of the head and hence generates no measurable signals in MEG.

orientation is the opposite between MEG and EEG. In contrast to the rodent brain, the human brain is folded in complex patterns of gyri and sulci. Therefore, only some parts of the brain are oriented parallel to the surface of the head (at the peak or the bottom of a gyrus), whereas others are oriented perpendicular to the surface of the head (cortical grey matter within the anterior and posterior walls of a gyrus).

Fig. 4-2A and B illustrates the orientation of dipole sources in the wall of a gyrus, like the anterior wall of the postcentral gyrus, where the primary somatosensory cortex is located (Brodmann area 3b). In this case, the orientation of the dipole source is tangential to the surface of the head, which leads to detectable magnetic flux (by MEG; Fig. 4-2B) into and out of the head on both sides of the dipole. The corresponding extracellular current leads to detectable electrical potential maxima (by EEG; Fig. 4-2A) at both ends of the dipole. As illustrated by the schematic views of the top of the head, both MEG and EEG record a bipolar field pattern, and the dipole source is located in between the measured field maxima.

Fig. 4-2C and D illustrates the orientation of dipole sources in the crown of a gyrus, again, like the postcentral gyrus, where another part of the somatosensory cortex is located (Brodmann area 1). In this case, the orientation of the dipole source is radial (perpendicular) to the surface of the head, which leads to an electrical potential maximum directly overlying the tip of the dipole. Although this signal is easily detectable by EEG (Fig. 4-2C), there is no measurable magnetic field difference (Fig. 4-2D), and hence MEG is blind to purely radially oriented dipole sources.

The neurophysiological basis of EEG and MEG signals has been outlined here only for excitatory input into deep layer 4 of the cortex. However, this is easily extended to excitatory input into superficial layers (by switching the signs of the potential differences and the direction of current flow), and also to inhibitory postsynaptic potentials (IPSPs) by again flipping the signs. Thus, in principle, all ongoing and evoked EEG and MEG activities can be understood on the same basis.

SOURCE LOCALIZATION WITH EEG AND MEG

Visual inspection of scalp maps of magnetic field or electrical potential distributions can lead to correct identification of the source, provided only a single brain region is active at any given point in time. This is almost true in the case of the very early part of a somatosensory evoked potential induced by electrical stimulation of a nerve trunk (e.g., in the case of median nerve stimulation, the N20).

In most situations, however, many parts of the brain are active simultaneously, and hence the resulting field distributions on the scalp superimpose. In this case, mathematical methods such as dipole source analysis can be used to sort out the contributions by the different sources. Although it is relatively straightforward how to calculate the scalp distribution that results from any given dipole source inside the head, the inverse problem, unfortunately, has no unique solution, since many different combinations of dipole sources can lead to the same scalp distribution. Commercially available software packages solve this problem, by allowing the user to introduce a priori constraints or assumptions. Examples of such assumptions include: (a) Only grey matter can generate measurable currents, and hence all white matter is excluded; (b) Activity in any brain region does not change abruptly from one instance to the next, and hence the analysis can combine adjacent time points into short segments; (c) Sometimes regions of interest for dipole locations can be narrowed down a priori according to neuroanatomical facts.

ADVANTAGES OF EEG AND MEG

Both techniques yield data on summed regional electrical brain activity, which is very close to the "language of the brain" and can be directly compared with subdural electrocorticography and depth recordings in neurosurgical patients [2, 11], as well as field potential recordings and intracellular recordings in animal models. Temporal resolution is at millisecond level and hence allows cross-correlations of signals to uncover network activity (coherence analysis, Granger causality, long-distance gamma synchronization, etc.). In the case of EEG, technical equipment is inexpensive, and by using EEG caps, the electrodes can be rapidly placed in a reliable manner, even allowing the subjects to move around while being recorded. With MEG systems, the measurement can start almost instantaneously after a brief localization of the head with respect to the sensor array (Dewar). Table 4-1 summarizes the basis and properties of EEG and MEG signals.

LIMITATIONS OF EEG AND MEG

As noninvasive recording techniques, EEG and MEG do not provide signals at the single cell level. Their spatial resolution (when using state-of-the-art dipole source analysis) is on the order of 1 cm, and the source analysis does not yield a unique solution. Thus, these techniques are limited when there is no a priori hypothesis about active regions. In turn, dipole source analysis is an ideal technique to test such hypotheses.

A limitation for EEG but not MEG is the lack of a truly inactive reference site on the body. Electrical potentials cannot be measured in absolute terms but only as potential

TABLE 4-1 **Comparison of EEG and MEG**

	EEG	MEG
Signal source	Extracellular currents due to EPSP and IPSP	Intracellular currents due to EPSP and IPSP
Readout	Field potentials at scalp surface	Magnetic fields outside head
Distortion by skull bones	Little on convexity of the skull, marked near base of skull	Not relevant
Artefacts due to head movements	Not relevant	Offsets in spatial coordinates
Positioning of reference electrode	Critical; best compromise for source analysis: average reference	Not relevant
Spatial analysis techniques	Dipole source analysis	Dipole source analysis
Tangential source	Between plus and minus	Between inwards and outwards
Radial source	Below maximum signal	Not possible
Deep source	Possible, but low precision	Not possible

Abbreviations: EPSP, excitatory postsynaptic potential; IPSP, inhibitory postsynaptic potential; MEG, magnetoencephalography.

differences between two electrodes. Therefore, placement of the reference electrode is critical for EEG recordings (no such problem exists for MEG). For dipole source analysis, the mean value across all electrodes is mostly used as reference (average reference), which is virtually situated in the middle of the head. When only linear signal transformations are used (such as for evoked potentials), the choice of reference plays only a minor role, since it only shifts the assignment of the value "zero" between different isopotential lines, but the structure of the field distribution remains unchanged. When nonlinear transformations are used (as in all spectral analyses), choice of reference site is critical, since spectral power density is automatically zero at that reference site.

Another limitation for the EEG is the anisotropy of the volume conductor due to different conductivities of different tissues leading to localization errors of dipolar sources [5, 12]. This problem is hardly relevant for the convexity of the brain, where skin, skull, CSF, and brain can be reasonably approximated as concentric spheres. But towards the base of the skull, there are major distortions by adjacent bones. These distortions can be overcome by realistic head models [26], but these models take time to be calculated even on modern computers. Again, MEG is not subject to these limitations.

There are some limitations specific to MEG that do not apply to EEG. The lack of sensitivity to radial sources has already been mentioned in Fig. 4-2D; this means that MEG never captures the entire electrical activity of the brain. In turn, the captured subset is often easier to analyse and interpret. Source localization by MEG is highly sensitive to movement artefacts, since the subject's head is not fixed to the MEG dewar. To overcome this limitation, standard methods have been developed that track the head position during MEG recording.

CONCLUSION AND OUTLOOK

It is fascinating to see how much functional magnetic resonance imaging (fMRI) using BOLD and ASL effects has influenced our concepts about the functions of the human brain. These techniques are noninvasive, widely available, can be applied to almost any psychophysical or even sociological experimental paradigm, and can be repeated in the same subject under different conditions. As a result, we now have much better macroscopic functional maps of all parts of the human brain with a relatively good spatial resolution. However, these maps rely on an epiphenomenon: the regulation of cortical perfusion by cortical activity. The physiology of excitation–perfusion coupling places intrinsic limitations on the spatial and temporal resolution of fMRI. Moreover, it is unclear how excitatory and inhibitory synaptic processes are reflected in fMRI signals, since both of them are associated with increased metabolic demand.

In order to make progress beyond the current "phrenology" of functional brain imaging, it is necessary to get closer to the type of signal processing that occurs within single cortical columns or neurons, and the long-range interactions between columns or neurons. Modern EEG and MEG provide excellent tools to address these questions; they can distinguish between excitation and inhibition, they allow time–frequency analyses of single regions and network interactions, and they can be used for short-duration (as evoked potentials or evoked fields) and long-duration phenomena (as ongoing EEG or MEG) [9, 15, 19, 21, 24]. The main limitation of dipole source analyses—nonuniqueness of solution of the inverse problem—can be overcome by using the wealth of spatial information that is already available from fMRI, and turning that spatial information into testable hypotheses about where a given function should lead to electrical signals. Once such signalling has been demonstrated at the regional level by EEG and MEG in humans, subsequent animal experiments can then fill in the necessary details at the cellular level. Without the intermediate step of EEG or MEG regional mechanistic data, it appears quite hopeless to try and search for the cellular level; the brain is simply too big for such an endeavour.

ACKNOWLEDGEMENT

The authors' work has been supported by DFG, BMBF, EU, and NIH.

REFERENCES

1. American EEG Society. American Electroencephalographic Society guidelines for standard electrode position nomenclature. J Clin Neurophysiol 1991;8:200–2.
2. Baumgärtner U, Vogel H, Ohara S, Treede RD, Lenz F. Dipole source analyses of laser evoked potentials obtained from subdural grid recordings from primary somatic sensory cortex. J Neurophysiol 2001;106:722–30.
3. Berger H. Über das Elektrenkephalogramm des Menschen. Arch Psychiatr 1929;87:527–70.
4. Cohen D. Magnetoencephalography: evidence of magnetic fields produced by alpha rhythm currents. Science 1968;161:784–6.
5. Cohen D, Cuffin BN, Yunokuchi K, Maniewski R, Purcell C, Cosgrove GR, Ives J, Kennedy JG, Schomer DL. MEG versus EEG localization test using implanted sources in the human brain. Ann Neurol 1990;28:811–7.
6. Cruccu G, Aminoff MJ, Curio G, Guerit JM, Kakigi R, Mauguiére F, Rossini PM, Treede RD, Garcia-Larrea L. Recommendations for the clinical use of somatosensory-evoked potentials. Clin Neurophysiol 2008;119:1705–19.
7. Dawson GD. A summation technique for the detection of small evoked potentials. Electroencephalogr Clin Neurophysiol 1954;6:65–84.

8. Ebner TJ, Chen G. Use of voltage-sensitive dyes and optical recordings in the central nervous system. Prog Neurobiol 1995;46:463–506.
9. Engel AK, Singer W. Temporal binding and the neural correlates of sensory awareness. Trends Cogn Sci 2001;5:16–25.
10. Forss N, Raij TT, Seppa M, Hari R. Common cortical network for first and second pain. Neuroimage 2005;24:132–42.
11. Frot M, Magnin M, Mauguière F, Garcia-Larrea L. Human SII and posterior insula differently encode thermal laser stimuli. Cereb Cortex 2007;17:610–20.
12. Güllmar D, Haueisen J, Reichenbach JR. Influence of anisotropic electrical conductivity in white matter tissue on the EEG/MEG forward and inverse solution: a high-resolution whole head simulation study. Neuroimage 2010;51:145–63.
13. Hari R. On brain's magnetic responses to sensory stimuli. J Clin Neurophysiol 1991;8:157–69.
14. Hauck M, Lorenz J, Engel AK. Attention to painful stimulation enhances gamma-band activity and synchronization in human sensorimotor cortex. J Neurosci 2007;27:9270–7.
15. Hipp JF, Engel AK, Siegel M. Oscillatory synchronization in large-scale cortical networks predicts perception. Neuron 2011;69:387–96.
16. Inui K, Tran TD, Qiu Y, Wang X, Hoshiyama M, Kakigi R. A comparative magnetoencephalographic study of cortical activations evoked by noxious and innocuous somatosensory stimulations. Neurosci 2003;120:235–48.
17. Jasper HH. The ten twenty electrode system of the International Federation. Electroencephalogr Clin Neurophysiol 1958;10:371–5.
18. Lantz G, Grave de Peralta R, Spinelli L, Seeck M, Michel CM. Epileptic source localization with high density EEG: how many electrodes are needed? Clin Neurophysiol 2003;114:63–69.
19. Leistner S, Sander T, Burghoff M, Curio G, Trahms L, Mackert BM. Combined MEG and EEG methodology for non-invasive recording of infraslow activity in the human cortex. Clin Neurophysiol 2007;118:2774–80.
20. Nir RR, Sinai A, Raz E, Sprecher E, Yarnitsky D. Pain assessment by continuous EEG: association between subjective perception of tonic pain and peak frequency of alpha oscillations during stimulation and at rest. Brain Res 2010;1344:77–86.
21. Ohara S, Crone NE, Weiss N, Lenz FA. Analysis of synchrony demonstrates 'pain networks' defined by rapidly switching, task-specific, functional connectivity between pain-related cortical structures. Pain 2006;123:244–53.
22. Ploner M, Gross J, Timmermann L, Pollok B, Schnitzler A. Pain suppresses spontaneous brain rhythms. Cereb Cortex 2006;16:537–40.
23. Slater R, Worley A, Fabrizi L, Roberts S, Meek J, Boyd S, Fitzgerald M. Evoked potentials generated by noxious stimulation in the human infant brain. Eur J Pain 2010;14:321–6.
24. Tiemann L, Schulz E, Gross J, Ploner M. Gamma oscillations as a neuronal correlate of the attentional effects of pain. Pain 2010;150:302–8.
25. Treede RD, Lorenz J Baumgärtner U. Clinical usefulness of laser-evoked potentials. Neurophysiol Clin 2003;33:303–14.
26. Wolters CH, Anwander A, Tricoche X, Weinstein D, Koch MA, MacLeod RS. Influence of tissue conductivity anisotropy on EEG/MEG field and return current computation in a realistic head model: a simulation and visualization study using high-resolution finite element modeling. Neuroimage 2006;30:813–26.

CHAPTER 5

The Time–Frequency Pattern of Pain Processing and Pain Modulation

Markus Ploner

This chapter reviews recent noninvasive neurophysiological studies on the brain mechanisms of pain. The chapter also focuses on frequency and time–frequency analyses of electroencephalographic (EEG) and magnetoencephalographic (MEG) recordings of neuronal activity associated with experimental and clinical pain. Time–frequency analyses of EEG and MEG data are briefly explained. The pattern of pain-related neuronal activity at different frequencies is reviewed, and their contribution to the experience of phasic and tonic experimental pain and ongoing clinical pain as well as their role in the modulation of pain is discussed. The chapter closes with a subjective appreciation of the current and future role of EEG and MEG in pain research.

Functional imaging studies have defined an extended network of brain areas associated with the experience of pain [1]. EEG and MEG studies as well as intracranial recordings have provided insights into the dynamics of pain processing within this network. EEG and MEG are noninvasive direct measures of neuronal function. Both methods detect signals that are mostly related to synchronous postsynaptic potentials of large populations of neurons. EEG detects electrical signals directly, whereas MEG records the magnetic fields that are induced by the electrical signals. As magnetic fields are not distorted by the cerebrospinal fluid, the skull, and the scalp, the spatial resolution of MEG is higher than that of EEG. However, the strength of both methods is their optimum temporal resolution, which allows for analysing neural processes in the range of milliseconds. EEG and MEG signals represent mixtures of neuronal activity at different frequencies. Most analyses refer to frequencies between 0.5 and 100 Hz where standard frequency bands have been defined and labelled with Greek letters (δ [<4 Hz], θ [4–8 Hz], α [8–13 Hz], β [14–40 Hz], and γ [>40 Hz]). The different frequency bands are not unequivocally related to certain brain areas or brain states. However, as a general rule, signals at higher frequencies reflect local neural processes, whereas lower frequency signals reflect integrative functions involving large brain networks [14]. For reviews of the basics of EEG and MEG, see [37] and [19].

PHASIC EXPERIMENTAL PAIN

Most EEG/MEG studies on pain refer to the processing of phasic experimental stimuli. In principle, EEG and MEG can record two types of responses to painful events. The two response types are phase-locked (evoked) and non-phase-locked (induced) responses (Fig. 5-1). Both response types differ in the temporal relationship between the event and the response. Latencies of evoked responses are fixed, whereas latencies of induced responses

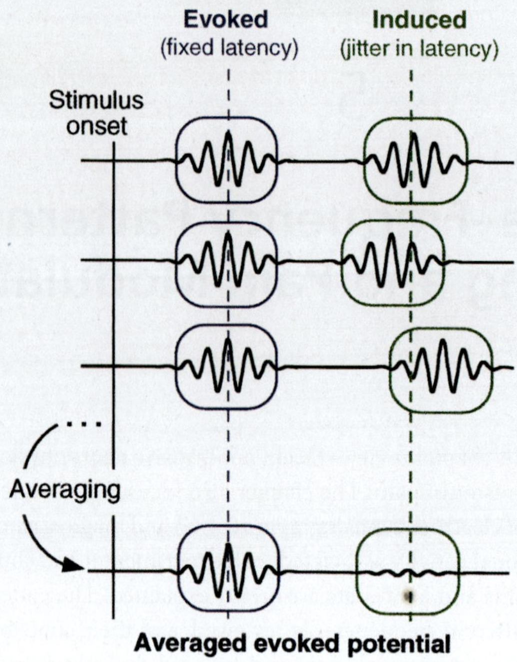

FIGURE 5-1 Phase-locked evoked and non-phase-locked induced responses to pain. (Adapted from Tallon-Baudry and Bertrand [55].)

differ between trials. Both response types can occur at the same time in the same brain area and are supposed to carry different functional information. The analysis of both response types needs different strategies. Evoked responses are analysed in the time domain using averaging techniques, which have been well established in neuroscience research for decades [30]. Applications of the evoked potential approach to the processing of pain will be reviewed in another chapter of this book. In contrast, induced responses may cancel out during averaging and are therefore analysed in the time–frequency domain. Data of single trials are transformed to time–frequency representations using methods like windowed Fourier transform or continuous wavelet transform (for review see [35, 44]). Averaging time–frequency representations across trials discloses both phase-locked evoked and non-phase-locked induced responses. Such analyses of induced responses are a younger research field than analyses of evoked responses, with most investigations performed during the last decade.

Time–frequency analyses disclosed that phasic painful stimuli are associated with a complex pattern of brain responses (Fig. 5-2). At frequencies below 10 Hz, a strong increase in neuronal activity is detected, which corresponds to the pain-evoked potential. Moreover, EEG and MEG studies consistently show a non-phase-locked suppression of neuronal activity around 10 and 20 Hz, that is, in the α and β frequency bands [2, 24, 34, 39, 40, 43]. Localization strategies revealed that suppressions occur in the bilateral sensorimotor areas as well as in the occipital cortex. Considering that at these frequencies and locations the brain exhibits prominent spontaneous neuronal oscillations, pain-induced decreases in neuronal activity are likely to reflect suppressions of spontaneous neuronal oscillations in sensory and motor systems. Since the level of spontaneous oscillations relates to the functional state and the excitability of sensory or motor systems [38, 53], this effect can be interpreted as a pain-induced global activation and increase in excitability of sensory and motor systems [39].

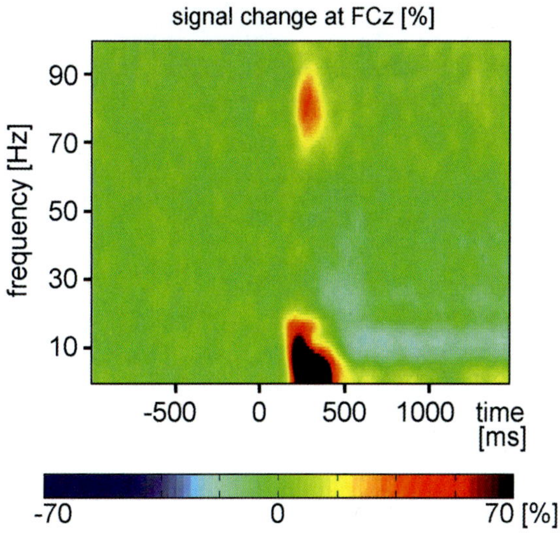

FIGURE 5-2 The time–frequency pattern of neuronal responses to phasic painful stimuli. Group mean time–frequency representation of neuronal activity at exemplary electrode FCz coded as percent signal change with respect to a prestimulus baseline. (From Schulz et al. [48].)

Most likely, the suppression of spontaneous oscillations reflects a physiological correlate of the involuntary attentional demands of pain, in the sense of an alerting mechanism.

Other recent studies have focused on pain-induced responses at higher frequencies. High-frequency oscillations in the γ frequency band, that is, between 30 and 100 Hz, have attracted considerable attention during the last decade [17, 61]. Gamma oscillations have been observed in lower-level sensory areas of animals and humans. Current theories propose that γ oscillations reflect neuronal interactions in local cortical networks, which encode sensory, motor, and cognitive variables [14]. Such local representations may promote neuronal interactions among distant brain regions that are mediated by diverse oscillations at lower, for example, β frequencies. Gamma oscillations may thereby closely relate to the behavioural relevance of internal or external events and promote their further processing in the brain [45]. If so, then this should particularly apply to pain, which is always behaviourally relevant, and should always receive preferential processing in the brain.

Indeed, recent EEG and MEG studies revealed that brief painful stimuli induce γ oscillations in the human somatosensory cortex [18, 21]. Latencies of responses were similar for induced γ oscillations and evoked responses. Thus, the painful stimuli elicit two different types of neuronal responses at the same time, which at least partly originate from the same brain areas. The search for the functional correlates of both neuronal responses showed that both responses increase with objective stimulus intensity and subjective pain intensity (Fig. 5-3A). To further elucidate their functional significance, responses to stimuli around pain threshold were analysed. These stimuli did not differ with respect to objective stimulus intensity, but only with respect to the subjective percept. The analysis showed that amplitudes of evoked responses did not differ between trials. In contrast, induced γ responses were significantly stronger for trials that were perceived as painful than for trials that were not (Fig. 5-3B) [18]. However, stimuli perceived as painful are also more salient. It may thus be the case that pain-induced γ oscillations reflect unspecific attentional processes rather than pain perception per se. A recent study applied an elegant paradigm to disentangle pain perception from saliency [62]. The results confirmed that pain-induced γ responses are closely related to the subjective perception of pain irrespective of its saliency (Fig. 5-3C).

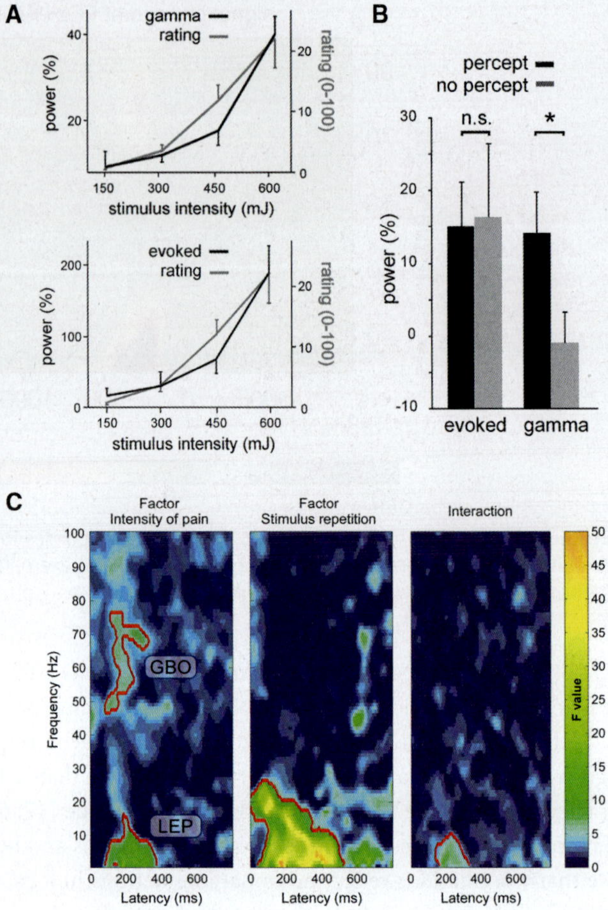

FIGURE 5-3 Gamma oscillations as a neuronal correlate of pain perception. **A:** Pain intensity, amplitudes of induced γ oscillations, and amplitudes of evoked potentials as a function of stimulus intensity. (Adapted from Gross et al. [18].) **B:** Amplitudes of induced γ oscillations and evoked potentials to differently perceived stimuli of equal stimulus intensity. (From Gross et al. [18].) **C:** Effect of pain intensity and stimulus repetition on neuronal activity. Laser-evoked potentials (LEP) were modulated by pain intensity and stimulus repetition, whereas γ band oscillations (GBO) were modulated only by pain intensity. In addition, a significant interaction between the two factors was found in the LEP cluster, indicating that the stimulus repetition reduced the strength of the relationship between pain intensity and LEP magnitude. (From Zhang et al. [62].)

Intriguingly, this close relationship between perception and neuronal activity was observed only for γ band responses, whereas all other features of the EEG were more closely related to saliency than to pain perception.

Another recent investigation further explored the functional significance of pain-induced γ oscillations [48]. In a simple paradigm, objectively similar potentially painful stimuli were applied to healthy human subjects. Single-trial pain ratings disclosed a remarkable variability across trials and subjects in the perception of identical stimuli. Variability of perception and behaviour is a well-known phenomenon, which is traditionally regarded as noise and therefore removed from analyses of brain activity. However, when the variability of pain perception was related to pain-evoked potentials and pain-induced γ oscillations, an interesting pattern was observed. Interindividual differences of perception were captured by pain-evoked potentials, whereas γ responses were particularly related to short-term intraindividual fluctuations of pain perception.

Taken together, at a very early stage of cortical processing, induced γ responses appear to be particularly related to the subjective experience of pain and its short-term modulations. Afferent nociceptive information from the external world, as reflected by the evoked responses, may be translated into a subjective percept taking into account current and previous experiences, attentional and emotional states, and behavioural demands. Gamma responses appear to represent a step further in this objective–subjective transformation process and may influence subsequent stimulus processing in the brain.

TONIC EXPERIMENTAL AND CHRONIC CLINICAL PAIN

As compared with the numerous EEG and MEG studies on phasic pain, few studies have addressed the brain processing of tonic and chronic pain. As the analysis of continuous neural processes is methodologically far more demanding than the analysis of phasic event-related phenomena, the neurophysiological assessment of tonic experimental and chronic clinical pain is still at a very early stage.

Because of the lack of the temporal component, continuous, tonic pain-related processes were analysed by using frequency domain rather than time–frequency domain approaches. However, investigations addressing tonic pain yielded very heterogeneous results. The most consistent result is a pain-associated decrease of neuronal activity in the α frequency band [6–8, 15, 26, 36, 51]. Other findings are increases of neuronal activity at δ [6, 7, 16, 26, 27] and β [3, 6, 8, 26, 51] frequencies. A single study found pain-related changes of neuronal γ oscillations, which were, however, at least partially due to muscle activity [15].

A few neurophysiological studies investigated changes in EEG activity related to chronic pain. They showed increases in θ [29, 46, 54] (Fig. 5-4), α [33], and β [20, 29, 46, 54] activity in patients suffering from chronic pain. Moreover, a link between chronic pain and abnormal neuronal γ oscillations has been proposed [13, 60], but no direct evidence for this has been presented so far.

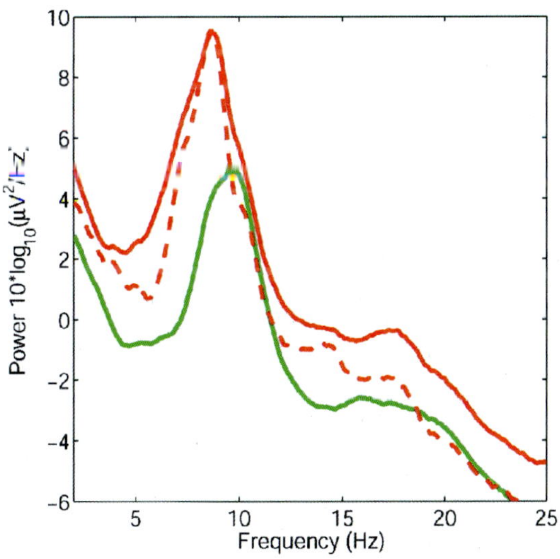

FIGURE 5-4 Spectral changes of brain activity in chronic pain patients. Average power spectra of EEG activity for a group of chronic pain patients (*red*) and healthy controls (*green*). The global EEG power was enhanced, and the dominant peak was shifted towards lower frequencies in the θ range in the patient group. The subgroup of six patients free from centrally acting medication showed the same effect (*dashed red line*). (From Sarnthein et al. [46].)

A crucial question is whether these phenomena directly reflect the subjective perception of pain or whether they rather reflect unspecific processes. Considering the unspecific suppression of α activity by phasic stimuli (mentioned earlier) and the debate on the specificity of pain-evoked potentials [28], most, if not all, of the observed EEG features could well represent unspecific phenomena, for example, related to the saliency of the painful stimulation. Novel paradigms are urgently needed to address this issue and to thereby help to translate the bulk of evidence on the processing of phasic pain to the clinically more relevant conditions of tonic and chronic pain.

PAIN MODULATION

A growing number of studies investigate the time–frequency patterns of the modulation of pain. The methods used to modulate pain are diverse. They include hypnosis [9, 11, 12, 58], music [22], attention [21], multisensory integration [31, 42], and emotional processes [50]. Most of these modulations represent top-down modulations. The results show changes of pain perception that were paralleled by changes in γ activity [21, 22, 42, 50] and by reverse changes in β activity [31, 42, 50].

Another approach did not assess the effects of attention on pain but assessed the effects of phasic painful stimuli on attentional performance and processing [56, 57]. By using a primary task paradigm, the interfering effect of pain on performance in a visual attention task has been investigated. The visual task was associated with γ oscillations in the visual system, whereas painful stimuli induced γ responses over somatosensory areas. Amplitudes of γ oscillations in both systems were negatively correlated. Intriguingly, the pain-induced changes in visual γ oscillations were correlated with pain-induced changes in visual task performance. These observations indicate that the attentional effects of pain are closely related to changes in neuronal γ oscillations in the human brain.

Taken together, these results are consistent with the idea that pain-related γ responses are sensitive to top-down modulations of the pain experience, whereas pain-evoked potentials may rather reflect the bottom-up characteristics of potentially painful events. However, no direct evidence for this hypothesis has been presented so far. Moreover, studies on the time–frequency pattern of pain modulations apply exclusively to phasic pain yet. Clinically more relevant modulations of tonic and chronic pain remain to be investigated.

CEREBRAL CONNECTIVITY

So far we have discussed the time–frequency pattern of local neuronal activity related to the experience of pain. However, considering the multitude of factors merging into a coherent pain percept, it seems natural that interactions across brain areas can shape the perception of pain. Interactions within the brain can be assessed at the levels of structural, functional, and effective connectivity [52]. The latter two phenomena are accessible to neurophysiological recordings. The limited spatial resolution and volume conduction effects, however, hamper the analysis of functional and effective connectivity from EEG and MEG recordings. Transformation of signals from electrode/sensor space to source space can at least partially overcome these limitations [47]. A first source-based MEG study indicated that the effective connectivity between brain areas carries behaviourally relevant information about pain [41], but further source-based analyses are urgently needed to understand the contribution of cerebral connectivity to the processing of pain at a high temporal resolution. Intracranial recordings, which have provided further insights into pain-related cerebral connectivity, will be reviewed in another chapter of this book.

PRACTICAL APPLICATIONS

The studies reviewed so far represent crucial insights into the cerebral mechanisms of pain. Such advances may, however, not only fascinate from a basic science perspective but also represent a step forward towards practical applications. Advances in our understanding of the brain processes underlying pain raise the question whether brain activity can be used to establish an objective neuronal marker of pain. Considering the complexity of pain-related brain processes, approaches that take into account complex temporal–spectral–spatial patterns of brain activity appear mandatory. In recent years, such computationally highly demanding multivariate approaches have attracted increasing attention. They have been applied to spatial patterns of brain activity assessed by functional magnetic resonance imaging to infer mental states or even hidden intentions from brain activity [23]. Most recently, such approaches have been used to decode the perception of pain from brain activity. A first EEG study applied multivariate approaches to decode intra- and interindividual differences in the perception of identical stimuli from the temporal–spectral pattern of brain activity [49]. The results revealed that it is indeed possible to decode how an individual perceives a potentially painful stimulus from brain activity, which has been corroborated by another recent EEG study [25]. Comparable results have been obtained by multivariate analyses of fMRI data [4, 5, 32, 59]. These approaches can potentially help to establish a neuronal marker of pain with implications for health care, for example, in patients who are no longer able to communicate. However, they also raise serious ethical issues [10].

OUTLOOK

The strength of EEG and MEG in pain research is twofold. Both methods represent direct measures of neuronal function, and they both have an optimum temporal resolution. These properties allow detecting and differentiating functionally and physiologically distinct neuronal phenomena, which may not be distinguished by other techniques. Furthermore, the analysis of neuronal oscillations and synchrony as measures of communication in the brain promises to add important and unique information to our knowledge about the neural correlates of pain in health and disease. Thus, electrophysiological methods should ideally complement the spatial and functional information provided by fMRI. The integration of the different methods is now emerging in nearly every neuroscientific field and should help to advance pain research in the near future.

However, many important questions remain to be addressed. First, evidence on the time–frequency pattern of neuronal activity in response to phasic stimuli needs to be complemented by studies on the clinically more relevant conditions of tonic and chronic pain. Second, new paradigms are needed to further disentangle neuronal activity directly related to the pain experience from unspecific activity related to processes like saliency. Third, analyses should take into account the full spatial–temporal–spectral complexity of the brain processes related to pain. Such approaches could adopt multivariate approaches, connectivity measures, and cross-frequency coupling of neuronal activations. Fourth, a standardization of analysis approaches would be desirable to make results comparable across studies and labs, and to enable the analysis, comparison, and replication of larger cohorts of subjects and patients. Refined and standardized paradigms and analyses thereby promise new substantial insights into the brain processes underlying the pain experience in health and chronic pain conditions as a major health care problem.

REFERENCES

1. Apkarian AV, Bushnell MC, Schweinhardt P. Representation of pain in the brain. In: McMahon SB, Koltzenburg M, Tracey I, Turk DC, editors. Wall and Melzack's textbook of pain. Philadelphia, PA: Elsevier; 2013. pp. 111–28.
2. Babiloni C, Babiloni F, Carducci F, Cincotti F, Rosciarelli F, Arendt-Nielsen L, Chen AC, Rossini PM. Human brain oscillatory activity phase-locked to painful electrical stimulations: a multi-channel EEG study. Hum Brain Mapp 2002;15:112–23.
3. Backonja M, Howland EW, Wang J, Smith J, Salinsky M, Cleeland CS. Tonic changes in alpha power during immersion of the hand in cold water. Electroencephalogr Clin Neurophysiol 1991;79:192–203.
4. Brodersen KH, Wiech K, Lomakina EI, Lin CS, Buhmann JM, Bingel U, Ploner M, Stephan KE, Tracey I. Decoding the perception of pain from fMRI using multivariate pattern analysis. NeuroImage 2012;63:1162–70.
5. Brown JE, Chatterjee N, Younger J, Mackey S. Towards a physiology-based measure of pain: patterns of human brain activity distinguish painful from non-painful thermal stimulation. PloS One 2011;6:e24124.
6. Chang PF, Arendt-Nielsen L, Chen AC. Dynamic changes and spatial correlation of EEG activities during cold pressor test in man. Brain Res Bull 2002;57:667–75.
7. Chang PF, Arendt-Nielsen L, Graven-Nielsen T, Svensson P, Chen AC. Comparative EEG activation to skin pain and muscle pain induced by capsaicin injection. Int J Psychophysiol 2004;51:117–26.
8. Chen AC, Rappelsberger P. Brain and human pain: topographic EEG amplitude and coherence mapping. Brain Topogr 1994;7:129–40.
9. Croft RJ, Williams JD, Haenschel C, Gruzelier JH. Pain perception, hypnosis and 40 Hz oscillations. Int J Psychophysiol 2002;46:101–8.
10. Davis KD, Racine E, Collett B. Neuroethical issues related to the use of brain imaging: can we and should we use brain imaging as a biomarker to diagnose chronic pain? Pain 2012;153:1555–9.
11. De Pascalis V, Cacace I. Pain perception, obstructive imagery and phase-ordered gamma oscillations. Int J Psychophysiol 2005;56:157–69.
12. De Pascalis V, Cacace I, Massicolle F. Perception and modulation of pain in waking and hypnosis: functional significance of phase-ordered gamma oscillations. Pain 2004;112:27–36.
13. De Ridder D, Elgoyhen AB, Romo R, Langguth B. Phantom percepts: tinnitus and pain as persisting aversive memory networks. Proc Natl Acad Sci USA 2011;108:8075–80.
14. Donner TH, Siegel M. A framework for local cortical oscillation patterns. Trends Cogn Sci 2011;15:191–9.
15. Dowman R, Rissacher D, Schuckers S. EEG indices of tonic pain-related activity in the somatosensory cortices. Clin Neurophysiol 2008;119:1201–12.
16. Ferracuti S, Seri S, Mattia D, Cruccu G. Quantitative EEG modifications during the cold water pressor test: hemispheric and hand differences. Int J Psychophysiol 1994;17:261–8.
17. Fries P. Neuronal gamma-band synchronization as a fundamental process in cortical computation. Annu Rev Neurosci 2009;32:209–24.
18. Gross J, Schnitzler A, Timmermann L, Ploner M. Gamma oscillations in human primary somatosensory cortex reflect pain perception. PLoS Biol 2007;5:e133.
19. Hansen P, Kringelbach M, Salmelin R. MEG: an introduction to methods. New York, NY: Oxford University Press; 2010.
20. Hargrove JB, Bennett RM, Simons DG, Smith SJ, Nagpal S, Deering DE. Quantitative electroencephalographic abnormalities in fibromyalgia patients. Clin EEG Neurosci 2010;41:132–9.
21. Hauck M, Lorenz J, Engel AK. Attention to painful stimulation enhances gamma-band activity and synchronization in human sensorimotor cortex. J Neurosci 2007;27:9270–7.
22. Hauck M, Metzner S, Rohlffs F, Lorenz J, Engel AK. The influence of music and music therapy on pain-induced neuronal oscillations measured by magnetencephalography. Pain 2013;154:539–47.
23. Haynes JD, Rees G. Decoding mental states from brain activity in humans. Nat Rev Neurosci 2006;7:523–34.
24. Hu L, Peng W, Valentini E, Zhang Z, Hu Y. Functional features of nociceptive-induced suppression of alpha band electroencephalographic oscillations. J Pain 2013;14:89–99.

25. Huang G, Xiao P, Hung YS, Iannetti GD, Zhang ZG, Hu L. A novel approach to predict subjective pain perception from single-trial laser-evoked potentials. NeuroImage 2013;81:283–93.
26. Huber MT, Bartling J, Pachur D, Woikowsky-Biedau S, Lautenbacher S. EEG responses to tonic heat pain. Exp Brain Res 2006;173:14–24.
27. Le Pera D, Svensson P, Valeriani M, Watanabe I, Arendt-Nielsen L, Chen AC. Long-lasting effect evoked by tonic muscle pain on parietal EEG activity in humans. Clin Neurophysiol 2000;111:2130–7.
28. Legrain V, Iannetti GD, Plaghki L, Mouraux A. The pain matrix reloaded: a salience detection system for the body. Prog Neurobiol 2011;93:111–24.
29. Llinas RR, Ribary U, Jeanmonod D, Kronberg E, Mitra PP. Thalamocortical dysrhythmia: a neurological and neuropsychiatric syndrome characterized by magnetoencephalography. Proc Natl Acad Sci USA 1999;96:15222–7.
30. Luck SJ. An introduction to the event-related potential technique. Cambridge, MA: MIT Press; 2005.
31. Mancini F, Longo MR, Canzoneri E, Vallar G, Haggard P. Changes in cortical oscillations linked to multisensory modulation of nociception. Eur J Neurosci 2013;37:768–76.
32. Marquand A, Howard M, Brammer M, Chu C, Coen S, Mourao-Miranda J. Quantitative prediction of subjective pain intensity from whole-brain fMRI data using Gaussian processes. NeuroImage 2010;49:2178–89.
33. Mo J, Maizels M, Ding M, Ahn AH. Does throbbing pain have a brain signature? Pain 2013;54(7):1150–5.
34. Mouraux A, Guerit JM, Plaghki L. Non-phase locked electroencephalogram (EEG) responses to CO_2 laser skin stimulations may reflect central interactions between Aδ- and C-fibre afferent volleys. Clin Neurophysiol. 2003;114:710–22.
35. Mouraux A, Iannetti GD. Across-trial averaging of event-related EEG responses and beyond. Magn Reson Imaging 2008;26:1041–54.
36. Nir RR, Sinai A, Moont R, Harari E, Yarnitsky D. Tonic pain and continuous EEG: prediction of subjective pain perception by alpha-1 power during stimulation and at rest. Clin Neurophysiol 2012;123:605–12.
37. Nunez PL, Srinivasan R. Eletric fields of the brain: the neurophysics of EEG. New York, NY: Oxford University Press; 2006.
38. Pfurtscheller G, Lopes da Silva FH. EEG event-related desynchronization (ERD) and event-related synchronization (ERS). In: Schomer DL, Lopes da Silva FH, editors. Niedermeyer's electroencephalography: basic principles, clinical applications, and related fields. Philadelphia, PA: Lippincott Williams & Wilkins; 2011. pp. 935–48.
39. Ploner M, Gross J, Timmermann L, Pollok B, Schnitzler A. Oscillatory activity reflects the excitability of the human somatosensory system. NeuroImage 2006;32:1231–6.
40. Ploner M, Gross J, Timmermann L, Pollok B, Schnitzler A. Pain suppresses spontaneous brain rhythms. Cereb Cortex 2006;16:537–40.
41. Ploner M, Schoffelen JM, Schnitzler A, Gross J. Functional integration within the human pain system as revealed by Granger causality. Hum Brain Mapp 2009;30:4025–32.
42. Pomper U, Hofle M, Hauck M, Kathmann N, Engel AK, Senkowski D. Crossmodal bias of visual input on pain perception and pain-induced beta activity. NeuroImage 2012;66C:469–78.
43. Raij TT, Forss N, Stancak A, Hari R. Modulation of motor-cortex oscillatory activity by painful Aδ- and C-fiber stimuli. NeuroImage 2004;23:569–73.
44. Roach BJ, Mathalon DH. Event-related EEG time-frequency analysis: an overview of measures and an analysis of early gamma band phase locking in schizophrenia. Schizophr Bull 2008;34:907–26.
45. Salinas E, Sejnowski TJ. Correlated neuronal activity and the flow of neural information. Nat Rev Neurosci 2001;2:539–50.
46. Sarnthein J, Stern J, Aufenberg C, Rousson V, Jeanmonod D. Increased EEG power and slowed dominant frequency in patients with neurogenic pain. Brain 2006;129:55–64.
47. Schoffelen JM, Gross J. Source connectivity analysis with MEG and EEG. Human Brain Mapp 2009;30:1857–65.
48. Schulz E, Tiemann L, Schuster T, Gross J, Ploner M. Neurophysiological coding of traits and states in the perception of pain. Cereb Cortex 2011;21:2408–14.
49. Schulz E, Zherdin A, Tiemann L, Plant C, Ploner M. Decoding an Individual's Sensitivity to pain from the multivariate analysis of EEG Data. Cereb Cortex 2012;22:1118–23.
50. Senkowski D, Kautz J, Hauck M, Zimmermann R, Engel AK. Emotional facial expressions modulate pain-induced beta and gamma oscillations in sensorimotor cortex. J Neurosci 2011;31:14542–50.
51. Shao S, Shen K, Yu K, Wilder-Smith EP, Li X. Frequency-domain EEG source analysis for acute tonic cold pain perception. Clin Neurophysiol 2012;123:2042–9.
52. Sporns O. Brain connectivity. Scholarpedia 2007;2:4695.

53. Steriade M, Llinas RR. The functional states of the thalamus and the associated neuronal interplay. Physiol Rev 1988;68:649–742.
54. Stern J, Jeanmonod D, Sarnthein J. Persistent EEG overactivation in the cortical pain matrix of neurogenic pain patients. NeuroImage 2006;31:721–31.
55. Tallon-Baudry C, Bertrand O. Oscillatory gamma activity in humans and its role in object representation. Trends Cogn Sci 1999;3:151–62.
56. Tiemann L, Schulz E, Gross J, Ploner M. Gamma oscillations as a neuronal correlate of the attentional effects of pain. Pain 2010;150:302–8.
57. Tiemann L, Schulz E, Winkelmann A, Ronel J, Henningsen P, Ploner M. Behavioral and neuronal investigations of hypervigilance in patients with fibromyalgia syndrome. PloS One 2012;7:e35068.
58. Valentini E, Betti V, Hu L, Aglioti SM. Hypnotic modulation of pain perception and of brain activity triggered by nociceptive laser stimuli. Cortex 2013;49:446–62.
59. Wager TD, Atlas LY, Lindquist MA, Roy M, Woo CW, Kross E. An fMRI-based neurologic signature of physical pain. N Engl J Med 2013;368:1388–97.
60. Walton KD, Llinas RR. Central pain as a thalamocortical dysrhythmia: a thalamic efference disconnection? In: Kruger L, Light AR, editors. Translational pain research: from mouse to man. Boca Raton, FL: CRC Press; 2010. pp. 301–14.
61. Wang XJ. Neurophysiological and computational principles of cortical rhythms in cognition. Physiol Rev 2010;90:1195–268.
62. Zhang ZG, Hu L, Hung YS, Mouraux A, Iannetti GD. Gamma-band oscillations in the primary somatosensory cortex—a direct and obligatory correlate of subjective pain intensity. J Neurosci 2012;32:7429–38.

CHAPTER 6

The Infrastructure of Brain Rhythms and Its Disruption in Pain

Alexis T. Baria

Take a look at any fMRI BOLD signal in the brain, and the most prominent feature is its rhythmic activity—it periodically fluctuates between high and low values. Unlike the common depiction of a single neuron that fires action potentials in the event of some stimulus and remains silent otherwise, you will never see a *silent* BOLD signal in a living brain. The fact is that rhythmic activity is ubiquitous in the brain and the rhythms can be measured when recording from vast populations of cells (as with fMRI, EEG, and local field potential [LFP]) all the way down to the single cell. These rhythms have been studied for a very long time, beginning with the discovery that rhythmic behaviour (such as breathing and locomotion) could exist without descending input from the brain. The idea that rhythms play a role in more complex operations such as cognition and perception, however, is relatively new, and somewhat more controversial. This chapter will thus go over some of the basic concepts behind the orchestrated rhythms in the brain, their relation to mental activity, and how they can be studied in *frequency space*. In particular, it will discuss the special properties of the brain's frequency spectrum that allow the many systems in the brain to communicate, and will go over how pain can be examined from this viewpoint.

BRAIN RHYTHMS AND NETWORK COMMUNICATION

The prevalent view of how the brain works suggests it is a reflexive system. That is, when it is perturbed by some outside force, different elements within the brain send messages back and forth to plan a response, and then it generates an output response signal. This is similar to the many spinal reflexes, like the knee jerk reflex one might experience at the doctor's office, as is with single neurons, which are often depicted as being mostly silent until perturbation from some external stimulus. This view illustrates the brain's default activity as quiet unless driven to react. This is only a half-truth, however, because while brain activity *is* influenced by exogenous forces, the vast majority of its energy is spent intrinsically, and in fact is never silent. Brain activity continuously ebbs and flows, periodically changing the distribution of its energy, whether you are thinking or not, dreaming or entirely unconscious, until you are no longer living. Thus, the brain is restless, and a growing number of scientists and clinicians are using this fact to understand the brain in new ways.

The most famous depiction of this view is probably that of the α wave, the most prominent EEG signal localized in the occipital cortex. This wave was discovered to constantly oscillate at about 10 Hz (the wave fluctuates 10 times/second), peaking around 150 μV, and change in amplitude when a subject kept their eyes closed [33]. From a certain standpoint, however, it is difficult to intuit what ongoing oscillations have to do with actions and mental processes that seemingly do not oscillate. Certainly, there do not appear to be any 10 Hz oscillations when closing one's eyes. To put it in the perspective of fMRI, a brain region may "activate" with a specific stimulus, but it never flat lines. The fact is that region is continuously "activating" (fluctuating between high and low blood oxygenation) regardless of whether the stimulus is there or not. Band-limited power of EEG signals behaves in the same manner, chugging along peaks and valleys in a way that is seemingly independent of behaviour or environmental stimuli. So what exactly is going on? The question has challenged neuroscientists for many decades, but the emerging answer is that oscillations reflect widespread modulation of activity that is driven by the system itself [26]. In other words, oscillations signify that certain groups of cells are working together to influence the activity of other groups of cells, which ultimately influences behaviour and perception. Such groups of cells (commonly referred to as systems or networks) are able to influence the actions of the others across long distances and at different temporal scales. The intricate interactions of the many brain rhythms play an important role in maintaining and interpreting information, and predicting environmental demands. The details of how this works is beyond the limited space allotted to this chapter, but we briefly describe it below.

The following is a simple illustration of how brain oscillations are defined by the communication of many networks. In actuality, the interactions are far more complex than described below, but hopefully this, and the corresponding Fig. 6-1, provides a good starting point to understand the concept. Imagine a small group of close, interconnected neurons that we will call "network A." Let us say the cells within it are *synchronized*, that is, they all fire together within a certain time window. The network is able to do this because (1) each neuron by itself exhibits phase-dependent excitability (there are periods of time when a perturbation is more likely to cause it to fire than others, due to the arrangement of channels along its membrane [26]), and (2) these periods of excitability can be shifted

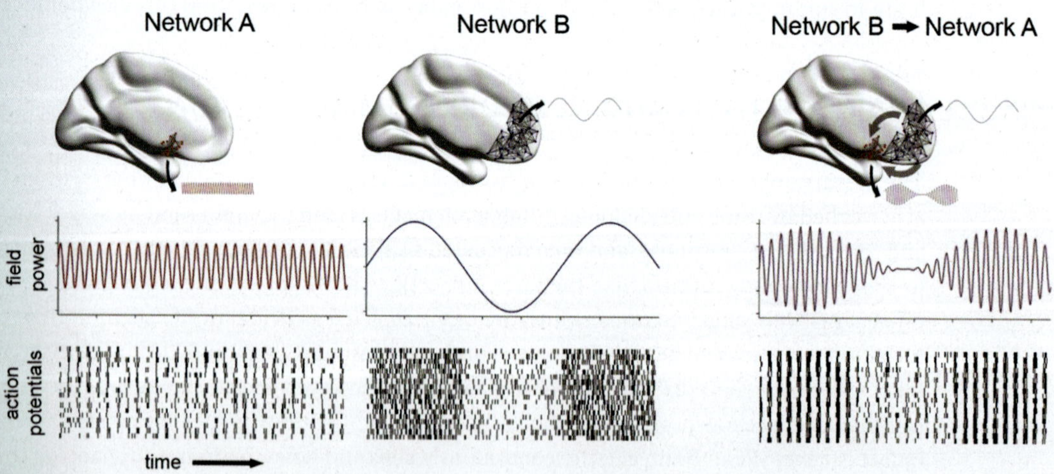

FIGURE 6-1 Brain rhythms indicate network synchrony. Left: Network A is small; thus, synchrony occurs within short time windows. The arrow points to an example of oscillatory behaviour that arises from network A. The waveform below is an enlarged view, demonstrating the rhythmic behaviour of the voltage field power generated by synchrony within the network. The raster plot on the bottom is temporally aligned to the field power wave. Each black mark indicates the firing of an action potential from a single unit (each row in the raster plot) from within the network. Notice, most action potentials occur around the peak of the waveform. Middle: Network B is much larger; thus, the field power generated by synchrony within it is much larger. Notice, the temporal windows by which single units within the network synchronize are much longer. Right: The influence of network B on A (cross-frequency coupling) results in increased high-frequency synchrony appearing periodically in long time windows.

by perturbations, for example, by an action potential transmitted from another physically connected cell. In general, the neurons within network A are able to synchronize because each cell can adjust to the intrinsic oscillatory behaviour of the others through their physical connections. Synchronization within network A can occur within very small time windows, or high frequencies, because the cells are close together and the transmission of action potentials along their axons is very fast. This synchronization generates a mean voltage field that fluctuates up and down—when the synchronization of the cells is tighter, the mean field generated by the network is higher. Because there are only a few cells generating the voltage field, the mean field oscillates around a relatively small value—on the scale of microvolts. Keep in mind this is far below the voltage needed to cause an action potential in a hyperpolarized cell, but it may be just enough to push a cell (or network of cells) near firing threshold to depolarize.

Now suppose there is a much bigger group of neurons, network B. Their mean distance is further from each other and thus they cannot synchronize within short time windows due to synaptic delays and limitations of axon conductance; their synchronization is defined by longer temporal windows (low frequencies). Because there are so many cells synchronizing within these longer time windows, their integrated activity generates bigger, slower fluctuations in the mean voltage field, which has some important implications. First, the stronger voltage field means it can have greater influence on the firing of other cells. This voltage field is still in microvolts, but it is much larger than that of network A, and thus it can push a cell (or network of cells) into firing that is even further from threshold. Second, the slow fluctuations of the field put it at higher strengths for longer periods of time; thus, its ability to push other cells into firing is temporally extended, compared with network A. Finally, both the larger strength and the lower frequency fluctuation of the field allow it to influence the behaviour of many more cells (or networks of cells), compared with network A. Overall, this means that these big, slow fluctuations can influence the behaviour of many cells, which may fire and fluctuate at much higher frequencies. This interaction is called "cross-frequency coupling" [10], and it is how networks communicate across different spatial and temporal scales. It is an important mechanism that enables parallel processing in the brain, and is the putative link between perception and behaviour occurring on relatively slow timescales to neural activity that is magnitudes faster. The short punch line of all this is that the larger, slower fluctuating networks have the power to influence the behaviour of the smaller, faster networks. But it does not stop there. In fact, there is some reciprocity of influence between smaller and bigger networks, and the intricate orchestration of this communication is a very important part of what allows us to perceive our environment, to learn, to make decisions—virtually everything we do. For more detailed and excellent reviews on the topic, see the following [8, 10, 14, 17].

The 1/*f* Frequency Power Spectrum

What is the infrastructure of rhythms that allows for the coordinated transfer of information, and thus communication, to occur across different systems in our brains? The question is easier to answer if one views brain activity in frequency space using a Fourier transform. This tool allows one to decompose fluctuating signals into components of sine waves with different frequencies (wavelengths, or time between peaks) and amplitudes (height of the wave). The amplitude of each sine wave can then be plotted as a function of its frequency, and the resulting plot is the *power spectrum* for the original signal. The power spectrum shown in Fig. 6-2 is typical of a BOLD signal in the brain, demonstrating the

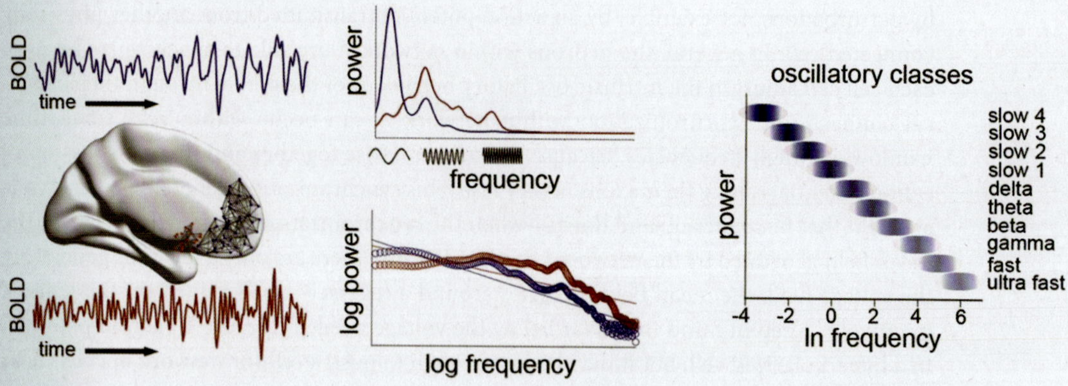

FIGURE 6-2 Brain rhythms can be examined in frequency space. Left: Typical fMRI BOLD signals are shown for different regions of the brain. Notice, the biggest fluctuations in the blue signal are slow relative to the big fluctuations in the red signal. Middle: These can be transformed into frequency space, where the signal is decomposed into sine waves with different wavelengths **(top middle)**. Bottom middle: Neural frequency spectra are characterized by the 1/*f* distribution of power. The frequency spectrum shown on the top is log transformed, and can be described by the linear fit, where a steeper slope in the line indicates a greater distribution of power towards lower-frequency activity. Right: Oscillatory classes within the neural frequency spectra are defined by the natural log of their mean frequency. Demarcations between classes are fuzzy, indicated by the overlaps in the plot. In general, the slower frequencies exhibit higher power, or greater amplitude, in their fluctuations.

highest power at the low frequencies. In other words, the biggest variance, or largest fluctuations in the signal, occur over longer periods of time, whereas smaller fluctuations occur relatively quickly. This relationship is presumed to exist at all spatial scales, and essentially is identical whether measured through LFPs that track activity in the micrometre range [24] or through EEG and fMRI [17] that track collective activity from many thousands to millions of cells across millimetres to centimetres of tissue. Interestingly, when plotted on the log scale, the power spectrum is roughly linear, and this distribution is referred to as "1/*f*," which has special implications for transfer of information within the brain, and will be discussed further below. But first let us quickly go over the rhythms within the distribution.

Typically, the power spectrum is divided up into different frequency bands, or boundaries demarcating specific rhythms that are associated with different functions and mechanisms, or drivers (Fig. 6-2). Examples of such mechanisms could be a network of cells, a specific part of the brain, or networks of cells across multiple brain structures. There are at least 10 frequency bands that make up the entire range of neural activity from <0.01 to >500 Hz, each one putatively generated by at least one distinct driver. However, the boundaries are not entirely clear-cut, as most frequencies of the brain power spectrum have been associated with an extensive number of behaviours and functions. Therefore, assigning a single driver to a specific rhythm is likely impossible. Attempts to localize drivers to frequency-specific rhythms show that the distribution is widespread, but anatomically distinct [1, 4, 5, 42]. The fact that many drivers can be linked to a single rhythm, and vice versa, is not a mistake. There is a specific order by which these 10 frequency bands (and thus mechanisms driving the activity within the bands) interact, allowing the brain to synchronize many of its systems at different timescales. If one divvies the power spectrum according to the mean frequency at each band, one will find the ratio between adjacent bands is *e*, or the base of the natural logarithm. Because *e* is an irrational number (roughly 2.17), this guarantees that the phase of the oscillators at each band will never overlap, resulting in fluctuating signals that are nonrepeating and weakly chaotic. In other words, adjacent frequency bands do not lock-step with each other, but constantly transition between unsynchronized and transiently synchronized states; the transient synchronization provides windows by which temporally independent mechanisms can communicate with each other. This is important because behaviour occurs across a range of timescales, from fractions of a second to several seconds, and precise timing of these behaviours is needed to successfully predict changes in the environment and navigate accordingly.

Now, back to the $1/f$ distribution of power that spans these frequency bands. The distribution arises from the intricate architecture of physical connections between cells and transmission delays that occur as action potentials travel longer distances [9]. The implication of the $1/f$ distribution of power is that a perturbation to low-frequency activity involving the synchrony of many cells (and thus high mean field power) will modify the activity in adjacent, higher frequency bands associated with fewer cells (which possess less mean field power). The low-frequency oscillations bias the extracellular membrane potential in local cortical regions, making it more likely that those local cells will fire synchronously [14]. Again, large brain networks with lots of energy influence local, small groups of networks over long expanses of space and time—low-frequency oscillating systems modulate high-frequency systems. And because the division of frequency bands in the power spectrum promotes quasistable interactions between systems (as mentioned above), this bouncing of interactions allows for parallel processing and cross-network communication. The main point of all of this is that the $1/f$ power distribution in the brain establishes a link between slow observable behaviour and fast neural activity [10].

Linking Slow Activity to Behaviour

Students are often introduced to neuroscience by demonstrating how single cells are related to behaviour—shine a light within the receptive field of a recorded neuron in the primary visual cortex, and one can hear a burst of sound from the recording equipment, representing an increase in the firing rate of action potentials. It is natural for students, then, to understand the brain–behaviour relationship within the context of single cells and fast, spiking activity. Establishing a causal link between slow, spontaneous oscillations and behaviour does not come so naturally, however. Yet, the evidence linking the two is quite strong, as human performance actually fluctuates at very low frequencies [35]. Another way to think about it is that performance is autocorrelated—how one performs in any one trial is similar to the recent preceding trials. Fluctuations in such behaviour can occur at roughly the same rate as infra-slow fluctuations (ISFs, 0.01–0.1 Hz) in the brain, and this property is preserved across a number of tasks [7, 22, 30]. For example, the phase (or the position along a waveform such as a *peak* or a *valley*) of EEG ISFs is highly correlated with the ability of subjects to perceive barely detectable visual stimuli, and detection is more reliable when ISFs are around the peak of their waveforms [31]. To bring back the $1/f$ distribution, this implies that when large groups of cells are synchronized, performance in this task is at a peak, presumably owing to enhanced communication between local visual networks and global cognitive networks.

RHYTHMS IN FMRI BOLD SIGNAL

Note, ISFs are just within the bandwidth of fMRI BOLD, suggesting perhaps that BOLD is more suitably illustrated as reflecting modulations to local neuronal activity rather than simply responding to local activity (as it is more commonly depicted). In fMRI research, we often model brain representations of behaviour according to the latter by employing a general linear model convolved with a hemodynamic response at a 6- to 12-second lag following a stimulus. This type of analysis implies one is interested in how the BOLD signal *responds* to the environment. Once again, from such a perspective we view the brain only as a *reflexive* system. Certainly, studying fMRI in this manner has provided much valuable information about brain function, and the evidence that BOLD signal does change in response to fast neuronal events is strong [23, 25]. But there is growing evidence that BOLD more accurately reflects a mixture of ongoing brain rhythms, as evidenced by simultaneous fMRI–LFP/EEG recordings [27, 28, 32, 37, 40]. Given this, it seems at least equally appropriate to examine fMRI signals from the viewpoint of their rhythmic behaviour, in frequency space.

It must be mentioned that the nonneural factors associated with BOLD fluctuations are quite extensive and include changes in oxygen consumption, microvascular architecture, blood flow, and movement artefact [6, 19]. The temporal fidelity of the hemodynamic response, which exhibits different waveforms in different brain areas [15], may also be a confounding factor when determining neural contribution to the signal. Regardless of how much neural activity is represented in BOLD, overwhelming evidence suggests that fMRI activity is of great functional relevance, and is sufficient for furthering our understanding about how the brain works. Interestingly, recent studies have shown that astrocyte networks are synchronized within the ISF frequency band [21, 38], and thus fluctuate at about the same frequency as BOLD. Up until recently, the function of these cells has largely been interpreted as supporting the physical structure of the brain, but perhaps large astrocyte networks are also granted the power to modulate activity of dispersed networks of neurons.

BRAIN RHYTHMS AND PAIN

So how do we relate all of this to pain? Chronic pain is characterized by its spontaneous onset and seemingly unexplainable persistence. Its qualities and descriptions vary from patient to patient, and the dynamics of its intensity are independent from the behaviour of the patient. For some reason, long after injuries have healed, this unpleasant experience sticks with some patients, and for them the gears of pain machinery continue to turn. As perception is a cortical phenomenon, chronic pain must be related to the mechanisms that drive the ongoing rhythms of the brain. Because of its complex nature, attempts to localize pain perception to a unitary brain region have failed. Although visual, somatosensory, and motor systems exhibit modality-specific and frequency-specific reactivity to stimuli, pain causes widespread modulations in power with acute stimulation [13, 36]. Gamma band oscillations in the primary somatosensory cortex are known to covary with acute pain perception [39, 41], and a multitude of studies have localized a "pain matrix" consisting mainly of the thalamus, primary somatosensory cortex, insula, anterior cingulate cortex, and periaqueductal gray that activates with painful stimuli. However, whether these changes in brain activity purely correspond to pain perception or are merely correlates of salience [41] presents a major challenge in pain research.

An emerging hypothesis suggests pain arises from the dynamic integration of information across many parts of the brain, which are embedded in its ongoing fluctuations [2, 11]. A recent study in our laboratory demonstrates this, showing that chronic pain changes oscillatory activity in the default mode network (DMN), and these disrupted oscillations are correlated with real-time spontaneous pain perception [3]. We divvied the power–frequency

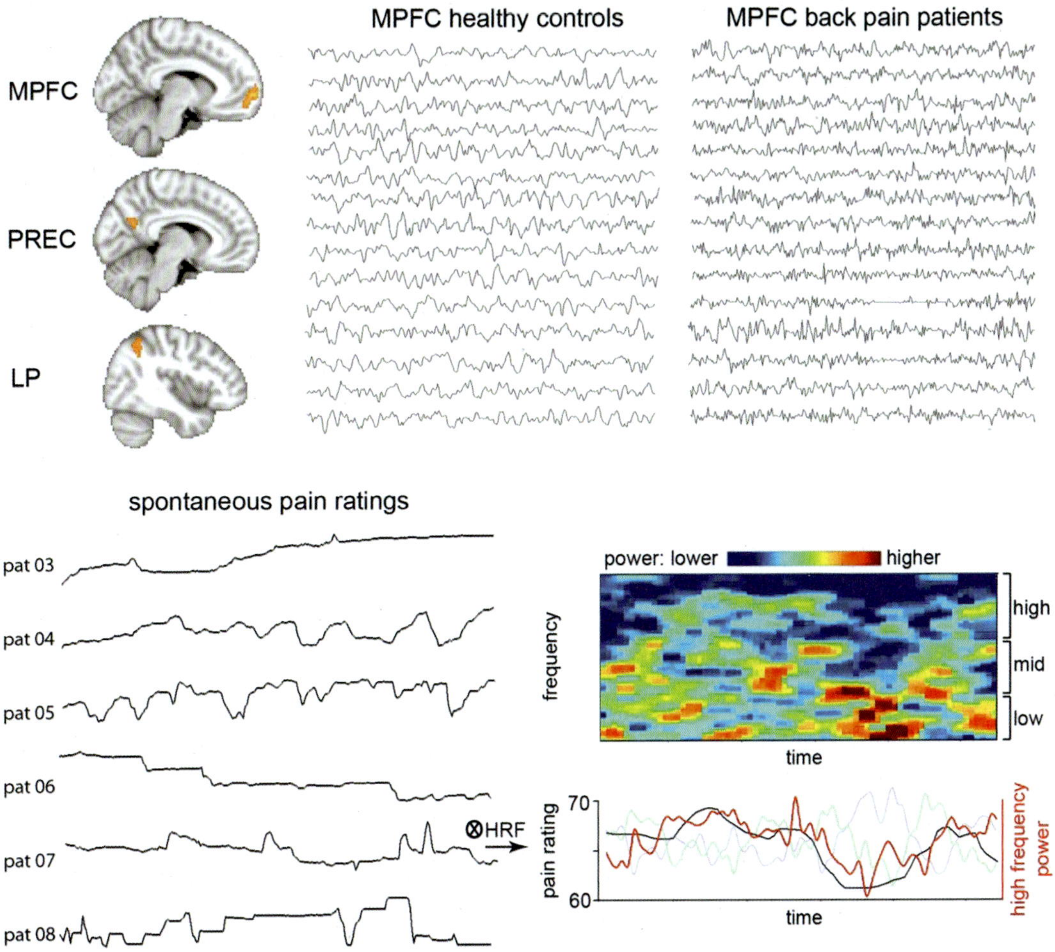

FIGURE 6-3 High-frequency BOLD fluctuations encode spontaneous pain. Top: Coloured regions in the brain indicate where high-frequency BOLD fluctuations are greater in patients with chronic back pain than in control subjects. Time series to the right are BOLD signals from the MPFC for individual subjects. Notice, the pain patients' signals fluctuate at a visibly higher frequency. Bottom: To the left are examples of spontaneous back pain ratings from individual patients. On the top right is the spectrogram of the MPFC BOLD signal for pat 07, demonstrating the progression of the distribution of frequency-specific power across time. The demarcations indicate the boundaries of three frequency bands studied separately: low, mid, and high. The power across time for the high-frequency band (*red line*) is shown in the plot directly below it. Notice, it is highly correlated with the pain rating of pat 07 (after convolving the pain rating with the hemodynamic response function). Power across time is shown for the other two frequency bands with faint lines.

spectrum into relatively low, medium, and high frequencies based off previous delineations of the fMRI BOLD signal [29]. When we compared high-frequency BOLD power in the chronic pain brain with healthy subjects, we found the greatest differences in the medial prefrontal, posterior cingulate, and bilateral parietal cortices (Fig. 6-3)—all major nodes of the DMN. As brain oscillations and network properties are inextricably related, we found these aberrant rhythms were correlated with increased communication between parts of the DMN and the insula and the secondary somatosensory cortex—regions associated with nociceptive processing. This suggests that nociceptive signals from ongoing pain had become integrated with parts of the brain that are responsible for evaluating one's current state of well-being. Finally, we found that the amplitude of high-frequency oscillations in the medial prefrontal cortex (MPFC), from second to second, corresponded to spontaneous surges in back pain ratings. In other words, when the high-frequency part of the BOLD signal increased from one time point to the next, so did the patient's spontaneous pain. These findings are in line with multiple studies demonstrating a shift in the power spectrum associated with chronic pain in diabetes [12], irritable bowel syndrome [18], multisomatoform disorder [34], fibromyalgia [20], and in multiple other etiologies [29].

More recently, we found predictive power in these brain fluctuations, and were able to identify patients who would respond to a placebo treatment for their back pain [16]. In a 2-week clinical trial of a placebo patch placed on the back of patients who had ongoing pain, we divided patients into placebo responders and nonresponders based off a median decrease in a visual analog scale (VAS) of their pain, ranging from 0 to 100. If a patient had a decrease in pain that was greater than the group absolute median change in pain, they were categorized as a responder. After comparing the frequency spectrum of BOLD signals across the brain for the two groups at baseline, we found that the responder group had bigger fluctuations at high frequencies in the dorsal MPFC. We further found that the frequency content of this region was about 80% accurate in predicting the pain outcome of a separate cohort of patients receiving the same treatment, validating that the findings may be generalized, at least within the chronic back pain population.

It is not surprising that chronic pain modulates the oscillatory activity of endogenous brain networks, which operate together as functionally defined, semi-independent systems. The ongoing and synchronous rhythms generated by these systems are a dynamic sum of the physiological activity giving rise to our subjective current state, or consciousness. Via a quasistable infrastructure, the $1/f$ power spectrum, the systems are orchestrated into playing together across spatial and temporal scales. Pain might be a product of dissonance in the orchestra—an unwanted interference in our consciousness. Here, we have seen how pain influences the rhythms of the brain (and vice versa). These *dissonant ripples* in the pained brain represent a disruption that is widespread across many regions. The growing evidence that pain perception is not localizable suggests, then, that studying network activity captured by the frequency–power spectrum will further our ability to identify how the brain represents pain.

REFERENCES

1. Andrews-Hanna JR, Reidler JS, Sepulcre J, Poulin R, Buckner RL. Functional-anatomic fractionation of the brain's default network. Neuron 2010;65(4):550–62.
2. Apkarian AV, Hashmi JA, Baliki MN. Pain and the brain: specificity and plasticity of the brain in clinical chronic pain. Pain 2011;152(3 Suppl):S49–64.
3. Baliki MN, Baria AT, Apkarian AV. The cortical rhythms of chronic back pain. J Neurosci 2011;31(39):13981–90.
4. Baria AT, Baliki MN, Parrish T, Apkarian AV. Anatomical and functional assemblies of brain BOLD oscillations. J Neurosci 2011;31(21):7910–9.
5. Baria AT, Mansour A, Huang L, Baliki MN, Cecchi GA, Mesulam MM, Apkarian AV. Linking human brain local activity fluctuations to structural and functional network architectures. NeuroImage 2013;73:144–55.
6. Birn RM, Diamond JB, Smith MA, Bandettini PA. Separating respiratory-variation-related fluctuations from neuronal-activity-related fluctuations in fMRI. NeuroImage 2006;31(4):1536–48.
7. Busch NA, Dubois J, VanRullen R. The phase of ongoing EEG oscillations predicts visual perception. J Neurosci 2009;29(24):7869–76.
8. Buzsaki G. Rhythms of the brain. New York, NY: Oxford University Press; 2006.
9. Buzsaki G, Draguhn A. Neuronal oscillations in cortical networks. Science 2004;304(5679):1926–9.
10. Canolty RT, Knight RT. The functional role of cross-frequency coupling. Trends Cogn Sci 2010;14(11):506–15.
11. Cauda F, Sacco K, D'Agata F, Duca S, Cocito D, Geminiani G, Migliorati F, Isoardo G. Low-frequency BOLD fluctuations demonstrate altered thalamocortical connectivity in diabetic neuropathic pain. BMC Neurosci 2009;10:138.

12. Cauda F, Sacco K, Duca S, Cocito D, D'Agata F, Geminiani GC, Canavero S. Altered resting state in diabetic neuropathic pain. PloS One 2009;4(2):e4542.
13. Chen AC, Herrmann CS. Perception of pain coincides with the spatial expansion of electroencephalographic dynamics in human subjects. Neurosci Lett 2001;297(3):183–6.
14. Frohlich F, McCormick DA. Endogenous electric fields may guide neocortical network activity. Neuron 2010;67(1):129–43.
15. Gonzalez-Castillo J, Saad ZS, Handwerker DA, Inati SJ, Brenowitz N, Bandettini PA. Whole-brain, time-locked activation with simple tasks revealed using massive averaging and model-free analysis. Proc Natl Acad Sci USA 2012;109(14):5487–92.
16. Hashmi JA, Baria AT, Baliki MN, Huang L, Schnitzer TJ, Apkarian AV. Brain networks predicting placebo analgesia in a clinical trial for chronic back pain. Pain 2012;153(12):2393–402.
17. He BJ, Zempel JM, Snyder AZ, Raichle ME. The temporal structures and functional significance of scale-free brain activity. Neuron 2010;66(3):353–69.
18. Hong JY, Kilpatrick LA, Labus J, Gupta A, Jiang Z, Ashe-McNalley C, Stains J, Heendeniya N, Ebrat B, Smith S, et al. Patients with chronic visceral pain show sex-related alterations in intrinsic oscillations of the resting brain. J Neurosci 2013;33(29):11994–2002.
19. Kim J, Van Dijk KR, Libby A, Napadow V. Frequency-dependent relationship between resting state fMRI signal power and head motion is localized within distributed association networks. Brain Connect 2014;4(1):30–9.
20. Kim JY, Kim SH, Seo J, Han SW, Nam EJ, Kim SK, Lee HJ, Lee SJ, Kim YT, Chang Y. Increased power spectral density in resting-state pain-related brain networks in fibromyalgia. Pain 2013;154(9):1792–7.
21. Kuga N, Sasaki T, Takahara Y, Matsuki N, Ikegaya Y. Large-scale calcium waves traveling through astrocytic networks in vivo. J Neurosci 2011;31(7):2607–14.
22. Lakatos P, Karmos G, Mehta AD, Ulbert I, Schroeder CE. Entrainment of neuronal oscillations as a mechanism of attentional selection. Science 2008;320(5872):110–3.
23. Lee JH, Durand R, Gradinaru V, Zhang F, Goshen I, Kim DS, Fenno LE, Ramakrishnan C, Deisseroth K. Global and local fMRI signals driven by neurons defined optogenetically by type and wiring. Nature 2010;465(7299):788–92.
24. Leopold DA, Murayama Y, Logothetis NK. Very slow activity fluctuations in monkey visual cortex: implications for functional brain imaging. Cereb Cortex 2003;13(4):422–33.
25. Lippert MT, Steudel T, Ohl F, Logothetis NK, Kayser C. Coupling of neural activity and fMRI-BOLD in the motion area MT. Magn Reson Imaging 28(8):1087–94.
26. Llinas RR. The intrinsic electrophysiological properties of mammalian neurons: insights into central nervous system function. Science 1988;242(4886):1654–64.
27. Logothetis NK, Pauls J, Augath M, Trinath T, Oeltermann A. Neurophysiological investigation of the basis of the fMRI signal. Nature 2001;412(6843):150–7.
28. Magri C, Schridde U, Murayama Y, Panzeri S, Logothetis NK. The amplitude and timing of the BOLD signal reflects the relationship between local field potential power at different frequencies. J Neurosci 2012;32(4):1395–407.
29. Malinen S, Vartiainen N, Hlushchuk Y, Koskinen M, Ramkumar P, Forss N, Kalso E, Hari R. Aberrant temporal and spatial brain activity during rest in patients with chronic pain. Proc Natl Acad Sci USA 2010;107(14):6493–7.
30. Mathewson KE, Gratton G, Fabiani M, Beck DM, Ro T. To see or not to see: prestimulus alpha phase predicts visual awareness. J Neurosci 2009;29(9):2725–32.
31. Monto S, Palva S, Voipio J, Palva JM. Very slow EEG fluctuations predict the dynamics of stimulus detection and oscillation amplitudes in humans. J Neurosci 2008;28(33):8268–72.
32. Mukamel R, Gelbard H, Arieli A, Hasson U, Fried I, Malach R. Coupling between neuronal firing, field potentials, and FMRI in human auditory cortex. Science 2005;309(5736):951–4.
33. O'Leary JL. Hans Berger on the electroencephalogram of man: the fourteen original reports on the electroencephalogram, Vol. 168. New York, NY: Elsevier; 1969.
34. Otti A, Guendel H, Wohlschlager A, Zimmer C, Noll-Hussong M. Frequency shifts in the anterior default mode network and the salience network in chronic pain disorder. BMC Psychiatry 2013;13:84.
35. Palva JM, Palva S. Roles of multiscale brain activity fluctuations in shaping the variability and dynamics of psychophysical performance. Prog Brain Res 2011;193:335–50.
36. Ploner M, Gross J, Timmermann L, Pollok B, Schnitzler A. Pain suppresses spontaneous brain rhythms. Cereb Cortex 2006;16(4):537–40.
37. Scheeringa R, Mazaheri A, Bojak I, Norris DG, Kleinschmidt A. Modulation of visually evoked cortical FMRI responses by phase of ongoing occipital alpha oscillations. J Neurosci 2011;31(10):3813–20.

38. Schulz K, Sydekum E, Krueppel R, Engelbrecht CJ, Schlegel F, Schroter A, Rudin M, Helmchen F. Simultaneous BOLD fMRI and fiber-optic calcium recording in rat neocortex. Nat Methods 2012;9:6.
39. Tiemann L, Schulz E, Gross J, Ploner M. Gamma oscillations as a neuronal correlate of the attentional effects of pain. Pain 2010;150(2):302–8.
40. Van de Ville D, Britz J, Michel CM. EEG microstate sequences in healthy humans at rest reveal scale-free dynamics. Proc Natl Acad Sci USA. 2010;107(42):18179–84.
41. Zhang ZG, Hu L, Hung YS, Mouraux A, Iannetti GD. Gamma-band oscillations in the primary somatosensory cortex—a direct and obligatory correlate of subjective pain intensity. J Neurosci 2012;32(22):7429–38.
42. Zuo XN, Di Martino A, Kelly C, Shehzad ZE, Gee DG, Klein DF, Castellanos FX, Biswal BB, Milham MP. The oscillating brain: complex and reliable. Neuroimage 2010;49(2):1432–45.

CHAPTER 7

Modelling the Brain as a Network

Guillermo Cecchi

Despite the highly complex behaviour of individual neurons and synaptic communication, and the average connectivity of neurons relative to the whole brain being quite small (at most 10^4 connections over a possible total of 10^{11}, i.e., a ratio of 10^{-7}), it is the intricate structure of connections between neurons, groups and classes of neurons, and areas that determines the daunting complexity of the brain. Even if we knew the precise connectivity for every single neuron, as we essentially do for *Caenorhabditis elegans* [67], the question still remains: what is the relationship between the parts (neurons, sets of neurons) and the whole (the brain)? That is, how do we understand neurons in the context of the brain and in the brain itself, given that it is composed of neurons?

The problem of understanding the relationship between the parts and the whole is not exclusive of neuroscience, and it is indeed as old as philosophy. In modern times it has pervaded almost every field of inquiry, including physics, ecology, sociology, economics, and literary theory. Prominently, in philosophy of language, the tension between the holistic and atomistic interpretations of meaning can be traced back at least to Frege [27], who introduced the *context principle*: the meaning of a word depends on the context of the sentence, and hence cannot be reduced to each single word-atom. Wittgenstein [69] later proposed the idea of language holism, stating that the meaning of a word requires not only the sentence as a context to be properly comprehended, but also the entire language. Radical holism, championed by Quine [66], posits that the proper context on which a single word's meaning can be expressed is that of the entirety of science, that is, the web of knowledge that a speaker and a listener share with society.

In neuroscience, this problem dates back to the very origins of the discipline. During the Nobel address, Golgi [33] decried the increasing popular theory of the neuron as the unit of neural function, right after Cajal presented the theory during his own address: *However opposed it may seem to the popular tendency to individualize the elements, I cannot abandon the idea of a unitary action of the nervous system, without bothering if, by that, I approach old conceptions.* Almost half a century later, Lashley proposed the notion that it is mass neuronal activity that defines the unit of neural function, represented by the idea of the n-gram: *The anatomic variability is so great as to preclude, I believe, any theory which assumes regularity and precision of anatomic arrangement. Such facts lead me to believe that theories of neuron interaction must be couched, not in terms of the activity of individual cells but in terms of mass relations among the cells. Even the simplest bit of behavior requires the integrated action of millions of neurons; the activity of any single neuron can have little influence on the whole, just as the path of an individual molecule of a gas has little influence on the gas pressure. It is questionable whether specific instances of behavior can ever be dealt with in terms of the activity of individual neurons; the complexity is too great. We shall probably have to use a different kind of model, a model which can be explained in principle by individual neuron action but which involves a somewhat different set of concepts and laws of action* [46].

These philosophical concepts, however, need to be transformed into analytic tools applicable to scientific disciplines, neuroscience among them. In this regard, graph theory and the related statistical network theory provide a mathematical framework to capture some of the intuitions behind the problem of the "parts and the whole." The basic mathematical object, a graph, is a collection of nodes and links between them, with possible additional attributes for both (such as orientation for links). The generality of this mathematical structure allows for a wide spectrum of possibilities of representation for nodes and links, from anatomically defined neurons and synapses (i.e., anatomical connectivity) to functionally defined activity clusters and intercluster coactivation (i.e., functional connectivity). Although it is possible to utilize anatomy to label brain-derived graphs, one of the main motivations to study systems with graph theoretic tools is the understanding that topology (how the nodes are connected with each other) is more robust than geometry (where the nodes are exactly located). Consider this example: It is highly relevant to know whether three connected excitatory neurons *A, B, C* are arranged in the feedback loop $A \rightarrow B \rightarrow C \rightarrow A$ or not, as their dynamical behaviour may be radically different. Knowing where they are located is only relevant to understand how they are connected to other neurons. Graph theory is precisely the study of topological regularities of systems represented as nodes and links, and encompasses a vast mathematical literature. The study of very large graphs is sometimes referred to as statistical network theory, and has gained significant attention in recent years owing to the availability of large networks created by science as well as technology. Returning to our loop example, graph theory provides us with tools to search for such a motif, and other possible ones, embedded in graphs, and to estimate how many of them to expect.

There is a vast literature on graph features and how to compute them, as well as on models of networks that display certain features and regularities, such as long-tailed distribution of connections per node [49]. Beyond the mathematical formalism, however, what is important about graphs in the context of neuroscience? Graphs can, evidently, represent the relationships between elements observed in neuroanatomy. The brain, however, as a system shaped by evolution to act and behave, is essentially determined by its dynamics. In turn, dynamics are only partially determined by connectivity: even a simple two-unit circuit can have very different behaviours depending on the sign of the connections, as well as the intrinsic dynamical properties of each unit (i.e., oscillator, integrator, rate-coded, graded, etc.). In this sense, it is more important to characterize the dynamics than the connectivity. As we will discuss in this chapter, graph (alternatively, network) theory can also provide a formal characterization of the dynamical state of the brain, on the basis of the ideas of functional connectivity and causal modelling.

CLASSES OF MODELS

The stimulus–response paradigm is arguably the most typical setting for neuroscientific experimentation, under the implicit assumption that the brain is a passive or reactive system whose purpose is to monitor external signals. However, a sizable body of literature has compared the brain's response to external stimuli to small modulations or disturbances of a quasi-dreamlike state even in wakefulness [38]. Experimental evidence indicates that ongoing brain activity (i.e., not elicited by stimuli), the reflection of a dynamic core [38, 23], has a structured temporal evolution [4]. Examples of such activity include the maintenance of a normal wakeful state and attentional and emotional biases, which are known to provide a strong top-down modulation of even early sensorial processing [26, 18]). Moreover, an

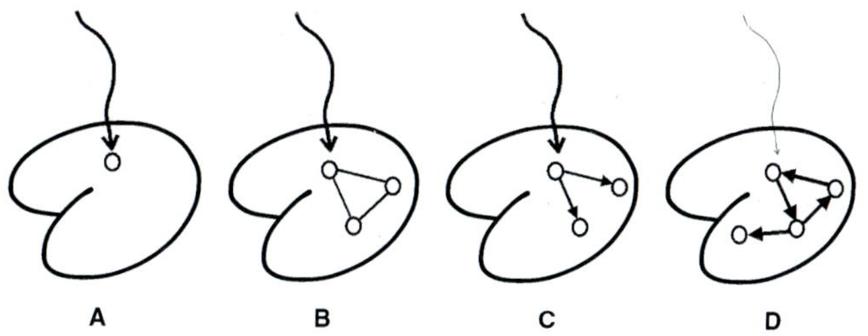

FIGURE 7-1 Increasing descriptive complexity of analytic approaches, where the incoming arrow symbolizes an external stimulation or task. **A:** Univariate, **B:** stimulus-driven correlation network, **C:** stimulus-driven causal network, and **D:** self-driven causal network modulated by stimulus.

explicit consideration of neural correlations—as opposed to external correlates—can lead to significant insights, such as the presence of otherwise undetectable collective states in local as well as distributed networks [60, 16]. The identification of the system known as the default-mode network [26, 54] has only made more urgent the need to analyze the validity of the dynamic core hypothesis: it postulates the presence of an extended network whose components evolve relatively slowly, and can be activated or deactivated en masse by an attention-demanding task, implying that brain function cannot be parsed as a set of separated modules implementing functions at well-defined segments of time. The association of the task-negative default-mode network, as identified by Raichle et al. [54], with a system of internal and external sensory monitors that is tuned down during attention [54] is another strong indication of a nontrivial interaction between the intrinsic timescale of the default mode and the less constrained one of the task.

The complexity of the brain's anatomy and physiology, therefore, begs the question: How can we analyze such a system? Any analytic framework implies a model of the system under study, which in its turn involves specific simplifications and assumptions, even though often times these are not made explicit. Let us consider a progression of analytic models for functional brain data, as represented in Fig. 7-1. While somewhat arbitrary, it will nevertheless be illuminating for the purpose of understanding the implications of modelling the brain as a graph. The most basic model is univariate, where an external stimulus (i.e., visual stimulation) or condition (i.e., REM sleep) is correlated with the activity of individual units or clusters (A); this is basically the approach of the General Linear Model (GLM). The field of functional brain imaging has been dominated by this analytic framework that focuses on the relationship between the activation of an area and the presence or absence of a task or stimulus, while ignoring temporal and spatial correlations that may influence local responses as much as the experimental paradigm [35]. Although the GLM approach has demonstrated its utility, and has resulted in many insights into brain function, it has limited applicability across a wide variety of experimental protocols, especially in the case of resting state and similar brain states [40]. Recently, the introduction of machine learning algorithms for fMRI analysis has demonstrated that there is a wealth of functional information in distributed patterns of activation, even though specific intervoxel interactions are usually not modelled [50, 48, 13].

The next model considers the effect of the stimulus or condition on a group of units identified through a network extraction approach (B). Model (A) will also produce a "network," that is, the units in that case are correlated with the stimulus, whereas in (B) the units are first correlated among them. This distinction is relevant because correlation, like other similar metrics to compute networks such as mutual information, is not transitive.

A simple example shows this: In a chain of correlated variables, $A\sim B$, $B\sim C$, $C\sim D$, it is quite generic to have a loss of correlation at each step (equivalently, information) such that there is no significant correlation between *A* and *D*. It may be possible, for instance, that two different stimuli or conditions cannot be discriminated on the basis of how correlated they are with individual brain units, and yet affect how those units are correlated with each other, therefore impacting the functional network. Conversely, maps of activation/deactivation typical of GLM do not necessarily imply that the encompassed units are correlated between themselves, as they may be being driven by a common input.

The simplest and most popular approaches to model interactions among different brain regions are based on the notion of functional connectivity [28]. Some of these approaches use pair-wise voxel correlations [24], whereas others use more sophisticated methods [15, 1, 11, 42] to generate networks of brain interactions. All these approaches suffer from the problem of spurious connections owing to confounding effects.

The approaches that attempt to alleviate this problem are termed as *effective* connectivity analysis methods [28]. These include dynamic causal modelling [29, 52], structural equation models (SEM) [51, 47, 10], graphical models [25, 19], and Granger causality analysis [34, 61, 59]. The SEM are based on a priori specification of all the potential interactions between the regions in the brain. Dynamic causal modelling, which is based on a nonlinear model of neuronal interactions, also requires a priori specification of the experimental hypothesis. To minimize the confounding effects, approaches such as partial correlations [58, 44] and partial mutual information [62, 57] have also been used for fMRI data analysis.

We can therefore think of the next model (C) as a variant of (B), albeit one with significant implications. If instead of estimating a correlation-based functional network, one computes a causal model such that there are units that predict other units, then this predictive structure itself may be altered or modulated by the stimulus or the condition of interest. Following the discussion above, we may not find changes in the correlation of a unit with the stimulus but how the unit affects other units, an effect that may be observed with a significant temporal delay. In this case, the model can be represented by a hybrid graph that includes directed links, indicating causation of the source node to the target node, and undirected links, when the nodes are correlated but causation cannot be inferred.

Early functional connectivity methods used correlation metrics [22, 24], which do not provide directional information for the links in the network. Delayed correlation analysis can be used to infer link directionality by including part of the temporal structure of voxel–voxel correlations [15], though this is not a robust method as it considers only pair-wise interactions. A more complete model was presented in [14], which introduced the idea of using a sparse regression framework to estimate an autoregressive model that best explained the measured fMRI time sequences. The idea of Granger causality is that a variable X is the cause of another Y if the past of X can be used to increase the predictability of the future of Y [34]; for practical reasons, autoregressive modelling is typically utilized to infer Granger causality. One limitation for the applicability of Granger causality to fMRI data is that autoregressive models at the voxel level are highly underconstrained, and therefore aggregation of voxels is required to reduce dimensionality and match it with the number of independent data samples [32]. However, this aggregation process can lead to severe artefacts [30].

As mentioned in the beginning of the chapter, the dynamics of the brain are only partially determined by connectivity: even a simple two-unit circuit can have very different behaviours depending on the sign of the connections, as well as the intrinsic dynamical properties of each unit (i.e., oscillator, integrator, rate-coded, graded, etc.). In this sense, it is more important to characterize the dynamics than the connectivity, and functional connectivity is a means to capture aspects of the dynamics. The final model (D) considers the brain as a dynamical system, whose behaviour includes a significant component of self-determined activity. This implies that, as it is the case for a typical nonlinear oscillator (e.g., a flip-flop), the response to a particular stimulus is conditional on its present state (e.g., the phase of the oscillator). In the case of linear autoregressive models, the model is completely determined by the regression matrices, which can be represented similarly to model (C); nonlinear models require further specifications.

It is evident, then, that an accurate description of functional data should include not only explicit dynamical components, but also a means to discover dynamical interactions, as opposed to just test the hypothesis of their significance based on a priori knowledge. Practical implementations of Granger causality analysis are generally based on multivariate autoregressive (MAR) modelling, since the Granger causality relationships are mostly determined by solving the model identification problem with a suitable MAR. Autoregressive modelling assumes that the state of a system at a certain time is a linear combination of the recent previous states. MARs can be applied in a purely data-driven manner, but require very good temporal data resolution. For this reason, it has mostly been applied to modalities such as EEG [9, 53, 2], MEG [20], and local field potential recordings [9, 37]. The application of Granger causality to fMRI data has been restricted to either pair-wise causality (bivariate analysis) as in [32] and [56] or analysis using a small number of prespecified regions of interest [61, 17, 21, 36]. Thus, for functional imaging data, the analysis either becomes susceptible to confounding effects or needs accurate specification of the key regions of interest and experimental hypothesis.

The work by Valdes-Sosa et al. [65] solved the model identification problem in Granger causality analysis using a variety of methods, including the use of the lasso regression [64]. They concluded that the performance of different techniques, as measured by the ROC curve area, does not differ significantly. While applying this technique to functional imaging, the fMRI data were aggregated into 116 regions—a step that was not really required for using their technique. Therefore, it was not possible to uncover certain key findings that we report in this chapter. The work by Garg et al. [30] developed a whole-brain method based on MAR, capturing the dynamics and spatial correlations of the brain using fMRI measurements from individual voxels, using also the lasso regression technique to solve the problem of underdetermination, given that they used the approximately 30,000 voxels of the original spatial resolution. In both cases, the estimated models identified causal relationships among brain areas or voxels, under the hypothesis that the structure of the information flow in the fMRI data reflects the flow of information in the underlying neural networks.

FEATURES AND REPRESENTATION

What features are relevant to measure in the context of functional brain networks? There are a large number of topological features that have been utilized and discussed in the literature. Among the most commonly used are *degree*, the number of links per node, *clustering*, the fraction of triangulations relative to the total possible ones, *minimal path*, the average minimal number of links needed to reach any node from each node, and *centrality*, the density of minimal paths connecting all nodes going through a particular one. These features, among a host of others, represent different simplified aspects of the network a high-dimensional mathematical object, and probe functional aspects whose importance

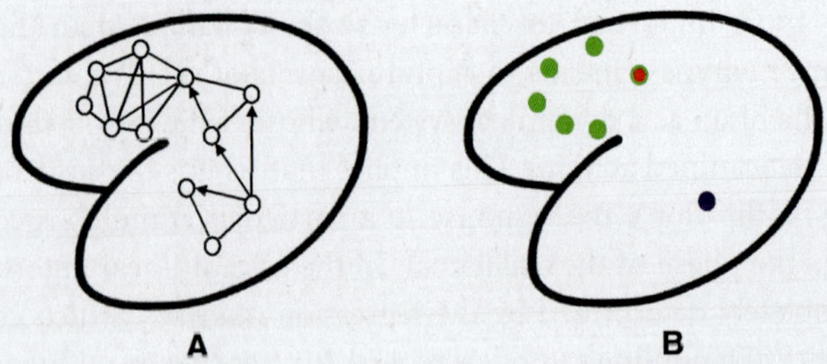

FIGURE 7-2 Geometric representation of topological features. **A:** Full representation of the network and **B:** simplified representation in a hybrid network: blue for high out-degree, green for high clustering, and red for centrality.

may depend on the neuroscientific questions to be asked. These features can be compiled as global "intensive" properties of the entire network, or as "extensive" ones mapped onto the brain anatomy (Fig. 7-2).

Beyond ready-made features, the identification of domain-specific features is essential in the application of machine learning techniques to high-dimensional data, and often contributes even more to the success of learning than the choice of a particular learning model. In neuroscience, particularly for brain imaging, the extraction of meaningful features is important to gain functional insights that a black-box approach cannot provide; this is emphatically the case for the infinite possibilities for features derived from network models. An illustrative example of how to combine complex feature extraction with neuroscientific insights is provided by a recent study on schizophrenia [16, 55]. The goal of this study was to identify predictive biomarkers from fMRI data of schizophrenic patients and control subjects performing a very simple, minimally demanding auditory task. Network theory is particularly relevant to the study of schizophrenia, as this condition seems to be difficult to attribute to a dysfunction of some particular brain areas, and hence delocalized. The failure to identify specific areas, as well as the controversy over which localized mechanisms are responsible for the symptoms associated with schizophrenia, have led researchers [8, 31, 41] to hypothesize that this disease may be better understood as a disruption of the emergent, collective properties of normal brain states, which can be better captured by functional networks. For this purpose, several topological features of the functional networks were compared across the normal and patient groups to ask the following questions: (1) what specific effects does schizophrenia have on the functional connectivity of brain networks? (2) Does schizophrenia affect functional connectivity in ways that are congruent with the effect it has on area-specific, task-dependent activations? (3) Is it possible to use functional connectivity to improve the classification accuracy of schizophrenic patients? The study showed that degree maps identify spatially clustered groups of voxels with statistically significant group differences; moreover, these highly significant voxel subsets are quite stable over different data subsets. In contrast, standard GLM contrast maps showed much weaker group differences as well as stability. Degree and clustering maps yield very informative features, with accuracies above 85%, whereas contrast maps could yield only accuracies slightly over 50% (chance). The result on classification accuracy was compounded by the observation that overall correlation strength was not significantly different between the groups, but the patient population exhibited stronger short-range correlations and weaker long-range (including interhemispheric) correlations. Moreover, the study also showed that the results depended critically on the identification of functional network features at the voxel level, as even sophisticated paradigm-driven functional parcellation techniques [63] did not reveal any statistically significant differences between the groups.

In the case of models based on causal or dynamic interactions, the definition of directionality in the functional connections requires more complex representations. The work by Cecchi et al. [15], for instance, proposed the utilization of different spatial maps for out- and in-degree for each voxel (total number of links point to other voxels, or other voxels pointing to it, respectively). This approach, however, can lead to an exponential explosion of features and motifs to be considered [42]. In contrast, Garg et al. proposed to study the "impulse response dynamics" represented by the autoregressive matrices in a whole-brain MAR analysis. This corresponds to identifying the voxels with the highest predictive power (equivalently the largest out-degree), such that the bulk of the temporal evolution of the brain can be accounted for [30]. The study showed that the model can be effectively visualized using the impulse response dynamics and the voxels with high prediction power form a large number of small spatially contiguous clusters exhibiting high intrasubject as well as intersubject consistency, that the results of the prediction power maps are consistent with previous results related to networks activated by the specific task, as well as networks related to the default-mode activity, and that the model recovered a global dynamical state dominated by two prominent streams, which originate in the posterior parietal cortex (as expected in the sensory-motor task studied) and the posterior cingulate/precuneus cortex. Moreover, these two streams span default-mode and task-specific networks, interact in several regions, including the insula, and suggest that the posterior cingulate is a central node of the default-mode network, in terms of its ability to predict the future evolution of the rest of the nodes. These results indicate that the method can be considered complementary to other functional connectivity methods. Moreover, given that "unfolding" of the dynamics through the impulse response function recovers a great percentage of the areas that are identified by GLM and the zero-lag correlation maps, the method clearly uncovers dynamical information not present in static maps.

STATISTICAL TESTING

The feature representation approaches mentioned earlier allow for univariate hypothesis testing by computing statistically significant differences in single global topological features (e.g., mean degree), maps (e.g., voxel-based degree), or multivariate testing on sets of topological features as well as spatial topological patterns. However, the intrinsic complexity of a network may require further controls. Consider the case of a network with a given mean degree and clustering: how can we test the hypothesis that these values indicate an underlying structure of the functional network? For this we need to resort to the notion of surrogate network, that is, a network that preserves some structure from the original one, corresponding to a null hypothesis [49]. The simplest such surrogate is the random or Erdos model: a network with the same number of nodes and links as the original one, but such that the specific nodes connected are chosen at random (Fig. 7-3, bottom left). This surrogation corresponds to the hypothesis that any measure we may have found is only due to having so many nodes and links, and can be tested by comparing the original measure with a distribution of the same measure over several surrogate instances. The Erdos surrogate can be used, for example, to test whether the degree distribution of the original network (e.g., long-tailed) is sufficiently different from random (approximately Gaussian).

A subtler surrogate is the Maslov network [45], created by randomizing the connections as in the Erdos model, but preserving the number of links in each node, and corresponds to the null hypothesis that what we observe in the original network is only a

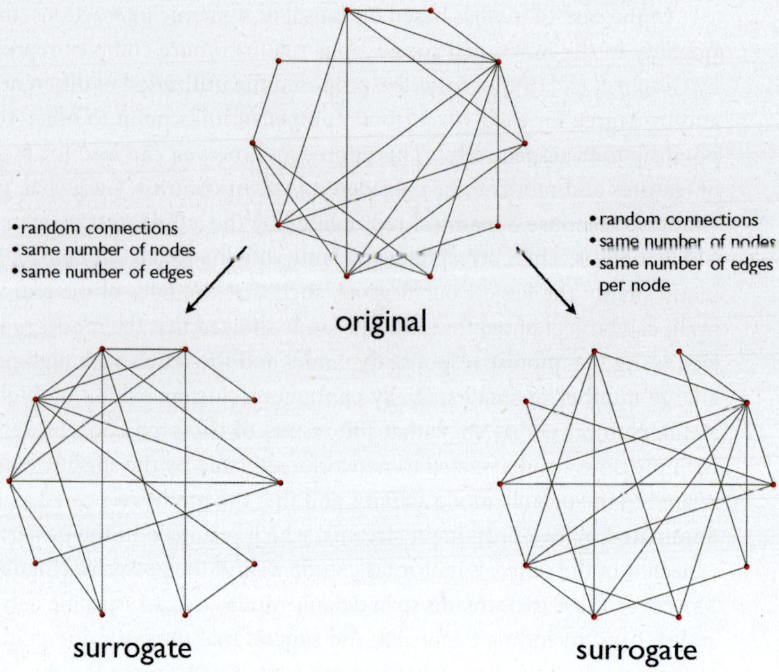

FIGURE 7-3 Surrogation for testing against a null hypothesis. Two possible surrogates create a network that preserves the number of nodes and edges from the original, with random connections **(lower left)**, and one that also preserves the total number of connections per node.

consequence of the specific degree distribution per node, regardless of any higher-order correlation between nodes. This model cannot be used, obviously, to test for structure in the degree distribution (it will be identical to the original one, by construction), but it is a good model to test how significant the clustering index is, as triangulations imply correlations between three nodes, absent in this surrogate. Evidently, it is possible to conceive other classes of surrogate networks, depending on the specific null hypothesis that we would like to test, but they may be more or less difficult to instantiate.

THEORETICAL IMPLICATIONS

It is often relevant to understand the potential implications of measured network features in terms of brain theory, beyond practical applications as, for instance, disease markers. Although this is a wide and expanding field, we will focus on one of the most common approaches to relate networks and function, namely, the theories on how network structure comes about. That is, given the observed features and regularities of a network, is there any theory that can explain these results based on a model to grow a network during development, or functionally sculpt it? The most popular growth models are the Erdos (ER) model already mentioned, the Strogatz–Watts (SW) small-world model [68], and the Barabasi–Alberts (BA) model [7]. The Erdos model can be understood as a growth process that starts with a fixed number of nodes, to which links are added by randomly choosing pairs of nodes. The ER model yields networks with short path length and low clustering. The SW model implies rewiring: A regular, long path length network with a high density of triangulations is rewired by choosing any link and reconnecting it at random. With only a

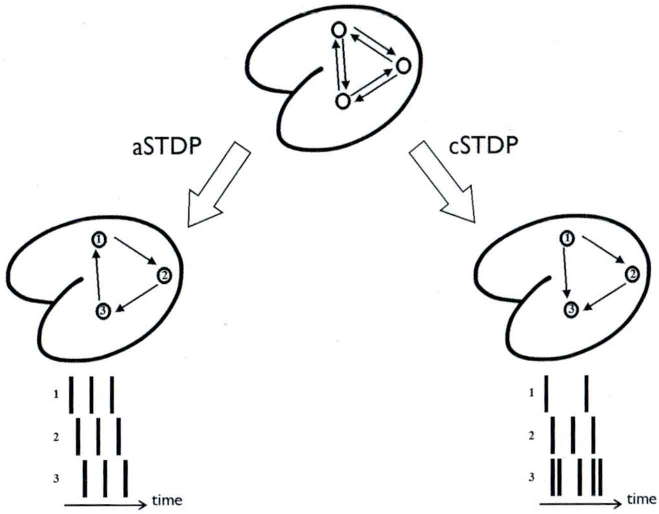

FIGURE 7-4 Theoretical implications of network motifs. Specific configurations, such as the feed-forward **(right)** or feedback patterns **(left)**, correspond with synaptic plasticity rules (classical STDP and anti-STDP, respectively).

few such rewiring steps, the initial network becomes "short" like ER, while preserving most triangulations, a phenomenon called "small world." The BA model involves the growth of an initial small number of nodes randomly connected; each new node is connected to some of the existing nodes, but with a probability proportional to how many links the existing nodes have. This creates a "rich-get-richer" process that can result in long-tailed, power-law degree distributions. There are many theoretical results for the three models and their several variants, which may avoid the task of actually generating instances of surrogate networks if one is interested in testing whether the original network is significantly similar to the model.

Models in which network connectivity is provided by established or hypothesized synaptic plasticity rules provide a perspective closer to neuroscience. An example is shown in Fig. 7-4: A network with an initial random connectivity is evolved under classical synaptic time-dependent plasticity (cSTDP), a neural plasticity rule experimentally observed [43]. This rule strengthens synapses that are active immediately before a somatic action potential (are "predictive"), and weakens those that are active immediately after (are "retrodictive"). This leads to a network with significantly fewer loops of any length than Erdos or Maslov surrogates [39], and consequently produces specific patterns of activity (Fig. 7-4, lower right). The less frequent but equally observed aSTDP, in which the synaptic weights are reversed with respect to cSTDP, similarly creates a network that has a significantly higher density of loops and accompanying activation patterns (lower left). A possible implication of this theory is that the paucity of feedback loops observed in fMRI functional networks with oriented links [42] may be explained as a consequence of the large-scale effect of cSTDP, although further experimental and simulation-based validation would be required.

Finally, let us consider the theoretical implications of the network perspective for the specific case of pain. As it is well established in the field, pain, in general, and chronic pain, in particular, cannot be ascribed to any one specific area of the brain, or even a small group thereof. Moreover, as a highly evolutionarily determined function, pain necessarily implicates lower-level, hedonic and emotional areas as well as higher-order cognitive processing [3]. Consistent with this hypothesis, Baliki et al. [6] showed that chronic pain disrupts the normal spatiotemporal structure of the default-mode network. However, this finding may still be explained in localized terms, as discussed earlier. In other words, it may still be possible that the main effect of chronic pain is to alter, for instance, the function of the precuneus, which would disrupt its interaction with other areas; this hypothetical situation would represent a network *effect*, but not a network *cause*. The work of Balenzuela et al. [5] partially addresses this issue, and illustrates how the network perspective can provide brain theoretical insights. They constructed functional networks using 90 brain regions from a Brodmann atlas on a group of chronic back pain (CBP) and healthy control subjects during resting state. Studying communities, that is, groups of areas strongly connected with each other, they observed an organization of six distinct modules with a similar structure in both CBP and controls, and modular disruptions in communities involving frontal and temporal regions. The differences involved changes in the community structure of the orbitofrontal cortex, the insula, and the posterior portion of the cingulate gyrus, and a higher cross-community connectivity strength of the anterior cingulate cortex in the CBP population. These results demonstrate that the functional disruption that accompanies chronic pain cannot, therefore, be simply explained as local alterations and imply that the condition, as much as normal pain processing, needs to be thought of, modelled, and experimentally studied as resulting from network interactions.

OUTLOOK

Clearly, modelling the brain as a network is only one among many possible approaches to understand such a rich system, and novel tools are required to capture the relationship between anatomy, physiology, and function in a way that is both descriptive and predictive. While we can find inspiration in physics and the development of thermodynamics and statistical mechanics as a successful example of the "parts" and the "whole," the complexity of even the most elementary components of neural systems precludes, at the moment, a similar first-principles approach to derive a formal mathematical framework. In the meantime, network theory can provide tools for practical use and for theoretical inquiry. Moreover, network theory is a very active area of research, and new developments such as data analysis based on the theory of persistent homology in algebraic topology [12] can help us move away from simplistic interpretations of brain function.

REFERENCES

1. Achard S, Salvador R, Whitcher B, Suckling J, Bullmore E. A resilient, low-frequency, small-world human brain functional network with highly connected association cortical hubs. J Neurosci 2006;26(1): 63–72.
2. Anderson CW, Stolz EA, Shamsunder S. Multivariate autoregressive models for classification of spontaneous electroencephalographic signals during mental tasks. IEEE Trans Biomed Eng 1998;45(3):277–86.
3. Apkarian AV, Sosa Y, Krauss BR, Thomas PS, Fredrickson BE, Levy RE, Harden RN, Chialvo DR. Chronic pain patients are impaired on an emotional decision-making task. Pain 2004;108(1–2):129–36.
4. Arieli A, Sterkin A, Grinvald A, Aertsen A. Dynamics of ongoing activity: explanation of the large variability in evoked cortical responses. Science 1996;273(5283):1868–71.
5. Balenzuela P, Chernomoretz A, Fraiman D, Cifre I, Sitges C, Montoya P, Chialvo DR. Modular organization of brain resting state networks in chronic back pain patients. Front Neuroinform 2010;4:116.
6. Baliki MN, Geha PY, Apkarian AV, Chialvo DR. Beyond feeling: chronic pain hurts the brain, disrupting the default-mode network dynamics. J Neurosci 2008;28(6):1398–403.
7. Barabasi AL, Albert R. Emergence of scaling in random networks. Science 1999;286(5439):509–12.
8. Bassett DS, Bullmore E, Verchinski BA, Mattay VS, Weinberger DR, Meyer-Lindenberg A. Hierarchical organization of human cortical networks in health and schizophrenia. J Neurosci 2008;28(37):9239–48.

9. Brovelli A, Ding M, Ledberg A, Chen Y, Nakamura R, Bressler SL. Beta oscillations in a large-scale sensorimotor cortical network: directional influences revealed by Granger causality. Proc Natl Acad Sci USA 2004;101(26):9849–54.
10. Buchel C, Friston KJ. Modulation of connectivity in visual pathways by attention: cortical interactions evaluated with structural equation modeling and fMRI. Cerebral Cortex 1997;7(8):768–78.
11. Bullmore E, Sporns O. Complex brain networks: graph theoretical analysis of structural and functional systems. Nature Rev Neurosci 2009;10(3):186–98.
12. Carlsson G. Topology and data. Bull Am Math Soc 2009;46(2):255–308.
13. Carroll MK, Cecchi GA, Rish I, Garg R, Rao AR. Prediction and interpretation of distributed neural activity with sparse models. NeuroImage 2009;44(1):112–22.
14. Cecchi GA, Garg R, Rao AR. Inferring brain dynamics using Granger causality on fMRI data. In: Proceedings of the 5th IEEE International Symposium on Biomedical Imaging. Paris, France: ISBI; May 14–17, 2008. pp. 604–7.
15. Cecchi GA, Rao AR, Centeno MV, Baliki M, Apkarian AV, Chialvo DR. Identifying directed links in large scale functional networks: application to brain fMRI. BMC Cell Biol 2007;8(Suppl 1):S5.
16. Cecchi GA, Rish I, Thyreau B, Thirion B, Plaze M, Paillere-Martinot M-L, Martelli C, Martinot J-L, Poline J-B. Discriminative network models of schizophrenia. In: Proceedings of the 23rd Annual Conference on Neural Information Processing Systems, Vol. 22. Vancouver, Canada: NIPS; 2009. pp. 250–62.
17. Chen H, Yang Q, Liao W, Gong Q, Shen S. Evaluation of the effective connectivity of supplementary motor areas during motor imagery using Granger causality mapping. NeuroImage 2009;47(4):1844–53.
18. Crist RE, Li W, Gilbert CD. Learning to see: experience and attention in primary visual cortex. Nature Neurosci 2001;4(5):519–25.
19. Dahlhaus R, Eichler M. Causality and graphical models in time series analysis. Oxf Stat Sci 2003:115–37.
20. Darvas F, Leahy RM. Functional imaging of brain activity and connectivity with MEG. In: Jirsa VK, McIntosh AR, editors. Handbook of brain connectivity. Berlin, Germany: Springer; 2007. pp. 201–20.
21. Deshpande G, LaConte S, James GA, Peltier S, Hu X. Multivariate Granger causality analysis of fMRI data. Hum Brain Mapp 2009;30(4):1361–73.
22. Dodel S, Herrmann JM, Geisel T. Functional connectivity by cross-correlation clustering. Neurocomputing 2002;44:1065–70.
23. Edelman GM, Tononi G. A Universe of consciousness: how matter becomes imagination. New York, NY: Basic books; 2000.
24. Eguiluz VM, Chialvo DR, Cecchi GA, Baliki M, Apkarian AV. Scale-free brain functional networks. Phys Rev Lett 2005;94(1):018102.
25. Eichler M. A graphical approach for evaluating effective connectivity in neural systems. Philos Trans R Soc Lond B Biol Sci 2005;360(1457):953–67.
26. Fox MD, Snyder AZ, Vincent JL, Corbetta M, Van Essen DC, Raichle ME. The human brain is intrinsically organized into dynamic, anticorrelated functional networks. Proc Natl Acad Sci USA 2005;102(27):9673–8.
27. Frege G. The foundations of arithmetic, 1884 [translated from the German by Austin JL]. Evanston, IL: Northwestern University Press; 1980.
28. Friston KJ. Functional and effective connectivity in neuroimaging: a synthesis. Hum Brain Mapp 1994;2(1–2):56–78.
29. Friston KJ, Harrison L, Penny W. Dynamic causal modeling. NeuroImage 2003;19(4):1273–302.
30. Garg R, Cecchi GA, Rao AR. Full-brain auto-regressive modeling (FARM) using fMRI. NeuroImage 2011;58(2):416–41.
31. Garrity AG, Pearlson GD, McKiernan K, Lloyd D, Kiehl KA, Calhoun VD. Aberrant "default mode" functional connectivity in schizophrenia. Am J Psychiatry 2007;164(3):450–7.
32. Goebel R, Roebroeck A, Kim DS, Formisano E. Investigating directed cortical interactions in time-resolved fMRI data using vector autoregressive modeling and Granger causality mapping. Magn Reson Imaging 2003;21(10):1251–61.
33. Golgi C. The neuron doctrine: theory and facts. Nobel Lecture 1906;1921:190–217.
34. Granger CW. Investigating causal relations by econometric models and cross-spectral methods. Econometrica 1969;37(3):424–38.
35. Grinband J, Wager TD, Lindquist M, Ferrera VP, Hirsch J. Detection of time-varying signals in event-related fMRI designs. NeuroImage 2008;43(3):509–20.
36. Harrison L, Penny WD, Friston K. Multivariate autoregressive modeling of fMRI time series. NeuroImage 2003;19(4):1477–91.
37. Kaminski M, Ding M, Truccolo WA, Bressler SL. Evaluating causal relations in neural systems: granger causality, directed transfer function and statistical assessment of significance. Biol Cybern 2001;85(2):145–57.

38. Koch C, Davis JL. Large-scale neuronal theories of the brain. London, UK: MIT Press; 1994.
39. Kozloski J, Cecchi GA. A theory of loop formation and elimination by spike timing-dependent plasticity. Front Neural Circuits 2010;4:7.
40. Li K, Guo L, Nie J, Li G, Liu T. Review of methods for functional brain connectivity detection using fMRI. Comput Med Imaging Graph 2009;33(2):131–9.
41. Liu Y, Liang M, Zhou Y, He Y, Hao Y, Song M, Yu C, Liu H, Liu Z, Jiang T. Disrupted small-world networks in schizophrenia. Brain 2008;131(Pt 4):945–61.
42. Ma'ayan A, Cecchi GA, Wagner J, Rao AR, Iyengar R, Stolovitzky G. Ordered cyclic motifs contribute to dynamic stability in biological and engineered networks. Proc Natl Acad Sci USA 2008;105(49):19235–40.
43. Markram H, Lubke J, Frotscher M, Sakmann B. Regulation of synaptic efficacy by coincidence of postsynaptic APs and EPSPs. Science 1997;275(5297):213–5.
44. Marrelec G, Krainik A, Duffau H, Pelegrini-Issac M, Lehericy S, Doyon J, Benali H. Partial correlation for functional brain interactivity investigation in functional MRI. NeuroImage 2006;32(1):228–37.
45. Maslov S, Sneppen K. Specificity and stability in topology of protein networks. Science 2002;296(5569):910–3.
46. McCulloch W. Embodiments of mind. Cambridge, MA: MIT Press; 1988 (1965).
47. Mclntosh A, Gonzalez-Lima F. Structural equation modeling and its application to network analysis in functional brain imaging. Hum Brain Mapp 1994;2(1–2):2–22.
48. Mitchell TM, Shinkareva SV, Carlson A, Chang KM, Malave VL, Mason RA, Just MA. Predicting human brain activity associated with the meanings of nouns. Science 2008;320(5880):1191–5.
49. Newman ME. The structure and function of complex networks. SIAM Review 2003;45(2):167–256.
50. Norman KA, Polyn SM, Detre GJ, Haxby JV. Beyond mind-reading: multi-voxel pattern analysis of fMRI data. Trends Cogn Sci 2006;10(9):424–30.
51. Pearl J. Graphs, causality, and structural equation models. Socio Meth Res 1998;27(2):226–84.
52. Penny WD, Stephan KE, Mechelli A, Friston KJ. Comparing dynamic causal models. NeuroImage 2004;22(3):1157–72.
53. Pereda E, Quiroga RQ, Bhattacharya J. Nonlinear multivariate analysis of neurophysiological signals. Prog Neurobiol 2005;77(1–2):1–37.
54. Raichle ME, MacLeod AM, Snyder AZ, Powers WJ, Gusnard DA, Shulman GL. A default mode of brain function. Proc Natl Acad Sci USA 2001;98(2):676–82.
55. Rish I, Cecchi G, Thyreau B, Thirion B, Plaze M, Paillere-Martinot ML, Martelli C, Martinot JL, Poline JB. Schizophrenia as a network disease: disruption of emergent brain function in patients with auditory hallucinations. PloS One 2013;8(1):e50625.
56. Roebroeck A, Formisano E, Goebel R. Mapping directed influence over the brain using Granger causality and fMRI. NeuroImage 2005;25(1):230–42.
57. Salvador R, Martinez A, Pomarol-Clotet E, Sarro S, Suckling J, Bullmore E. Frequency based mutual information measures between clusters of brain regions in functional magnetic resonance imaging. NeuroImage 2007;35(1):83–88.
58. Salvador R, Suckling J, Schwarzbauer C, Bullmore E. Undirected graphs of frequency-dependent functional connectivity in whole brain networks. Philos Trans R Soc Lond B Biol Sci 2005;360(1457):937–46.
59. Sato JR, Morettin PA, Arantes PR, Amaro Jr E. Wavelet based time-varying vector autoregressive modelling. Comput Stat Data Anal 2007;51(12):5847–66.
60. Schneidman E, Berry MJ II, Segev R, Bialek W. Weak pairwise correlations imply strongly correlated network states in a neural population. Nature 2006;440(7087):1007–12.
61. Seth AK. Causal connectivity of evolved neural networks during behavior. Network 2005;16(1):35–54.
62. Sun FT, Miller LM, D'Esposito M. Measuring interregional functional connectivity using coherence and partial coherence analyses of fMRI data. NeuroImage 2004;21(2):647–58.
63. Thirion B, Flandin G, Pinel P, Roche A, Ciuciu P, Poline JB. Dealing with the shortcomings of spatial normalization: multi-subject parcellation of fMRI datasets. Hum Brain Mapp 2006;27(8):678–93.
64. Tibshirani R. Regression shrinkage and selection via the lasso. J Roy Stat Soc B 1996;73(3):267–88.
65. Valdes-Sosa PA, Sanchez-Bornot JM, Lage-Castellanos A, Vega-Hernandez M, Bosch-Bayard J, Melie-Garcia L, Canales-Rodriguez E. Estimating brain functional connectivity with sparse multivariate autoregression. Philos Trans Roy Soc Lond Biol Sci 2005;360(1457):969–81.
66. Quine WVO. Two dogmas of empiricism. Phil Rev 1951;60:20–43.
67. Varshney LR, Chen BL, Paniagua E, Hall DH, Chklovskii DB. Structural properties of the Caenorhabditis elegans neuronal network. PLoS Comput Biol 2011;7(2):e1001066.
68. Watts DJ, Strogatz SH. Collective dynamics of 'small-world' networks. Nature 1998;393(6684):440–2.
69. Wittgenstein L. Philosophical investigations. Hoboken, NJ: John Wiley & Sons; 2010.

CHAPTER 8

Pain and Machine Learning

Guillermo Cecchi

WHAT IS MACHINE LEARNING?

Machine learning is an expanding field, ever encompassing new areas wherein basic researchers, clinicians, and technologists discover the utility of its tools [24]. Because of this expansion, its boundaries can be somewhat fuzzy and can overlap with statistics, computer science, computational neuroscience, and even abstract mathematics [12]. In the context of brain science, however, the more common interpretation is that machine learning is a tool that makes sense of large datasets with hundreds to millions of variables, and often with a significantly small number of samples [1, 13, 31]. The "machine" aspect of machine learning is not relevant for the purpose of this chapter; however, it is remarkable that the exponential growth of computer power in recent years is one of the engines driving machine learning's expansion. For most practical applications, the availability of resources is such that compute time is vanishing as an analysis constraint, allowing for instances of human-like capabilities in tasks, such as face recognition and quiz games [14, 18].

However, what concerns us is the "learning" aspect of machine learning, that is, the algorithms that help us make sense of the data. But why do we have to learn? In classical statistical analysis, the assumed provenance of data is some (parametric or nonparametric) distribution, with expected discriminations (e.g., patients vs. controls) performed at the group level to test whether the corresponding distributions are significantly different. In contrast, at the core of machine learning is the idea of asking whether an *individual* sample can be discriminated on a case-by-case basis. This approach, usually called predictive modelling, provides an alternative description of the structure of the data and is also particularly relevant for practical applications, such as the context of clinical settings. In its simplest and most generic form, a predictive model is a transformation from the space of features to a discrete label. The space of features may be of high dimensionality, for instance a vector whose components are several thousand voxels activations, and the discrete labels *condition* and *control*. Learning a predictive model for a labeled dataset implies setting its parameters so that it can reliably transform the input features of each sample into the correct label.

In the next sections, we will present a brief overview of the main ingredients of machine learning for practical applications; many excellent references are available for readers interested in deeper technical aspects [16, 24].

SUPERVISED LEARNING

The first step to formalize the notions described above involves transforming the given dataset into a mathematical structure. This process of transforming raw data is called feature engineering, and it is a crucial aspect of the process: without the right representation, no algorithm will be able to give us a satisfying answer. Most machine learning techniques use vectors as the mathematical structure representing the data. Each sample, for example a brain scan, will be represented by an n-dimensional vector $\vec{x}_k$, whose components x_{ki} are usually called features. The features may be readily interpretable, for example, voxel activations, or highly abstracted transformations of the raw data, for example, random projections to higher dimensional spaces. To each sample vector $\vec{x}_k$, there is an associated target variable $\vec{y}_k$. In classification settings mentioned earlier, the target variable is discrete and can be considered a label. However, more generically, this variable may be continuous and multidimensional, in which case the problem becomes one of *regression*. The problem of classification/regression is therefore finding a model that maps the input vector $\vec{x}$ into the label/vector $\vec{y}$; following the example of the brain scan, the output may be the labels "stimulus A" and "stimulus B" for classification, or a vector representation of the stimuli (e.g., pixel values of a screen) for regression. Once the assignment of input features and out labels is set, what remains is to estimate the model. This is where the supervised nature of the process is enforced: Most models are parametric, that is, degrees of freedom can be tuned, so that the output for a given input can be made closer to its corresponding label. In other words, this parameter adjustment is the *learning* in machine learning.

For classification problems, there are not too many alternative measures of performance, which typically consist of a balance between false positives and false negatives when the model is tested. In the case of regression, however, there are different ways to measure how similar the predicted and expected vectors are, such as Euclidean and non-Euclidean distances, as well as different impositions on the predicted vectors themselves given a priori knowledge of the expected vectors, such as positivity or sparsity. The latter, in fact, may also be utilized in a classification setting, if the model includes an intermediate vectorial representation of the output before they are collapsed into discrete labels.

The goal of learning is to obtain the best possible performance, subject eventually to additional constraints. Mathematically, this can be expressed as an optimization problem equivalent to finding the minimum of a loss function $L = L(X,Y,\Theta)$ (similar to energy in physics) that depends on the input X and labels Y for the entire training set, and the model's parameters Θ. The second component of the "art" of machine learning after feature engineering is a choice of model in conjunction with a choice of loss function; for this there are no magic recipes. Just as with features, the models may be, among other things, more or less easily interpretable, or computationally demanding. Regarding interpretation, the choice to be made in the context of neuroscience depends on whether the main goal is to gain scientific understanding or to develop clinically oriented methodologies. The issue of computability, on the other hand, is highly determined by the first choice: Finding the minimum of the loss function corresponding to the "best" model may be an intractable problem with arbitrarily long compute times, and therefore in most cases a compromise is needed between the model's performance, estimation, and interpretation. There is an ever-growing list of classification models to choose from, as well as variants that can be posited for any particular application, as long as the loss function can be expressed and its minimum computed. We will discuss later two very popular models, k-Nearest Neighbours (kNN) and Support Vector Machines (SVM), to illustrate these choices.

VALIDATION

Learning the parameters of a predictive model is only part of the problem, as how it is learned and validated is equally important. The setting in which the parameters are set by adjusting them so as to match the labels of the samples is called supervised learning; as opposed to group testing, the validity of a predictive model is usually determined by how well it can classify individual samples; but the question is, which samples? Does it matter if the samples were used to set the parameters of the model? The answer is yes: The models typically used in machine learning have many parameters, and it is therefore quite easy to fall into the trap of overfitting. To understand this, let us consider a simple example of a linear regression: While the underlying relationship between two variables may be linear, the measurement noise may make it look more complex. We can succeed in fitting almost perfectly the given samples with a polynomial of high enough order (and consequently with more parameters) for the given samples, but a new sample will be mapped artificially as a high-order polynomial instead of a linear relationship. In other words, an overfit solution does not generalize. To avoid this issue, a standard practice in machine learning is to implement what is called cross-validation: The predictive model is learned using a subset of the samples, and its performance after learning validated on a different subset, not used in any way during the learning stage. Thus, the problem of poor generalization due to overfitting is directly folded into the validation scheme, and in a "realistic" manner as, ultimately, a predictive model should be applicable to situations in which the labels are not known, and the data never seen before. There are several specific cross-validation schemes such as partitioning the data into a number of folds for learning and testing, or leaving just one sample out for testing and using the rest of the data to learn.

CLASSIFICATION MODELS

We will illustrate the general discussion on predictive models presented earlier with two common classification models, kNN and SVM. The kNN algorithm is one of the simplest models for classification and regression. In kNN classification, a test sample is classified by a majority vote of the labels of its immediate neighbours in the vectorial feature space. This model has no parameters to be learned during training, as the number of neighbours k is fixed in advance. However, choosing k as well as the distance measure in the feature space (Euclidean, City-block, etc.) still gives degrees of freedom to explore the best model. It makes sense to choose k as an odd number to avoid ties, and in fact it may be set to $k = 1$, so that the label of a test sample will be that of its nearest neighbour. Similarly, for kNN regression, the output for a test sample is an average of the output vectors of its k neighbours. If $k > 1$, this average may be estimated in different ways, for instance by weighing each neighbour's output vector by the distance to the test sample in the feature space. The advantages of kNN are its simplicity and ease of computation, making it extremely fast. On the other hand, the model is impervious to the possible nonlocal structure of the data, for example, if the data do not live on well-defined "clusters," and may also be highly susceptible to the particular choice of k and distance measure [38].

SVM is a model based on the hypothesis that the feature vectors from two classes can be separated by a hyperplane in a sufficiently high-dimensional space. The hyperplane is chosen by the algorithm so as to maximize the separation of the classes, defining the "widest avenue" between the corresponding clouds of data points. Consider the following example: Two classes are represented by two-dimensional features, with the data clouds forming vertical stripes so that the horizontal feature completely separates the classes. If the original data are such that these two parallel stripes appear rotated in the feature space, none of the original features can discriminate the classes, but a properly rotated line will; SVM provides an algorithm to find such a line, or hyperplane in general, if it exists. The separating hyperplane is estimated with the training set, such that the class of a point is determined by which side of the hyperplane it is. The best separation is attained by the hyperplane that is farthest away from the nearest data point of any class during training, as the wider the separation, the higher the chance that test data will be labeled correctly.

There are several variants of SVMs, including regression and nonlinear kernels. Glossing over the technical details, SVM regression can be understood by considering that the data points that actually define the separating hyperplane are those closest to the boundary; therefore, the "incomplete" data points that define a function that needs to be regressed can be considered as the points that determine the hyperplane in a classification scheme. The hyperplane that results in this case is in fact a functional regression. To understand the use of SVM with nonlinear kernels, we need to point out that by definition, a hyperplane is determined by all the points $\vec{x}$ whose dot product with a given vector is a constant, $\vec{x} \cdot \vec{n} = c$, where $\vec{n}$ represents the vector perpendicular to the plane. Points on one side of the divide will have always a positive dot product with $\vec{n}$, whereas it will always be negative for points on the other side, determining thus the class identity of any test sample. The dot product can be generalized to kernel functions $K(\vec{x},\vec{n})$ with specific properties that match expected properties of the feature space, such as Radial Basis Functions or Polynomial kernels [22].

Note, finally, that, at least for linear kernel SVMs, the models can be reasonably interpreted. Consider the case of brain activation in imaging; a good SVM model implies that there is a certain combination of activation values across the brain, that is, a *pattern* that associates the brain state with a class, and its opposite with the complementary class. The vector representing the hyperplane is precisely this pattern, which can be "devectorized" and laid out on the volume of the brain for further neuroscientific scrutiny [26].

UNSUPERVISED LEARNING

The goal of unsupervised learning is to find intrinsic structure in the data that can be further exploited for either classification or analysis and modelling. This structure is expressed as a transformation of the input vectors into a set of discrete labels or a new (typically lower dimensional) vector space, similar to what a supervised learning model does, but using as training only the input vectors and generic constraints on the structure itself.

Unlike supervised learning, in which the loss function is defined by how well the model predicts, labels, or infers a vector output, the loss function $L = L(X,\hat{X},\Theta)$ is determined by how much *distortion* on X is introduced by the transformation $\hat{X}$, and how "noncompliant" the structure Θ is with respect to the constraints imposed on it. This can be better understood by discussing the simplest and most popular supervised learning technique, Principal Component Analysis (PCA) and the related Singular Value Decomposition (SVD). The goal of this algorithm is to express the original data as a linear combination of orthonormal vectors (i.e., forming a basis of the space), so that a given data point can be represented as $\vec{x} = \sum_{i=1,N} c_i\vec{v}_i$, where c is the weight on the component $\vec{v}$, or, equivalently, the coordinate on the new dimensions. With enough components, this representation may be exact, that is, without distortion; however, one of the main applications of PCA is dimensionality reduction: by approximating the input with a small number of components (i.e., dimensions), $\hat{\vec{x}} = \sum_{i=1,n} c_i \vec{v}_i$, PCA ensures that the distance (in Euclidean sense) $\| \hat{\vec{x}} - \vec{x} \|$ is the minimal possible for the given reduction (N to n) and condition on the structure (orthonormality). As mentioned earlier, besides dimensionality reduction, PCA can also provide for interpretation, as the components have the same dimensionality as the original data, and therefore can be scrutinized in the same way as the separating hyperplane in SVM.

Many dimensionality reduction algorithms, often called matrix factorization, can be understood as variations on the conditions imposed on distortion and structure. Two popular examples are Independent Component Analysis (ICA) and Nonnegative Matrix Factorization (NMF). The condition of orthonormality on the components of PCA is equivalent to their pairwise correlation being zero, that is, they are decorrelated. However, decorrelation does not mean statistical independence, as, for instance, two signals may be uncorrelated at zero lag, but correlated at a delay; ICA is a matrix factorization that imposes statistical independence between the components, usually estimated by minimization of their mutual Shannon information. This technique has been widely applied in various domains, including functional imaging [7].

Similarly, NMF is a matrix factorization that imposes nonnegativity of the coordinates and the components. This constraint can provide for a better interpretation of the components when the original data can only be properly understood as non-negative, for instance in the case of firing probabilities or frequencies. In most practical applications, NMF also tends to produce *sparse* components, that is, vectors with nonzero weights concentrated in a small number of elements. When applied to functional imaging, NMF typically results in components that are spatially localized [21], a property that may be desirable for purposes of interpretations as well as classification/regression, as we will discuss in the next section.

PREDICTIVE MODELLING AND SPARSIFICATION IN BRAIN IMAGING

The use of machine learning is particularly relevant for brain imaging applications, as they generate data with high dimensionality and with information contained in distributed patterns. In the absence of formal neuronal theories of global brain function, however, the analysis of functional magnetic resonance imaging (fMRI) has been frequently reduced to modelling the relationship between specific image voxels and the associated mental tasks. The highest priority of early fMRI analysis was the interpretation of analyses to infer relevant voxels, usually involving testing hypotheses that related localized regions of interests (ROIs) to function. Over time, the putative regions became more localized and hypothesized functions more specific, such that, for instance, different brain regions were associated with viewing a face versus viewing a house. However, Haxby et al. [17] published a seminal paper in which models built solely from submaximally responding voxels were able to discriminate between mental states using SVM, underscoring both the extent of distribution of brain function and the need for models that accurately predict mental states from fMRI data. Since then, a diverse collection of sophisticated predictive modelling methods have been introduced to the fMRI literature [10, 26], achieving impressive prediction performance that has surprised many neuroscientists. However, although predictive accuracy is vital to model assessment, it is important to keep in mind the ultimate objective of fMRI data analysis that underscores neuroscientific discovery, and thus include model interpretability as a necessary evaluation criterion.

In statistical data analysis, proper variable selection is as critical for prediction as for interpretation [35]; therefore, one development that has contributed to strong predictive performance is sparse modelling, in which resulting models use information from only a relatively small subset of predictive variables. Standard predictive models from fMRI data are built using individual image voxels as predictors and single time point (time to response or TR) volumes as examples [25], leading to datasets typically consisting of a large number (e.g., 10^4) of predictors but many fewer examples (e.g., 10^2–10^3). Learning statistical models from such data is particularly challenging since it is easy to overfit the training data and produce models that generalize poorly, as previously discussed. However, the overfitting problem can be tempered by reducing the dimensionality of the data, and thus prediction performance can be significantly improved by employing methods that identify the relevant predictive variables or combinations of them. Many predictor selection techniques (e.g., as in [25]) use a straightforward filtering approach, treating the selection stage as separate from the modelling stage, but sparse modelling approaches combine the selection and modelling states into one process, sometimes called embedded selection. Other methods, such as ICA [7], use dimensionality reduction to extract new predictors by linearly combining voxels.

Sparse modelling methods, such as LASSO [35] (for regression) and Sparse PCA [36] (for dimensionality reduction), compare favourably to nonsparse methods on prediction performance, since they incorporate multivariate information into the selection process and, in some cases, through their incremental nature facilitate the optimization of predictors. Sparse regression is related to the concept of regularization: When there are not enough independent samples to estimate a model, it is often convenient or even necessary to impose specific constraints on the solution. A classic example of this is Moore–Penrose's (M–R) pseudo-inverse [20]. To solve a regression problem $X = AY$, where X, Y are data matrices, it is required to invert the matrix X so that $A = X^{-1}Y$. If there are not enough data points, the matrix will be noninvertible, which means that an infinite number of matrices will produce a product "close enough" to the identity, $X^{\text{“}-1\text{”}} X \sim I$; the M–R pseudo-inverse corresponds to choosing among these the one with minimal Euclidean norm, usually referred as L_2. However, this is not the only restriction that may be imposed; for instance, it would be convenient to find the matrix with the minimal number of nonzero entries, so as to match that number with the number of independent samples. This is equivalent to asking for the minimal L_0, which, unfortunately, is computationally intractable. A related problem, the minimization of $L_1(M) = \sum_{i,j} |M_{ij}|$, turns out to be tractable and yields in most practical cases results similar to those expected from L_0 minimization, that is, a very small number of nonzero entries in the matrix. This is the core idea behind the LASSO algorithm [35].

In principle, a sound fMRI model should exclude all irrelevant voxels while retaining all relevant ones, and the set of selected voxels will be reliable or robust, that is, consistent across multiple well-designed experiments exploring a task. Therefore, a voxel selection method such as LASSO should both facilitate the optimization of the number of included voxels and produce robust models. Although the prediction performance of a model is a good measure of model validity, Zou and Hastie [40] suggest that prediction performance alone does not guarantee validity. They prove that in datasets in which many relevant predictors are correlated with each other, such as genetics data, existing sparse techniques will tend to include only one representative predictor from each cluster of correlated predictors.

The authors introduce a new algorithm, the Elastic Net, which they demonstrate matches, and in some cases surpasses, the prediction performance of sparse methods such as LASSO, yet can achieve the grouping effect of assigning similar weights to correlated predictors. Elastic Net even offers the implementer the ability to adjust the degree to which the grouping effect is enforced through one of its input parameters, while the other parameter controls the model sparseness, that is, the number of voxels selected. Since activity levels of individual voxels are known to correlate highly with each other, some sparse modelling methods, such as LASSO, might fail to include all of the relevant voxels, but Elastic Net in such cases appears to fulfil interpretability goals of voxel selection while still surpassing the prediction performance of traditional nonsparse methods. To reconcile traditional fMRI analysis approaches, which were guided by the intuition that functional units are localized regions rather than voxels, with the success of models of spatially distributed activity, we can hypothesize that the true neural response will be marked by distributed patterns of localized clusters of activity. The Elastic Net parameter controlling the grouping effect is a particularly interesting variable for testing this hypothesis. Since nearby voxels tend to be highly correlated with each other, it is reasonable to assume that as this grouping parameter is adjusted to increase the degree to which groups of correlated voxels are included, the model would feature more localized clusters, and hence the "scattering," or "spatial distribution," of the model voxels (formally defined later) would decrease.

Elastic Net was first applied and evaluated for fMRI data [8], resulting in a number of findings: (1) optimizing the number of voxels included in the model via cross-validation on the data instead of choosing a fixed number of voxels is vital to prediction and, by facilitating this optimization, Elastic Net outperforms the traditional regression method of Ordinary Least Squares (OLS) in prediction performance; (2) for a fixed grouping parameter, better predictive performance of cross-validated models is positively correlated with increased spatial distribution; (3) increasing the grouping parameter tends to increase the robustness of a model; (4) models do become less spatially distributed as the grouping parameter is increased; and (5) equally predictive models can still be markedly different in terms of their spatial distribution.

In fMRI analysis, the core goal underlying predictive modelling is production of a model that can be interpreted to pinpoint all relevant voxel activity and exclude all irrelevant activity. Therefore, it is crucial not to lose sight of the interpretation of the resulting models in the quest to optimize prediction performance. Innumerable techniques have been developed for choosing an appropriate set of voxels from which to build models. Not surprisingly, these techniques are most often evaluated on the basis of the prediction performance of the resulting models. As our results confirm, selecting a set of voxels that optimizes prediction performance is indeed critical for model interpretation. When fixed numbers of voxels are chosen, the resulting models are frequently overfit to training data, and therefore implicate many voxels that are actually irrelevant. Since these spurious voxels will tend to be randomly distributed throughout the brain, these models might misrepresent more general neuroscientific characteristics, for instance by overestimating the spatial distribution of response. Elastic Net is able to select an optimal number of voxels by automatically selecting voxels as part of the modelling process and computing the full regularization path, which facilitates cross-validation. When choosing a validated set of voxels, the true importance of spatial distribution becomes clear; the most predictive models draw on information from the most distributed regions of the brain. Still, in conjunction with the inferior yet impressive predictive performance of random voxels, the findings of Carroll et al. [8] underscore that the highly distributed nature of neural response necessitates the use of multivariate methods, not tied to localized regions, which can be validated by prediction performance. However, overemphasizing prediction performance can be counterproductive. Models that function as highly predictive "black boxes" might be useful for neuroengineering "mind reading" efforts, but for informing neuroscience, these models should also be reliable and valid. At the least, we would expect useful models to incorporate the same, or very similar, sets of voxels when trained on data from different experimental runs of the same paradigm. Elastic Net goes beyond other sparse modelling approaches by facilitating, with only one additional parameter, an increase in model robustness without compromising prediction performance. Examining the findings more closely by manipulating the grouping parameter, the authors observed that neural response is marked by clusters of correlated voxel activity. Existing sparse methods, which effectively use a very low grouping value, will tend to include only one voxel from each cluster; the voxel chosen is in effect arbitrary due to minor fluctuations in the dataset. By selecting more voxels from within these clusters that are redundant for prediction yet relevant to the task, Elastic Net with a higher grouping value achieves more robust, and hence valid, models. However, even with the spatial relaxation provided by Elastic Net over pure LASSO, alternative models can achieve an almost identical prediction performance [29]: the only possible way to avoid this model degeneracy is to introduce further functional constraints, including local and global neural dynamics, and perhaps challenge the idea that brain function arises from sufficiently repeatable spatiotemporal patterns.

MACHINE LEARNING FOR PAIN

Although pain is not the only nor the most prominent of human experiences, it is particularly incumbent upon pain researchers to demonstrate that the subjective quality of the pain experience can be objectively quantified, as well as related to specific brain structures and processes that underlie perception. The idea that pain perception is irreducibly subjective and hence incommunicable has held sway in the scientific community and among philosophers. Dennett [11] has argued, on the basis of modern neuroscientific understanding, that due to its subjective nature, and in contrast to visual perception, pain cannot be captured in computational models. Moreover, the official definition of pain as accepted by the International Association for the Study of Pain is that it is "an unpleasant sensory and emotional experience," and that "pain is always subjective" [23].

However, a line of research starting with Weber [39] and culminating with Stevens' [34] law of magnitude perception has demonstrated that statistical properties of pain can be quantified and modelled using simple equations [28]. Currently, statistics of pain are most commonly quantified with questionnaire-based tools, and these remain the main instruments with which the efficacy of pain therapies is studied in clinical trials. More objective measurements, both in terms of the applicability and consistency in describing individual subjects, and in terms of physiological grounding, are required to advance the field of pain research. Predictive modelling, as already discussed, is an approach that can provide answers in these two dimensions; one of the first applications of predictive modelling was presented in [29]. Studying subjects reporting their perceived pain intensity upon stimulation with a lower back thermal patch, the authors used the Elastic Net algorithm to learn highly predictive models of subjective pain perception from fMRI data, often achieving correlation values close to 0.8 between the predicted and actual pain ratings. In practically all cases, EN outperformed significantly the OLS regression, indeed making use of regularization to prevent overfitting. The use of regularization allowed the authors to explore models with higher dimensionality, by incorporating several past TRs as features on which to predict the subjective responses. Using the information of up to eight TRs provides consistent and often significant improvement in predictive accuracy. Moreover, using such temporal information may provide new insights into the brain mechanisms related to pain perception, since sparse temporal models discover highly predictive and thus functionally relevant brain activity patterns that are left undetected by more traditional, nontemporal models. The authors conclude that (a) the use of sparse predictive modelling for pain perception analysis reveals that fMRI signals possess considerably higher information than expected by a simple linear regression approach; (b) functional dynamics can also considerably increase the amount of information about the subject's performance, as opposed to single TR, or "instantaneous" approaches, and (c) the sparse, temporal models reveal functional areas that are not identified by nontemporal approaches, and yet can be highly predictive and thus functionally relevant.

In a related study, Brown et al. [5] applied an SVM classifier on fMRI data to assess whether global patterns of activity can discriminate between painful and nonpainful stimulation, in the absence of direct subjective report. Healthy individuals were presented with painful and nonpainful thermal stimuli; during training, a group of subjects and their reports were used to learn the model, which was then tested to predict whether the two conditions could be identified solely on the basis of fMRI data on unused subjects. The whole-brain SVM classifier performed with accuracy close to 85%, with most of the weight of the separating hyperplane concentrated in pain-processing areas, including the primary somatosensory cortex, secondary somatosensory cortex, insular cortex, primary motor cortex, and cingulate cortex. To test the significance of this global pattern of activity as the basis of the discrimination, as opposed to specific "pure pain" areas, the authors tested whether individual regions of interest provided for similar classification accuracy. Interestingly, the authors observed that, using also an SVM classifier restricted to the secondary somatosensory cortex, it was possible to obtain a classification accuracy statistically significantly higher than chance, higher than any other individual area, but lower than that obtained by the global, whole-brain activation pattern.

In a follow-up study to [29], Cecchi et al. [9] modelled the time evolution of acute thermal pain perception as a dynamical system described by differential equations. They showed that simple and interpretable first- and second-order differential equations with very few parameters accurately model time variability of pain perception in humans elicited by thermal stimulation patterns of varying complexity. The equations can be used to infer with high accuracy (90%) the *full temporal response* of individuals in modelling conditions that include access to the stimulus temperature, and in "mind reading" set-ups, that is, when pain perception is solely inferred from functional images of the brain aided by the derived equations and using Elastic Net constrained regression (75% accuracy). The results show that acute thermal pain perception applied to healthy skin follows simple quantitative deterministic patterns. The dynamic model is derived from a behaviourally relevant interpretation of pain perception as a warning signal that quickly reports immediate threat of injury (temperature above threshold), and approaching danger (rapid temperature increases), and can also as easily discount the threat once it goes away or is expected to do so (temperature decreases).

The model, using few parameters, can reproduce with high accuracy the dynamical transformation from stimulus to perception. The model also has high predictive accuracy, and accounts for subjects' variability with simple and interpretable mechanisms.

Moreover, it provides a summary of a relatively complex behaviour, whose physiological correlates and mechanisms can be directly investigated through pharmacological manipulation and the design of targeted stimulus conditions. Temporal processing is ubiquitous in sensory systems, including the somatosensory pathway [15, 19]. However, it is only in a few cases that spatiotemporal transformations can be functionally interpreted, beyond generic sharpening for enhanced localization [27], or information compression [30]. The perceptual dynamics captured by the model cannot be reduced to peripheral processing. In fact, as previously reported [3], the BOLD response to a similar task reveals a rich temporal structure across several cortical and subcortical areas compatible with the time scale of the perceptual ratings, such that the dynamics of pain perception may result from the emergent interaction of extensive networks. Moreover, given its ultimately nonlinear nature, the model further predicts dynamical features of pain perception that may have unexpected behavioural relevance. The utilization of the analytic model within the "mind reading" setup highlights its predictive efficacy, and provides an additional validation step. A further reason for using the combined model, besides simply inferring pain from fMRI, is to go beyond the limitation of simple linear inference models such as Elastic Net, while keeping the nonlinear model simple, tractable, and interpretable. Given the nature of brain processes, it is reasonable to expect the true relationship between the high-dimensional fMRI signal and pain ratings to be a complex nonlinear one. However, fitting an ad hoc nonlinear model (e.g., a neural network) to such high-dimensional data to predict pain rating directly could be computationally much more challenging than fitting a linear one. On the other hand, given an accurate analytical model linking temperature to pain, we may exploit its advantages in our combined nonlinear method, first obtaining an estimate of the temperature from fMRI data via simple and computationally efficient linear regression, and then using a nonlinear model predicting pain from temperature. Although the combined predictive model involves inferring temperature as a hidden variable, it outperforms the direct EN model because it captures (at least the temperature-to-pain part of) the nonlinear relationship between fMRI and pain perception.

The completely data-driven selection of voxels used for the previously described predictive models is specific to the individual and not easily transferable across subjects, probably because the models are not constrained by a priori information [9, 29]. Moreover, even with the addition of grouping, sparse regression tends to select very small numbers of voxels, and therefore normalizing across subjects becomes difficult. To circumvent these limitations, Wager et al. [37] developed an fMRI-based signature pattern that predicts pain intensity at the level of the individual person. They used machine learning analyses to identify a pattern of fMRI activity across brain regions associated with thermal pain. The pattern included the thalamus, the posterior and anterior insulae, the secondary somatosensory cortex, the anterior cingulate cortex, the periaqueductal grey matter, and other regions. The authors also showed the specificity of this pain signature by comparing its responses with warm stimuli, as well as nonphysical pain conditions, more specifically social pain. In all cases, sensitivity and specificity were highly statistically significant, ranging from 75% to over 90%. Moreover, the response of the pain signature was significantly reduced by the administration of an analgesic, demonstrating a direct connection with physiological mechanisms. It is important to remark that by a careful preselection of the areas that could be considered as part of the pain system, this study obtained a universal model, such that the areas and activation intensities in this "signature," forming a high-dimensional vector, can be directly compared with the same *for an individual*, in order to infer whether the particular individual is perceiving pain or not.

By aligning the mathematical formalism closer to the actual complex nature of brain function, machine learning approaches based on distributed pattern analysis and sparse regression have provided results showing that there is a possible path to link perceptual, emotional, and cognitive behaviours in general, and pain in particular, with neurophysiology. Considering that these results are based on what can only be considered a coarse measure of brain activity such as fMRI, the development of novel techniques with increasing spatial and temporal resolution will only make the need to implement more adequate analysis techniques even more pressing that it currently is [1]. This will require machine learning techniques that include more realistic constraints beyond sparsity and spatial distribution, incorporating at least models of local neuronal dynamics [6], short-term plasticity [33], and nonlocal connectivity as measured by Diffusion Tensor Imaging [4] as well as from the vast accumulated knowledge of neuroanatomical architectural patterns [2, 32]. From a computational perspective, the challenge will be to make these models computationally tractable, whereas from a neuroscientific point of view more efforts will be required to abstract the features that uniquely determine the behaviour of extended neural systems. Be it as it may, the future of pain research, and neuroscience in general, will be necessarily tied to machine learning and computational modelling.

REFERENCES

1. Ahrens MB, Orger MB, Robson DN, Li JM, Keller PJ. Whole-brain functional imaging at cellular resolution using light-sheet microscopy. Nat Methods 2013;10(5):413–20.
2. Alexander GE, DeLong MR, Strick PL. Parallel organization of functionality segregated circuits linking basal ganglia and cortex. Ann Rev Neurosci 1986;9(1):357–81.
3. Baliki MN, Geha PY, Apkarian AV. Parsing pain perception between nociceptive representation and magnitude estimation. J Neurophysiol 2009;101(2):875–87.
4. Baria AT, Mansour A, Huang L, Baliki MN, Cecchi GA, Mesulam MM, Apkarian AV. Linking human brain local activity fluctuations to structural and functional network architectures. NeuroImage 2013;73:144–55.
5. Brown JE, Chatterjee N, Younger J, Mackey S. Towards a physiology-based measure of pain: patterns of human brain activity distinguish painful from non-painful thermal stimulation. PloS One 2011;6(9):e24124.
6. Cabral J, Fernandes HM, Van Hartevelt TJ, James AC, Kringelbach ML, Deco G. Structural connectivity in schizophrenia and its impact on the dynamics of spontaneous functional networks. Chaos 2013;23(4):046111.
7. Calhoun VD, Liu J, Adali T. A review of group ICA for fMRI data and ICA for joint inference of imaging, genetic, and ERP data. NeuroImage 2009;45(1 Suppl):S163–72.
8. Carroll MK, Cecchi GA, Rish I, Garg R, Rao AR. Prediction and interpretation of distributed neural activity with sparse models. NeuroImage 2009;44(1):112–22.
9. Cecchi GA, Huang L, Hashmi JA, Baliki M, Centeno MV, Rish I, Apkarian AV. Predictive dynamics of human pain perception. PLoS Comput Biol 2012;8(10):e1002719.
10. Cox DD, Savoy RL. Functional magnetic resonance imaging (fMRI) "brain reading": detecting and classifying distributed patterns of fMRI activity in human visual cortex. NeuroImage 2003;19(2 Pt 1):261–70.
11. Dennett DC. Why you can't make a computer that feels pain. Synthese 1978;38(3):415–56.
12. Edelsbrunner H, Harer J. Computational topology: an introduction. Providence, RI: American Mathematical Society; 2010.
13. Feinberg DA, Moeller S, Smith SM, Auerbach E, Ramanna S, Gunther M, Glasser MF, Miller KL, Ugurbil K, Yacoub E. Multiplexed echo planar imaging for sub-second whole brain FMRI and fast diffusion imaging. PloS One 2010;5(12):e15710.
14. Ferrucci D, Brown E, Chu-Carroll J, Fan J, Gondek D, Kalyanpur AA, Lally A, Murdock JW, Nyberg E, Prager J, et al. Building Watson: an overview of the DeepQA Project. AI Magazine 2014;31:59–79.
15. Fu W. Penalized regression: the bridge versus the lasso. J Comput Graph Stat 1998;7(3):397–416.
16. Hastie T, Tibshirani R, Friedman J. The elements of statistical learning: data mining, inference and prediction. New York, NY: Springer-Verlag; 2009.
17. Haxby JV, Gobbini MI, Furey ML, Ishai A, Schouten JL, Pietrini P. Distributed and overlapping representations of faces and objects in ventral temporal cortex. Science 2001;293(5539):2425–30.

18. Hinton GE, Osindero S, Teh YW. A fast learning algorithm for deep belief nets. Neural Comput 2006;18(7): 1527–54.
19. Hoerl A, Kennard R. Ridge regression. In: Encyclopedia of statistical sciences, Vol. 8. New York, NY: Wiley; 1988. pp. 129–36.
20. Horn RA, Johnson CR. Matrix analysis. Cambridge, MA: Cambridge University Press; 2012.
21. Lohmann G, Volz KG, Ullsperger M. Using non-negative matrix factorization for single-trial analysis of fMRI data. NeuroImage 2007;37(4):1148–60.
22. Magnin B, Mesrob L, Kinkingnehun S, Pelegrini-Issac M, Colliot O, Sarazin M, Dubois B, Lehericy S, Benali H. Support vector machine-based classification of Alzheimer's disease from whole-brain anatomical MRI. Neuroradiology 2009;51(2):73–83.
23. Merskey H, Bogduk N. Classification of chronic pain, IASP Task Force on Taxonomy. Seattle, WA: International Association for the Study of Pain Press; 1994.
24. Mitchell T. Machine learning. Maidenhead, UK: McGraw-Hill; 1997.
25. Mitchell T, Hutchinson R, Niculescu R, Pereira F, Wang X, Just M, Newman S. Learning to decode cognitive states from brain images. Mach Learn 2004;57:145–75.
26. Norman KA, Polyn SM, Detre GJ, Haxby JV. Beyond mind-reading: multi-voxel pattern analysis of fMRI data. Trends Cogn Sci 2006;10(9):424–30.
27. Phillips JR, Johnson KO, Hsiao SS. Spatial pattern representation and transformation in monkey somatosensory cortex. Proc Natl Acad Sci USA 1988;85:1317–21.
28. Price DD. Psychological and neural mechanisms of pain. New York, NY: Raven Press; 1988.
29. Rish I, Cecchi GA, Baliki M, Apkarian AV. Sparse regression models of pain perception. In: Yao YY, editor. Proceedings of the Brain Informatics, Vol. 6334. Toronto, Canada: Brain Informatics International Conference; 2010. pp. 212–23.
30. Romo R, Salinas E. Touch and go: decision-making mechanisms in somatosensation. Annu Rev Neurosci 2001;24:107–37.
31. Schwartz DA, Lebedev MA, Hanson TL, Dimitrov DF, Lehew G, Meloy J, Rahangam S, Subramanian V, Ifft PJ, Li Z, et al. Chronic, wireless recordings of large-scale brain activity in freely moving rhesus monkeys. Nat Methods 2014;11:670–6.
32. Sherman SM, Guillery RW. The role of the thalamus in the flow of information to the cortex. Philos Trans R Soc Lond B Biol Sci 2002;357(1428):1695–708.
33. Solovey G, Miller KJ, Ojemann JG, Magnasco MO, Cecchi GA. Self-regulated dynamical criticality in human ECoG. Front Integr Neurosci 2012;6:44.
34. Stevens SS. On the psychophysical law. Psychol Rev 1957;64(3):153–81.
35. Tibshirani R. Regression shrinkage and selection via the Lasso. J Roy Stat Soc B 1996;58(1):267–88.
36. Ulfarsson M, Solo V. Sparse variable principal component analysis with application to fMRI. In: Proceedings of the 4th IEEE International Symposium on Biomedical Imaging. Arlington, VA: IEEE; 2007. pp. 460–3.
37. Wager TD, Atlas LY, Lindquist MA, Roy M, Woo CW, Kross E. An fMRI-based neurologic signature of physical pain. N Engl J Med 2013;368(15):1388–97.
38. Wang X, Hutchinson R, Mitchell TM. Training fMRI classifiers to detect cognitive states across multiple human subjects. In: Thrun S, Saul LK, Scholkopf B, editors. Proceedings of the Neural Information Processing Systems, Vol. 16. London, UK: MIT Press; 2003, pp. 709–16.
39. Weber EH. The sense of touch [translated by Ross HE and Murray DJ]. London, UK: Academic Press; 1978.
40. Zou H, Hastie T. Regularization and variable selection via the elastic net. J Roy Stat Soc B 2005;67(2):301–20.

CHAPTER 9

Modulation of Acute and Chronic Pain by Noninvasive Stimulation: Advances and Future Potential

Jean-Pascal Lefaucheur, Camilo Diaz Cruz, and Felipe Fregni

Following the first reports of treatment of chronic, drug-resistant pain by motor cortex stimulation (MCS) using surgically implanted electrodes [136, 137], many efforts have been made to show that pain relief could also be achieved via noninvasive transcranial stimulation. First analgesic effects produced by repeated application of single pulses of transcranial magnetic stimulation (TMS) delivered over the primary motor cortex (M1) were reported in a patient with chronic neuropathic pain [91]. Then, more reliable results were obtained when repetitive TMS (rTMS) became available to stimulate the cortex at frequencies closer to those used in MCS, such as 10 Hz [66]. Since this preliminary report, numerous studies have confirmed the value of rTMS to relieve various types of pain, including experimental acute provoked pain and chronic pain of neuropathic or non-neuropathic origin (review and analysis in [59, 61, 79, 81, 106]). Analgesic effects have also been reported by using another technique of noninvasive transcranial stimulation, known as transcranial direct current stimulation (tDCS) [36, 37].

Various aspects of acute and chronic pain modulation following noninvasive cortical stimulation via rTMS and tDCS techniques have been discussed in several recent reviews [4, 38, 73, 86, 93, 95, 103, 115, 144, 145]. Although recent meta-analyses have confirmed that noninvasive brain stimulation is associated with significant reductions in pain, these studies showed modest pooled effect sizes, and some of these meta-analyses show significant heterogeneity. Given this heterogeneity, it is important to understand the mechanisms of action of cortical stimulation on pain along with its therapeutic efficacy. In this chapter, we will focus on this aspect of MCS research, highlighting the results of neuroimaging studies and how neuroimaging methods may be useful to optimize effects of MCS.

GENERAL PRINCIPLES OF NONINVASIVE CORTICAL STIMULATION

Although magnetic fields are delivered at scalp level, the real effect of TMS is to induce intracerebral electrical stimulation, according to Faraday's law of electromagnetic induction. The strength–duration relationship of membrane properties makes fibres of passage more excitable than local cell bodies at the stimulation site for all types of brain stimulation techniques commonly used in therapeutics [87, 104, 105]. The axons recruited by cortical stimulation can be short fibres of intracortical interneurons, as well as longer afferent or efferent fibres connected with distant structures, resulting in either antidromic or orthodromic volleys of action potentials. Finally, orthodromic activation may lead to long-term postsynaptic excitation or inhibition in cortical or deep brain structures connected to the stimulation target. Thus, the mechanisms of action of rTMS cannot be restricted to local cortical excitation or inhibition, but should rather be modelled in terms of excitatory or inhibitory neural circuit activation with potentially remote effects [60, 65].

The mechanism of action of tDCS differs from that of rTMS, since tDCS is purely a neuromodulation technique, while rTMS exerts both neurostimulatory and neuromodulatory effects [62]. Neurostimulation means that stimulation intensity exceeds the threshold for triggering action potentials that propagate in neural circuits. Neuromodulation means that stimulation intensity is not high enough to generate action potentials, but can modulate nerve excitability by increasing or decreasing axon membrane potential (depolarization or hyperpolarization).

Long-lasting changes of cortical excitability and activity can be induced by tDCS, reversibly, painlessly, and safely [100, 101]. In fact, tDCS causes polarity-dependent shifts of the resting membrane potential and consequently could change neuronal excitability at the site of stimulation and in the connected areas. If the stimulation lasts long enough, tDCS induces after-effects, which are thought to depend on synaptic plasticity changes related to transient activation of glutamatergic NMDA receptors [80, 102]. In fact, tDCS is able to produce a cascade of events at the cellular and molecular levels, potentially involving a variety of neurotransmitter systems [88].

Finally, it should be mentioned that rTMS and tDCS effects may largely vary according to different methodological aspects, such as the type and orientation of the stimulation coil or the waveform of the magnetic pulse regarding TMS; the polarity and montage of the electrodes regarding tDCS; and the intensity of stimulation, the orientation of the cortical axons in the induced electrical field, and the plasticity and "receptivity" of the brain circuits prior to the stimulation regarding both techniques [62]. All these observations easily explain why it is so difficult to model the mechanisms of action of noninvasive cortical stimulation, to predict its effectiveness when applied to different categories of patients, and to determine the best parameters of stimulation, including the optimal target to stimulate. Under these conditions, it is tempting to think that the effectiveness of the stimulation can be improved by the use of neuroimaging techniques. In the context of the treatment of pain, we will first review the data provided by neuroimaging to better understand the involved mechanisms of action and the perspectives of using neuroimaging to optimize the therapeutic efficacy.

MECHANISMS OF ACTION OF CORTICAL STIMULATION IN THE BRAIN

Brain imaging studies show that implanted MCS leads to regional cerebral blood flow changes in the thalamus, the insula, and upper brainstem structures [41, 42, 112, 113]. These structures are potentially involved in thermal sensation processing [23, 27], and thereby they could mediate the associated effects of MCS on spontaneous pain and thermonociceptive stimuli perception [31, 74, 76]. Brain imaging studies also showed that tDCS applied over the motor cortex was associated with significant activation in distant brain regions such as the supplementary motor area, the posterior parietal cortex, or the thalamus [57, 58]. As with rTMS, the analgesic effects of tDCS may involve distant neural structures and, depending on the site of stimulation, tDCS modulation could occur in various neural circuits, involved in sensori-discriminative, cognitive, or emotional aspects of chronic pain.

Early studies by Tsubokawa et al. [136, 137] suggest that MCS could act through a reduction in pain-related thalamic hyperactivity in thalamic relays or interfere with abnormal thalamothalamic or thalamocortical oscillations, via corticothalamic projections or rather antidromic modulation of thalamocortical pathways and connections between thalamic nuclei. Recent neuroimaging studies confirm that the integrity of the thalamocortical tract (TCT) is required to mediate the antinociceptive effects of 5- and 10-Hz rTMS [43, 109]. The connections between pyramidal cells and afferent fibres from thalamic nuclei are thought to have an important role in the control of nociception [141]. This hypothesis was further supported by the demonstration of an improvement in sensory discrimination in pain patients treated by epidural MCS [31]. High-frequency rTMS delivered to the motor cortex can also modulate the perception of innocuous thermal stimuli or acute provoked pain applied in the painful region of patients with neuropathic pain [74, 76]. Sensory discrimination improvement appeared to be specific for thermo-nociceptive signals conveyed by the spinothalamic tract. This precludes a mechanism of pain relief due to the reinforcement of the lemniscal "gate control" over the nociceptive system. The functional integrity of the lemniscal system is essential to the efficacy of spinal cord stimulation [129], but not to that of MCS [42].

However, it has been demonstrated that MCS could also activate descending pathways, leading to reinforced or restored inhibitory control of nociceptive transmission in the dorsal horns of the spinal cord, as shown by neuronal recordings in animal models [121, 126] and by the increase in nociceptive spinal (R3) reflexes in some pain patients when MCS is switched ON [42, 112]. These descending controls could take place in various brainstem or spinal cord nuclei and be involved in the process of pain relief resulting from MCS. This hypothesis is reinforced by the low rate of efficacy observed in patients with brainstem stroke or spinal cord lesion in response to motor cortex rTMS [70] or implanted MCS [40, 138].

Brain imaging studies [41, 42, 112, 113] also show that MCS could activate superficial or deep brain structures involved in the affective, cognitive, and emotional aspects of pain, such as the cingulate and orbitofrontal cortices. Using single-photon emission computed tomography, Tamura et al. [132] further demonstrated that beneficial effects of motor cortex rTMS on capsaicin-induced acute pain correlated with an activation of the caudal part of the anterior cingulate cortex (ACC) and an inhibition of the medial prefrontal cortex.

Given the results of MCS on descending inhibitory control along with its interaction with opioid drugs, it is likely that MCS has a direct or indirect effect on opioidergic activity. Recent imaging studies showed that MCS enhanced the release of endogenous opioids in various brain structures, and this was correlated with pain relief when the release was observed in the cingulate cortex and periaqueductal grey matter [82]. The fact that the injection of naloxone, an opioid receptor antagonist, could significantly decrease the analgesic effects induced by high-frequency rTMS of the motor cortex confirmed the involvement of endogenous opioid systems in these effects [28]. In various types of acutely provoked experimental pain, naloxone was also found to block the analgesic effect produced by rTMS delivered at 20 Hz over the contralateral parietal cortex [3] or at 10 Hz over the left dorsolateral prefrontal cortex (DLPFC) [133, 134]. Furthermore, a preliminary report of a study assessing μ-opioid system during positron emission tomography (PET) in a chronic pain patient undergoing tDCS of motor cortex confirmed and extended these results. In this study, although there was no change in the baseline clinical pain after a single session of tDCS, there was a significant modulation of the μ-opioidergic system along with changes in pain threshold; suggesting that modulation of this system is the first step to induce future clinical changes in baseline pain [30]. Finally, an elevation of serum β-endorphin concentration was found in patients with phantom limb pain treated by a series of five daily sessions of rTMS delivered at 20 Hz over the motor cortex that produced long-lasting pain relief [2].

In terms of neurotransmitters, the mechanisms of action of MCS could also involve inhibitory GABAergic transmission. Intracortical GABAergic circuits can be assessed by a paired-pulse TMS technique, which measures the percentage of intracortical inhibition (ICI) of motor-evoked potentials (MEPs). This ICI is reduced in patients with neuropathic pain, but could be restored after a single session of high-frequency rTMS of the motor cortex, in correlation with the degree of pain relief [71]. This result was confirmed by studies of other types of pain [90] or based on other types of TMS protocols [78], or even following tDCS [8]. All these observations support a role played by a reinforcement of intracortical GABAergic inhibition induced by MCS. An increased ICI was also found to be associated with the analgesic effects of rTMS delivered at high frequency over the left DLPFC after capsaicin application on hand skin of healthy subjects [34]. The increase in ICI following high-frequency subthreshold rTMS in chronic pain patients is opposite to what is observed in naïve healthy subjects [83, 111]. Interestingly, motor cortex inhibition is associated with the existence of 20 Hz cortical oscillations that are abolished in the presence of chronic or provoked pain [52, 116]. By restoring such oscillatory activity in M1, MCS could restore defective inhibitory mechanisms.

Thus, the mechanisms of action of cortical stimulation in pain probably involve the activation or functional modulation of various neural structures and pathways, including orthodromic activation of corticofugal pathways and antidromic activation of thalamocortical pathways.

ANALGESIC EFFECTS OF RTMS DELIVERED TO THE MOTOR CORTEX

Numerous studies have reported rTMS effects on various types of acute provoked pain, but results are conflicting [95]. M1 remains the most studied target of cortical stimulation to modulate provoked pain in healthy volunteers in the line of the results obtained in chronic pain patients. Analgesic effects of motor cortex rTMS appear to depend on various parameters such as stimulation pattern or frequency of the fibre type recruited by the protocol of provoked pain (Aδ or C fibres). However, the most robust effect appears to be a reduced susceptibility to cold pain induced by high-frequency rTMS of M1 in healthy subjects [95].

Results regarding the ability of motor cortex rTMS to produce analgesic effects in patients with chronic neuropathic pain syndrome are more consistent. First, it was shown that the relief of spontaneous ongoing pain in those patients was obtained when rTMS was administered to the motor cortex corresponding to the painful zone at "high frequency" (10–20 Hz) rather than at "low frequency" (0.5–1 Hz) [5, 67, 123].

Second, optimal analgesic effects were found to be delayed by a few days and to last for about a week after a single motor cortex rTMS session [68, 122]. This time course is similar to what is observed for chronic epidural MCS: clinical changes are delayed for several days after switching the stimulator ON or OFF or after modifying the parameters of stimulation [96–98]. Expression of secondary messengers and time-consuming processes of synaptic plasticity in cortical circuitry may explain why the effects are delayed and why they last and are stabilized beyond the time of stimulation.

However, the analgesic effects resulting from a single rTMS session are too short-lived to achieve a durable control of chronic pain. Since rTMS-induced analgesic effects are rather modest and short-lasting, rTMS was not considered a therapeutic method [24], but instead a preoperative tool to assess whether or not the surgical implantation of MCS should be performed and to predict its outcome in clinical practice [77]. Nevertheless, repeated rTMS sessions are able to produce cumulative effects [55, 110]. Beyond their use to help patients in waiting for surgical MCS implantation [69], repeated rTMS sessions could be performed to control various chronic pain syndromes for a prolonged period [64], although the strategy of maintenance therapy remains to be validated [90]. In the management of chronic pain syndromes, rTMS could also be used in combination with physical therapy or medications, as recently illustrated [114].

Most studies have shown the efficacy of rTMS in the management of neuropathic pain conditions, but motor cortex rTMS was also shown to produce analgesic effects in other pain conditions, such as complex regional pain syndrome type I (CRPS-I) [114] and fibromyalgia [90, 110]. This latter condition was also found to be responsive to motor cortex tDCS.

ANALGESIC EFFECTS OF TDCS DELIVERED TO THE MOTOR CORTEX

From a technical point of view, tDCS is easier to perform than rTMS. As rTMS, tDCS has been applied to modulate the perception of acute provoked pain in experimental studies [95]. These studies support the analgesic potential of tDCS that can be further reinforced by pharmacological procedures. Both anodal and cathodal tDCS procedures (despite having theoretically opposite effects on cortical excitability, as high- and low-frequency rTMS) were found to be efficacious on provoked pain. However, it seems that cathodal tDCS is more effective than anodal tDCS in reducing provoked pain, in contrast to what was observed with spontaneous chronic pain [95]. In fact, there are probably huge differences in the pattern and mechanisms of pain relief produced by cortical stimulation between acute pain provoked in healthy subjects and chronic pain presented by patients. This may relate to the influence of disease-related processes of cortical plasticity on the neural circuits potentially activated by cortical stimulation.

Actually, in chronic pain syndromes, a few sham-controlled studies have been published to date, all showing positive results for anodal tDCS. In the first published study, patients with pain due to spinal cord injury were randomized to receive sham or active anodal tDCS over the left or right M1 (2 mA, 20 minutes) for 5 consecutive days [36]. Pain was reduced significantly after anodal stimulation, but not after sham stimulation. A second study of the same group showed that the same protocol of stimulation (anodal tDCS over M1) produced a similar decrease in pain perception in patients with fibromyalgia [37]. Pain relief was maximal at the end of the week of stimulation and was still significant 3 weeks later. The same team reported several other studies on this topic showing in particular that anodal tDCS over the left M1 produced more prolonged clinical improvement beyond the time of stimulation, up to 2 months after a series of 10 daily sessions [139], with a better impact on sleep efficiency [120], compared with anodal tDCS over the left DLPFC. However, in patients with fibromyalgia receiving a multidisciplinary protocol of rehabilitation concomitantly with weekly sessions of anodal tDCS over M1, the clinical improvement in terms of quality of life was not clearly improved following active rather than sham stimulation [119]. One potential explanation for these results is the frequency of stimulation—weekly rather than daily.

The same team reported a modest pain reduction in a pilot series of seven patients with chronic refractory pelvic pain of various origins following anodal tDCS applied over the motor cortex for only 2 consecutive days [33]. They also found that the combination of transcutaneous electrical nerve stimulation with anodal tDCS of M1 has a superior analgesic effect compared with tDCS alone in another pilot series of eight patients with chronic neuropathic pain affecting the upper limbs [11]. Bolognini et al. [12] recently reported that anodal tDCS of M1 reduced phantom limb pain, whereas cathodal tDCS of the posterior parietal cortex decreased nonpainful phantom sensations. In a series of patients with chronic pain related to disabling multiple sclerosis, another team reported that anodal but not sham tDCS applied over the motor cortex for 5 consecutive days could significantly reduce pain scores and improve quality of life up to 3 weeks beyond the period of stimulation [94]. Finally, Dasilva et al. [26] give evidence that patients with chronic migraine could have a positive, but delayed, response to anodal tDCS of M1. Case reports also have suggested that anodal tDCS of M1 may induce analgesic effects in cancer pain [128], orofacial pain [7], or itching pain associated with syringomyelia [56]. All these findings provide initial evidence of a beneficial effect of anodal tDCS applied over M1 in various types of chronic pain, thus encouraging further trials in larger series of patients. However, one must acknowledge some negative results of M1 tDCS reported in patients with chronic low back pain [107] or longstanding neuropathic pain due to spinal cord injury [143].

Although tDCS induces plastic modifications in M1 that may be similar to that induced by rTMS, these two techniques have fundamental differences in their mechanisms of action. Given tDCS mechanisms in modulating likelihood of neuronal firing, this technique is suitable to be combined with behavioural interventions that can reinforce and potentiate tDCS effects on specific neural networks. In fact, a recent trial investigated the combination of tDCS and visual illusion—a behavioural technique that can induce pain relief in patients with spinal cord injury. In this trial, the combination therapy induced a significantly larger pain reduction compared with each technique alone [130].

Interestingly, it has been demonstrated that chronic MCS with surgically implanted epidural electrodes was more efficacious when the contacts placed over M1 were selected as cathodes [48, 49]. This observation cannot be considered as opposite to the preferential analgesic efficacy of anodal tDCS because the physical characteristics and mechanisms of action of tDCS differed from those of implanted epidural MCS. In fact, epidural MCS probably shares more similar neurostimulation properties with rTMS than with tDCS to produce analgesic effects [67].

OTHER CORTICAL TARGETS

Cortical targets other than the motor cortex have been proposed in the treatment of neuropathic pain using implanted MCS, especially the postrolandic somatosensory cortex [20, 21, 29]. However, in line with Tsubokawa's work, most research teams have found that stimulation using precentral contacts was more efficacious than stimulation using postcentral ones, when the MCS lead was positioned perpendicular to the central sulcus. The results of a study that used navigated rTMS confirmed that only the stimulation of M1, but not of adjacent cortical regions (such as the postcentral gyrus [S1] and the premotor or supplementary motor area), could provide a significant relief of neuropathic pain [47].

In contrast, 1 Hz rTMS applied over the right secondary somatosensory cortex (S2) was found to reduce chronic visceral pain due to chronic pancreatitis [35]. In this latter study, the rTMS target was also defined by means of a navigation system. The same team has recently reported the results of a Phase 2, sham-controlled clinical trial assessing the effects of daily sessions of 1 Hz rTMS over the right S2 for 10 days in patients with chronic pancreatitis and severe visceral pain [39]. They found a significant reduction in pain after real rTMS that lasted for at least 3 weeks following treatment. Nevertheless, stimulation over the anterior bank of the central sulcus remains the preferred targeting strategy for analgesic cortical stimulation, at least for chronic implanted stimulation.

Besides precentral and postcentral stimulations, several rTMS studies aimed at modulating the perception of experimental pain have also explored the possibility of targeting cortical areas involved in cognitive and emotional aspects of pain, such as the DLPFC. For example, Graff-Guerrero et al. [44] showed in a large series of healthy volunteers that rTMS applied over the right DLPFC could increase the tolerance to cold-induced pain. However, the potential therapeutic value of the DLPFC target for analgesia is rather based on effects reported in patients with chronic pain syndrome, such as fibromyalgia. First, Sampson et al. [124] reported a complete resolution of fibromyalgia-associated pain in four women treated for depression by low-frequency (1 Hz) rTMS applied to the right DLPFC. Pain relief was unrelated to antidepressant effects. More recently, Short et al. [127] showed durable and clinically relevant pain reduction, preceding an improvement in depression symptoms in a series of 20 patients with fibromyalgia, who received 4000 rTMS pulses at 10 Hz over the left DLPFC for 2 weeks.

A reduction in pain, not explained by the antidepressant effects, was also shown by Avery et al. [9] in patients with drug-resistant depression and pain who received high-frequency (10 Hz) rTMS delivered over the left DLPFC. Similarly, Reid and Pridmore [117] reported the efficacy of repeated sessions of 20 Hz rTMS delivered to the left DLPFC in a depressive patient with drug-resistant facial pain due to teeth removal. Pain decreased by 42% during the 2nd week of stimulation and maintained 4 weeks after the end of treatment, unrelated to mood changes.

The DLPFC target was also evaluated in patients with various forms of headaches. O'Reardon et al. [108] observed in two patients that DLPFC stimulation used to treat a major depressive episode could also reduce daily headaches. Brighina et al. [19] further showed in a controlled trial that a series of 12 daily sessions of high-frequency rTMS delivered over the left DLPFC could ameliorate chronic migraine, during and in the month after the treatment compared with the month before treatment.

Finally, patients with neuropathic pain could also benefit from DLPFC stimulation. Borckardt et al. [15] performed three real and three sham sessions of 10 Hz rTMS over the left DLPFC in four patients with chronic neuropathic pain. Real rTMS produced a significant improvement in average daily pain in three of the four participants, independently of changes in mood. More recently, Sampson et al. [125] applied 15 sessions of 1-Hz rTMS (1600 stimulations/session) to the right DLPFC in nine subjects with refractory neuropathic pain over 3 weeks. Four patients improved by more than 50% in pain ratings up to the end of the 3-month follow-up. Both left DLPFC stimulation at high frequency and right DLPFC stimulation at low frequency could be valuable to produce analgesic effects, as it was already well demonstrated for the antidepressant effects.

The DLPFC target has also been used in more transient pain syndromes, such as postoperative pain. In a sham-controlled study of 20 patients who underwent gastric bypass surgery, Borckardt et al. [13] found that a single session of high-frequency (10 Hz) rTMS applied immediately after surgery over the left DLPFC for a total of 4000 pulses was associated with a 40% reduction in total morphine use during the first 2 days after surgery, regardless of the effects of rTMS on mood ratings. This reduction corresponded to the effect of active rTMS minus that of sham stimulation. This finding has been replicated by the same team [14]. More recently, these authors found that anodal tDCS applied to the left DLPFC could reduce analgesia requirements and subjective pain ratings after a procedure of endoscopic retrograde cholangiopancreatography [16]. The same team also reported that a combination of cathodal tDCS of the right DLPFC with anodal tDCS of M1 could reduce patient-controlled analgesia (opioid medication) in the postsurgical time following total knee arthroplasty surgery [18]. However, one must acknowledge the absence of any significant analgesic effect of either cathodal or anodal tDCS of the left DLPFC to control postoperative pain in a recent series of patients following lumbar spine surgery [32].

Further studies are still needed before considering the DLPFC as a valuable target for cortical stimulation in pain patients. In particular, these studies should specify the side and frequency (or polarity) of stimulation according to the type of pain syndrome.

Besides the motor (precentral) cortical target, other cortical areas are emerging as potential targets for relieving the various existing pain syndromes. Therefore, in the future, the main challenge for the pain specialist may be to define the best cortical target and stimulation technique to treat a given patient, according to his or her own understanding of the pathophysiological pain mechanisms involved in that particular patient. In any case, this issue should benefit from neuroimaging technique advances.

NEUROIMAGING PERSPECTIVES FOR TREATING PAIN BY NONINVASIVE CORTICAL STIMULATION

The mechanisms underlying the efficacy of rTMS applied over M1 for pain control have remained elusive. In an attempt to solve this uncertainty, studies have combined rTMS with functional brain imaging techniques, and one possible explanation has emerged: rTMS triggers both local and remote neurophysiologic effects along widespread pain-related neural networks [118].

Within this context, PET and functional magnetic resonance imaging (fMRI) studies have shown an increase in the regional cerebral blood flow (rCBF) in restricted brain areas after the application of noxious stimuli. This change in rCBF has been used as an indirect measurement of cortical activation. Those brain regions most frequently involved include S2, the bilateral insula, ACC, the ventrolateral and medial thalamus, S1, the posterior parietal cortex, and the prefrontal cortex [142]. As aforementioned, Tamura et al. [132] found an increase in rCBF in the ACC and a decrease in the right medial prefrontal cortex that were both significantly correlated with the reduction in the intensity of capsaicin-induced acute pain reported by healthy volunteers after 1-Hz rTMS over M1. However, it has to be noted that an experimental model of acute pain was used and that a difference in the modulation of sensory perception by cortical stimulation between pain patients and healthy subjects has been acknowledged [95]. Therefore, the results obtained in that study may not be generalizable to the population of chronic pain patients.

Besides the use of neuroimaging to understand mechanisms of MCS in reducing pain, this technique can also be used to optimize the effects of MCS. We reviewed two methods of using neuroimaging to optimize the application of MCS in chronic pain: neuroimaging as a predictor for best responders and neuroimaging to guide targeting of MCS.

The utility of structural imaging of fibre tracts to predict the response to rTMS in the management of chronic pain has been investigated. Two studies have addressed the hypothesis suggesting that the efficacy of rTMS for patients with central poststroke pain (CPSP) may be predictable on the basis of fibre tracking.

In the first one, Goto et al. [43] performed fibre tracking of the corticospinal tract (CST) and TCT using diffusion tensor imaging (dTI) in 13 patients with CPSP. The primary outcome was the delineation ratio (DR, defined as the ratio of the cross section of the affected side to that of the unaffected side) of the CST and the TCT. One single 5-Hz rTMS session was given to all patients over M1 representation of the painful area. Five subjects had a reduction of more than 30% of their baseline pain and were thus classified as responders, whereas the remaining eight had a decrease of less than 30% or no decrease at all and were regarded as nonresponders. The rTMS-responsive group had a higher DR for both tracts (especially for TCT) than the rTMS-nonresponsive group. The authors concluded that the effectiveness of rTMS over M1 is diminished when delineation of the TCT is poor presumably because the effects of cortical stimulation cannot reach the thalamus if this tract is severely impaired. Furthermore, these results suggest that the structural integrity of the CST may be critical for obtaining pain reduction when delivering rTMS over M1 [43].

In a second study, 10 patients with CPSP underwent dTI and fMRI to evaluate the integrity of the anterior and superior TCTs and the activation pattern of pain networks, respectively [109]. One daily 10-Hz rTMS session was delivered over M1 corresponding to the painful area over 5 consecutive days. Participants were divided into responders ($n = 6$) and nonresponders ($n = 4$), depending on whether their pain score had decreased or increased/not changed, respectively. In responders, the superior TCTs of the infarcted hemisphere were well delineated, whereas in nonresponders the same tract showed extreme deterioration in the damaged hemisphere, compared with the undamaged one. Comparison of fMRI images obtained pre-rTMS and post-rTMS showed remarkably decreased activity in S2, insula, prefrontal cortex, putamen, and cerebellum in the responder group after rTMS. No apparent differences were found in the nonresponder group. These results suggest that the analgesic effects of rTMS may be associated with modulation of neural activity in a diffuse pain network that includes areas distant to the stimulated region. Furthermore, this study is consistent with the previous observation that the analgesic effects of rTMS in patients with CPSP may be facilitated when the superior TCT is still spared after an ischemic insult, as this tract allows the stimulated cortex to transmit the neuromodulatory effects to the thalamus [109].

Although the findings of both studies suggest that the efficacy of rTMS for CPSP could be predicted through fibre tracking of the "rTMS pain relief pathway," none of them included a control group for comparison. This is a critical limitation to be corrected in future trials if firm conclusions are to be drawn.

Another important issue is targeting. The efficacy of rTMS likely depends on targeting accuracy, at least regarding M1 stimulation. Actually, high-frequency rTMS may fail to produce significant analgesia when it is not focally applied with a circular coil [122]. In a series of 60 patients with chronic neuropathic pain of various origins and locations, Lefaucheur et al. [70] found that facial pain better improved than hand pain when the hand motor area was stimulated. In another study, rTMS was found more effective when the stimulation site was adjacent to the cortical representation of the painful zone rather than within the painful zone itself [72]. In contrast to the heterotopic efficacy of rTMS, the efficacy of chronic electrical stimulation of the cortex using epidural electrodes implanted over M1 is homotopic [96–98]. Targeting differences between these techniques are likely due to differences in the geometry of the induced electric field. Because fibres are more prone to be stimulated than cell bodies, it is critical to consider the relationships between the magnitude and polarity of the current and the depth and orientation of the fibres that are amenable to activation within the cortical layers [49, 84, 85]. Analgesic effects are likely mediated via the activation of horizontal fibres in the superficial layers of the precentral gyrus [75, 99]: epidural stimulation and rTMS may differ by the way they recruit such fibres.

Several considerations strongly support the use of image-guided navigation systems in the practice of rTMS [63], even for targeting the motor cortex in the aim of treating pain. First, the orientation of the figure-eight-shaped coil usually used to perform motor cortex rTMS crucially influences the direction of the current induced into the cortex and then the nature of the circuits activated by the stimulation. It has been demonstrated that when the current is induced into the brain from anterior to posterior (according to the direction of a monophasic TMS pulse or to the second, most effective phase of a biphasic TMS pulse), TMS can generate late I-waves, similarly to cathodal electrical stimulation, and this orientation is the one associated with pain relief [6]. Therefore, between-study variability of the clinical effects produced by rTMS can be due, at least in part, to the inaccuracy of TMS coil positioning and handling.

Several methods of TMS coil positioning have been described [46, 131]. The most conventional one is based on the definition of a targeted cortical region as situated at a "standard" scalp distance to the location of M1 ("function-guided procedure") [131]. The reference point in M1 is usually the "hand motor hotspot," which is the scalp site where TMS is able to produce MEPs of maximal amplitude in a contralateral hand muscle. The "standard" function-guided procedure locates the DLPFC 5 cm anterior to the "hand motor hotspot," the premotor cortex (PMC) 2–3 cm anterior, and S1 3 cm posterior. However, these anatomical definitions are empiric and do not take into account the large intersubject variability in brain morphology and the functional changes that disease can produce in cortical representations. This may result in wrong coil placement as demonstrated by the few studies in which the "standard" and "navigated" procedures were compared [1, 45]. This situation opened large perspectives to the use of navigation systems, allowing TMS targeting to be based on more reliable anatomical grounds, provided by the integration of brain imaging data.

Image-guided navigation integrates data provided by structural MRI, fMRI, or PET. Either individual data obtained in the subject who undergoes TMS ("individual approach") or normalized data taken from previous group studies ("probabilistic approach") can be used. However, the "gold standard" technique includes a real-time frameless stereotaxic system to position the coil over the cortical target, which is previously determined on individual brain imaging data. Such a system usually integrates high-resolution structural T1-weighted MRI slices to perform a 3D reconstruction of the head and brain anatomy. An infrared camera system detects reflectors mounted on the subject's head and fixed to the magnetic coil. A referencing procedure using cranial landmarks is first performed to coregister the head and the coil in the coordinate system of the brain MRI. When this coregistration is achieved, the system allows the visualization of the location and orientation of the coil over the head and the resulting electric field density within the cortex in real time on a computer screen.

First, navigation systems are valuable to improve the reproducibility (repeatability) of coil placement, including the optimal coil orientation, within and between the sessions. This is particularly important for rTMS protocols with repeated daily sessions for several weeks. Image-guided targeting in real time is clearly more precise than cranial landmarks plotted on a lycra swimming cap. Second, navigation systems are valuable to optimize the accuracy of target location for cortical stimulation, according to patients' imaging data. Since the principle of cortical stimulation is to activate given neural circuits, fibre tracking information provided by dTI could be of particular interest in the context of a navigated strategy of cortical stimulation, as aforementioned [43, 109]. However, only a few studies have really used image-guided navigation to perform rTMS of M1 in pain patients [47, 78].

Another procedure of TMS coil or tDCS electrode positioning is based on the "international 10–20 system" of electroencephalographic (EEG) electrode placement. This procedure offers the advantage to be based on a worldwide used method of labelling scalp points, allowing very good between-study reproducibility in theory. Even greater perspectives are opened for physiological or therapeutic studies by the combination of navigated TMS and EEG [135]. EEG studies have also provided information about changes in neural oscillations associated with tDCS [50, 51, 54]. However, regarding tDCS, modelling first the spatial distribution of the magnitude and direction of the current density into the brain resulting from the stimulation is a major challenge [92]. These parameters are strongly influenced by the geometry and position of the electrodes and their montage [22, 25]. This point is of particular interest because new studies are based on a new tDCS design, called high-definition tDCS (HD-tDCS) [17, 89, 140]. With this method, four cathodes are placed equidistant (7 cm) from each other and from the anode, which serves as the active electrode. This montage increases the spatial selectivity of the stimulation. For example, anodal HD-tDCS delivered to the left M1 was shown to decrease cold detection and pain thresholds, to increase warm sensory thresholds, but to not alter heat pain thresholds [17]. Such antinociceptive effect of anodal HD-tDCS runs counter to the inefficacy of "standard" anodal tDCS in all previous studies performed in healthy subjects [10, 53], but fits well with the proved analgesic effect of anodal (but not of cathodal) tDCS of M1 observed in patients with chronic pain, of either neuropathic or non-neuropathic origin. This observation illustrates the crucial influence of the technique on cortical stimulation effects. In this context, the use of neuroimaging guidance may be an important element for a better standardization of noninvasive cortical stimulation protocols.

CONCLUSION

Significant analgesic effects of rTMS and tDCS have been found in many studies of patients with chronic pain of various origins, even when the placebo effect was appropriately controlled. Concerning rTMS, high-frequency M1 stimulation was shown to reduce pain scores by 20–45% following active stimulation and by less than 10% following sham stimulation. Regarding individual results, 35–60% of the published patients have been considered as good responders to rTMS (more than 30% pain relief following active rTMS). Concerning tDCS, repeated daily sessions of anodal tDCS over M1 used alone as an alternative technique to rTMS were found to decrease pain scores by 58%, which is a larger result compared with most of rTMS studies.

Analgesic effects were obtained whatever the origin of pain, and it is not possible to determine an overall order of efficacy of noninvasive cortical stimulation with respect to pain diagnoses. Good results have also been reported with either rTMS or tDCS administered over M1, S2, or DLPFC in chronic pain syndromes that are not typically "neuropathic," such as visceral pain, cancer pain, migraine, fibromyalgia, or CRPS-I.

However, the strategies using noninvasive cortical stimulation to treat chronic pain syndromes still remain to be optimized. Increasing the total number of pulses per session and repeating the sessions for several days or weeks is surely able to enhance and prolong rTMS-induced analgesia. The influence of various parameters of stimulation (including target localization and electrode montage) in the production of tDCS-induced analgesic effects also needs to be assessed in future studies. Regardless of the method of cortical stimulation, the methods for determining the most suitable site of cortical stimulation remain an open question. Finally, future investigation should also address the issues of interindividual variability of the analgesic effects provided by cortical stimulation, priming influence of various analgesic medications, and characterization of the significant predictors of efficacy. Various neuroimaging techniques could be valuable to provide such information and to be integrated into the practice of rTMS to produce analgesic effects.

REFERENCES

1. Ahdab R, Ayache SS, Brugières P, Goujon C, Lefaucheur JP. Comparison of "standard" and "navigated" procedures of TMS coil positioning over motor, premotor and prefrontal targets in patients with chronic pain and depression. Neurophysiol Clin 2010;40:27–36.
2. Ahmed MA, Mohamed SA, Sayed D. Long-term antalgic effects of repetitive transcranial magnetic stimulation of motor cortex and serum beta-endorphin in patients with phantom pain. Neurol Res 2011;33:953–8.
3. Amassian VE, Vergara MS, Somasundaram M, Maccabee PJ, Cracco RQ. Induced pain is relieved by repetitive stimulation (rTMS) of human parietal lobe through endorphin release. Electroencephalogr Clin Neurophysiol 1997;103:179.
4. Andrade DC, Borges I, Bravo GL, Bolognini N, Fregni F. Therapeutic time window of non-invasive brain stimulation for pain treatment: inhibition of maladaptive plasticity with early intervention. Expert Rev Med Devices 2013;10:339–52.
5. André-Obadia N, Peyron R, Mertens P, Mauguière F, Laurent B, Garcia-Larrea L. Transcranial magnetic stimulation for pain control: double-blind study of different frequencies against placebo, and correlation with motor cortex stimulation efficacy. Clin Neurophysiol 2006;117: 1536–44.
6. André-Obadia N, Mertens P, Gueguen A, Peyron R, Garcia-Larrea L. Pain relief by rTMS: differential effect of current flow but no specific action on pain subtypes. Neurology 2008;71:833–40.
7. Antal A, Paulus W. A case of refractory orofacial pain treated by transcranial direct current stimulation applied over hand motor area in combination with NMDA agonist drug intake. Brain Stimul 2011;4:117–21.
8. Antal A, Terney D, Kühnl S, Paulus W. Anodal transcranial direct current stimulation of the motor cortex ameliorates chronic pain and reduces short intracortical inhibition. J Pain Symptom Manag 2010;39:890–903.
9. Avery DH, Holtzheimer PE III, Fawaz W, Russo J, Neumaier J, Dunner DL, Haynor R, Claypoole KH, Wajdik C, Roy-Byrne P. Transcranial magnetic stimulation reduces pain in patients with major depression: a sham-controlled study. J Nerv Ment Dis 2007;195:378–81.
10. Bachmann CG, Muschinsky S, Nitsche MA, Rolke R, Magerl W, Treede RD, Paulus W, Happe S. Transcranial direct current stimulation of the motor cortex induces distinct changes in thermal and mechanical sensory percepts. Clin Neurophysiol 2010;121:2083–9.
11. Boggio PS, Amancio EJ, Correa CF, Cecilio S, Valasek C, Bajwa Z, Freedman SD, Pascual-Leone A, Edwards DJ, Fregni F. Transcranial DC stimulation coupled with TENS for the treatment of chronic pain: a preliminary study. Clin J Pain 2009;25:691–5.
12. Bolognini N, Olgiati E, Maravita A, Ferraro F, Fregni F. Motor and parietal cortex stimulation for phantom limb pain and sensations. Pain 2013;154:1274–80.
13. Borckardt JJ, Weinstein M, Reeves ST, Kozel FA, Nahas Z, Smith AR, Byrne TK, Morgan K, George MS. Postoperative left prefrontal repetitive transcranial magnetic stimulation reduces patient-controlled analgesia use. Anesthesiology 2006;105:557–62.
14. Borckardt JJ, Reeves ST, Weinstein M, Smith AR, Shelley N, Kozel FA, Nahas Z, Byrne KT, Morgan K, George MS. Significant analgesic effects of one session of postoperative left prefrontal cortex repetitive transcranial magnetic stimulation: a replication study. Brain Stimul 2008;1:122–7.
15. Borckardt JJ, Smith AR, Reeves ST, Madan A, Shelley N, Branham R, Nahas Z, George MS. A pilot study investigating the effects of fast left prefrontal rTMS on chronic neuropathic pain. Pain Med 2009;10:840–9.
16. Borckardt JJ, Romagnuolo J, Reeves ST, Madan A, Frohman H, Beam W, George MS. Feasibility, safety, and effectiveness of transcranial direct current stimulation for decreasing post-ERCP pain: a randomized, sham-controlled, pilot study. Gastrointest Endosc 2011;73:1158–64.
17. Borckardt JJ, Bikson M, Frohman H, Reeves ST, Datta A, Bansal V, Madan A, Barth K, George MS. A pilot study of the tolerability and effects of high-definition transcranial direct current stimulation (HD-tDCS) on pain perception. J Pain 2012;13:112–20.

18. Borckardt JJ, Reeves ST, Robinson SM, May JT, Epperson TI, Gunselman RJ, Schutte HD, Demos HA, Madan A, Fredrich S, et al. Transcranial direct current stimulation (tDCS) reduces postsurgical opioid consumption in total knee arthroplasty (TKA). Clin J Pain 2013;29:925–8.
19. Brighina F, Piazza A, Vitello G, Aloisio A, Palermo A, Daniele O, Fierro B. rTMS of the prefrontal cortex in the treatment of chronic migraine: a pilot study. J Neurol Sci 2004;227:67–71.
20. Canavero S. Cortical stimulation for central pain. J Neurosurg 1995;83:1117.
21. Canavero S, Bonicalzi V. Therapeutic extradural cortical stimulation for central and neuropathic pain: a review. Clin J Pain 2002;18:48–55.
22. Cano T, Morales-Quezada JL, Bikson M, Fregni F. Methods to focalize non-invasive electrical brain stimulation: principles and future clinical development for the treatment of pain. Expert Rev Neurother 2013;13:465–7.
23. Casey KL, Minoshima S, Morrow TJ, Koeppe RA. Comparison of human cerebral activation pattern during cutaneous warmth, heat pain, and deep cold pain. J Neurophysiol 1996;76:571–81.
24. Cruccu G, Aziz TZ, Garcia-Larrea L, Hansson P, Jensen TS, Lefaucheur JP, Simpson BA, Taylor RS. EFNS guidelines on neurostimulation therapy for neuropathic pain. Eur J Neurol 2007;14:952–70.
25. DaSilva AF, Volz MS, Bikson M, Fregni F. Electrode positioning and montage in transcranial direct current stimulation. J Vis Exp 2011;(51):2744.
26. Dasilva AF, Mendonca ME, Zaghi S, Lopes M, Dossantos MF, Spierings EL, Bajwa Z, Datta A, Bikson M, Fregni F. tDCS-induced analgesia and electrical fields in pain-related neural networks in chronic migraine. Headache 2012;52:1283–95.
27. Davis KD, Kwan CL, Crawley AP, Mikulis DJ. Functional MRI study of thalamic and cortical activations evoked by cutaneous heat, cold, and tactile stimuli. J Neurophysiol 1998;80:1533–46.
28. de Andrade DC, Mhalla A, Adam F, Texeira MJ, Bouhassira D. Neuropharmacological basis of rTMS-induced analgesia: the role of endogenous opioids. Pain 2011;152:320–6.
29. De Ridder D, De Mulder G, Verstraeten E, Sunaert S, Moller A. Somatosensory cortex stimulation for deafferentation pain. Acta Neurochir 2007;97(Suppl):67–74.
30. DosSantos MF, Love TM, Martikainen IK, Nascimento TD, Fregni F, Cummiford C, Deboer MD, Zubieta JK, Dasilva AF. Immediate effects of tDCS on the μ-opioid system of a chronic pain patient. Front Psychiatry 2012;3:93.
31. Drouot X, Nguyen JP, Peschanski M, Lefaucheur JP. The antalgic efficacy of chronic motor cortex stimulation is related to sensory changes in the painful zone. Brain 2002;125:1660–4.
32. Dubois PE, Ossemann M, de Fays K, De Bue P, Gourdin M, Jamart J, Vandermeeren Y. Postoperative analgesic effect of transcranial direct current stimulation in lumbar spine surgery: a randomized control trial. Clin J Pain 2013;29:696–701.
33. Fenton BW, Palmieri PA, Boggio P, Fanning J, Fregni F. A preliminary study of transcranial direct current stimulation for the treatment of refractory chronic pelvic pain. Brain Stimul 2009;2:103–7.
34. Fierro B, De Tommaso M, Giglia F, Giglia G, Palermo A, Brighina F. Repetitive transcranial magnetic stimulation (rTMS) of the dorsolateral prefrontal cortex (DLPFC) during capsaicin-induced pain: modulatory effects on motor cortex excitability. Exp Brain Res 2010;203:31–8.
35. Fregni F, DaSilva D, Potvin K, Ramos-Estebanez C, Cohen D, Pascual-Leone A, Freedman SD. Treatment of chronic visceral pain with brain stimulation. Ann Neurol 2005;58:971–2.
36. Fregni F, Boggio PS, Lima MC, Ferreira MJ, Wagner T, Rigonatti SP, Castro AW, Souza DR, Riberto M, Freedman SD, et al. A sham-controlled, phase II trial of transcranial direct current stimulation for the treatment of central pain in traumatic spinal cord injury. Pain 2006;122:197–209.
37. Fregni F, Gimenes R, Valle AC, Ferreira MJ, Rocha RR, Natalle L, Bravo R, Rigonatti SP, Freedman SD, Nitsche MA, et al. A randomized sham-controlled proof-of-principle study of transcranial direct current stimulation for the treatment of pain in fibromyalgia. Arthritis Rheum 2006;54:3988–98.
38. Fregni F, Freedman S, Pascual-Leone A. Recent advances in the treatment of chronic pain with non-invasive brain stimulation techniques. Lancet Neurol 2007;6:188–91.
39. Fregni F, Potvin K, Dasilva D, Wang X, Lenkinski RE, Freedman SD, Pascual-Leone A. Clinical effects and brain metabolic correlates in non-invasive cortical neuromodulation for visceral pain. Eur J Pain 2011;15:53–60.
40. Fujii M, Ohmoto Y, Kitahara T, Sugiyama S, Uesugi S, Yamashita T, Shiroyama Y, Ito H. Motor cortex stimulation therapy in patients with thalamic pain. Neurol Surg 1997;25:315–9.
41. Garcia-Larrea L, Peyron R. Motor cortex stimulation for neuropathic pain: from phenomenology to mechanisms. Neuroimage 2007;37(Suppl 1):S71–9.
42. Garcia-Larrea L, Peyron R, Mertens P, Gregoire MC, Lavenne F, Le Bars D, Convers P, Mauguière F, Sindou M, Laurent B. Electrical stimulation of motor cortex for pain control: a combined PET-scan and electrophysiological study. Pain 1999;83:259–73.

43. Goto T, Saitoh Y, Hashimoto N, Hirata M, Kishima H, Oshino S, Tani N, Hosomi K, Kakigi R, Yoshimine T. Diffusion tensor fiber tracking in patients with central post-stroke pain; correlation with efficacy of repetitive transcranial magnetic stimulation. Pain 2008;140:509–18.
44. Graff-Guerrero A, González-Olvera J, Fresán A, Gómez-Martín D, Méndez-Núñez JC, Pellicer F. Repetitive transcranial magnetic stimulation of dorsolateral prefrontal cortex increases tolerance to human experimental pain. Cogn Brain Res 2005;25:153–60.
45. Herwig U, Padberg F, Unger J, Spitzer M, Schönfeldt-Lecuona C. Transcranial magnetic stimulation in therapy studies: examination of the reliability of "standard" coil positioning by neuronavigation. Biol Psychiatry 2001;50:58–61.
46. Herwig U, Schönfeldt-Lecuona C, Wunderlich AP, von Tiesenhausen C, Thielscher A, Walter H, Spitzer M. The navigation of transcranial magnetic stimulation. Psychiatry Res 2001;108:123–31.
47. Hirayama A, Saitoh Y, Kishima H, Shimokawa T, Oshino S, Hirata M, Kato A, Yoshimine T. Reduction of intractable deafferentation pain by navigation-guided repetitive transcranial magnetic stimulation of the primary motor cortex. Pain 2006;122:22–7.
48. Holsheimer J, Lefaucheur JP, Buitenweg JR, Goujon C, Nineb A, Nguyen JP. The role of intra-operative motor evoked potentials in the optimization of chronic cortical stimulation for the treatment of neuropathic pain. Clin Neurophysiol 2007;118:2287–96.
49. Holsheimer J, Nguyen JP, Lefaucheur JP, Manola L. Cathodal, anodal or bifocal stimulation of the motor cortex in the management of chronic pain. Acta Neurochir 2007;97(Suppl):57–66.
50. Jacobson L, Ezra A, Berger U, Lavidor M. Modulating oscillatory brain activity correlates of behavioral inhibition using transcranial direct current stimulation. Clin Neurophysiol 2012;123:979–84.
51. Jensen MP, Sherlin LH, Askew RL, Fregni F, Witkop G, Gianas A, Howe JD, Hakimian S. Effects of non-pharmacological pain treatments on brain states. Clin Neurophysiol 2013;124:2016–24.
52. Juottonen K, Gockel M, Silén T, Hurri H, Hari R, Forss N. Altered central sensorimotor processing in patients with complex regional pain syndrome. Pain 2002;98:315–23.
53. Jürgens TP, Schulte A, Klein T, May A. Transcranial direct current stimulation does neither modulate results of a quantitative sensory testing protocol nor ratings of suprathreshold heat stimuli in healthy volunteers. Eur J Pain 2012;16:1251–63.
54. Keeser D, Padberg F, Reisinger E, Pogarell O, Kirsch V, Palm U, Karch S, Möller HJ, Nitsche MA, Mulert C. Prefrontal direct current stimulation modulates resting EEG and event-related potentials in healthy subjects: a standardized low resolution tomography (sLORETA) study. Neuroimage 2011;55:644–57.
55. Khedr EM, Kotb H, Kamel NF, Ahmed MA, Sadek R, Rothwell JC. Longlasting antalgic effects of daily sessions of repetitive transcranial magnetic stimulation in central and peripheral neuropathic pain. J Neurol Neurosurg Psychiatry 2005;76:833–8.
56. Knotkova H, Portenoy RK, Cruciani RA. Transcranial direct current stimulation (tDCS) relieved itching in a patient with chronic neuropathic pain. Clin J Pain 2013;29:621–2.
57. Kwon YH, Ko MH, Ahn SH, Kim YH, Song JC, Lee CH, Chang MC, Jang SH. Primary motor cortex activation by transcranial direct current stimulation in the human brain. Neurosci Lett 2008;435:56–9.
58. Lang N, Siebner HR, Ward NS, Lee L, Nitsche MA, Paulus W, Rothwell JC, Lemon RN, Frackowiak RS. How does transcranial DC stimulation of the primary motor cortex alter regional neuronal activity in the human brain? Eur J Neurosci 2005;22:495–504.
59. Lefaucheur JP. The use of repetitive transcranial magnetic stimulation (rTMS) in chronic neuropathic pain. Neurophysiol Clin 2006;36:117–24.
60. Lefaucheur JP. Principles of therapeutic use of transcranial and epidural cortical stimulation. Clin Neurophysiol 2008;119:2179–84.
61. Lefaucheur JP. Use of repetitive transcranial magnetic stimulation in pain relief. Expert Rev Neurother 2008;8:799–808.
62. Lefaucheur JP. Methods of therapeutic cortical stimulation. Neurophysiol Clin 2009;39:1–14.
63. Lefaucheur JP. Why image-guided navigation becomes essential in the practice of transcranial magnetic stimulation. Neurophysiol Clin 2010;40:1–5.
64. Lefaucheur JP. Is rTMS a therapeutic option in chronic pain syndrome? Insights from the treatment of fibromyalgia. Pain 2011;152:1447–8.
65. Lefaucheur JP. Neurophysiology of cortical stimulation. Int Rev Neurobiol 2012;107:57–85.
66. Lefaucheur JP, Nguyen JP, Drouot X, Pollin B, Keravel Y, Harf A. Chronic pain treated by rTMS of motor cortex. Electroencephalogr Clin Neurophysiol 1998;107:92.
67. Lefaucheur JP, Drouot X, Keravel Y, Nguyen JP. Pain relief induced by repetitive transcranial magnetic stimulation of precentral cortex. NeuroReport 2001;12:2963–5.

68. Lefaucheur JP, Drouot X, Nguyen JP. Interventional neurophysiology for pain control: duration of pain relief following repetitive transcranial magnetic stimulation of the motor cortex. Neurophysiol Clin 2001;31:247–52.
69. Lefaucheur JP, Drouot X, Ménard-Lefaucheur I, Nguyen JP. Neuropathic pain controlled for more than a year by monthly sessions of repetitive transcranial magnetic cortical stimulation, Neurophysiol Clin 2004;34:91–5.
70. Lefaucheur JP, Drouot X, Ménard-Lefaucheur I, Zerah F, Bendib B, Cesaro P, Keravel Y, Nguyen JP. Neurogenic pain relief by repetitive transcranial magnetic cortical stimulation depends on the origin and the site of pain. J Neurol Neurosurg Psychiatry 2004;75:612–6.
71. Lefaucheur JP, Drouot X, Ménard-Lefaucheur I, Keravel Y, Nguyen JP. Motor cortex rTMS improves defective intracortical inhibition in patients with chronic neuropathic pain: correlation with pain relief. Neurology 2006;67:1568–74.
72. Lefaucheur JP, Hatem S, Nineb A, Ménard-Lefaucheur I, Wendling S, Keravel Y, Nguyen JP. Somatotopic organization of the analgesic effects of motor cortex rTMS in neuropathic pain. Neurology 2006;67:1998–2004.
73. Lefaucheur JP, Antal A, Ahdab R, Ciampi de Andrade D, Fregni F, Khedr EM, Nitche M, Paulus W. The use of repetitive transcranial magnetic stimulation (rTMS) and transcranial direct current stimulation (tDCS) to relieve pain. Brain Stimul 2008;1:337–44.
74. Lefaucheur JP, Drouot X, Ménard-Lefaucheur I, Keravel Y, Nguyen JP. Motor cortex rTMS in chronic neuropathic pain: pain relief is associated with thermal sensory perception improvement. J Neurol Neurosurg Psychiatry 2008;79:1044–9.
75. Lefaucheur JP, Holsheimer J, Goujon C, Keravel Y, Nguyen JP. Descending volleys generated by efficacious epidural motor cortex stimulation in patients with chronic neuropathic pain. Exp Neurol 2010;223:609–14.
76. Lefaucheur JP, Jarry G, Drouot X, Ménard-Lefaucheur I, Keravel Y, Nguyen JP. Motor cortex rTMS reduces acute pain provoked by laser stimulation in patients with chronic neuropathic pain. Clin Neurophysiol 2010;121:895–901.
77. Lefaucheur JP, Ménard-Lefaucheur I, Goujon C, Keravel Y, Nguyen JP. Predictive value of rTMS in the identification of responders to epidural motor cortex stimulation therapy for pain. J Pain 2011;12:1102–11.
78. Lefaucheur JP, Ayache SS, Sorel M, Farhat WH, Zouari HG, Ciampi de Andrade D, Ahdab R, Ménard-Lefaucheur I, Brugières P, et al. Analgesic effects of repetitive transcranial magnetic stimulation of the motor cortex in neuropathic pain: influence of theta burst stimulation priming. Eur J Pain 2012;16:1403–13.
79. Leung A, Donohue M, Xu R, Lee R, Lefaucheur JP, Khedr EM, Saitoh Y, André-Obadia N, Rollnik J, Wallace M, et al. rTMS for suppressing neuropathic pain: a meta-analysis. J Pain 2009;10:1205–16.
80. Liebetanz D, Nitsche MA, Tergau F, Paulus W. Pharmacological approach to the mechanisms of transcranial DC-stimulation-induced after-effects of human motor cortex excitability. Brain 2012;125:2238–47.
81. Lima MC, Fregni F. Motor cortex stimulation for chronic pain: systematic review and meta-analysis of the literature. Neurology 2008;70:2329–37.
82. Maarrawi J, Peyron R, Mertens P, Costes N, Magnin M, Sindou M, Laurent B, Garcia-Larrea L. Motor cortex stimulation for pain control induces changes in the endogenous opioid system. Neurology 2007;69:827–34.
83. Maeda F, Keenan JP, Tormos JM, Topka H, Pascual-Leone A. Modulation of corticospinal excitability by repetitive transcranial magnetic stimulation. Clin Neurophysiol 2000;111:800–5.
84. Manola L, Roelofsen BH, Holsheimer J, Marani E, Geelen J. Modelling motor cortex stimulation for chronic pain control: electrical potential field, activating functions and responses of simple nerve fibre models. Med Biol Eng Comput 2005;43:335–43.
85. Manola L, Holsheimer J, Veltink P, Buitenweg JR. Anodal vs cathodal stimulation of motor cortex: a modeling study. Clin Neurophysiol 2007;118:464–74.
86. Marlow NM, Bonilha HS, Short EB. Efficacy of transcranial direct current stimulation and repetitive transcranial magnetic stimulation for treating fibromyalgia syndrome: a systematic review. Pain Pract 2013;13:131–45.
87. McIntyre CC, Grill WM. Extracellular stimulation of central neurons: influence of stimulus waveform and frequency on neuronal output. J Neurophysiol 2002;88:1592–604.
88. Medeiros LF, de Souza IC, Vidor LP, de Souza A, Deitos A, Volz MS, Fregni F, Caumo W, Torres IL. Neurobiological effects of transcranial direct current stimulation: a review. Front Psychiatry 2012;3:110.
89. Mendonca ME, Santana MB, Baptista AF, Datta A, Bikson M, Fregni F, Araujo CP. Transcranial DC stimulation in fibromyalgia: optimized cortical target supported by high-resolution computational models. J Pain 2011;12:610–7.
90. Mhalla A, Baudic S, Ciampi de Andrade D, Gautron M, Perrot S, Teixeira MJ, Attal N, Bouhassira D. Long-term maintenance of the analgesic effects of transcranial magnetic stimulation in fibromyalgia. Pain 2011;152:1478–85.
91. Migita K, Uozumi T, Arita K, Monden S. Transcranial magnetic coil stimulation of motor cortex in patients with central pain. Neurosurgery 1995;36:1037–40.

92. Miranda PC, Lomarev M, Hallett M. Modeling the current distribution during transcranial direct current stimulation. Clin Neurophysiol 2006;117:1623–9.
93. Moreno-Duarte I, Morse LR, Alam M, Bikson M, Zafonte R, Fregni F. Targeted therapies using electrical and magnetic neural stimulation for the treatment of chronic pain in spinal cord injury. Neuroimage 2014;85(3):1003–13.
94. Mori F, Codecà C, Kusayanagi H, Monteleone F, Buttari F, Fiore S, Bernardi G, Koch G, Centonze D. Effects of anodal transcranial direct current stimulation on chronic neuropathic pain in patients with multiple sclerosis. J Pain 2010;11:436–42.
95. Mylius V, Borckardt JJ, Lefaucheur JP. Non-invasive cortical modulation of experimental pain. Pain 2012;153:1350–63.
96. Nguyen JP, Lefaucheur JP, Decq P, Uchiyama T, Carpentier A, Fontaine D, Brugières P, Pollin B, Fève A, Rostaing S, et al. Chronic motor cortex stimulation in the treatment of central and neuropathic pain: correlations between clinical, electrophysiological and anatomical data. Pain 1999;82:245–51.
97. Nguyen JP, Lefaucheur JP, Keravel Y. Motor cortex stimulation. In: Simpson BA, editor. Pain research and clinical management, Vol. 15, Electrical stimulation and the relief of pain. Amsterdam, the Netherlands: Elsevier; 2003. pp. 197–209.
98. Nguyen JP, Lefaucheur JP, Raoul S, Roualdes V, Péréon Y, Keravel Y. Motor cortex stimulation for the treatment of neuropathic pain. In: Krames ES, Hunter Peckham P, Rezai AR, editors. Neuromodulation. Amsterdam, the Netherlands: Elsevier; 2009. pp. 515–26.
99. Nguyen JP, Nizard J, Keravel Y, Lefaucheur JP. Invasive brain stimulation for the treatment of neuropathic pain. Nat Rev Neurol 2011;7:699–709.
100. Nitsche MA, Paulus W. Excitability changes induced in the human motor cortex by weak transcranial direct current stimulation. J Physiol (London) 2000;527:633–9.
101. Nitsche MA, Paulus W. Sustained excitability elevations induced by transcranial DC motor cortex stimulation in humans. Neurology 2001;57:1899–901.
102. Nitsche MA, Fricke K, Henschke U, Schlitterlau A, Liebetanz D, Lang N, Henning S, Tergau F, Paulus W. Pharmacological modulation of cortical excitability shifts induced by transcranial direct current stimulation in humans. J Physiol (London) 2003;553:293–301.
103. Nizard J, Lefaucheur JP, Helbert M, de Chauvigny E, Nguyen JP. Non-invasive stimulation therapies for the treatment of refractory pain. Discov Med 2012;14:21–31.
104. Nowak LG, Bullier J. Axons, but not cell bodies, are activated by electrical stimulation in cortical gray matter, I: evidence from chronaxie measurements. Exp Brain Res 1998;118:477–88.
105. Nowak LG, Bullier J. Axons, but not cell bodies, are activated by electrical stimulation in cortical gray matter, II: evidence from selective inactivation of cell bodies and axon initial segments. Exp Brain Res 1998;118:489–500.
106. O'Connell NE, Wand BM, Marston L, Spencer S, De Souza LH. Non-invasive brain stimulation techniques for chronic pain. Cochrane Database Syst Rev 2010;(9):CD008208.
107. O'Connell NE, Cossar J, Marston L, Wand BM, Bunce D, De Souza LH, Maskill DW, Sharp A, Moseley GL. Transcranial direct current stimulation of the motor cortex in the treatment of chronic nonspecific low back pain: a randomized, double-blind exploratory study. Clin J Pain 2013;29:26–34.
108. O'Reardon JP, Fontecha JF, Cristancho MA, Newman S. Unexpected reduction in migraine and psychogenic headaches following rTMS treatment for major depression: a report of two cases. CNS Spectr 2007;12:921–5.
109. Ohn SH, Chang WH, Park CH, Kim ST, Lee JI, Pascual-Leone A, Kim YH. Neural correlates of the antinociceptive effects of repetitive transcranial magnetic stimulation on central pain after stroke. Neurorehabil Neural Repair 2012;26:344–52.
110. Passard A, Attal N, Benadhira R, Brasseur L, Saba G, Sichere P, Perrot S, Januel D, Bouhassira D. Effects of unilateral repetitive transcranial magnetic stimulation of the motor cortex on chronic widespread pain in fibromyalgia. Brain 2007;130:2661–70.
111. Peinemann A, Lehner C, Mentschel C, Münchau A, Conrad B, Siebner HR. Subthreshold 5-Hz repetitive transcranial magnetic stimulation of the human primary motor cortex reduces intracortical paired-pulse inhibition. Neurosci Lett 2000;296:21–4.
112. Peyron R, Garcia-Larrea L, Deiber MP, Cinotti L, Convers P, Sindou M, Mauguière F, Laurent B. Electrical stimulation of precentral cortical area in the treatment of central pain: electrophysiological and PET study. Pain 1995;62:275–86.
113. Peyron R, Faillenot I, Mertens P, Laurent B, Garcia-Larrea L. Motor cortex stimulation in neuropathic pain. Correlations between analgesic effect and hemodynamic changes in the brain: a PET study. Neuroimage 2007;34:310–21.

114. Picarelli H, Teixeira MJ, de Andrade DC, Myczkowski ML, Luvisotto TB, Yeng LT, Fonoff ET, Pridmore S, Marcolin MA. Repetitive transcranial magnetic stimulation is efficacious as an add-on to pharmacological therapy in complex regional pain syndrome (CRPS) type I. J Pain 2010;11:1203–10.
115. Plow EB, Pascual-Leone A, Machado A. Brain stimulation in the treatment of chronic neuropathic and non-cancerous pain. J Pain 2012;13:411–24.
116. Raij TT, Forss N, Stancák A, Hari R. Modulation of motor-cortex oscillatory activity by painful Aδ- and C-fiber stimuli. Neuroimage 2004;23:569–73.
117. Reid P, Pridmore S. Improvement in chronic pain with transcranial magnetic stimulation. Aust N Z J Psychiatry 2001;35:252.
118. Reithler J, Peters JC, Sack AT. Multimodal transcranial magnetic stimulation: using concurrent neuroimaging to reveal the neural network dynamics of noninvasive brain stimulation. Prog Neurobiol 2011;94:149–65.
119. Riberto M, Marcon Alfieri F, Monteiro de Benedetto Pacheco K, Dini Leite V, Nemoto Kaihami H, Fregni F, Rizzo Battistella L. Efficacy of transcranial direct current stimulation coupled with a multidisciplinary rehabilitation program for the treatment of fibromyalgia. Open Rheumatol J 2011;5:45–50.
120. Roizenblatt S, Fregni F, Gimenez R, Wetzel T, Rigonatti SP, Tufik S, Boggio PS, Valle AC. Site-specific effects of transcranial direct current stimulation on sleep and pain in fibromyalgia: a randomized, sham-controlled study. Pain Pract 2007;7:297–306.
121. Rojas-Piloni G, Martínez-Lorenzana G, Condés-Lara M, Rodríguez-Jiménez J. Direct sensorimotor corticospinal modulation of dorsal horn neuronal C-fiber responses in the rat. Brain Res 2010;1351:104–14.
122. Rollnik JD, Wüstefeld S, Däuper J, Karst M, Fink M, Kossev A, Dengler R. Repetitive transcranial magnetic stimulation for the treatment of chronic pain—a pilot study. Eur Neurol 2002;48:6–10.
123. Saitoh Y, Hirayama A, Kishima H, Shimokawa T, Oshino S, Hirata M, Tani N, Kato A, Yoshimine T. Reduction of intractable deafferentation pain due to spinal cord or peripheral lesion by high-frequency repetitive transcranial magnetic stimulation of the primary motor cortex. J Neurosurg 2007;107:555–9.
124. Sampson S, Rome JD, Rummans TA. Slow-frequency rTMS reduces fibromyalgia pain. Pain Medicine 2006;7:115–8.
125. Sampson SM, Kung S, McAlpine DE, Sandroni P. The use of slow-frequency prefrontal repetitive transcranial magnetic stimulation in refractory neuropathic pain. J ECT 2011;27:33–7.
126. Senapati AK, Huntington PJ, Peng YB. Spinal dorsal horn neuron response to mechanical stimuli is decreased by electrical stimulation of the primary motor cortex. Brain Res 2005;1036:173–9.
127. Short EB, Borckardt JJ, Anderson BS, Frohman H, Beam W, Reeves ST, George MS. Ten sessions of adjunctive left prefrontal rTMS significantly reduces fibromyalgia pain: a randomized, controlled pilot study. Pain 2011;152:2477–84.
128. Silva G, Miksad R, Freedman SD, Pascual-Leone A, Jain S, Gomes DL, Amancio EJ, Boggio PS, Correa CF, Fregni F. Treatment of cancer pain with non-invasive brain stimulation. J Pain Symptom Manag 2007;34:342–5.
129. Sindou MP, Mertens P, Bendavid U, García-Larrea L, Mauguière F. Predictive value of somatosensory evoked potentials for long-lasting pain relief after spinal cord stimulation: practical use for patient selection. Neurosurgery 2003;52:1374–83.
130. Soler MD, Kumru H, Pelayo R, Vidal J, Tormos JM, Fregni F, Navarro X, Pascual-Leone A. Effectiveness of transcranial direct current stimulation and visual illusion on neuropathic pain in spinal cord injury. Brain 2010;133:2565–77.
131. Sparing R, Buelte D, Meister IG, Paus T, Fink GR. Transcranial magnetic stimulation and the challenge of coil placement: a comparison of conventional and stereotaxic neuronavigational strategies. Hum Brain Mapp 2008;29:82–96.
132. Tamura Y, Okabe S, Ohnishi T, N Saito D, Arai N, Mochio S, Inoue K, Ugawa Y. Effects of 1-Hz repetitive transcranial magnetic stimulation on acute pain induced by capsaicin. Pain 2004;107:107–15.
133. Taylor JJ, Borckardt JJ, Canterberry M, Li X, Hanlon CA, Brown TR, George MS. Naloxone-reversible modulation of pain circuitry by left prefrontal rTMS. Neuropsychopharmacology 2013;38:1189–97.
134. Taylor JJ, Borckardt JJ, George MS. Endogenous opioids mediate left dorsolateral prefrontal cortex rTMS-induced analgesia. Pain 2012;153:1219–25.
135. Thut G, Miniussi C. New insights into rhythmic brain activity from TMS-EEG studies. Trends Cogn Sci 2009;13:182–9.
136. Tsubokawa T, Katayama Y, Yamamoto T, Hirayama T, Koyama S. Chronic motor cortex stimulation for the treatment of central pain. Acta Neurochir (Wien) 1991;52(Suppl):137–9.
137. Tsubokawa T, Katayama Y, Yamamoto T, Hirayama T, Koyama S. Treatment of thalamic pain by chronic motor cortex stimulation. Pacing Clin Electrophysiol 1991;14:131–4.

138. Tsubokawa T, Katayama Y, Yamamoto T, Hirayama T, Koyama S. Chronic motor cortex stimulation in patients with thalamic pain. J Neurosurg 1993;78:393–401.

139. Valle A, Roizenblatt S, Botte S, Zaghi S, Riberto M, Tufik S, Boggio PS, Fregni F. Efficacy of anodal transcranial direct current stimulation (tDCS) for the treatment of fibromyalgia: results of a randomized, sham-controlled longitudinal clinical trial. J Pain Manag 2009;2:353–61.

140. Villamar MF, Wivatvongvana P, Patumanond J, Bikson M, Truong DQ, Datta A, Fregni F. Focal modulation of the primary motor cortex in fibromyalgia using 4×1-ring high-definition transcranial direct current stimulation (HD-tDCS): immediate and delayed analgesic effects of cathodal and anodal stimulation. J Pain 2013;14:371–83.

141. Villanueva L, Fields HL. Endogenous central mechanisms of pain modulation. In: Villanueva L, Dickenson AH, Ollat H, editors. Progress in pain research and management, Vol. 31, The pain system in normal and pathological states: a primer for clinicians. Seattle, WA: IASP Press; 2004. pp. 223–46.

142. Wager TD, Atlas LY, Lindquist MA, Roy M, Woo CW, Kross E. An fMRI-based neurologic signature of physical pain. N Engl J Med 2013;368:1388–97.

143. Wrigley PJ, Gustin SM, McIndoe LN, Chakiath RJ, Henderson LA, Siddall PJ. Longstanding neuropathic pain after spinal cord injury is refractory to transcranial direct current stimulation: a randomized controlled trial. Pain 2013;154:2178–84.

144. Zaghi S, Thiele B, Pimentel D, Pimentel T, Fregni F. Assessment and treatment of pain with non-invasive cortical stimulation. Restor Neurol Neurosci 2011;29:439–51.

145. Zaghi S, Heine N, Fregni F. Brain stimulation for the treatment of pain: a review of costs, clinical effects, and mechanisms of treatment for three different central neuromodulatory approaches. J Pain Manag 2009;2:339–52.

CHAPTER 10

Spinal Cord fMRI to Study Pain Processing in Humans

Christian Sprenger and Christian Büchel

While numerous brain regions exhibit considerable species-specific differences, the spinal cord displays a high degree of structural similarity across vertebrates, pointing at its uniform functional relevance for the vertebrate's organism. As the spinal cord is the site where a substantial amount of information enters and leaves the CNS, it takes a key position related to a number of basic functions of the CNS, such as motor responses, autonomic functions, and the processing and forwarding of somatosensory and nociceptive signals. In the context of pain, the spinal cord is of peculiar interest for several reasons. The dorsal horn of the spinal cord contains the first synapse of the pain pathway, which is a site of important nociceptive modulation, either by descending systems from the brainstem or by local propriospinal mechanisms. Furthermore, a link between the nociceptive system and the autonomic nervous system can be found in the spinal cord, and cross-modal interactions, for instance with itch, can be observed. The cord is a well-known site for central sensitization and pain chronification processes, and it most likely plays an important role in the context of different pain syndromes. As the neurophysiological assessment of spinal cord function is difficult in humans, most knowledge about spinal cord pain processing is derived from neurophysiological experiments in animals. However, in the last decade, studying spinal nociceptive processing in humans became possible through noninvasive imaging techniques. This is especially important in view of the known limitations of animal research, such as the difficulty of studying modulatory effects of higher cognitive functions on basic pain processing.

CHALLENGES IN SPINAL fMRI AND SOLUTION APPROACHES

While fMRI of the brain is well established, with more than 20,000 papers published (2013), fMRI of the spinal cord can still be considered in a development phase, with a limited number of publications and research institutes employing this technique. First reports of spinal fMRI already appeared in the 1990s [55, 66], and although the results display lower reproducibility compared with the brain [6, 23], fMRI of the spinal cord has been shown to be feasible in both humans and animals and has provided important insights into human physiology [16, 21, 36, 42, 50].

fMRI of the spinal cord is more challenging than that of the brain [23, 27, 52]. First, the spinal cord has a very small cross-sectional diameter (at the level of the sixth cervical segment about 12 mm in the left–right and 8 mm in the anterior–posterior direction [31]) with an even smaller embedded grey matter structure. To reliably distinguish blood oxygenation level–dependent (BOLD) responses within the four quadrants of the spinal cord, a high in-plane resolution (typically about 1×1 mm^2) is indispensable. As the signal-to-noise ratio (SNR) is a direct function of the voxel volume, investigators usually increase the slice thickness (typically about 5 mm). Increased slice thickness can be tolerable or even advantageous with regard to the columnar histological organization of the grey matter structure within the spinal cord but creates the risk of generating partial volume effects between the spinal cord and the CSF, and also between the grey and white matter structure within the spinal cord. Consequently, most spinal fMRI studies use axial slice orientation perpendicular to the spinal cord, which offers high in-plane resolution. Alternatively, a sagittal slice orientation can be used, which allows covering the spinal cord with only a few slices. However, this approach usually employs a lower spatial resolution.

Second, compared with the brain, there is a much higher inhomogeneity of the magnetic flux density in the region of the vertebral column. Static magnetic field inhomogeneities are caused by differences of the magnetic susceptibilities between adjacent tissues, especially between the vertebral bodies and the vertebral disks [14, 35]. The observed artefacts are typically periodic signal dropouts due to intravoxel dephasing along the rostrocaudal axis and distortions in echo-planar imaging (EPI) images. Therefore, optimizing the shimming procedure to reduce B0 inhomogeneities is crucial in spinal fMRI [17, 24]. Additional dynamic field inhomogeneities are induced by the periodically changing amount of air in the measured volume during the respiratory cycle [63].

An elegant solution to minimize signal dropouts due to static field inhomogeneities is the "z-shim" approach [17]. It is realized by a slice-specific gradient offset that individually reduces the T_2^*-relevant intravoxel dephasing and therefore also increases the overall signal intensity within the spinal cord. Another proposed approach is to acquire several thin slices and then average them together [24], which reduces morphology-induced intravoxel dephasing and related signal dropouts, albeit with the cost of longer repetition time (TR). Another approach to circumvent inhomogeneity-related artefacts is the use of T2-weighted fast spin-echo sequences [29, 56]. Fast spin-echo protocols can produce images with less distortion, but are at the same time considerably less BOLD sensitive than T_2^*-weighted images [3, 6, 44]. The involvement of an additional contrast mechanism in fast spin-echo sequences by extravascular protons was discussed [57].

Compared with the brain, static image SNR is lower in the spinal cord [13], which contributes to the reduced BOLD sensitivity of spinal fMRI. The reasons for reduced static SNR are, mainly, lower sensitivity of receiver coils in this region and the above-mentioned susceptibility artefacts. Compared with the static SNR, temporal SNR, defined as the ratio of the voxel's mean signal intensity over a given time period and its standard deviation, is an even better indicator of the sensitivity of the experimental system to detect BOLD changes in an fMRI experiment [45]. However, in addition, the temporal SNR is typically considerably reduced in spinal fMRI experiments compared with the brain (about 40% in [13]). This reduction results from the low static SNR and the considerable signal variability over time owing to the influence of physiological noise, which is of greater magnitude at the spinal level compared with the brain.

There are several physiological sources contributing to the strong signal variability at the spinal level in a complex manner, among which cardiac- and respiratory-related effects, including their interactions and secondary effects, such as CSF pulsations seem to be most important. For instance, the CSF pulsation is a consequence of the transient increase in intracranial blood volume during the cardiac cycle, leading to a highly variable signal in the subarachnoid space in the low frequency range [20]. The spinal cord itself moves in a craniocaudal oscillatory fashion during the cardiac cycle with a maximal caudal displacement of 0.5–1 mm [41]. The precise physiological noise characteristics in spinal fMRI were the object of several studies [5, 8, 20, 28, 46, 63, 64]. To reduce artefacts related to physiological movements, some of the spinal fMRI studies used cardiac gating [2, 54], flow rephasing, and/or spatial saturation pulses during the acquisition of the images [16, 21, 50]. Furthermore, external physiological measurements such as the recording of respiratory-related chest movements, ECG, or pulsoxymetric pulse curve to capture the cardiac cycle, and a subsequent physiological noise modelling during the data analysis are crucial for spinal fMRI [8, 32, 46]. Different approaches have been developed over time to account for the influence of physiological noise during the statistical analysis [8, 15, 26, 30, 64]. Of these approaches, the finite-impulse-response (FIR) function-based selective averaging approach of Deckers et al. [15] and the Fourier expansion–based RETROICOR approach by Glover et al. [8, 26] are currently frequently applied. A detailed introduction to physiological noise modelling for spinal fMRI is beyond the scope of this chapter and can be found elsewhere [8, 32].

Besides cardiac, respiratory, and CSF-related effects, movements of voluntary muscles are a particular challenge in spinal fMRI. Movements of neck muscles, for example, have a much stronger influence on the functional images compared with the brain. They not only constitute the dominating part of the image volume but can also cause considerable deformation of the spinal cord. Immobilization collars or vacuum mats are therefore a useful measure to minimize changes in neck position [65]. Finally, task-related motion represents a particular risk in spinal fMRI as even small movements within the submillimeter range correlated with the experimental factor of interest can produce a pattern of false-positive activity or obscure true BOLD responses. This has to be considered when designing the experimental paradigm.

HEMODYNAMIC RESPONSE IN THE SPINAL CORD

Given that fMRI relies on the BOLD effect, and the well-known fact that the hemodynamic response function varies across the brain [1], questions arise about the characteristics of the BOLD response in the spinal cord. Although the complex mechanisms underlying the BOLD contrast in the brain are still not fully clarified, there is no doubt that similar basic contrast mechanisms also apply to the spinal cord. On the basis of the fine vascular architecture and the orientation of blood vessels within the spinal cord [60], responses are expected to be at least distinguishable in the four quadrants of the spinal cord [23] even if the precise localization of expected BOLD responses is a subject of debate [13, 37, 62, 67]. Early animal studies measuring blood flow in the spinal cord using microelectrodes reported a similar regulation of blood flow within the grey matter of spinal cord compared with the brain and showed localized responses spatially close to neuronal activity [40, 43]. More recently, intrinsic optical imaging studies measuring neural activity in the dorsal horn evoked by peripheral nerve stimulation confirmed the assumption of a circumscribed hemodynamic response in the spinal cord [7, 49].

fMRI STUDIES INVESTIGATING NOCICEPTIVE PROCESSING IN THE SPINAL CORD

In a pioneering rodent spinal fMRI study, Pórszász et al. [48] observed MR signal alterations after subcutaneous injection of formalin into the hind paw in the ipsilateral lumbar spinal cord in the segments L4–L5, temporally corresponding to the animal's pain-related licking behaviour. In subsequent studies, similar responses in the rodent's dorsal horn could be detected by employing different kinds of noxious stimulation, such as capsaicin injection or electrical stimulation [33, 34, 37–39]. Lilja et al. [34], for example, reported BOLD responses in the ipsilateral lumbar dorsal horn of rats that received electrical stimulation of the hind paw. The magnitude and extent of the observed responses in the spinal cord clearly mirrored the intensity of electrical stimulation. Interestingly, the observed spinal BOLD responses could be significantly suppressed by systemic administration of morphine, and, furthermore, this suppression could be reversed by administration of the unselective opioid antagonist naloxone. In a different series of experiments, Zhao et al. [67–69] showed that BOLD responses to noxious stimulation can be reliably detected in the dorsal horn at different spinal levels. Additionally, they were able to show that local injections of lidocaine, inducing a blockage of peripheral nerve transmission, abolished all stimulation-induced fMRI signals and that intravenous administration of lidocaine likewise reduced the observed responses [69]. Lawrence et al. [33] investigated neuronal activity in the rat cervical and lumbar spinal cord by using functional MRI and immunohistochemistry. *C-fos*-stained cells were predominantly found between the spinal segments L4 and L6, and C5–C7 after noxious electrical stimulation of the hind paw and forepaw, respectively. Importantly, they observed an overall good correspondence between pain-related neuronal activities determined by functional MRI and by *c-fos* labelling, which is, furthermore, in accordance with early autoradiographic data [12, 47]. Taken together, these studies demonstrate that spinal fMRI in rodents at high field strength is a reliable tool to visualize nociception in the spinal cord, providing insights in accordance with basic neurophysiological concepts of pain processing regarding spatial distribution and laterality and even suited for investigating pharmacological modulations of spinal pain processing.

Yoshizawa et al. [66], in the first published spinal fMRI study in humans, investigated neuronal activity in the cervical spinal cord in response to a hand-closing task in healthy volunteers. This study was able to demonstrate an ipsilateral BOLD increase in the ventral and intermediate grey matter structure in corresponding spinal segments. On the basis of this encouraging work, other groups started to investigate neuronal responses to somatosensory and nociceptive stimuli in the human spinal cord. For the first demonstration of spinal responses to painful stimulation, Backes et al. [2] used electrical stimulation of the median nerve and cardiac-gated fMRI with both a sagittal and a transverse slice orientation. In the sagittal plane, signal increases could be detected in five of seven volunteers in the cervical segments C4–T1, whereas in the transverse imaging plane, signal responses could be found only in two of six volunteers. Subsequently, Stroman et al. [11, 22, 53, 58] investigated in a number of studies the feasibility of imaging somatosensory and nociceptive processing in the human spinal cord by employing a T2-weighted single-shot fast spin-echo protocol. Ghazni et al. [22], for instance, reported responses to tactile stimulation with two different von Frey filaments (2 and 15 g) throughout the spinal cord, brainstem, and thalamus. Surprisingly, the responses in the ipsilateral cervical dorsal horn were stronger for the 2 g von Frey filament compared with the 15 g, which was interpreted as descending inhibition from brainstem nuclei.

Using a segmented gradient echo EPI sequence, Summers et al. [59] observed spinal cord BOLD responses, which were significantly stronger for noxious laser stimuli (activating predominantly Aδ fibres) than for innocuous soft brushing (activating predominantly Aβ fibres). This was the first study to assess false-positive detection rates in the spinal cord obtained by a separate measurement while volunteers were at rest. Importantly, the number of activated voxels in response to laser stimulation was found to exceed the false-positive level. While this study found bilateral responses to both stimuli, more recent studies provided evidence for a predominant ipsilateral BOLD response to noxious stimulation in the

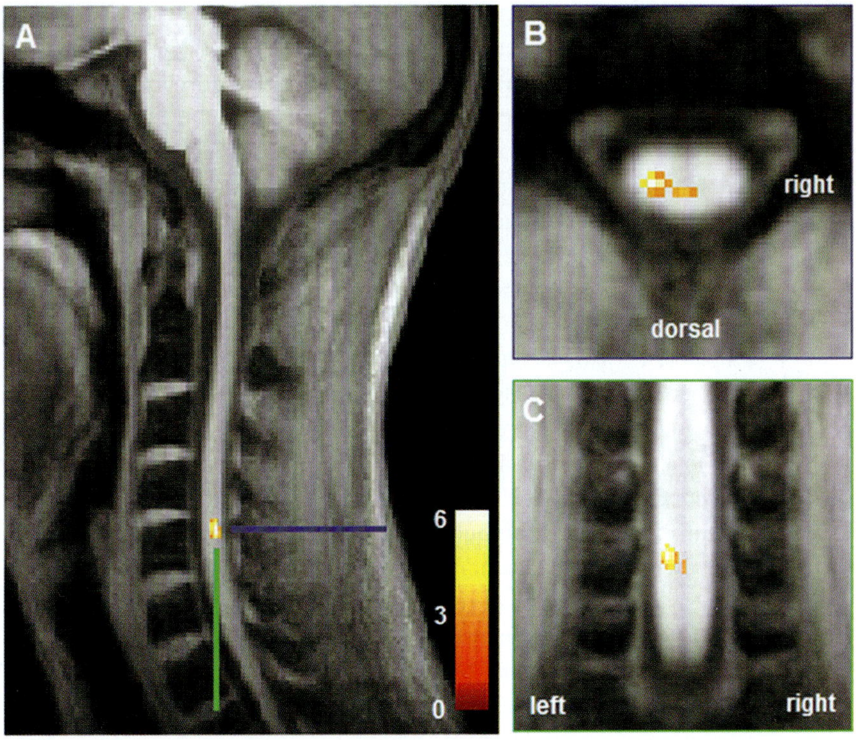

FIGURE 10-1 Pain-related BOLD responses in the spinal cord [50]. Pain-related BOLD responses are overlaid on the mean structural T1-weighted image of all participants. Painful thermal stimuli were applied with a 30×30 mm^2 Peltier thermode to the left radial forearm (dermatome C6). **A:** The sagittal section allows an identification of the spinal level of the BOLD response. The blue and the green lines indicate the transverse and coronal level of **(B)** and **(C)**, respectively. The color bar indicates *t*-values. **B** and **C:** The BOLD response is located ipsilateral to the side of stimulation in the dorsal horn of the spinal cord. The visualization threshold is set to an uncorrected level of $P < 0.005$.

spinal cord [9, 16, 42, 50] (see Fig. 10-1). Brooks et al. [9] reported responses in the ipsilateral half of the spinal cord, which were significantly stronger compared with the contralateral half for both painful thermal and nonpainful tactile stimulation. In a recent study, Nash et al. [42] were able to demonstrate BOLD responses not only corresponding to the side of stimulation but also following a segmental pattern in the spinal cord. Noxious thermal stimulation of the deltoid and thenar region led to activations at clearly distinguishable craniocaudal levels of the spinal cord. Not only are these findings in accordance with the neuroanatomy of the nociceptive system, but they also confirm findings from spinal animal fMRI studies at high field strength [34, 67], and are furthermore in line with neurophysiological studies employing different methodological approaches to characterize the spinal response to noxious stimulation [7, 12, 19, 40, 47, 49]. They therefore suggest that functional MRI of basic features of pain processing such as laterality and intensity in the human spinal cord is feasible, and highlight the possibility of noninvasively imaging endogenous pain modulation at the level of the spinal cord.

Using a placebo cream paradigm in combination with painful thermal stimulation and spinal fMRI, Eippert et al. [16] were able to demonstrate how descending pain modulation can emerge already at the level of the dorsal horn in humans. Thermal stimulation of the left radial forearm generated a BOLD response in the ipsilateral dorsal horn in the spinal segment C6 that was significantly reduced when participants believed that they would be treated with a strongly acting analgesic cream. Together with previous imaging studies (see Chapter 19), the involvement of all key regions of the descending pain modulatory system in placebo analgesia was hence demonstrated. It became obvious that psychological factors, which are known predictors of pain chronification, have the ability to influence nociceptive processing already at the level of the spinal cord, which in turn has been extensively characterized in the animal as a site for central sensitization processes. The results therefore establish an important new link. In line with this, a recent study by Geuter and Büchel [21] showed that negative expectations can also influence nociceptive responses in the spinal cord. While there is evidence that the psychological and neuronal mechanisms underlying nocebo hyperalgesia are distinct from placebo analgesia [4], the expectation of receiving a supposedly pain-facilitating capsaicin cream enhances spinal cord responses to noxious stimulation. Reassuringly, both studies used the same site of stimulation and observed the main effect of pain approximately at the same site in the ipsilateral part of the spinal cord. Due to a refined acquisition technique [17], BOLD responses were clearly stronger in the study of Geuter and Büchel [21], though. However, the modulation of the spinal cords' processing of nociceptive stimuli seems not to be limited to expectation-related mechanisms. In a recent study, we demonstrated that also simple distraction from pain by a working memory task is capable of reducing pain-related neuronal activity in the spinal cord [50]. High levels of distraction by working memory load led not only to reduced pain perception but also to reduced spinal cord BOLD responses. As the behavioural effect could be partially inhibited by application of the opioid receptor blocker naloxone [50], pain modulation by attentional mechanisms appears to be partially opioid dependent, similar to placebo analgesia (see Chapter 19). Together, these results suggest the assumption that modulation of pain-related activity in the spinal cord by descending influences from supraspinal centres could be a common mechanism underlying different types of endogenous pain modulation [61] serving a recurrent hierarchical system that allows for biological adaptability in the sense of predictive coding [10]. In such a framework, the dorsal horn of the spinal cord can be viewed as one site where incoming nociceptive signals are matched with top-down predictions. This highlights the necessity of studying the functional interplay between the brain and the spinal cord for a more comprehensive understanding of pain processing.

FUTURE DIRECTIONS

While for fMRI of the brain widely accepted standards regarding most relevant issues from data acquisition up to reporting results exist, fMRI of the spinal cord is still under development. To strengthen the basis for spinal cord BOLD fMRI and to increase its reproducibility, the main tasks are related to a better characterization of the foundational physiological phenomena in the spinal cord, improved MRI acquisition protocols, and the optimization and standardization of data analysis strategies. For example, a more thorough description of the neurovascular coupling at the spinal level, which might differ from that in the brain [43], would help to better model the relationship between neuronal activity, vascular response, physiological noise, and the MR signal.

Ongoing improvements in spinal fMRI can be expected by technically refining the acquisition technique. This refers to the employment of more elaborated shimming approaches [17, 18] or repeated recordings of field maps [63], the employment of optimized pulse sequences such as the application of spiral k-space trajectories [25, 42] or multiband EPI, CSF-suppression strategies, saturation bands, or slice-specific gradient offsets [17] to reduce image artefacts. The development of specifically dedicated MR coils and usage of higher field strengths might further help to improve the sensitivity, although despite increasing SNR, higher field strength also increases image artefacts such as distortions and signal dropouts.

With regard to the analysis of spinal fMRI data, it will be important to optimize and standardize preprocessing strategies adapted to the peculiarities of the anatomical region. Currently, there is no standard anatomical template of the spinal cord, and normalization approaches used for the brain are less suited for spinal cord data. Furthermore, the location of spinal segments varies in relation to the vertebral bodies. In order to allow for a comparison of results between different studies, the use of a standardized anatomical space or at least an unambiguous assignment of the activations to the spinal segments is indispensable.

Finally, with the progress in spinal cord fMRI over the last few years, interest in targeting its functional interaction with the brain has also increased. Studies investigating the functional connectivity between the brain and the spinal cord would be very informative with regard to key issues of endogenous pain modulation and its alteration in pathological conditions. To this end, we recently developed a practical approach that allows the consecutive acquisition of the brain and the cervical spinal cord within one measurement employing two fields of view and a dynamic update of linear shim terms and resonance frequency [18] (see Fig. 10-2). Such a specialized acquisition protocol provides benefits compared

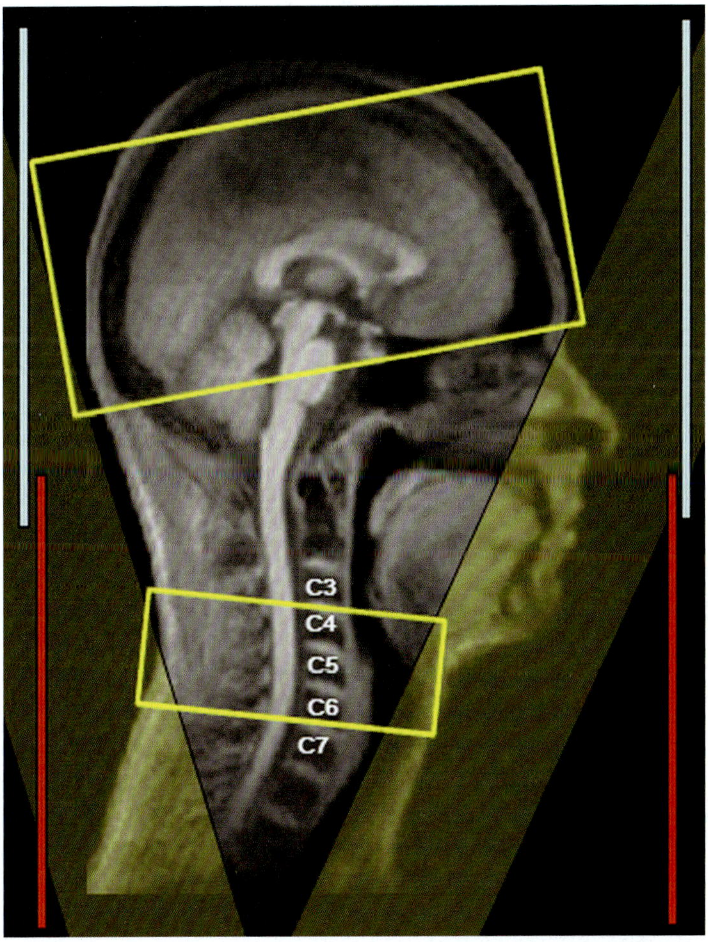

FIGURE 10-2 Illustration of the geometric setup for combined measurements of the brain and the spinal cord. The two subvolumes *(yellow)* with different image resolutions are individually positioned to the brain and the spinal cord, respectively. The green and the red lines indicate the locations of the head coil *(green)* and neck coil *(red)* relative to the volunteer. Saturation pulses *(transparent yellow)* are applied anterior and posterior to the spinal cord in a V-shaped manner.

with a coverage of the entire head and neck region [13] as geometric parameters such as slice thickness, in-plane resolution, and plane tilting can be individually adapted to the requirements of each region and hence also the timing (i.e., receiver bandwidth, echo spacing, echo time) can be optimized. As the optimal shimming parameters usually differ considerably between the brain and the spinal cord, which can cause significant image artefacts (see above), we additionally implemented a dynamic update of linear shim terms applying the optimized shim currents during the acquisition of the respective region. This approach allows acquiring optimized EPI of both regions within an appropriate TR suited to study the functional interplay between the brain and the spinal cord in future studies [18, 51].

REFERENCES

1. Aguirre GK, Zarahn E, D'esposito M. The variability of human, BOLD hemodynamic responses. NeuroImage 1998;8:360–9.
2. Backes WH, Mess WH, Wilmink JT. Functional MR imaging of the cervical spinal cord by use of median nerve stimulation and fist clenching. Am J Neuroradiol 2001;22:1854–9.
3. Bandettini PA, Wong EC, Jesmanowicz A, Hinks RS, Hyde JS. Spin-echo and gradient-echo EPI of human brain activation using BOLD contrast: a comparative study at 1.5 T. NMR Biomed 1994;7:12–20.
4. Benedetti F, Amanzio M, Vighetti S, Asteggiano G. The biochemical and neuroendocrine bases of the hyperalgesic nocebo effect. J Neurosci 2006;26:12014–22.
5. Bosma RL, Stroman PW. Assessment of data acquisition parameters, and analysis techniques for noise reduction in spinal cord fMRI data. Magn Reson Imaging 2014;32(5):473–81.
6. Bouwman CJC, Wilmink JT, Mess WH, Backes WH. Spinal cord functional MRI at 3 T: gradient echo echo-planar imaging versus turbo spin echo. NeuroImage 2008;43:288–96.
7. Brieu N, Beaumont E, Dubeau S, Cohen-Adad J, Lesage F. Characterization of the hemodynamic response in the rat lumbar spinal cord using intrinsic optical imaging and laser speckle. J Neurosci Methods 2010;191:151–7.
8. Brooks JC, Beckmann CF, Miller KL, Wise RG, Porro CA, Tracey I, Jenkinson M. Physiological noise modelling for spinal functional magnetic resonance imaging studies. Neuroimage 2008;39:680–92.
9. Brooks JC, Kong Y, Lee MC, Warnaby CE, Wanigasekera V, Jenkinson M, Tracey I. Stimulus site and modality dependence of functional activity within the human spinal cord. J Neurosci 2012;32:6231–9.
10. Büchel C, Geuter S, Sprenger C, Eippert F. Placebo analgesia: a predictive coding perspective. Neuron 2014;81: 1223–39.
11. Cahill CM, Stroman PW. Mapping of neural activity produced by thermal pain in the healthy human spinal cord and brain stem: a functional magnetic resonance imaging study. Magn Reson Imaging 2011;29:342–52.
12. Coghill RC, Price DD, Hayes RL, Mayer DJ. Spatial distribution of nociceptive processing in the rat spinal cord. J. Neurophysiol 1991;65:133–140.
13. Cohen-Adad J, Gauthier CJ, Brooks JCW, Slessarev M, Han J, Fisher JA, Rossignol S, Hoge RD. BOLD signal responses to controlled hypercapnia in human spinal cord. NeuroImage 2010;50:1074–84.
14. Cooke FJ, Blamire AM, Manners DN, Styles P, Rajagopalan B. Quantitative proton magnetic resonance spectroscopy of the cervical spinal cord. Magn Reson Med 2004;51:1122–8.
15. Deckers RH, van Gelderen P, Ries M, Barret O, Duyn JH, Ikonomidou VN, Fukunaga M, Glover GH, de Zwart JA. An adaptive filter for suppression of cardiac and respiratory noise in MRI time series data. NeuroImage 2006;33: 1072–81.
16. Eippert F, Finsterbusch J, Bingel U, Büchel C. Direct evidence for spinal cord involvement in placebo analgesia. Science 2009;326:404.
17. Finsterbusch J, Eippert F, Büchel C. Single, slice-specific z-shim gradient pulses improve T2*-weighted imaging of the spinal cord. NeuroImage 2012;59:2307–15.
18. Finsterbusch J, Sprenger C, Büchel C. Combined T2*-weighted measurements of the human brain and cervical spinal cord with a dynamic shim update. NeuroImage 2013;79:153–61.
19. Fitzgerald M. The contralateral input to the dorsal horn of the spinal cord in the decerebrate spinal rat. Brain Res 1982;236:275–87.
20. Friese S, Hamhaber U, Erb M, Klose U. B-waves in cerebral and spinal cerebrospinal fluid pulsation measurement by magnetic resonance imaging. J Comput Assist Tomogr 2004;28:255–62.
21. Geuter S, Büchel C. Facilitation of pain in the human spinal cord by nocebo treatment. J Neurosci 2013;33: 13784–90.

22. Ghazni NF, Cahill CM, Stroman PW. Tactile sensory and pain networks in the human spinal cord and brain stem mapped by means of functional MR imaging. AJNR Am J Neuroradiol 2010;31:661–7.
23. Giove F, Garreffa G, Giulietti G, Mangia S, Colonnese C, Maraviglia B. Issues about the fMRI of the human spinal cord. Magn Reson Imaging 2004;22:1505–16.
24. Glover GH. 3D z-shim method for reduction of susceptibility effects in BOLD fMRI. Magn Reson Med 1999;42:290–9.
25. Glover GH, Law CS. Spiral-in/out BOLD fMRI for increased SNR and reduced susceptibility artifacts. Magn Reson Med 2001;46:515–22.
26. Glover GH, Li TQ, Ress D. Image-based method for retrospective correction of physiological motion effects in fMRI: RETROICOR. Magn Reson Med 2000;44:162–7.
27. Govers N, Béghin J, Van Goethem JWM, Michiels J, van den Hauwe L, Vandervliet E, Parizel PM. Functional MRI of the cervical spinal cord on 1.5 T with fingertapping: to what extent is it feasible? Neuroradiology 2007;49:73–81.
28. Greitz D, Franck A, Nordell B. On the pulsatile nature of intracranial and spinal CSF-circulation demonstrated by MR imaging. Acta Radiol 1993;34:321–8.
29. Hennig J, Nauerth A, Friedburg H. RARE imaging: a fast imaging method for clinical MR. Magn Reson Med 1986;3:823–33.
30. Hu X, Le TH, Parrish T, Erhard P. Retrospective estimation and correction of physiological fluctuation in functional MRI. Magn Reson Med 1995;34:201–12.
31. Ko H-Y, Park JH, Shin YB, Baek SY. Gross quantitative measurements of spinal cord segments in human. Spinal Cord 2004;42:35–40.
32. Kong Y, Jenkinson M, Andersson J, Tracey I, Brooks JCW. Assessment of physiological noise modelling methods for functional imaging of the spinal cord. NeuroImage 2012;60:1538–49.
33. Lawrence J, Stroman PW, Bascaramurty S, Jordan LM, Malisza KL. Correlation of functional activation in the rat spinal cord with neuronal activation detected by immunohistochemistry. NeuroImage 2004;22:1802–7.
34. Lilja J, Endo T, Hofstetter C, Westman E, Young J, Olson L, Spenger C. Blood oxygenation level-dependent visualization of synaptic relay stations of sensory pathways along the neuroaxis in response to graded sensory stimulation of a limb. J Neurosci 2006;26:6330–6.
35. Maieron M, Iannetti GD, Bodurka J, Tracey I, Bandettini PA, Porro CA. Functional responses in the human spinal cord during willed motor actions: evidence for side- and rate-dependent activity. J Neurosci 2007;27:4182–90.
36. Mainero C, Zhang W-T, Kumar A, Rosen BR, Sorensen AG. Mapping the spinal and supraspinal pathways of dynamic mechanical allodynia in the human trigeminal system using cardiac-gated fMRI. NeuroImage 2007;35:1201–10.
37. Majcher K, Tomanek B, Jasinski A, Foniok T, Stroman PW, Tuor UI, Kirk D, Hess G. Simultaneous functional magnetic resonance imaging in the rat spinal cord and brain. Exp Neurol 2006;197:458–64.
38. Majcher K, Tomanek B, Tuor UI, Jasinski A, Foniok T, Rushforth D, Hess G. Functional magnetic resonance imaging within the rat spinal cord following peripheral nerve injury. NeuroImage 2007;38:669–76.
39. Malisza KL, Stroman PW. Functional imaging of the rat cervical spinal cord. J Magn Reson Imaging 2002;16:553–8.
40. Marcus ML, Heistad DD, Ehrhardt JC, Abboud FM. Regulation of total and regional spinal cord blood flow. Circ Res 1977;41:128–34.
41. Mikulis DJ, Wood ML, Zerdoner OA, Poncelet BP. Oscillatory motion of the normal cervical spinal cord. Radiology 1994;192:117–21.
42. Nash P, Wiley K, Brown J, Shinaman R, Ludlow D, Sawyer A-M, Glover G, Mackey S. Functional magnetic resonance imaging identifies somatotopic organization of nociception in the human spinal cord. Pain 2013;154:776–81.
43. Nix W, Capra NF, Erdmann W, Halsey JH. Comparison of vascular reactivity in spinal cord and brain. Stroke J Cereb Circ 1976;7:560–3.
44. Parkes LM, Schwarzbach JV, Bouts AA, Deckers RHR, Pullens P, Kerskens CM, Norris DG. Quantifying the spatial resolution of the gradient echo and spin echo BOLD response at 3 tesla. Magn Reson Med 2005;54:1465–72.
45. Parrish TB, Gitelman DR, LaBar KS, Mesulam MM. Impact of signal-to-noise on functional MRI. Magn Reson Med 2000;44:925–32.
46. Piché M, Cohen-Adad J, Nejad MK, Perlbarg V, Xie G, Beaudoin G, Benali H, Rainville P. Characterization of cardiac-related noise in fMRI of the cervical spinal cord. Magn Reson Imaging 2009;27:300–10.
47. Porro CA, Cavazzuti M, Galetti A, Sassatelli L, Barbieri GC. Functional activity mapping of the rat spinal cord during formalin-induced noxious stimulation. Neuroscience 1991;41:655–65.

48. Pórszász R, Beckmann N, Bruttel K, Urban L, Rudin M. Signal changes in the spinal cord of the rat after injection of formalin into the hindpaw: characterization using functional magnetic resonance imaging. Proc Natl Acad Sci USA 1997;94:5034–9.
49. Sasaki S, Yazawa I, Miyakawa N, Mochida H, Shinomiya K, Kamino K, Momose-Sato Y, Sato K. Optical imaging of intrinsic signals induced by peripheral nerve stimulation in the in vivo rat spinal cord. NeuroImage 2002;17:1240–55.
50. Sprenger C, Eippert F, Finsterbusch J, Bingel U, Rose M, Büchel C. Attention modulates spinal cord responses to pain. Curr Biol 2012;22:1019–22.
51. Sprenger C, Finsterbusch J, Büchel C. Spinal cord-midbrain functional connectivity is related to perceived pain intensity: a combined spino-cortical fMRI study. J Neurosci 2015;35:4248–57.
52. Stroman PW. Magnetic resonance imaging of neuronal function in the spinal cord: spinal FMRI. Clin Med Res 2005;3:146.
53. Stroman PW, Kornelsen J, Bergman A, Krause V, Ethans K, Malisza KL, Tomanek B. Noninvasive assessment of the injured human spinal cord by means of functional magnetic resonance imaging. Spinal Cord 2004;42:59–66.
54. Stroman PW, Krause V, Malisza KL, Frankenstein UN, Tomanek B. Functional magnetic resonance imaging of the human cervical spinal cord with stimulation of different sensory dermatomes. Magn Reson Imaging 2002;20:1–6.
55. Stroman PW, Nance PW, Ryner LN. BOLD MRI of the human cervical spinal cord at 3 tesla. Magn Reson Med 1999;42:571–6.
56. Stroman PW, Ryner LN. Functional MRI of motor and sensory activation in the human spinal cord. Magn Reson Imaging 2001;19:27–32.
57. Stroman PW, Tomanek B, Krause V, Frankenstein UN, Malisza KL. Functional magnetic resonance imaging of the human brain based on signal enhancement by extravascular protons (SEEP fMRI). Magn Reson Med 2003;49:433–9.
58. Stroman PW, Tomanek B, Krause V, Frankenstein UN, Malisza KL. Mapping of neuronal function in the healthy and injured human spinal cord with spinal fMRI. NeuroImage 2002;17:1854–60.
59. Summers PE, Ferraro D, Duzzi D, Lui F, Iannetti GD, Porro CA. A quantitative comparison of BOLD fMRI responses to noxious and innocuous stimuli in the human spinal cord. NeuroImage 2010;50:1408–15.
60. Thron AK. Vascular anatomy of the spinal cord: neurological investigations and clinical syndromes. New York, NY: Springer Verlag; 1988.
61. Tracey I, Mantyh PW. The cerebral signature for pain perception and its modulation. Neuron 2007;55:377–391.
62. Turner R. How much cortex can a vein drain? Downstream dilution of activation-related cerebral blood oxygenation changes. NeuroImage 2002;16:1062–67.
63. Verma T, Cohen-Adad J. Effect of respiration on the B0 field in the human spinal cord at 3T. Magn Reson Med 2014:72(6)1629–36.
64. Xie G, Piché M, Khoshnejad M, Perlbarg V, Chen J-I, Hoge RD, Benali H, Rossignol S, Rainville P, Cohen-Adad J. Reduction of physiological noise with independent component analysis improves the detection of nociceptive responses with fMRI of the human spinal cord. NeuroImage 2012;63:245–52.
65. Yiannakas MC, Kearney H, Samson RS, Chard DT, Ciccarelli O, Miller DH, Wheeler-Kingshott CAM. Feasibility of grey matter and white matter segmentation of the upper cervical cord in vivo: a pilot study with application to magnetisation transfer measurements. NeuroImage 2012;63:1054–9.
66. Yoshizawa T, Nose T, Moore GJ, Sillerud LO. Functional magnetic resonance imaging of motor activation in the human cervical spinal cord. Neuroimage 1996;4:174–82.
67. Zhao F, Williams M, Meng X, Welsh DC, Coimbra A, Crown ED, Cook JJ, Urban MO, Hargreaves R, Williams DS. BOLD and blood volume-weighted fMRI of rat lumbar spinal cord during non-noxious and noxious electrical hindpaw stimulation. NeuroImage 2008;40:133–47.
68. Zhao F, Williams M, Meng X, Welsh DC, Grachev ID, Hargreaves R, Williams DS. Pain fMRI in rat cervical spinal cord: an echo planar imaging evaluation of sensitivity of BOLD and blood volume-weighted fMRI. NeuroImage 2009;44:349–62.
69. Zhao F, Williams M, Welsh DC, Meng X, Ritter A, Abbadie C, Cook JJ, Reicin AS, Hargreaves R, Williams DS. fMRI investigation of the effect of local and systemic lidocaine on noxious electrical stimulation-induced activation in spinal cord. Pain 2009;145:110–9.

CHAPTER 11

Neuroimaging the Genomics of Pain Processing

Ulrike Bingel and Jeffrey S. Mogil

INTERINDIVIDUAL VARIABILITY

The significant interindividual variability in pain behaviour and its contributing factors remains a pervasive clinical challenge and has generated intense scientific investigations in this field. Recent studies indicate that our genes considerably influence nociceptive information processing, how our nociceptive system copes with peripheral injury, and the individual response to analgesic treatments. Neuroimaging studies of pain are beginning to link such genetic influences with physiological processes in the human brain. This chapter reviews the pioneering endeavours of neuroimaging pain genes in humans and indicates potential future directions.

Experimental studies using standardized pain stimuli confirm remarkable individual differences in thresholds, tolerance, and psychophysical ratings [64]; for review, see [55]. These interindividual differences are reflected in simultaneously obtained measures of brain activity [1, 10, 16]. The correlation of brain activity with pain report makes artefacts or scale misuse unlikely and permits brain activity to serve as an intermediate phenotype of pain behaviour, with the important caveat that no brain areas are specific for nociceptive processing [58]. Studies of chronic pain conditions that develop after specific traumatic or infectious events (e.g., chronic back pain after disc herniation, postherpetic neuralgia after herpes zoster) reveal that only a small proportion of patients develop chronic pain [15, 74, 76]. Significant variability has also been documented for the individual response to analgesic treatments, including opioids, placebo, and other analgesics [2, 10, 75, 80].

This chapter aims to (a) provide a brief introduction to the genetic variability in human pain behaviour; (b) highlight the initial experiments in the emerging field of neuroimaging investigations of pain genes; and (c) offer a perspective on how genetic information may be successfully combined with modern neuroimaging techniques in the future. A comprehensive overview of the vast and rapidly evolving field of pain genetics in both animals and humans and applied methodologies is beyond the scope of this chapter. For comprehensive recent reviews of this field, see [19, 26, 46, 55] and the *Pain Genes Database* [42].

HERITABILITY OF PAIN TRAITS IN HUMANS

Ethnic and familial aggregation of pain behaviour and several clinical pain conditions have repeatedly been reported in the literature [21, 23, 40, 41, 84]. The heightened pain sensitivity in subjects with a parental history of chronic pain is associated with differential responses to naloxone compared with controls, suggesting differences in endogenous opioid function [11]. Unfortunately, epidemiological and familial aggregation studies do not rule out the contribution of shared environmental factors.

In humans, twin studies have helped to estimate the relative importance of genetic factors over shared environments in explaining the observed familial aggregation. Twin studies of various clinical pain conditions (e.g., lower back pain, neck pain, fibromyalgia, osteoarthritis, pelvic pain) report robust albeit variable genetic contributions of up to 70% [5, 7, 25, 32, 37, 49, 68, 90]. For these clinical pain conditions, it is often difficult to differentiate whether the heritability refers to the propensity to develop the painful condition or the amount of pain patients experience once the condition has manifested. One might imagine, for example, very different sets of genes affecting the risk of developing osteoarthritis, which is often painful, versus the risk of osteoarthritis pain itself. Twin studies of experimental pain are easier to interpret in this respect, and confirm a significant genetic contribution to pain sensitivity, as indicated in pain thresholds, suprathreshold pain ratings, and pain tolerance [65, 66]. Notably, experimental pain sensitivity has been shown to be predictive of the susceptibility to clinical (e.g., persistent postoperative) pain and the response to treatment [22, 33, 70, 86].

However, one important lesson learned from rodent studies is that different pain modalities (e.g., thermal, chemical, mechanical) are genetically distinct, with variability in each being produced by different sets of genes [56, 57]. Recent studies suggest that this principle might also apply to humans [9, 63, 65], although this remains controversial [62].

THE PAIN SYSTEM

Fig. 11-1 illustrates the core neuroanatomical features underlying nociceptive information processing, pain perception, and its modulation. Even this oversimplified view highlights the multitude of regions in which genes and their products potentially contribute to variation in the pain phenotype. Briefly, the following key components of the pain processing system should be considered when evaluating the potential influence of genetic variability: the *primary afferent nociceptive neurons* including their different components, especially certain types of ion channels, their interactions with the *immune system* (e.g., inflammation), various areas within the *spinal cord* and the *brain* including *afferent* and *descending pain modulatory pathways*, and their interaction with other brain areas not primarily accessed by nociceptive input but involved in the contextual modulation of pain. From a neurochemical perspective, genetic variation of the endogenous opioid system but also of other systems, including the dopaminergic, adrenergic, serotonergic, and cannabinoid systems (for an extensive review, see [52, 71]), is likely to affect pain behaviour. Finally, glial cells have recently been highlighted as key contributors to pathological and chronic pain mechanisms [35, 53].

THE NEUROIMAGING OF PAIN AND PAIN GENES

Modern functional neuroimaging techniques including electrophysiological and metabolic measures, in combination with elegant experimental designs, have revolutionized our understanding of the CNS processes underlying pain perception and its modulation in

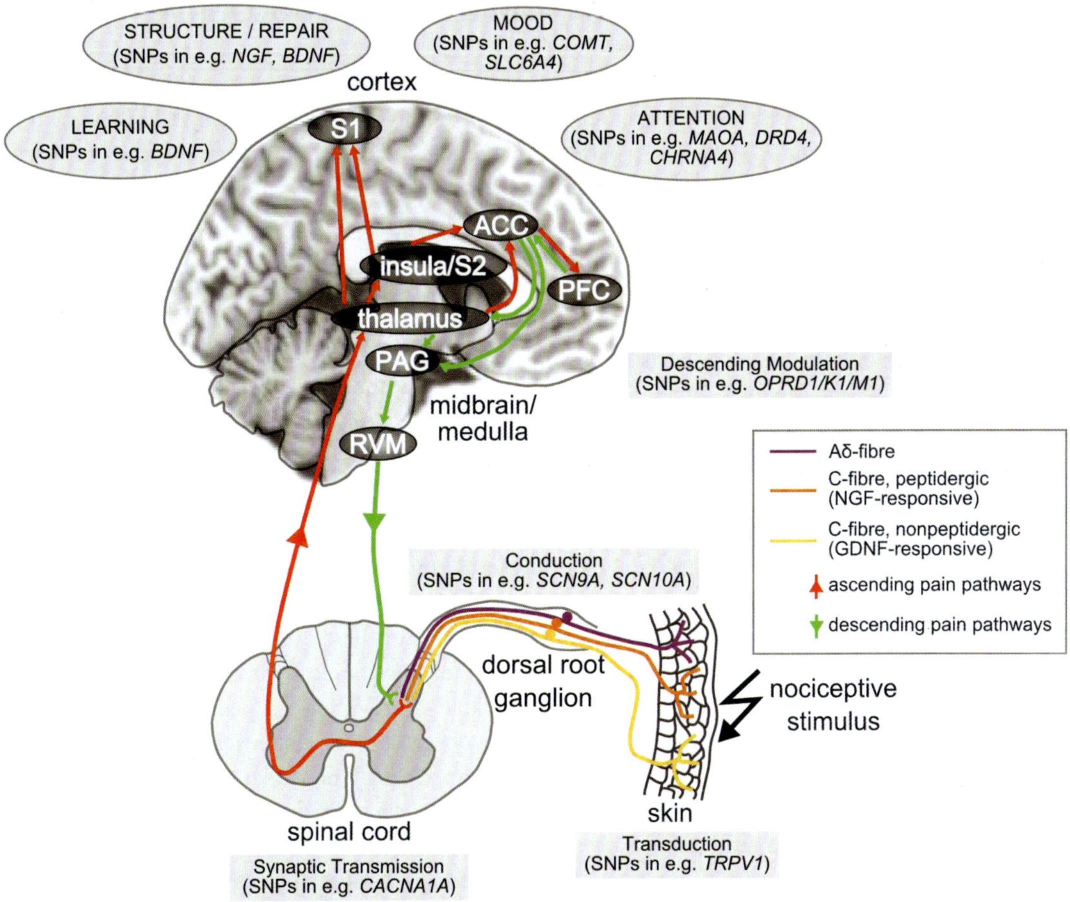

FIGURE 11-1 The pain system and potential sites for genetic variability (see text for details). ACC, anterior cingulate cortex; BDNF, brain-derived neurotrophic factor; CACNA1A, calcium channel, voltage-dependent, P/Q type, alpha 1A subunit; CHRNA4, cholinergic receptor, nicotinic, alpha 4; COMT, catechol-*O*-methyltransferase; DRD4, dopamine receptor D4; GDNF, glial cell–derived neurotrophic factor; MAO A, monoamine oxidase A; NGF, nerve growth factor; OPRD1, opioid receptor, delta 1; OPRK1, opioid receptor, kappa 1; OPRM1, opioid receptor, mu 1; PAG, periaqueductal grey; PFC, prefrontal cortex; RVM, rostral ventromedial medulla; S1, primary somatosensory cortex; S2, secondary somatosensory cortex; SCN9A, sodium channel, voltage-gated, type IX, alpha subunit; SCN10A, sodium channel, voltage-gated, type X, alpha subunit; SNPs, single-nucleotide polymorphisms; TRPV1, transient receptor potential cation channel, subfamily V, member 1.

humans. Recently, more emphasis is being directed towards investigating the distinct neural mechanisms of pathological pain conditions (for reviews see [6, 12, 60, 82].

Combining neuroimaging approaches with information regarding individual genetic properties of the pain system provides the opportunity to relate variation in specific genes to measures of the morphology and/or the functionality of pain-related structures. These trait (genetic) and state (imaging) biomarkers of the individual pain phenotype may close a knowledge gap at the systems level of how genes and their products contribute to the individual pain phenotype (experience) in a context-specific manner. Ultimately, such an approach promises to provide a better understanding of the *individual* neurobiology of the pain experience, and to pave the way for future therapeutic approaches that are patient-specific.

NEUROIMAGING PAIN GENOMICS: METHODOLOGICAL CONSIDERATIONS

From a diagnostic and therapeutic perspective, it might be useful to use brain imaging data to identify characteristic brain patterns in phenomenologically similar pain patients that reflect different (e.g., genetically determined) pathophysiological entities that may predict the individual response to drugs or other treatments. This approach, which has already been used successfully in other chronic diseases such as Parkinson disease [85], could be helpful not only in pharmacological studies but also in validating findings from quantitative sensory testing [78] to provide a better overall characterization of different pain syndromes.

Several methodological caveats need to be considered when using neuroimaging to identify the genetic contributions to pain processing in humans. First, the appropriate imaging modality has to be chosen. This selection depends on both the proposed effect of the genetic variation and the particular aspects of pain processing to be studied. Functional magnetic resonance imaging (fMRI), for instance, is an ideal tool to assess the contribution of both cortical and subcortical brain areas, and most recently also spinal regions, to the processing of acute (phasic) painful stimuli. In combination with connectivity analyses such as Psychophysiological Interactions or Dynamic Causal Modelling, valuable information about the context-/gene-dependent interplay of these areas can be derived [28, 50]. However, fMRI provides only low sensitivity for low-frequency events such as occasional fluctuations of chronic pain, and is less capable of providing a signal for tonic pain. Positron emission tomography (PET) allows the observation of responses to tonic stimuli, but requires the application of a radioactive substance, which precludes repetitive or longitudinal investigations. To further elaborate the issue of spontaneous or ongoing (tonic) pain, a shift in applied methodology may be needed, as addressed in recent studies using arterial spin labelling perfusion imaging [48, 73], perhaps a more appropriate tool for assessing the genetic contribution to key clinical pain symptoms. Another novel, potentially valuable technique is proton magnetic resonance spectroscopy that allows quantifying neural responses to pain by assessing concentrations of neurotransmitters such as glutamine and glutamate [31, 59].

Second, statistical issues need to be resolved, for example, the question of how to determine the ideal sample size of participants and their properties. Inherent to this question in the context of pain genetics is the expected effect size of a specific genetic variant on pain or brain behaviour. One possibility to increase the effect magnitude is a careful subject selection, especially if we are interested in the contribution of specific single-nucleotide polymorphisms (SNPs) or other genetic variants to pain processing. In general, the more homogeneous the population, the smaller the error variance and the more focused the effect. Most importantly, the effect size of the variation in phenotype of a particular gene needs to be considered. In order to obtain a sample of carriers that are homozygous for a certain allele, it might be necessary to screen a large group of subjects. For example, Oertel et al. [67] examined 750 volunteers but included only 15 wild types and 9 homozygous carriers of the μ-opioid receptor variant OPRM1 118A>G in their study.

Finally, it is of critical importance to choose an appropriate pain model to study the influence of specific SNPs on pain processing and its modulation, as variability within different pain modalities (e.g., thermal, chemical, mechanical) appears to be mediated by different genes entirely [56, 59]. Also, the majority of currently employed pain assays both in animals and in humans measure responses to experimenter-evoked pain, whereas the key clinical complaint is ongoing and spontaneous pain. This again needs to be considered when trying to translate genetic findings in animals and healthy volunteers into patient groups. By carefully choosing the characteristics of the sample and experimental design, and by controlling for potentially confounding variables, it seems possible to obtain valid results even from comparably small samples with functional imaging.

WHICH GENES ARE KEY?

The power of combining functional imaging with genetics obviously hinges on which genes are selected for study. Although genome-wide association study (GWAS) and exome sequencing methodologies have now begun to be used for the study of chronic pain [3, 4, 13, 27, 29, 39, 44, 61, 69, 72, 87], the very large numbers of subjects required for multigenic approaches present an insurmotable monetary barrier to studies involving imaging. Thus, imaging genetic studies will likely continue to be single-gene association studies for the most part, adding yet more importance to the decision of which gene to study.

There are, unfortunately, no easy answers to the question. A small number of genes have been studied for their association with pain traits far more than any others; as of 2012, the 10 most common were (in order): *COMT* (catechol-*O*-methyltransferase), *OPRM1* (μ-opioid receptor), *GCH1* (GTP cyclohydrolase), *HLA* (human lymphocyte antigen), *SLC6A4* (the serotonin transporter), *HTR2A* (the serotonin 2A receptor), *IL1* (interleukin-1), *IL1RN* (interleukin-1 receptor antagonist), *TRPV1* (transient receptor potential, V1), and *TNF* (tumor necrosis factor) [55]. Although in the case of *GCH1*, the gene was discovered using an unbiased transcriptome (i.e., microarray) search in rats [81], all other genes on this list were chosen because of the already well-known function of their protein products. As such, there is no strong reason to believe that any one of these genes is somehow more important (e.g., in terms of trait variance explained) than any others that are either known or presently unknown to be associated with pain. The emerging consensus is that variance in most complex traits is mediated by very small contributions from very large numbers of genes, and that much of the variability lies "hidden" in gene–gene and gene–environment interactions [14]. In the best-known example, adult human height, over 200 associated genetic loci have been found, but their additive effects account for only ≈10% of the variance [43]. In a just-published GWAS of schizophrenia [77], the authors estimate that 8300 SNPs contribute to risk of the disorder, together accounting for 32% of the variance in liability. Of course, there are a number of disease traits where single genes account for overwhelming percentages of the variance as well. Just how many genes affect chronic pain is completely unknown at the present time.

Another important caveat applying to known genetic associations with pain is that their replicability is tremendously poor. An instructive example is *COMT*, the most commonly studied "pain gene." It is well known that the $V^{158}M$ variant (see below) was shown to be associated with experimental muscle pain in 2003 [91]. In 2005, a haplotype of four SNPs within *COMT* was shown to be associated with experimental pain (multiple modalities averaged) and the incidence of temporomandibular disorder [20], but the $V^{158}M$ variant itself was not significantly associated. As of 2012, we count 19 positive findings of association (with any SNP or haplotype of *COMT*) with experimental or clinical pain, and 24 reports of no association. This suggests that either the positive associations are false [34] or, more likely, *COMT*'s true role in pain is complex and modality-specific [8].

We trust that with time, the best gene candidates for neuroimaging genetics studies will become clearer. For the moment, however, all choices should be considered arbitrary.

SEMINAL STUDIES OF NEUROIMAGING PAIN GENOMICS

To our knowledge, thus far only a handful of studies have tried to link variations in SNPs suspected of relevance in pain processes with neuroimaging.

The pioneering study in this subfield was performed by Zubieta et al. [91], who used PET and the μ-opioid receptor-selective radiotracer [^{11}C]carfentanil to study the influence of the well-studied *COMT* V^{158}M polymorphism on endogenous opioidergic neurotransmission. This was studied at rest (baseline) and in response to pain in an experimental model of sustained jaw pain. They found that individuals homozygous for the met^{158} allele of the *COMT* V^{158}M polymorphism show lower regional μ-opioidergic neurotransmission at baseline and in response to the tonic painful stimulus in several brain areas, particularly the thalamus, basal ganglia, and the nucleus accumbens. These effects coincided with a higher sensitivity to pain (as assessed by the amount of saline injected into the masseter muscle needed to achieve comparable pain perception), higher affective pain ratings, as well as a more negative internal state. These effects on the endogenous opioid system, which may underlie, at least partially, interindividual differences in the response to pain and other stressful stimuli, are thought to result from downstream effects of the altered dopaminergic neurotransmission associated with the varying levels of COMT activity. These findings are at least in part supported by two recent studies investigating blood oxygenation level–dependent (BOLD) responses to phasic pain stimuli depending on the *COMT* V^{158}M polymorphism [45, 54]. Although neither study confirmed a heightened pain sensitivity on the behavioural level, they report stronger BOLD responses to painful stimuli in homozygous Met carriers compared with heterozygotes or homozygotes of the Val allele. Loggia et al. reported stronger BOLD responses after the repeated exposure to high-intensity heat pain stimuli in Met/Met compared with Val/Val subjects in several brain areas, including the PAG, lingual gyrus, cerebellum, hippocampal formation, and the precuneus. The Mobascher et al. study found stronger BOLD responses to laser pain stimuli in an area of the anterior cingulate cortex that is often found to correlate with perceived pain intensity. Taken together, these two studies support the notion that genetic variations in *COMT* modulate the central processing of painful stimuli, if not pain perception per se (Fig. 11-2).

Love et al. studied the influence of genetic variations within the oxytocin gene (*OXT*) on dopamine-related stress responses using [^{11}C]raclopride PET in combination with sustained deep muscle pain. However, no influence of the *OXT* polymorphism on any psychophysical measures specifically related to pain, or changes in affective state induced by the painful stimulus was observed [47].

A study by Oertel et al. [67] elegantly illustrates how the combination of genetic information, fMRI, and a pharmacological challenge allows for more detailed insights into the mechanisms underlying dose- and context-specific drug effects on different components of the pain experience, as well as their interindividual variability. The authors investigated the differential effects of escalating doses of the opioid alfentanil on the sensory and affective processing of painful stimuli in subjects stratified by the μ-opioid receptor gene (*OPRM1*) variant N40D (A118G).

Increasing alfentanil doses led to linearly decreasing BOLD responses to pain in primary sensory brain regions such as the primary and secondary somatosensory cortices and the posterior insula. In contrast, brain regions known to process the affective dimensions of pain (amygdala, anterior insula) displayed a concentration-independent behaviour and no pain-related activations at the lowest alfentanil dose. This dual effect of alfentanil is

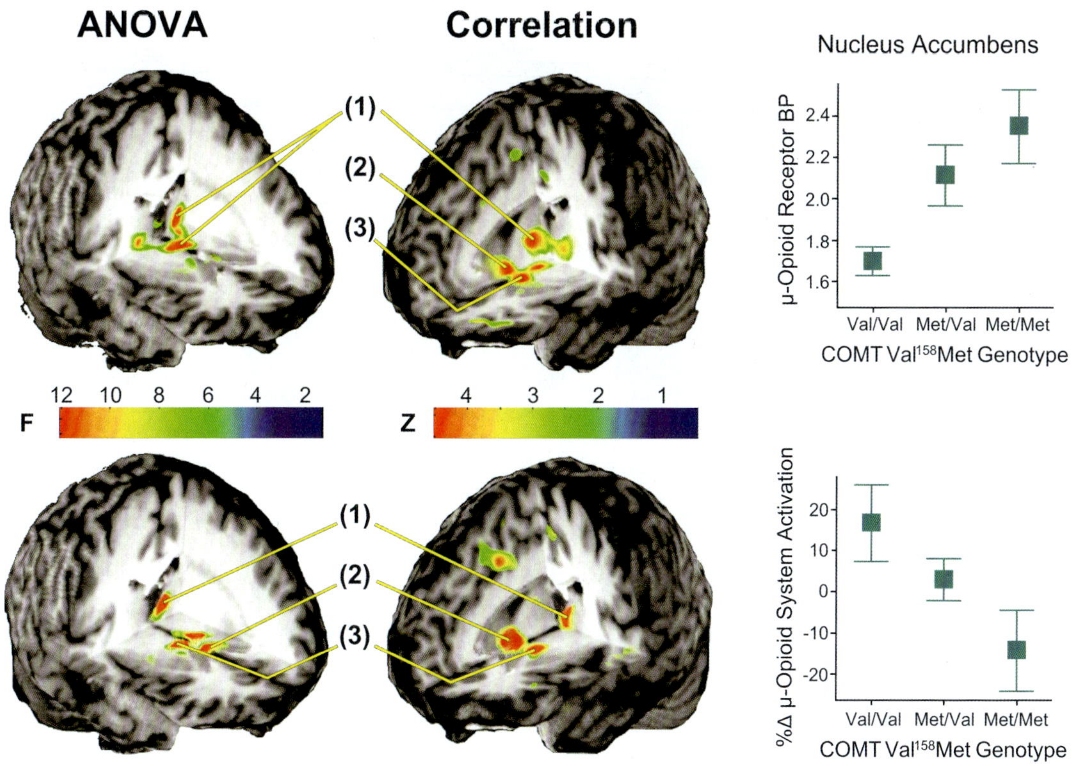

FIGURE 11-2 Influence of the *COMT* V^{158}M polymorphism on endogenous opioidergic neurotransmission in response to sustained pain. (Adapted from Zubieta et al. [91], with permission.) **Upper left:** Three-dimensional display of significant ANOVA results for the effects of COMT *val*^{158}*met* genotypes on baseline μ-opioid receptor binding potential (BP). Significant effects of genotype on baseline BP were observed in the anterior and posterior thalamus (1). Near the multiple comparisons threshold, possible effects were observed bilaterally in the nucleus accumbens and ventral pallidum and in the contralateral thalamic pulvinar. **Lower left:** ANOVA results for the effects of COMT *val*^{158}*met* genotypes on μ-opioid system activation during sustained pain stress. Significant effects were observed in the anterior and posterior thalamus (1), nucleus accumbens (2), ventral pallidum (3), and subthalamic nucleus, bilaterally. ANOVA *F* scores are represented by the pseudocolour scale between the two images. **Upper right:** Correlations between COMT activity conferred by the COMT *val*^{158}*met* polymorphisms and baseline μ-opioid receptor BP. COMT activity was coded as follows: −1, *met/met*; 0, *val/met*; −1, *val/val*. Significant correlations were obtained in the anterior thalamus (1), nucleus accumbens (2), and adjacent ventral pallidum (3) ipsilateral to pain. Mean ± SD of nucleus accumbens (ipsilateral) BP values are shown. **Lower right:** Correlations between COMT activity and μ-opioid system activation were obtained in the posterior thalamus (1) ipsilateral to the challenge, nucleus accumbens (2), and ventral pallidum (3), bilaterally, and the contralateral amygdala and adjacent temporal cortex. The subthalamic nuclei, bilaterally, registered levels of statistical significance approaching the multiple comparisons threshold. Mean ± SD values for the percentage change in the magnitude of μ-opioid system activation in the nucleus accumbens are shown. *Z* scores for the correlations are represented by the pseudocolour scale between the two right images. Threshold for display of results was set at $P < 0.01$ for all analyses.

in line with the common clinical observation that low doses of opioid analgesics reduce the affective but not the sensory dimension of pain. Of note, only the influence on the somatosensory component was modulated by the μ-opioid receptor gene polymorphism, with less pronounced effects in *OPRM1* 118G carriers, while the effect on affective brain areas showed no genotype difference [67] (Fig. 11-3).

An interesting new study by the Peyron group [17] used fMRI to study empathic responses in patients with congenital insensitivity to pain (CIP) to provide insight into the fascinating question of whether we can "share pain we never felt." This addresses the contribution of two proposed mechanisms underlying empathic feelings. One is the phenomenon

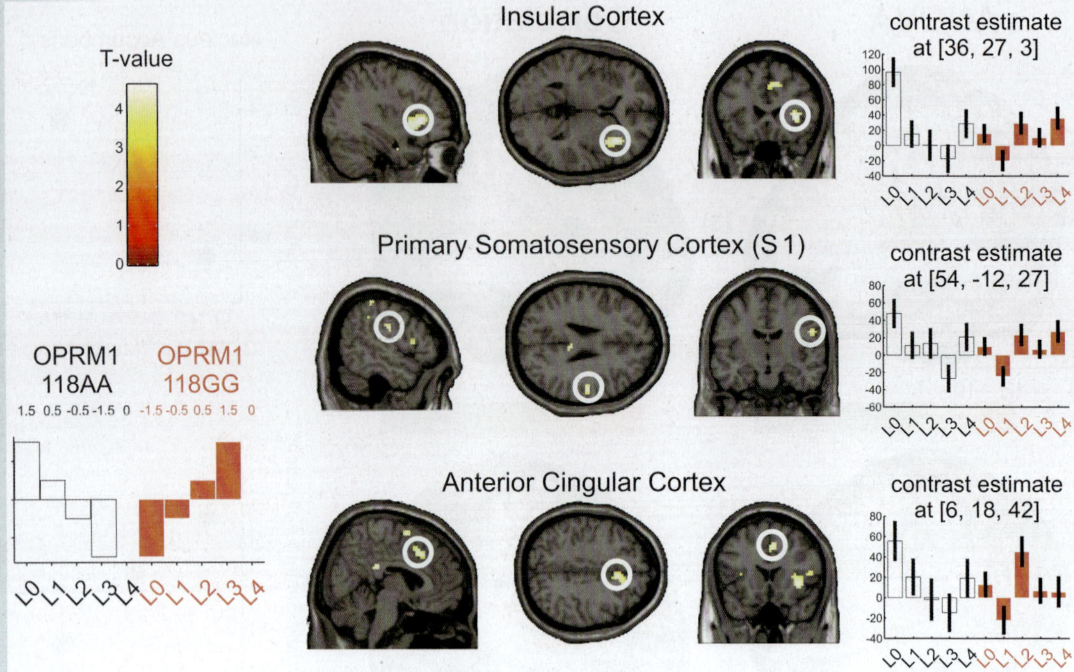

FIGURE 11-3 Differential effects of increasing doses of the opioid alfentanil on the sensory and affective processing of painful stimuli in carriers and noncarriers of μ-opioid receptor variant N40D. (Adapted from Oertel et al. [67], with permission). The influence of μ-opioid receptor variant N40D on the concentration-dependent decrease of brain activation in response to nasal CO_2 stimulation was existent only in regions of the right brain hemisphere with a predominantly linear or at most intermediate decrease of brain activation (contrast 1.5 0.5 −0.5 −1.5 0 −1.5 −0.5 0.5 1.5 0 at $P < 0.001$ uncorrected). The right column visualizes the contrast estimates at the location with the highest *t*-value within these regions of noncarriers of μ-opioid receptor variant N40D (OPRM1 118AA; solid white columns) and of carriers of μ-opioid receptor variant N40D (OPRM1 118GG; solid *red* columns).

of automatic activation of brain areas representing a specific sensation (e.g., pain), called "mirror matching" or "embodied simulation." The other is "perspective taking," referring to higher-level cognitive processes that enable us to understand others' emotions. In contrast to the initial hypothesis, patients who have never felt pain in the past produce "normal" activation in pain neural circuits, specifically the anterior insula and the mid-cingulate, when observing pain in others. However, in the patient group, only the empathy trait correlated with the additional involvement of the ventromedial prefrontal and the posterior cingulate cortex, depending on whether somatosensory or emotional aspects of pain were to be assessed. This finding suggests that in CIP patients, empathy for pain in others relies on the engagement of these midline structures known to be relevant in emotional perspective taking to assess someone else's feeling. This would in part compensate for the patients' lack of automatic "embodied simulation."

Recently, neuroimaging studies have also started to link genetic traits to specific chronic pain conditions. On the basis of the observation that serotonin (5-HT)-3 receptor antagonists alleviate symptoms of irritable bowel syndrome (IBS), Kilpatrick et al. [38] studied the influence of an SNP in the *HTR3A* gene, −42C>T (C178T) on brain activity, anxiety, and IBS severity. The authors found that the wild-type (CC) genotype was associated with increased amygdala responsiveness during both emotional and nonemotional tasks compared with carriers of the T allele, which was paralleled by higher levels of anxiety and IBS severity.

FUTURE DIRECTIONS

The joint venture of imaging and pain genetics is still in its infancy, but it promises many fascinating directions to pursue.

Coping with Nociceptive Input at Various Stages of the Pain Neuraxis

How the individual responds to repetitive painful events or injury is likely to represent a key factor of the development of chronic pain states. As indicated in Fig. 11-1, genetic variations at multiple sites in the nociceptive system and its modulatory control regions can account for the phenotype of increased pain sensitivity, including mechanisms of sensitization in the nociceptive system, disinhibition of endogenous pain control, and the emotional/attentional augmentation of pain. Combining information of the genetic variability that affects these distinct components with the neuroimaging of the human brain and the spinal cord [24, 79] has the potential to elucidate the contribution of peripheral, spinal, and central mechanisms to an increased sensitivity to pain or ongoing pain.

Individual Variation in the Ability for Endogenous Pain Modulation

The question of how the individual copes with painful stimulation is closely linked to the individual ability for endogenous pain control. As predicted by animal research, neuroimaging studies strongly support the concept that the interaction of cingulo-frontal regions with specific brainstem nuclei represents a major pathway of descending endogenous pain modulation in humans [83]. Even though the relationship between different mechanisms of pain modulation is far from being understood, there is evidence suggesting a substantial interindividual variability in the ability to engage different mechanisms of endogenous pain control [80] and an association between the individual capacity for pain control and the susceptibility to chronic pain states [89]. Recent studies have begun to link variability in endogenous pain control, such as placebo analgesia, to genetic traits [30]. Combining neuroimaging with information about SNPs affecting the variety of neurotransmitters involved in endogenous pain control, including the opioidergic (e.g., *OPRM1*, *OPRD1*), dopaminergic (e.g., *COMT*, *DRD4*), adrenergic (e.g., *ADRB2*), serotonergic (e.g., *SLC6A4*), and cannabinoid (e.g., *CNR1*) systems, will, hopefully, help to unravel the distinct contribution of these systems to endogenous pain control and to understand aberrant functioning in clinical pain states.

Structural Differences

Individual pain sensitivity and the capacity for pain modulation may depend not only on genetic variation in the *functional* characteristics of this system (e.g., in neurochemical processes) but also on the *structural* characteristics, such as the proportion of different brain areas and the strength of their structural connections, as, for instance, shown for placebo analgesia [80]. Recent studies suggest that chronic pain states are associated with structural changes in the brain. Most brain regions that showed differences in grey matter volume are key antinociceptive areas, such as the cingulate and prefrontal cortex and the brainstem (for review, see [51]). Although the detailed underlying cellular substrate as well as the reversibility of these structural changes with successful pain treatment remains to be elucidated, these studies support the notion that time-dependent reorganization on a structural level may contribute to the process of pain chronification. The degree of this process is most likely influenced by genes involved in the development, survival, and repair of nociceptive neurons (e.g., genes for TrKA, NGF, and BDNF); inflammatory responses; and the supporting function of glial cells. Combining high-resolution morphometric measures (e.g., voxel-based morphometry) or tractography, which uses diffusion-weighted images to trace fibre bundles in the human brain (for review, see [36]), with information on SNPs that influence the growth and development of the nervous system in healthy controls and patients with distinct pain phenotypes may not only reveal new insights into the underpinnings of individual differences in pain behaviour, but may also identify patients at risk for chronic pain.

OUTLOOK

The linkage of nature- and nurture-driven influences on behaviour and brain function will become a major research topic in pain research for the foreseeable future. However, the combination of neuroimaging and pain genetics represents a true interdisciplinary challenge. Variations in candidate genes need to be carefully chosen on the basis of replicated and well-characterized effects, ideally in both animal and human studies. That being said, we encourage investigators not to focus only on commonly studied variants, as there is no real reason to believe they are more important (e.g., by explaining more trait variance) than less-studied (and indeed, as yet unstudied) genes. The application of recent advances in pain imaging, including functional, structural, and molecular measures along the whole ascending and descending neuronal axes of pain, should be carefully tailored to the proposed function of the candidate gene. If successful, this marriage of neuroimaging and genetic investigations is likely to greatly expand our insight into the neurobiology contributing to the *individual* pain experience in health and disease. This understanding may aid the development of personalized therapeutic approaches to target both acute and chronic pain states.

ACKNOWLEDGEMENT

This work was supported by grants from BMBF (UB) and the Louise and Alan Edwards Foundation (JSM).

REFERENCES

1. Abbruzzese G, Ratto S, Favale E, Abbruzzese M. Proprioceptive modulation of somatosensory evoked potentials during active or passive finger movements in man. J Neurol Neurosurg Psychiatry 1981;44(10):942–9.
2. Amanzio M, Pollo A, Maggi G, Benedetti F. Response variability to analgesics: a role for non-specific activation of endogenous opioids. Pain 2001;90(3):205–15.
3. Anttila V, Stefansson H, Kallela M, Todt U, Terwindt GM, Calafato MS, Nyholt DR, Dimas AS, Freilinger T, Muller-Myhsok B, et al. Genome-wide association study of migraine implicates a common susceptibility variant on 8q22.1. Nat Genet 2010;42(10):869–73.
4. Anttila V, Winsvold BS, Gormley P, Kurth T, Bettella F, McMahon G, Kallela M, Malik R, de Vries B, Terwindt G, et al. Genome-wide meta-analysis identifies new susceptibility loci for migraine. Nat Genet 2013;45(8):912–7.
5. Arguelles LM, Afari N, Buchwald DS, Clauw DJ, Furner S, Goldberg J. A twin study of posttraumatic stress disorder symptoms and chronic widespread pain. Pain 2006;124(1–2):150–7.

6. Baliki MN, Petre B, Torbey S, Herrmann KM, Huang L, Schnitzer TJ, Fields HL, Apkarian AV. Corticostriatal functional connectivity predicts transition to chronic back pain. Nat Neurosci 2012;15(8):1117–9.
7. Battie MC, Videman T, Levalahti E, Gill K, Kaprio J. Heritability of low back pain and the role of disc degeneration. Pain 2007;131(3):272–80.
8. Belfer I, Segall SK, Lariviere WR, Smith SB, Dai F, Slade GD, Rashid NU, Mogil JS, Campbell CM, Edwards RR, et al. Pain modality- and sex-specific effects of COMT genetic functional variants. Pain 2013;154(8):1368–76.
9. Bhalang K, Sigurdsson A, Slade GD, Maixner W. Associations among four modalities of experimental pain in women. J Pain 2005;6(9):604–11.
10. Bornhovd K, Quante M, Glauche V, Bromm B, Weiller C, Buchel C. Painful stimuli evoke different stimulus-response functions in the amygdala, prefrontal, insula and somatosensory cortex: a single-trial fMRI study. Brain 2002;125(Pt 6):1326–36.
11. Bruehl S, Chung OY. Parental history of chronic pain may be associated with impairments in endogenous opioid analgesic systems. Pain 2006;124(3):287–94.
12. Bushnell MC, Ceko M, Low LA. Cognitive and emotional control of pain and its disruption in chronic pain. Nat Rev Neurosci 2013;14(7):502–11.
13. Chasman DI, Schürks M, Anttila V, de Vries B, Schminke U, Launer LJ, Terwindt GM, van den Maagdenberg AM, Fendrich K, Völzke H, et al. Genome-wide association study reveals three susceptibility loci for common migraine in the general population. Nat Genet 2011;43(7):695–8.
14. Chatterjee N, Wheeler B, Sampson J, Hartge P, Chanock SJ, Park J-H. Projecting the performance of risk prediction based on polygenic analyses of genome-wide association studies. Nat Genet 2013;45(4):400-5, e401–3.
15. Cluff RS, Rowbotham MC. Pain caused by herpes zoster infection. Neurol Clin 1998;16(4):813–32.
16. Coghill RC, McHaffie JG, Yen YF. Neural correlates of interindividual differences in the subjective experience of pain. Proc Natl Acad Sci USA 2003;100(14):8538–42.
17. Danziger N, Faillenot I, Peyron R. Can we share a pain we never felt? Neural correlates of empathy in patients with congenital insensitivity to pain. Neuron 2009;61(2):203–12.
18. Day RO. Variability in response to NSAID. Agents Actions 1985;17(Suppl):15–19.
19. Diatchenko L, Nackley AG, Tchivileva IE, Shabalina SA, Maixner W. Genetic architecture of human pain perception. Trends Genet 2007;23(12):605–13.
20. Diatchenko L, Slade GD, Nackley AG, Bhalang K, Sigurdsson A, Belfer I, Goldman D, Xu K, Shabalina SA, Shagin D, et al. Genetic basis for individual variations in pain perception and the development of a chronic pain condition. Hum Mol Genet 2005;14(1):135–43.
21. Edwards CL, Fillingim RB, Keefe F. Race, ethnicity and pain. Pain 2001;94(2):133–7.
22. Edwards RR. Individual differences in endogenous pain modulation as a risk factor for chronic pain. Neurology 2005;65(3):437–43.
23. Edwards RR, Doleys DM, Fillingim RB, Lowery D. Ethnic differences in pain tolerance: clinical implications in a chronic pain population. Psychosom Med 2001;63(2):316–23.
24. Eippert F, Finsterbusch J, Bingel U, Buchel C. Direct evidence for spinal cord involvement in placebo analgesia. Science 2009;326(5951):404.
25. Fejer R, Hartvigsen J, Kyvik KO. Heritability of neck pain: a population-based study of 33,794 Danish twins. Rheumatology (Oxford) 2006;45(5):589–94.
26. Foulkes T, Wood JN. Pain genes. PLoS Genet 2008;4(7):e1000086.
27. Freilinger T, Anttila V, de Vries B, Malik R, Kallela M, Terwindt GM, Pozo-Rosich P, Winsvold B, Nyholt DR, van Oosterhout WP, et al. Genome-wide association analysis identifies susceptibility loci for migraine without aura. Nat Genet 2012;44(7):777–82.
28. Friston KJ, Buechel C, Fink GR, Morris J, Rolls E, Dolan RJ. Psychophysiological and modulatory interactions in neuroimaging. Neuroimage 1997;6(3):218–29.
29. Galvan A, Skorpen F, Klepstad P, Knudsen AK, Fladvad T, Falvella FS, Pigni A, Brunelli C, Caraceni A, Kaasa S, et al. Multiple Loci modulate opioid therapy response for cancer pain. Clin Cancer Res 2011;17(13):4581-4587.
30. Hall KT, Lembo AJ, Kirsch I, Ziogas DC, Douaiher J, Jensen KB, Conboy LA, Kelley JM, Kokkotou E, Kaptchuk TJ. Catechol-*O*-methyltransferase val[158]met polymorphism predicts placebo effect in irritable bowel syndrome. PloS ONE 2012;7(10):e48135.
31. Harris RE, Sundgren PC, Pang Y, Hsu M, Petrou M, Kim SH, McLean SA, Gracely RH, Clauw DJ. Dynamic levels of glutamate within the insula are associated with improvements in multiple pain domains in fibromyalgia. Arthritis Rheum 2008;58(3):903–7.
32. Hestbaek L, Iachine IA, Leboeuf-Yde C, Kyvik KO, Manniche C. Heredity of low back pain in a young population: a classical twin study. Twin Res 2004;7(1):16–26.

33. Hsu YW, Somma J, Hung YC, Tsai PS, Yang CH, Chen CC. Predicting postoperative pain by preoperative pressure pain assessment. Anesthesiology 2005;103(3):613–8.
34. Ioannidis JPA. Why most published research findings are false. PLoS Med 2005;2(8).
35. Ji RR, Berta T, Nedergaard M. Glia and pain: is chronic pain a gliopathy? Pain 2013;154(Suppl 1):S10–28.
36. Johansen-Berg H, Behrens TE. Just pretty pictures? What diffusion tractography can add in clinical neuroscience. Curr Opin Neurol 2006;19(4):379–85.
37. Kato K, Sullivan PF, Evengard B, Pedersen NL. Importance of genetic influences on chronic widespread pain. Arthritis Rheum 2006;54(5):1682–6.
38. Kilpatrick LA, Labus JS, Coveleskie K, Hammer C, Rappold G, Tillisch K, Bueller JA, Suyenobu B, Jarcho JM, McRoberts JA, et al. The HTR3A polymorphism c. −42C>T is associated with amygdala responsiveness in patients with irritable bowel syndrome. Gastroenterology 2011;140(7):1943–51.
39. Kim H, Ramsay E, Lee H, Wahl S, Dionne RA. Genome-wide association study of acute post-surgical pain in humans. Pharmacogenomics 2009;10(2):171–9.
40. Komiyama O, Kawara M, De Laat A. Ethnic differences regarding tactile and pain thresholds in the trigeminal region. J Pain 2007;8(4):363–9.
41. Komiyama O, Wang K, Svensson P, Arendt-Nielsen L, Kawara M, De Laat A. Ethnic differences regarding sensory, pain, and reflex responses in the trigeminal region. Clin Neurophysiol 2009;120(2):384–9.
42. Lacroix-Fralish ML, Ledoux JB, Mogil JS. The Pain Genes Database: an interactive web browser of pain-related transgenic knockout studies. Pain 2007;131(1–2):3 e1–4.
43. Lango Allen H, Estrada K, Lettre G, Berndt SI, Weedon MN, Rivadeneira F, Willer CJ, Jackson AU, Vedantam S, Raychaudhuri S, et al. Hundreds of variants clustered in genomic loci and biological pathways affect human height. Nature 2010;467(7317):832–8.
44. Ligthart L, de Vries B, Smith AV, Ikram MA, Amin N, Hottenga J-J, Koelewijn SC, Kattenberg VM, de Moor MHM, Janssens AC, et al. Meta-analysis of genome-wide association for migraine in six population-based European cohorts. Eur J Hum Genet 2011;19(8):901–7.
45. Loggia ML, Jensen K, Gollub RL, Wasan AD, Edwards RR, Kong J. The catechol-*O*-methyltransferase (COMT) val^{158}met polymorphism affects brain responses to repeated painful stimuli. PLoS ONE 2011;6(11):e27764.
46. Lotsch J. Genetic variability of pain perception and treatment—clinical pharmacological implications. Eur J Clin Pharmacol 2011;67(6):541–51.
47. Love TM, Enoch MA, Hodgkinson CA, Pecina M, Mickey B, Koeppe RA, Stohler CS, Goldman D, Zubieta JK. Oxytocin gene polymorphisms influence human dopaminergic function in a sex-dependent manner. Biol Psychiatry 2012;72(3):198–206.
48. MacIntosh BJ, Pattinson KT, Gallichan D, Ahmad I, Miller KL, Feinberg DA, Wise RG, Jezzard P. Measuring the effects of remifentanil on cerebral blood flow and arterial arrival time using 3D GRASE MRI with pulsed arterial spin labelling. J Cereb Blood Flow Metab 2008;28(8):1514–22.
49. Markkula R, Jarvinen P, Leino-Arjas P, Koskenvuo M, Kalso E, Kaprio J. Clustering of symptoms associated with fibromyalgia in a Finnish Twin Cohort. Eur J Pain 2009;13(7):744–50.
50. Marreiros AC, Kiebel SJ, Friston KJ. Dynamic causal modelling for fMRI: a two-state model. Neuroimage 2008;39(1):269–78.
51. May A. Chronic pain may change the structure of the brain. Pain 2008;137(1):7–15.
52. Millan MJ. Descending control of pain. Prog Neurobiol 2002;66(6):355–474.
53. Milligan ED, Watkins LR. Pathological and protective roles of glia in chronic pain. Nat Rev Neurosci 2009;10(1):23–36.
54. Mobascher A, Brinkmeyer J, Thiele H, Toliat MR, Steffens M, Warbrick T, Musso F, Wittsack HJ, Saleh A, Schnitzler A, et al. The val^{158}met polymorphism of human catechol-*O*-methyltransferase (COMT) affects anterior cingulate cortex activation in response to painful laser stimulation. Mol Pain 2010;6:32.
55. Mogil JS. Pain genetics: past, present and future. Trends Genet 2012;28(6):258–66.
56. Mogil JS, Wilson SG, Bon K, Lee SE, Chung K, Raber P, Pieper JO, Hain HS, Belknap JK, Hubert L, et al. Heritability of nociception I: responses of 11 inbred mouse strains on 12 measures of nociception. Pain 1999;80(1–2):67–82.
57. Mogil JS, Wilson SG, Bon K, Lee SE, Chung K, Raber P, Pieper JO, Hain HS, Belknap JK, Hubert L, et al. Heritability of nociception II. 'Types' of nociception revealed by genetic correlation analysis. Pain 1999; 80(1–2):83–93.
58. Mouraux A, Diukova A, Lee MC, Wise RG, Iannetti GD. A multisensory investigation of the functional significance of the "pain matrix". Neuroimage 2011;54(3):2237–49.
59. Mullins PG, Rowland LM, Jung RE, Sibbitt WL Jr. A novel technique to study the brain's response to pain: proton magnetic resonance spectroscopy. NeuroImage 2005;26(2):642–6.

60. Mutso AA, Radzicki D, Baliki MN, Huang L, Banisadr G, Centeno MV, Radulovic J, Martina M, Miller RJ, Apkarian AV. Abnormalities in hippocampal functioning with persistent pain. J Neurosci 2012;32(17):5747–56.
61. Nakajima M, Takahashi A, Kou I, Rodriguez-Fontenla C, Gomez-Reino JJ, Furuichi T, Dai J, Sudo A, Uchida A, Fukui N. New sequence variants in HLA class II/III region associated with susceptibility to knee osteoarthritis identified by genome-wide association study. PLoS ONE 2010;5(3):e9723.
62. Neddermeyer TJ, Fluhr K, Lotsch J. Principle components analysis of pain thresholds to thermal, electrical, and mechanical stimuli suggests a predominant common source of variance. Pain 2008;138(2):286–91.
63. Neziri AY, Curatolo M, Nuesch E, Scaramozzino P, Andersen OK, Arendt-Nielsen L, Juni P. Factor analysis of responses to thermal, electrical, and mechanical painful stimuli supports the importance of multi-modal pain assessment. Pain 2011;152(5):1146–55.
64. Nielsen CS, Price DD, Vassend O, Stubhaug A, Harris JR. Characterizing individual differences in heat-pain sensitivity. Pain 2005;119(1–3):65–74.
65. Nielsen CS, Stubhaug A, Price DD, Vassend O, Czajkowski N, Harris JR. Individual differences in pain sensitivity: genetic and environmental contributions. Pain 2008;136(1–2):21–29.
66. Norbury TA, MacGregor AJ, Urwin J, Spector TD, McMahon SB. Heritability of responses to painful stimuli in women: a classical twin study. Brain 2007;130(Pt 11):3041–9.
67. Oertel BG, Preibisch C, Wallenhorst T, Hummel T, Geisslinger G, Lanfermann H, Lotsch J. Differential opioid action on sensory and affective cerebral pain processing. Clin Pharmacol Ther 2008;83(4):577–88.
68. Page WF, Hoaglund FT, Steinbach LS, Heath AC. Primary osteoarthritis of the hip in monozygotic and dizygotic male twins. Twin Res 2003;6(2):147–51.
69. Painter JN, Anderson CA, Nyholt DR, Macgregor S, Lin J, Lee SH, Lambert A, Zhao ZZ, Roseman F, Guo Q, et al. Genome-wide association study identifies a locus at 7p15.2 associated with endometriosis. Nat Genet 2011;43(1):51–4.
70. Pan PH, Coghill R, Houle TT, Seid MH, Lindel WM, Parker RL, Washburn SA, Harris L, Eisenach JC. Multifactorial preoperative predictors for postcesarean section pain and analgesic requirement. Anesthesiology 2006;104(3):417–25.
71. Pertwee RG. Cannabinoid receptors and pain. Prog Neurobiol 2001;63(5):569–611.
72. Peters MJ, Broer L, Willemen HL, Eiriksdottir G, Hocking LJ, Holliday KL, Horan MA, Meulenbelt I, Neogi T, Popham M, et al. Genome-wide association study meta-analysis of chronic widespread pain: evidence for involvement of the 5p15.2 region. Ann Rheum Dis 2013;72(3):427–36.
73. Petersen ET, Zimine I, Ho YC, Golay X. Non-invasive measurement of perfusion: a critical review of arterial spin labelling techniques. Br J Radiol 2006;79(944):688–701.
74. Peul WC, Brand R, Thomeer RT, Koes BW. Influence of gender and other prognostic factors on outcome of sciatica. Pain 2008;138(1):180–91.
75. Preston SJ, Arnold MH, Beller EM, Brooks PM, Buchanan WW. Variability in response to nonsteroidal anti-inflammatory analgesics: evidence from controlled clinical therapeutic trial of flurbiprofen in rheumatoid arthritis. Br J Clin Pharmacol 1988;26(6):759–64.
76. Puolakka K, Ylinen J, Neva MH, Kautiainen H, Hakkinen A. Risk factors for back pain-related loss of working time after surgery for lumbar disc herniation: a 5 year follow-up study. Eur Spine J 2008;17(3):386–92.
77. Ripke S, O'Dushlaine C, Chambert K, Moran JL, Kahler AK, Akterin S, Bergen SL, Collins AL, Crowley JJ, Fromer M, et al. Genome-wide association analysis identifies 13 new risk loci for schizophrenia. Nature genetics 2013;45:1150–9.
78. Rolke R, Magerl W, Campbell KA, Schalber C, Caspari S, Birklein F, Treede RD. Quantitative sensory testing: a comprehensive protocol for clinical trials. Eur J Pain 2006;10(1):77–88.
79. Sprenger C, Eippert F, Finsterbusch J, Bingel U, Rose M, Buchel C. Attention modulates spinal cord responses to pain. Curr Biol 2012;22(11):1019–22.
80. Stein N, Sprenger C, Scholz J, Wiech K, Bingel U. White matter integrity of the descending pain modulatory system is associated with interindividual differences in placebo analgesia. Pain 2012;153(11):2210–17.
81. Tegeder I, Costigan M, Griffin RS, Abele A, Belfer I, Schmidt H, Ehnert C, Nejim J, Marian C, Scholz J, et al. GTP cyclohydrolase and tetrahydrobiopterin regulate pain sensitivity and persistence. Nat Med 2006;12(11):1269–77.
82. Tracey I, Bushnell MC. How neuroimaging studies have challenged us to rethink: is chronic pain a disease? J Pain 2009;10(11):1113–20.
83. Tracey I, Dickenson A. SnapShot: pain perception. Cell 2012;148(6):1308–1308.e2.
84. Turk DC, Flor H, Rudy TE. Pain and families, I: etiology, maintenance, and psychosocial impact. Pain 1987;30(1):3–27.
85. van der Vegt JP, van Nuenen BF, Bloem BR, Klein C, Siebner HR. Imaging the impact of genes on Parkinson's disease. Neuroscience 2009;164(1):191–204.

86. Werner MU, Duun P, Kehlet H. Prediction of postoperative pain by preoperative nociceptive responses to heat stimulation. Anesthesiology 2004;100(1):115–9; discussion 115A.
87. Williams FMK, Scollen S, Cao D, Memari Y, Hyde CL, Zhang B, Sidders B, Ziemek D, Shi Y, Harris J, et al. Genes contributing to pain sensitivity in the normal population: an exome sequencing study. PLoS Genet 2012;8(12):e1003095.
88. Wolff BB, Kantor TG, Jarvik ME, Laska E. Response of experimental pain to analgesic drugs. 3. Codeine, aspirin, secobarbital, and placebo. Clin Pharmacol Ther 1969;10(2):217–28.
89. Yarnitsky D. Conditioned pain modulation (the diffuse noxious inhibitory control-like effect): its relevance for acute and chronic pain states. Curr Opin Anaesthesiol 2010;23(5):611–5.
90. Zondervan KT, Cardon LR, Kennedy SH, Martin NG, Treloar SA. Multivariate genetic analysis of chronic pelvic pain and associated phenotypes. Behav Genet 2005;35(2):177–88.
91. Zubieta J-K, Heitzeg MM, Smith YR, Bueller JA, Xu K, Xu Y, Koeppe RA, Stohler CS, Goldman D. COMT val^{158}met genotype affects mu-opioid neurotransmitter responses to a pain stressor. Science 2003;299(5610):1240–3.

SECTION 3

Technology: Animal Neuroimaging

CHAPTER 12

fMRI Pain-Related Brain Measures in Rodents

Jaymin Upadhyay, David Borsook, and Lino Becerra

In the preclinical setting, pain and the effectiveness of analgesic treatments have been routinely assessed using multiple screening assays that include behaviour, electrophysiology, autoradiography, or genetic tests and manipulations. Pain, by its very nature, is a brain "experience," and chronic pain alters brain circuits functionally, structurally, and chemically. This chapter focuses on the implementation of preclinical functional brain imaging assays as a means to the brain's pain state. Further, we briefly explore how this methodology can inform upon a known or novel analgesic mechanism. Recent findings derived from the clinical pain imaging field with parallel advancements in the preclinical domain give impetus to utilizing brain imaging technology within the pain therapeutic area. There is a clear need to implement translational measures to evaluate novel pharmacological compounds that cannot be directly administered to humans in their early development. We summarize the types of preclinical brain imaging readouts relevant to pain as well as the inherent challenges associated with the technology.

STRUCTURAL PROPERTIES AND ORGANIZATION IN HUMAN AND RODENT BRAINS

No matter what the species, the brain is structurally partitioned, yet interconnected, to perform specific functions that support processing of sensory input and its behavioural consequences (e.g., emotional and other responses). In the case of the sensorimotor system, the structural organization and axonal projection between the sensory and motor cortices are parallel between humans and rodents [28]. This is despite the fact that the relevance or type of sensory input (skin vs. whiskers) differs between the two species. Such similarities can be found in other brain systems as well (e.g., auditory, visual, or memory) and therefore rodents are often an ideal model species to understand brain function and structure in conjunction with behaviour. Nonetheless, key differences do exist between humans and rodents, be it structure size relative to the rest of the brain (e.g., hypothalamus) or, in the case of the neocortex, the surface area. For the neocortex, specifically, the greater surface area in humans is linked with the ability to perform more complex mental processes such as spatial reasoning, perception, or language. Given that pain, especially in its chronic form, is both a sensorimotor and a complex perceptual experience, the neocortical difference between species must be kept in mind when evaluating pain perception in rodents and projecting this information to a human population. However, subcortical processes including brainstem, basal ganglia structures such as the accumbens, and thalamus are better conserved across species, and are now well known to be involved in the complexities of pain processing.

PARALLEL PAIN PATHWAYS IN HUMANS AND RODENTS

Pain, be it in the context of a mechanism of protection or a pathological state, is an evolutionary old process that has been preserved between rodents and humans. Taking also into consideration the preservation of functional organization of the brain between the two species [4, 19, 23, 31], it may be expected that functional imaging studies utilizing similar experimental pain protocols in rodents or humans yield analogous findings within supraspinal pain processing pathways. A clear example of this commonality is the activation observed within the ascending (reticular formation, ventroposterior lateral thalamus to somatosensory cortices) and descending (periaqueductal gray to rostral ventral medulla) pain pathways following acute, noxious stimulation (e.g., thermal or electrical) in naïve rodents and healthy human volunteers [9, 33, 36]. Given the basic presence of translatable, acute pain responses, a preclinical brain imaging study that utilizes such an approach can be very informative with respect to how novel and known mechanisms modulate ascending and descending pathways, but, importantly, how the mechanism is likely to behave in humans. In fact, preclinical studies where opioids (remifentanil [20]) or sodium channel blockers (lidocaine [39]) are assessed show similar pharmacodynamic effects in the brain compared with the corresponding clinical work [25, 35]. However, even in a rather straightforward experimental paradigm involving acute pain, differences can be observed between responses in naïve rodents (caudate–putamen deactivation) and healthy human volunteers (caudate–putamen activation), and one needs to use caution in the interpretation of preclinical findings and how they may project to a clinical population, particularly when additional variables (e.g., treatment) are experimentally introduced [24, 27]. Such differences as that identified in the caudate–putamen may stem from differences in brain activity and connectivity or cerebrovascular differences between humans and rodents.

AWAKE OR ANAESTHETIZED

In order to obtain a robust fMRI signal without substantial motion artefact, rodents are kept in an anaesthetized state, often using isoflurane, ketamine/medetomidine or α-chloralose. Although motion artefact is substantially diminished by the use of an anaesthetic, it can be argued that the animal, naïve or one that models a specific type of pain, does not have a normal brain state even when very low levels of anaesthesia (e.g., 0.5–1.0% isoflurane) are used and cardiovascular changes caused by the anaesthetic are controlled for [18, 30] (Fig. 12-1). In an experimental paradigm where a pharmacological treatment is evaluated, drug–anaesthetic interactions may preclude a straightforward interpretation of data [15]. This caution should particularly be considered if an analgesic effect is derived by central or central + peripheral drug action. Previous work has determined that positive or negative ketamine-induced "evoked" blood oxygenation level–dependent (BOLD) responses in the retrosplenial cortex among other structures can be measured following the use of α-chloralose or isoflurane, respectively. An anaesthetic itself yields a diminished BOLD response to noxious stimulation, and this could underlie a lack of treatment effect compared with saline or baseline conditions that could be observed, thus yielding a false-negative

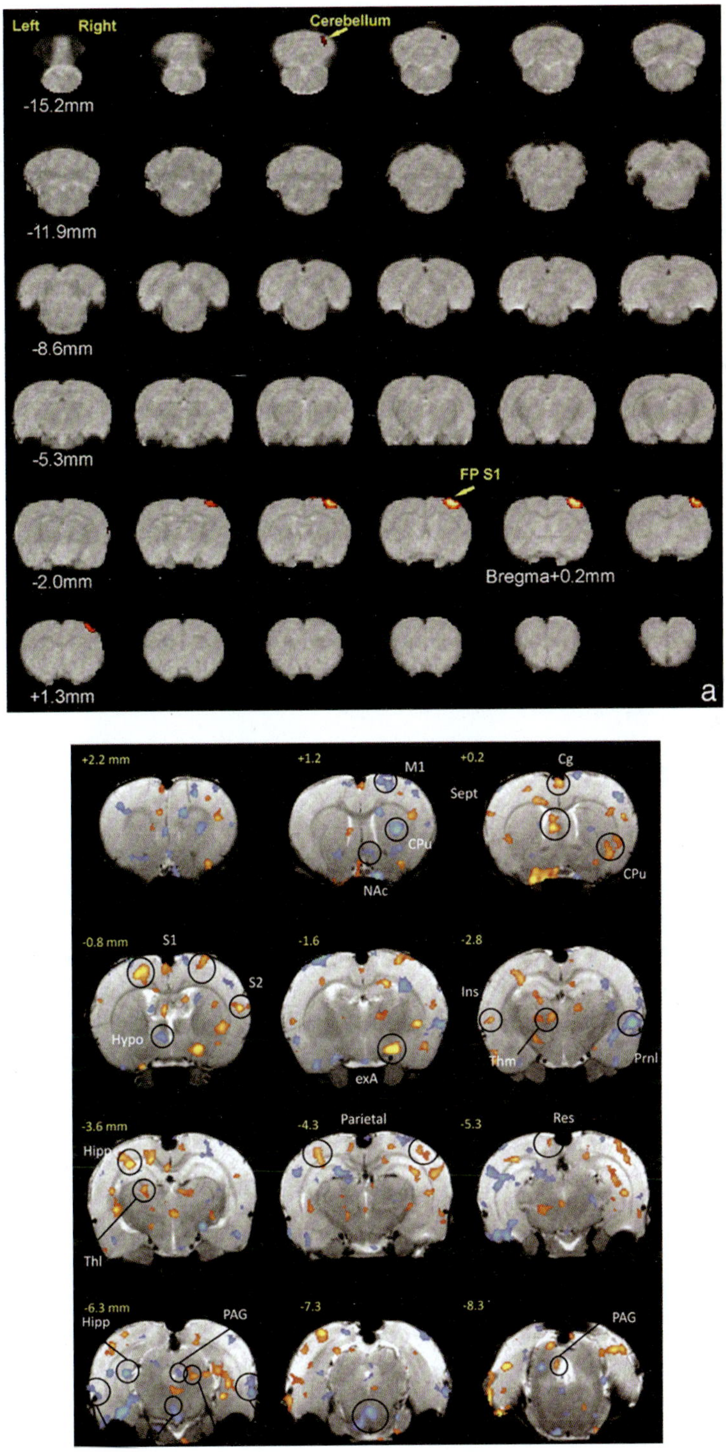

FIGURE 12-1 Activation to evoked pain in awake and anaesthetized rats. The top panel depicts activation to electrical stimulation to anaesthetized animals [22], whereas the bottom panel depicts activity to thermal stimulation in awake animals [2]. The limited areas of activity under anaesthesia could be due in part to the presence of an anaesthetic as well as the stimulation type. These factors as well as others explained in the text should be taken into account when performing imaging studies of pain in rodents.

result [26]. The presence of anaesthetics can also induce nonlinear responses to evoked stimuli, and this effect will compromise the interpretation of, for instance, dose responses in drug studies. To avoid the above-mentioned anaesthesia-related confounds, compensatory approaches have been established, such as graded stimuli and measurement of the difference, but more animals are required to achieve enough statistical power. In that regard, the use of an exogenous contrast agent such as *u*ltrasmall *s*uper*p*aramagnetic *i*ron *o*xide (USPIO) could enhance the observed signal and reduce the number of animals needed [37, 38]. Nevertheless, this would affect the cost and logistics of the preclinical study.

Current studies have administered noxious stimulation to awake rodents during acquisition of fMRI data in order to circumvent confounds induced by anaesthetic use [2, 6]. However, such an experimental factor could lead to the enhancement of stress perceived by the animal, a potential state of learned helplessness that could affect the measured brain activity, diminished throughput or "lost" datasets due to head motion artefact, and potentially more complex fMRI analysis procedures needed for addressing head motion artefact. A solution for this approach is to utilize fairly short stimuli (less than 5 seconds), in which the animal perceives the pain but is not prompted to escape it. Whether anaesthetized or awake evoked fMRI preclinical studies are carried out, the animals' physiology should be properly monitored with a view to avoiding unnecessary mortality. For translational models, human–animal equivalence, whether anaesthetized or not, should be further established along the lines of some reports [2–5]. Further validation is clearly needed.

PAIN MODELS AND fMRI

There are numerous preclinical models that aim to mimic clinical chronic pain condition, such as neuropathic pain caused by peripheral nerve compression (e.g., spinal nerve ligation, spared nerve injury, and chronic constriction injury models) or arthritic pain caused by cartilage degradation (medial meniscus tear [MMT] or monosodium iodoacetate models). Aside from brain imaging, there are several reasons to believe that there is general utility of these animals in preclinical work aiming to characterize a specific type of pain or a mechanism in a chronic pain state spanning several weeks. These reasons include, but are not limited to: (a) behavioural pain efficacy observed for a standard of care (celecoxib) in a relevant preclinical model (MMT model of OA); (b) up- or downregulation of soluble biomarkers (IL-1β) that regulate pain at the molecular level; (c) presence of peripheral and central sensitization; and (d) observed modulations in motivation and drive.

Within the last 5–10 years, pain researchers, including those who utilize brain imaging methodologies, have provided objective data that better elucidate what brain structures or networks underlie and sustain chronic pain, and in turn, which networks to target in preclinical and clinical studies in order to induce a potential analgesic effect. From clinical imaging studies involving chronic pain patients, a strong argument can be made for the behaviour within emotional and reward networks rather than those that mediate sensation that better define the etiology of a chronic pain state [1, 13, 14, 21]. Considering that it is not trivial to objectively evaluate emotion and reward processes in a preclinical pain setting, particularly from behavioural measures alone, brain imaging methodologies are crucial to probing emotional and reward circuitry. Recent studies involving preclinical neuropathic and osteoarthritic pain states provide such examples [16, 17, 32]. Moreover, what is often impossible to back-translate to the preclinical imaging settings is the full complexity of the clinical condition. Genetic and environmental factors, past and ongoing consumption of medications, manner in which pain was induced, and comorbidities (e.g., depression) are just some of the contributing factors that not only define the clinical pain condition but also affect brain function and structure [34].

EVOKED PAIN fMRI AND RESTING-STATE fMRI MEASUREMENTS IN ANAESTHETIZED AND AWAKE STATES

By incorporating evoked pain fMRI (E-fMRI) measurements in preclinical imaging studies, it is possible to directly induce responses in ascending and descending pain pathways in the brain (Fig. 12-2). Given that such studies are primarily carried out while the animals are fully intact, the methodology lends itself to longitudinal study designs. By combining E-fMRI with more invasive approaches, one could theoretically take further advantage of the preclinical model [7, 10, 29]. For example, fMRI-based changes in brain activity due to an enhanced pain state could be used to constrain a specific network or structure to be assessed via *in vivo* microscopy approaches where dendritic morphology can be assessed. A common choice of noxious stimulation is electrical in nature and often delivered to the hind paw or forepaw [8, 12, 22]. The advantages of utilizing electrical stimulation include fast on and off states, ease of stimulus delivery, and the well-established brain response signature in rodents—mainly, activation in the somatosensory cortices and deactivation in the caudate–putamen. In a more limited number of studies, noxious thermal and mechanical (von Frey) stimuli have been utilized, where the activation and deactivation patterns are in line with pain responses driven by noxious stimulation.

E-fMRI methodology enables a manner in which to perturb, in real time, activity in ascending and descending pain pathways that may be normal or altered by a pain condition. It could be argued that such evoked responses are not inducing a brain response that is specific to a single preclinical or clinical chronic pain condition. Alternatively, fMRI-based, resting-state brain connectivity can be measured in either anaesthetized or awake

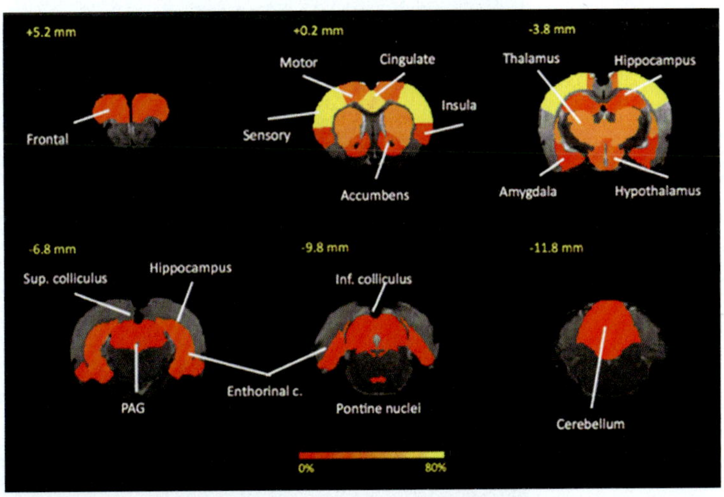

FIGURE 12-2 Summary figure of reported brain activation with pain. The figure summarizes percentage of reported activity of certain brain structures following acute pain stimuli. The cingulate and sensorimotor areas are most often reported as active as other areas. Among subcortical areas, the thalamus is the most common activated structure [7].

animal experimental paradigms (Fig. 12-3). Here, the aim is to measure correlation or disturbances in correlation between two or more hypothesized brain structures. If robust changes in correlation are observed between a naïve/sham rodent cohort and preclinical model, it can be assumed that the change in correlation is driven by the induction and sustainment of chronic pain. The respective benefits and limitations stemming from anaesthetized and awake animal E-fMRI paradigms in larger part hold true for resting-state fMRI (RS-fMRI) measurements. However, some limiting factors, particularly for awake imaging, may be less of an issue. While it is still a stressful state for animals to remain awake and constrained in the MRI scanner, following several habituation training sessions, animal constrain becomes less burdensome as determined by less movement, but also by the presence of global physiological signals (e.g., respiratory rate) that are within the range of when an animal is in a normal, awake behaving state [11]. From a data acquisition standpoint, RS-fMRI data are comparatively less complex than E-fMRI studies where peripheral stimulation equipment is needed. However, from a data analysis standpoint, RS-fMRI data have comparatively more degrees of freedom or ways in which the data can be analyzed and subsequently interpreted. Nonetheless, if an effect driven by pain, treatment, or a combination of the two is robust enough, the result and interpretation should

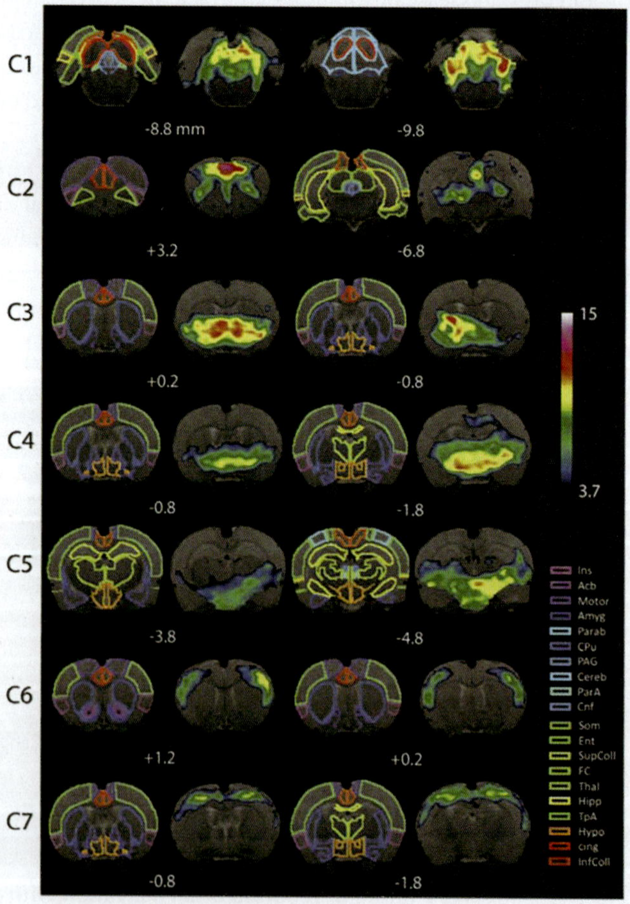

FIGURE 12-3 Robust, reproducible resting-state networks (RSNs) in brains of awake rodents. The figure displays sample RSN maps for awake rodents. Similar results have been reported by others, and there seems to be a defined set of networks in rodents, some of which resemble the human ones [4, 19].

converge irrespective of the analysis-processing stream that is utilized. Moreover, in a RS-fMRI study, more subjects per cohort may be needed given the variability of the method compared with E-fMRI paradigms.

CONCLUSIONS

Whether E-fMRI or RS-fMRI methods are incorporated into preclinical pain imaging studies, the fMRI readout can be crucial in defining dose–response or exposure–response relationships for an analgesic or potential analgesic effect. If dose–response or exposure–response relationships have been assessed from other assays (e.g., behavioural measures), then confirming such exposures with objective preclinical imaging data would be crucial. The latter is true whether the mechanism being evaluated is central, peripheral, or both.

REFERENCES

1. Baliki MN, Mansour A, Baria AT, Huang L, Berger SE, Fields HL, Apkarian AV. Parceling human accumbens into putative core and shell dissociates encoding of values for reward and pain. J Neurosci 2013;33(41):16383–93.
2. Becerra L, Chang PC, Bishop J, Borsook D. CNS activation maps in awake rats exposed to thermal stimuli to the dorsum of the hindpaw. NeuroImage 2011;54(2):1355–66.
3. Becerra L, Navratilova E, Porreca F, Borsook D. Analogous responses in the nucleus accumbens and cingulate cortex to pain onset (aversion) and offset (relief) in rats and humans. J Neurophysiol 2013;110(5):1221–6.
4. Becerra L, Pendse G, Chang PC, Bishop J, Borsook D. Robust reproducible resting state networks in the awake rodent brain. PloS ONE 2011;6(10):e25701.
5. Becerra L, Upadhyay J, Chang PC, Bishop J, Anderson J, Baumgartner R, Schwarz AJ, Coimbra A, Wallin D, Nutile L, et al. Parallel buprenorphine phMRI responses in conscious rodents and healthy human subjects. J Pharmacol Exp Ther 2013;345(1):41–51.
6. Bifone A, Gozzi A. Neuromapping techniques in drug discovery: pharmacological MRI for the assessment of novel antipsychotics. Expert Opin Drug Discov 2012;7(11):1071–82.
7. Borsook D, Becerra L. CNS animal fMRI in pain and analgesia. Neurosci Biobehav Rev 2011;35(5):125–43.
8. Bosshard SC, Grandjean J, Schroeter A, Baltes C, Zeilhofer HU, Rudin M. Hyperalgesia by low doses of the local anesthetic lidocaine involves cannabinoid signaling: an fMRI study in mice. Pain 2012;153(7):1450–8.
9. Bushnell MC, Duncan GH, Hofbauer RK, Ha B, Chen JI, Carrier B. Pain perception: is there a role for primary somatosensory cortex? Proc Natl Acad Sci USA 1999;96(14):7705–9.
10. Desai M, Kahn I, Knoblich U, Bernstein J, Atallah H, Yang A, Kopell N, Buckner RL, Graybiel AM, Moore CI, et al. Mapping brain networks in awake mice using combined optical neural control and fMRI. J Neurophysiol 2011;105(3):1393–405.
11. Ferris CF, Smerkers B, Kulkarni P, Caffrey M, Afacan O, Toddes S, Stolberg T, Febo M. Functional magnetic resonance imaging in awake animals. Rev Neurosci 2011:22(6):665–74.
12. Ghazni NF, Cahill CM, Stroman PW. Tactile sensory and pain networks in the human spinal cord and brain stem mapped by means of functional MR imaging. AJNR Am J Neuroradiol 2010;31(4):661–7.
13. Harris RE, Napadow V, Huggins JP, Pauer L, Kim L, Hampson J, Sundgren PC, Foerster B, Petrou M, Schmidt-Wilcke T, et al. Pregabalin rectifies aberrant brain chemistry, connectivity, and functional response in chronic pain patients. Anesthesiology 2013;119(6):1453–64.
14. Hashmi JA, Baliki MN, Huang L, Baria AT, Torbey S, Hermann KM, Schnitzer TJ, Apkarian AV. Shape shifting pain: chronification of back pain shifts brain representation from nociceptive to emotional circuits. Brain 2013;136(Pt 9):2751–68.
15. Hodkinson DJ, de Groote C, McKie S, Deakin JF, Williams SR. Differential effects of anaesthesia on the phMRI response to acute ketamine challenge. Br J Med Med Res 2012;2(3):373–85.
16. Hooker BA, Tobon G, Baker SJ, Zhu C, Hesterman J, Schmidt K, Rajagovindan R, Chandran P, Joshi SK, Bannon AW, et al. Gabapentin-induced pharmacodynamic effects in the spinal nerve ligation model of neuropathic pain. Eur J Pain 2014;18(2):223–37.
17. Jones KL, Finn DP, Governo RJ, Prior MJ, Morris PG, Kendall DA, Marsden CA, Chapman V. Identification of discrete sites of action of chronic treatment with desipramine in a model of neuropathic pain. Neuropharmacology 2009;56(2):405–13.

18. Liang Z, King J, Zhang N. Intrinsic organization of the anesthetized brain. J Neurosci 2012;32(30):10183–91.
19. Liang Z, King J, Zhang N. Uncovering intrinsic connectional architecture of functional networks in awake rat brain. J Neurosci 2011;31(10):3776–83.
20. Liu CH, Greve DN, Dai G, Marota JJ, Mandeville JB. Remifentanil administration reveals biphasic phMRI temporal responses in rat consistent with dynamic receptor regulation. NeuroImage 2007;34(3):1042–53.
21. Loggia ML, Berna C, Kim J, Cahalan CM, Gollub RL, Wasan AD, Harris RE, Edwards RR, Napadow V. Disrupted brain circuitry for pain-related reward/punishment in fibromyalgia. Arthritis Rheum 2014;66(1):203–12.
22. Lowe AS, Beech JS, Williams SC. Small animal, whole brain fMRI: innocuous and nociceptive forepaw stimulation. NeuroImage 2007;35(2):719–28.
23. Lu H, Zou Q, Gu H, Raichle ME, Stein EA, Yang Y. Rat brains also have a default mode network. Proc Natl Acad Sci USA 2012;109(10):3979–84.
24. Mishra AM, Ellens DJ, Schridde U, Motelow JE, Purcaro MJ, DeSalvo MN, Enev M, Sanganahalli BG, Hyder F, Blumenfeld H. Where fMRI and electrophysiology agree to disagree: corticothalamic and striatal activity patterns in the WAG/Rij rat. J Neurosci 2011;31(42):15053–64.
25. Schenk LA, Sprenger C, Geuter S, Buchel C. Expectation requires treatment to boost pain relief: an fMRI study. Pain 2014;155(1):150–7.
26. Shih YY, Chang C, Chen JC, Jaw FS. BOLD fMRI mapping of brain responses to nociceptive stimuli in rats under ketamine anesthesia. Med Eng Phys 2008;30(8):953–8.
27. Shih, YY, Chen CC, Shyu BC, Lin ZJ, Chiang YC, Jaw FS, Chen YY, Chang C. A new scenario for negative functional magnetic resonance imaging signals: endogenous neurotransmission. J Neurosci 2009;29(10):3036–44.
28. Smith JB, Alloway KD. Rat whisker motor cortex is subdivided into sensory-input and motor-output areas. Front Neural Circ 2013;7:4.
29. Tian P, Teng IC, May LD, Kurz R, Lu K, Scadeng M, Hillman EM, De Crespigny AJ, D'Arceuil HE, Mandeville JB, et al. Cortical depth-specific microvascular dilation underlies laminar differences in blood oxygenation level-dependent functional MRI signal. Proc Natl Acad Sci USA 2010;107(34):15246–51.
30. Tsurugizawa T, Uematsu A, Uneyama H, Torii K. Effects of isoflurane and alpha-chloralose anesthesia on BOLD fMRI responses to ingested L-glutamate in rats. Neuroscience 2010;165(1):244–51.
31. Upadhyay J, Baker SJ, Chandran P, Miller L, Lee Y, Marek GJ, Sakoglu U, Chin CL, Luo F, Fox GB, et al. Default-mode-like network activation in awake rodents. PloS ONE 2011;6(11):e27839.
32. Upadhyay J, Baker SJ, Rajagovindan R, Hart M, Chandran P, Hooker BA, Cassar S, Mikusa JP, Tovcimak A, Wald MJ, et al. Pharmacological modulation of brain activity in a preclinical model of osteoarthritis. NeuroImage 2013;64:341–55.
33. Upadhyay J, Pendse G, Anderson J, Schwarz AJ, Baumgartner R, Coimbra A, Bishop J, Knudsen J, George E, Grachev I, et al. Improved characterization of BOLD responses for evoked sensory stimuli. NeuroImage 2010;49(3):2275–86.
34. von Hehn CA, Baron R, Woolf CJ. Deconstructing the neuropathic pain phenotype to reveal neural mechanisms. Neuron 2012;73(4):638–52.
35. Wise RG, Williams P, Tracey I. Using fMRI to quantify the time dependence of remifentanil analgesia in the human brain. Neuropsychopharmacology 2004;29(3):626–35.
36. Zhao F, Williams M, Bowlby M, Houghton A, Hargreaves R, Evelhoch J, Williams DS. Qualification of fMRI as a biomarker for pain in anesthetized rats by comparison with behavioral response in conscious rats. NeuroImage 2014;84:724–32.
37. Zhao F, Williams M, Meng X, Welsh DC, Coimbra A, Crown ED, Cook JJ, Urban MO, Hargreaves R, Williams DS. BOLD and blood volume-weighted fMRI of rat lumbar spinal cord during non-noxious and noxious electrical hindpaw stimulation. NeuroImage 2008;40(1):133–47.
38. Zhao F, Williams M, Meng X, Welsh DC, Grachev ID, Hargreaves R, Williams DS. Pain fMRI in rat cervical spinal cord: an echo planar imaging evaluation of sensitivity of BOLD and blood volume-weighted fMRI. NeuroImage 2009;44(2):349–62.
39. Zhao F, Williams M, Welsh DC, Meng X, Ritter A, Abbadie C, Cook JJ, Reicin AS, Hargreaves R, Williams DS. fMRI investigation of the effect of local and systemic lidocaine on noxious electrical stimulation-induced activation in spinal cord. Pain 2009;145(1–2):110–9.

CHAPTER 13

Combining Neuroimaging with Electrophysiology in Animal Studies

Li Min Chen

Modern brain imaging such as functional MRI (fMRI) has revolutionized our view about pain, allowing an opportunity to investigate neural mechanisms of pain by measuring simultaneously across multiple brain regions in functions related to the perception and modulation of pain in health and diseases. The fundamental tenet in these imaging studies is that fMRI signal (e.g., blood oxygenation level–dependent [BOLD]) changes parallel neural activity. The precise relationships between fMRI signal and neuronal activity (also called neurovascular coupling), however, are not fully understood and are active research topics, but we know that neuronal spiking and synaptic activity, excitatory or inhibitory, all contribute to blood flow demand being detected by fMRI signals. Much of the existing knowledge comes mainly from studies in visual system in physiological conditions by assessing the relationships between changes in neuronal electrophysiological signals (spiking and local field potentials) and MRI signal amplitude. Few studies have examined the spatial relationships between these two types of signal, neither in pathological conditions. Specifically in the pain research field, wide applications of fMRI not only identified brain regions that are responsible for the multidimensional experience of pain perception, but also revealed widespread alterations in brain function and structure in various chronic pain conditions. However, accurate interpretations of these MRI findings and a full appreciation of their clinical and behavioural implications require knowledge of the MRI activity of the underlying neuronal constituents, given BOLD fMRI signal measures indirectly ensemble properties and activities of relatively large neuron populations [17, 36, 40]. Such information is difficult, and indeed is often impossible to obtain in human subjects for both technical and ethical reasons, but can be acquired from animal studies. In contrast, fMRI in animals allows one to directly compare neuronal activity and MRI activity, and ultimately provides the much-needed information about the physiological basis of the fMRI signals.

In my laboratory, we have taken such an approach by combining high-resolution fMRI (at 9.4 T), microelectrode recording, and histology, and have focused our studies on understanding the processes of painful and nonpainful touch inputs in normal and pathological conditions in early somatosensory cortices (areas around the central and lateral sulci) in lightly anaesthetized squirrel monkeys. Information provided by each method is independent and complementary, and provides a more comprehensive view about cortical processing. In this chapter, I mainly review findings derived from studies in the S1 cortex (areas 3a, 3b, and 1/2) in two experimental settings: nociceptive and tactile processes in normal (input-intact) condition and tactile process in deafferentation (input-deprived) condition. Deafferentation study is motivated by the observations of rarely detected S1 cortex activation in chronic pain conditions, yet numerous reports on plastic change in structure and somatotopic map. In our study, deafferentation is introduced by unilateral dorsal column lesion at high cervical level, a procedure that selectively disrupts the pathway important for fine discriminative touch. We started our deafferentation study with this model system because it has been well studied with other invasive methods (microelectrode mapping and immunohistological evaluation). Although we did not specifically test the effects of disruption of nociceptive pathways on pain response, we believe understanding the effects of deafferentation on fMRI signal and its relationship with neuronal activity has implications for other deafferentation conditions, including some types of chronic pain.

fMRI STUDY OF NOCICEPTION IN NONHUMAN PRIMATES: MISSING LINK BETWEEN ANIMAL AND HUMAN DATA

Studying nociception in monkeys is advantageous in several aspects. First, the monkey brain closely resembles the human brain, compared with those of rodents. For example, rather than single areas of the S1 and the S2 cortices in rodents, the S1 and S2 regions in primates including humans comprise several functionally and anatomically distinct subregions. Out of these well-established four subregion structures in primates, only area 3b is regarded as the homologous region as S1 region in rodents [26]. Similar functional organization differences are known to exist in other high-order pain processing regions such as those along the lateral sulcus [27–29]. Thus, information derived from monkey studies provides the important missing link between rodent and human data. Second, the achievable high-spatial resolution fMRI images in monkeys [12, 20, 23–25] allow the examination of pain network at the submillimeter scale. At ultrahigh MRI field (e.g., 9.4 T), signal– and contrast–noise ratios increase significantly, which permits high-resolution fMRI studies at the submillimeter scale [7, 9, 12, 22, 34, 35]. This achievement is critical for understanding brain function and pain processing [35, 39] as fine-scale columnar structures are believed to be the building blocks and basic information processing units of the cerebral cortical function. fMRI activation maps not only allow us to examine the nociceptive responses at various network scales (e.g., modular organization within one area and across areas), but also help tremendously in selecting target regions for the time-consuming electrophysiological mapping and recording studies, particularly in areas in which we have little prior knowledge.

fMRI AND OPTICAL IMAGING OF INTRINSIC SIGNAL REVEALED DIFFERENTIAL CORTICAL REPRESENTATIONS OF THERMAL NOCICEPTION AND TOUCH IN S1 CORTEX

The role of the S1 cortex in pain perception has long been debated to this day [4, 30, 46, 47]. The doubt about the role of the S1 cortex in pain perception comes mainly from three observations: inconsistent detection of fMRI activations in human S1 cortex, particularly in chronic pathological pain conditions; the small number of nociceptive neurons identified in corresponding areas 3a, 3b, and 1/2 in monkeys [18, 19, 42, 51]; and failure to evoke or diminish pain sensation by stimulating or ablating the S1 cortex. On the basis of our own data, we believe that several factors have contributed to these observations. The first one is the use of relatively large fMRI signal voxels on sampling signals originating from functionally heterogeneous neuronal populations. The second factor relates to the compromised fMRI response detection in pathological conditions such as deafferentation. Findings derived from our high-resolution fMRI studies support our speculation about the first factor. I focus my discussion on the S1 cortex because it is a flat cortical region that allows detailed spatial comparison among maps obtained with fMRI, microelectrode mapping and recordings, and histology.

Under light anaesthesia (0.5–1% isoflurane), we found that nociceptive heat stimulation (47.5°C pulse in 24 seconds duration) of digits evoked robust (~0.8% BOLD signal change), widely distributed, and reproducible fMRI activations at topographically appropriate regions in areas 3a, 3b, and 1/2 of S1 and anterior M1 cortices (Fig. 13-1A, D, E, and H) [8]. In contrast, fMRI activations elicited by innocuous tactile stimuli are more constrained spatially; located at somatotopically appropriate regions in areas 3b and 1 (Fig. 13-1B and F; see the colour-coded microelectrode penetrations in Fig. 13-1D and H). These differential activation patterns to nociceptive heat versus touch are present across monkeys. Fig. 13-1 shows data from two representative animals (for the entire figure, see Figure 4 in Chen et al. [8]).

Occasionally, we also detected tactile stimulus-related BOLD signal changes in area 3a in some monkeys (e.g., D2 activation in area 3a shown in Fig. 13-1B). By characterizing the receptive field and preferred stimulus properties of neurons at each microelectrode penetration site (colour dots in Fig. 13-1C and G), we determined the cortical territories of each digit representation in each cortical area and their interareal borders (dotted lines in Fig. 13-1C and G). Careful examination of the activation maps and BOLD time courses at each cortical area led to two main findings in the S1 cortex. First, the spatial relationships between heat pain and tactile fMRI activations varied across areas. fMRI tactile activations in areas 3b and 1/2 correlate spatially quite well with the digit representations defined by microelectrode recordings. In strong contrast, heat activation does not overlap with tactile responses. Heat activation locates at the centre of area 3b–area 1 border region, and tactile activation locates at the centre of area 3b strip. In area 1/2, the foci of heat nociceptive

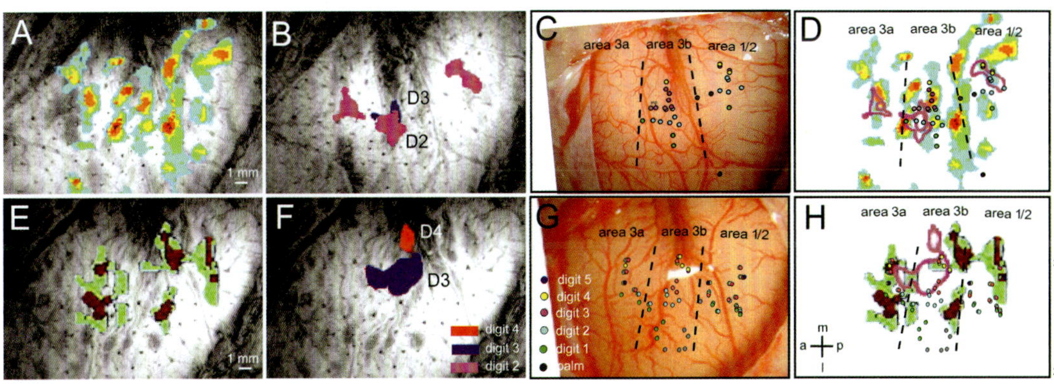

FIGURE 13-1 Comparison of nociceptive] heat and tactile fMRI activations within S1 cortex in two representative monkeys. **A, E:** Colour-coded activation probability maps illustrate the frequency of detected activations (in each run) to 47.5°C nociceptive heat stimulation of digits within each imaging session. Activation in each run was thresholded at < 0.0001 (uncorrected). **B, F:** Composite digit tactile activation maps of the same animals. Letters indicate the stimulated digits associated with the activation. **C, G:** Digit representation maps as determined electrophysiologically by microelectrode mapping. Receptive field properties of neurons at each penetration (Colour dots) were colour coded for different digits. Dotted lines indicate the estimated interareal borders. **D, H:** Overlays of nociceptive heat and tactile fMRI activation patterns and electrophysiological maps in each animal. Colour-coded scale bars indicate the number of activated runs of the total of scanned runs **(far right)**. a, anterior; p, posterior; m, middle; l, lateral. Scale bars, 1 mm. (Modified from Figure 4 in Chen et al. [8].)

activation only partially overlapped with that of tactile activation. Different from areas 3b and 1/2, area 3a responded preferentially to nociceptive heat stimuli. Second, BOLD signal changes to heat stimulation in areas 3a and 1 peaked earlier than that of area 3b (Fig. 13-2C). This area 3a/area 1 to area 3b information flow direction is reversed from the area 3b-to-area 1 flow for processing tactile inputs. Certainly, the differential interareal information processing flows for heat versus tactile need to be further tested with electrophysiological recordings. Thus far, targeted microelectrode recordings conducted in our laboratory indeed identified nociceptive neurons at each fMRI activation cluster we examined ([8, 10] and unpublished observations).

Extending previous neuroimaging findings in monkey S1 cortex [10, 21, 43, 44], our high-resolution fMRI studies illustrated a spatially more complex and segregated, and temporally more dynamic interareal network for processing nociceptive heat information. The complexity in spatial and temporal features very likely contributes to the variation in fMRI signals; this results in inconsistent detection of pain-related fMRI signal changes in the S1 cortex in human studies, in which functionally and anatomically distinct four-region structure is treated as a single entity. For instance, from the detection point of view, if a large proportion of fMRI voxels were sampling signals originating from a mixture of different S1 subregions or regions mixed with nociceptive and innocuous neurons, then the net detectable fMRI signal changes would likely change drastically, depending on the location of those voxels and the composition of different stimulus-preferred neuron clusters across subjects. The editorial by Davis [17] illustrated very well one aspect of the above-mentioned complex, the possible relationships between a single fMRI voxel and underlying anatomical and functional substitutes. As expected, if we reduced the fMRI voxel size to a fine scale (e.g., the submillimeter scale in our study) with which activities that originated from distinct functional cortical columns or regions are separable, then the detection and reproducibility of fMRI activation evoked by painful stimuli would increase drastically. In fact, these were our observations in both monkey and human high-resolution fMRI studies. In monkeys, fMRI signal changes to nociceptive heat, cold (unpublished data), and innocuous touch were consistently detected across imaging runs, imaging sessions, and across animals. In humans, by applying high-resolution fMRI (1×1 mm^2 in-plane resolution) at 7 T, we constantly detected pain-related signal changes in area 3a and other subregions in the S1 cortex (Stringer EA, Gore JC, and Chen LM, unpublished observation).

Using the high-resolution fMRI activation maps as guides for microelectrode recording, we have identified nociceptive neurons at each fMRI activation focus (in areas 3a, 3b,

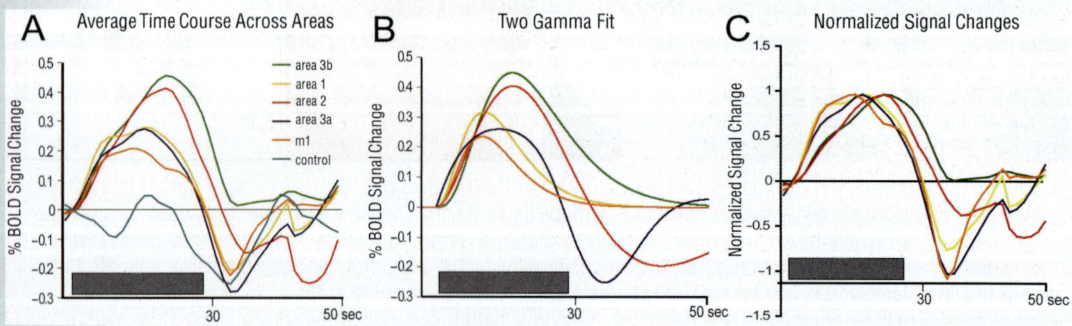

FIGURE 13-2 Comparison of average BOLD time courses and two γ fittings across animals in different cortical areas. **A:** Plot of average time courses of BOLD signal changes in each area. **B:** Two γ curve fits of raw average BOLD time courses from all cases. **C:** Plot of normalized BOLD signal changes across areas. Grey bars: stimulus presentation period. (Adapted from Chen et al. [8].)

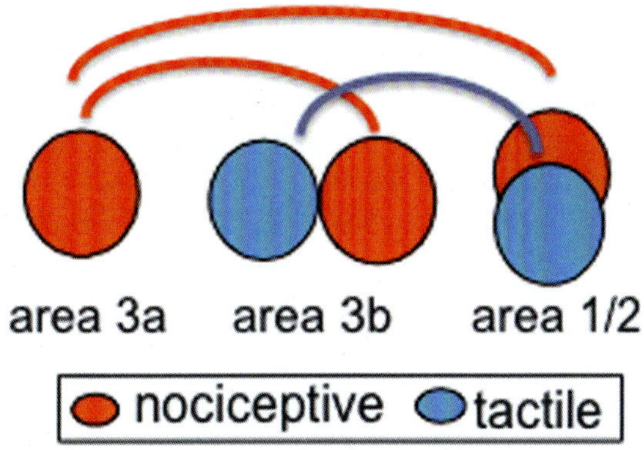

FIGURE 13-3 Model for cortical processing of nociception and touch within S1 cortex.

and 1, and S2) we have examined so far. Our so far successful recording experience confirms the speculation by Treede et al. [45] about the possible searching bias caused by the mapping stimulus of probe tapping in the majority of previous studies [18, 19, 31–33]. Ongoing studies in our laboratory aim to explore and characterize the response properties of nociceptive neurons in cortical areas where nociception-related fMRI signals were detected.

To summarize, evidence obtained from our fMRI and optical imaging experiments support involvements of areas 3a, 3b, and 1/2 of the S1 cortex in processing heat [8, 21, 43], mechanical [10], and cold [52] nociceptive inputs. Local heat nociceptive processing network within S1 appears to be apart from that of innocuous tactile processing. On the basis of our observations of spatial segregations of heat and tactile fMRI activations and the early-peaked heat fMRI signal changes in area 3a, we propose that nociceptive heat and tactile inputs are processed by different interareal circuitries within the S1 cortex. Area 3a–area 1/2 circuitry is for nociceptive heat, whereas area 3b–area 1/2 is for innocuous touch. The proposed model for the representation of heat nociception is illustrated in Fig. 13-3. On the basis of observation of overlapping mechanical and tactile activations within areas 3b and 1 [10], we also hypothesize that mechanical and heat nociceptive inputs are likely processed by different groups of neurons and local circuitries within and across S1 subareas. To date, however, clear experimental data for a labelled-line nociceptive processing are available only for the peripheral system (for a recent review, see [37]). Thus, whether the different circuitries identified within and across S1 subareas are nociceptive specific and receive functionally specific thalamic inputs remains to be determined. More neuronal electrophysiological and anatomical connectivity data are necessary to support (or disapprove) the proposed networks for differential representation of heat and mechanical pain in primates [14–16, 46].

RESTING-STATE FMRI SIGNALS REVEAL DIFFERENT INTERAREAL FUNCTIONAL CONNECTIVITY OF AREAS 3A AND 3B

Building upon the evidence for segregated nociceptive versus tactile activation processing circuitries within S1, we next asked the question of whether these nociceptive regions are actually functionally connected. We used the well-documented indicator for functional connectivity, interregional correlation of low-frequency fMRI signals at resting state, to probe the functional connection between areas of 3a, 3b, and 1/2. Numerous studies have demonstrated the power and usefulness of the resting-state fMRI signals for probing intrinsic functional connectivity among brain regions in humans and monkeys [2, 3, 48]. Using this measure, we found that the areas 3b and 3a exhibited differential connectivity patterns (Fig. 13-4). Area 3b connects strongly to area 1/2, but not area 3a, whereas area 3a connects strongly to area 1/2 (comparing D and G with E and H in Fig. 13-4). Importantly, the interareal functional connectivity pattern is somatotopically specific (e.g., D2 tip to D2 tip), a feature indicating its functional relevance for spatial localization and discrimination of sensory inputs. Subsequent microelectrode recording studies indeed reveal synchronized spiking activity among those regions exhibiting strong resting-state fMRI signal [5, 49].

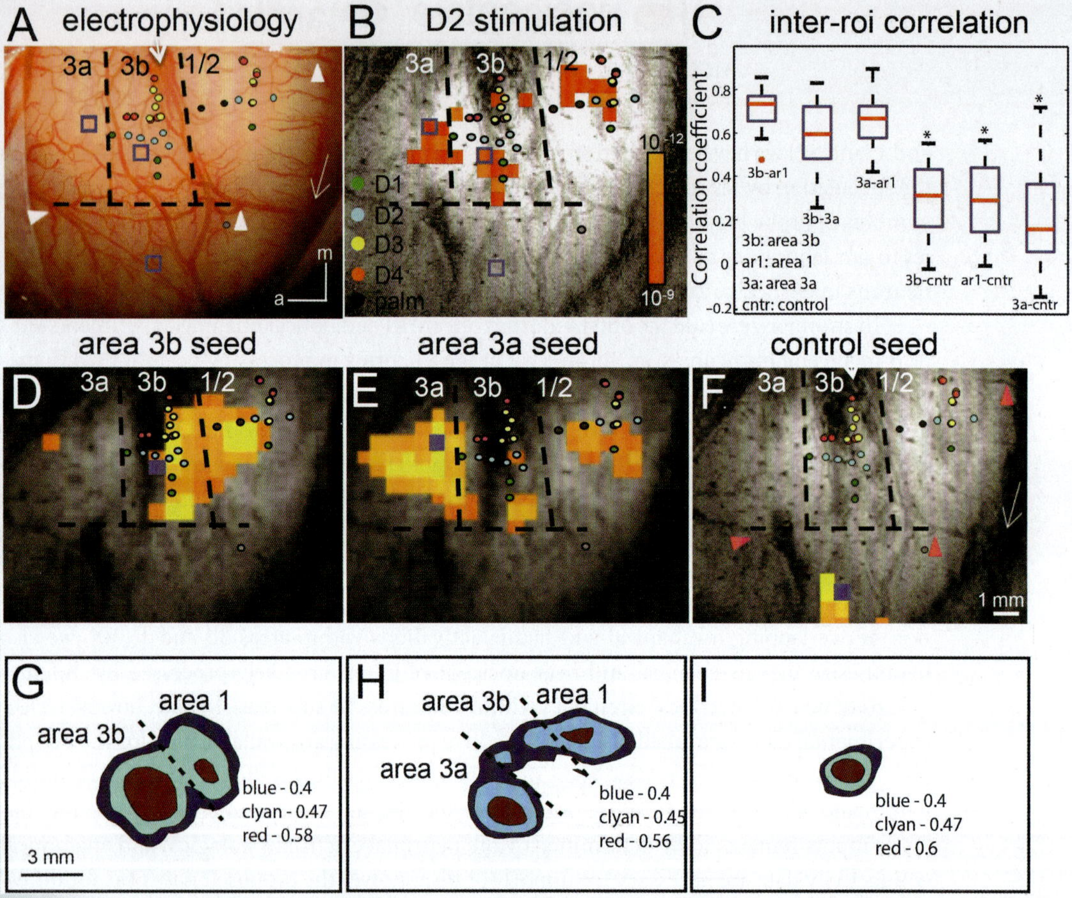

FIGURE 13-4 Resting-state fMRI connectivity within S1 cortex of squirrel monkeys. One case is shown in **(A,B)**, **(D–F)**; population data in **(C)** and **(G–I)**. **A:** Electrophysiological map of digit region. Coloured dots: see legend, digits 1–4, palm. Dotted lines: estimated interareal borders between areas 3a, 3b, and 1, and between hand/face. White arrows: the central and lateral sulci. Blue boxes: areas 3a, 3b, and 3b face seed regions. White arrowheads: vessel markers used for alignment with image in **(F)** (*pink arrowheads*). **B:** BOLD activation in response to vibrotactile stimulation of D2 tip. Activated voxels are observed in areas 3a, 3b, and 1. Correlation maps were thresholded at $r > 0.7$ with a peak correlation value of 0.9. **C:** Boxplot of correlation coefficient values between area 3b and area 1 (3b–1), area 3b and area 3a (3b–3a), area 3a and area 1 (3a–1), and with control locations (3b–cntr, 1–cntr, 3a–cntr). **D–F:** BOLD correlation maps in resting state. Seed voxels (*solid blue boxes*) were placed in the digit regions in area 3b **(C)**, area 3a **(D)**, and face regions in area 3b **(E)** for voxel-wise correlation analysis. **G–I:** Cross-animal (or population) correlation maps of seeds in area 3b **(G)**, area 3a **(H)**, and face **(I)** regions. Correlations are a summary of 18 runs (i.e., each map based on 18 seeds, seeds overlay D2, D3, or D4 digit tip) conducted in 10 animals. To average across animals, seed voxels were used to align all the cross-animal images. Correlation maps are centred on the seed region. Because seed location is relative to the imaging field of view across animals, there are some deviations in spatial location between average correlation map and individual cases. (Adapted from Figure 1 in Orban [40] and Wang et al. [49].)

Examination of the local intrinsic anatomical connection pattern also identified preferential connections of areas 3b and 1 [1, 38, 49]. For the first time, our study establishes an anatomical and electrophysiological basis for resting-state fMRI (<0.1 Hz) networks within the S1 cortex at a local millimeter-based scale.

PROPOSED MODELS FOR CORTICAL PROCESSING OF NOCICEPTION AND TOUCH WITHIN S1 CORTEX

We proposed an interareal selective circuitry model for heat and touch inputs processing within the S1 cortex on the basis of the findings from stimulus-evoked and resting-state fMRI experiments. This model, illustrated in Fig. 13-3, suggests the following information processing features within the S1 cortex: (1) heat pain processing circuitry within the S1 cortex is composed of regions in areas 3a, 3b, and 1/2 (red circles), and in a topographic manner. Touch circuitry is independent of heat pain circuitry, which consists of areas 3b and 1 (blue circles). (2) There is a general anterior-to-posterior information processing hierarchy (colour lines) for both heat pain and touch. (3) Area 3a-to-area 1/2 connection is the dominant pathway for pain within the S1 cortex. Area 3a could be the first relay station for processing heat nociceptive inputs as proposed by Craig [13]. We recognized that more *in vivo* microelectrode recording and mapping studies in monkeys are needed to fully construct the circuitry and to understand the flow for nociceptive information integration within the S1 cortex. Further studies in humans are also needed to determine the functional relevance of these interareal local networks within the S1 cortex in pain perception.

EFFECTS OF DEAFFERENTATION ON BOLD, LOCAL FIELD POTENTIAL, AND SPIKING ACTIVITY IN S1 CORTEX: IMPLICATION FOR DETECTING S1 CORTEX NOCICEPTIVE RESPONSE IN CHRONIC PAIN CONDITIONS

To understand the effects of deafferentation on fMRI signal, neuronal electrophysiological activity, and the relationships between these two types of signals, we conducted a series of experiments on squirrel monkeys undergoing unilateral dorsal column lesion. Dorsal column lesion of spinal cord at the cervical level is a relatively clear experimental condition because it selectively disrupts ascending afferents carrying discriminative fine touch information to the S1 cortex as demonstrated previously. This model allows us to quantify the effects of deafferentation on fMRI signals change in activation size and magnitude, neuronal activity of spiking and local field potential (LFP), and the spatial and magnitude correlations between changes in these two types of signals in a very well controlled deafferentation condition. Specifically, we evaluated the effectiveness of lesion (the percentage of dorsal column afferents disruption) by quantifying the number of spared tracer intake fibre terminals at the dorsal column nuclei in the brain stem (for details see [6, 41]). Comparing fMRI responses obtained before and after lesions that resulted in 78–99% afferent disruption in monkeys, we found at input-deprived area 3b that (1) the detection rate of fMRI response to identical tactile stimulation drops about 30%; (2) the fMRI responsive region is enlarged; and (3) spatially, the detected fMRI activation centre shifted away from its original representation location, resulting in the reorganization of digit maps. Compared with the digit representation maps determined by neuronal activity, (4) fMRI response at the input-deprived region is larger in size. After lesion, (5) response magnitude of fMRI and multiunit firing activity to 8 Hz stimulation reduce significantly. These findings indicate that the input-deprived (deafferentated) cortex exhibited weaker, spatially shifted and more defused fMRI signal changes. Neurons at those input-deprived cortical regions exhibited a similar reduction in multiunit activity to external drive in area 3b. The extent of activity reduction, however, varied across areas. Neuronal spiking activity in area 1 is significantly weaker than that in area 3b. Most importantly, simultaneous recordings of the spiking and LFPs from those input-deprived regions (but reactivated regions, definition is provided in [50]) revealed that a reduction in multiunit spiking activity did not parallel similar changes in LFPs, suggesting a disproportionally enhanced synaptic contribution to fMRI signal changes at the input-deprived cortex.

Figs. 13-5 and 13-6 illustrate examples for the above-described changes in areas 3b and 1 [11, 41]. In this particular animal, much of the input-deprived digit regions (D2–D5) in areas 3b and 1 were unresponsive electrophysiologically at 8 weeks following spinal cord

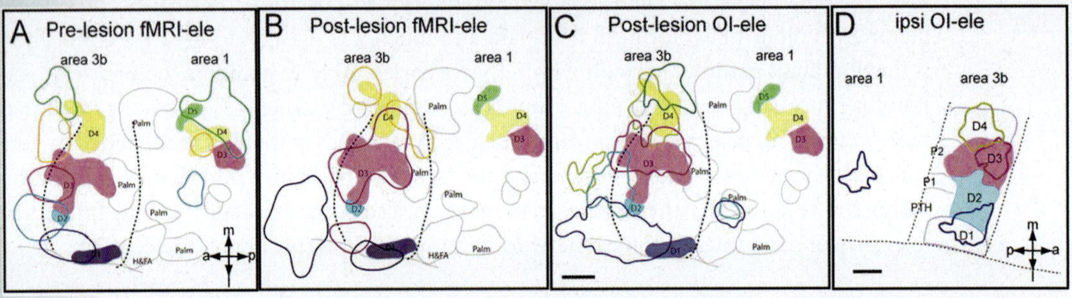

FIGURE 13-5 Comparisons of fMRI, optical imaging, and electrophysiology maps of digit activation after dorsal column lesion in contralateral and ipsilateral areas 3b and 1 in one monkey. **A:** Overlay of prelesion fMRI and postlesion electrophysiology maps of digits. Colour outlines indicate location and size of fMRI activations, whereas colour patches present location and size of neuronal responses. **B:** Spatial comparison of postlesion fMRI and postlesion electrophysiology digit maps. **C:** Spatial comparison of postlesion optical imaging (OI) and postlesion electrophysiology digit maps. **D:** Overlay of optical imaging and electrophysiology maps of digits D1–D4 in the ipsilateral areas 3b and 1 of the same animals. CS, central sulcus. Dotted black lines denote estimated interareal borders. Scale bar: 1 mm. a, anterior; p, posterior; l, lateral; m, medial. (Modified from Figure 9 in Chen et al. [11].)

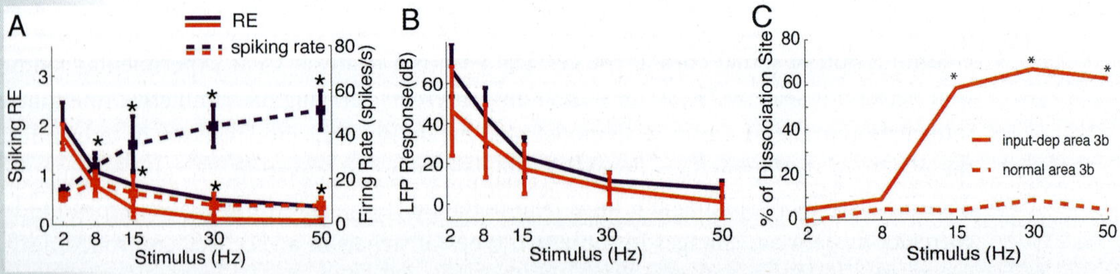

FIGURE 13-6 Group quantification of spiking **(A)** and LFP **(B)** responses in area 3b as function of stimulus frequency and summary of percentage of spike–LFP dissociation in control and input-deprived deafferentated cases **(C)**. **A:** The mean response efficacies (RE, *solid lines*) to different stimulus frequencies declined progressively in deafferentated area 3b, and were significantly lower than those of normal cases ($^*P < 0.05$, except for 2 Hz stimulus). The firing rates of normal cortex are also significantly higher than those of deafferentated cortex. **B:** The mean power of evoked LFP in area 3b also decreased with increasing stimulus frequency. The LFP signal was persistently and robustly modulated by the tactile stimulation under all conditions, and there is no difference between signals in normal versus deafferentated cortex ($P > 0.05$). **C:** Summary of spike–LFP dissociation as function of stimulus frequency in area 3b of normal and input-deprived (plasticity subjects). With increasing stimulation frequency, the LFP response became more frequently dissociated with spiking activity in plasticity cases. $^*P < 0.05$. (Modified from Figure 6 in Wang et al. [50].)

lesion at the D2 level, with islands of neurons with enlarged receptive fields and weak responses. Compared with the prelesion digit activation fMRI map (colour outlines in Fig. 13-5A), there were apparent spatial shifts in the remaining digit responses towards the palm (color outlines in Fig. 13-5B–C) and interareal border of areas 3b and 1. D1 (dark blue outline), D3 (magenta outline), and D4 (yellow outline) fMRI activations were located at somatotopically appropriate sites, but the sizes of the activation sites were larger than normal (particularly for D4, Fig. 13-5B). Unlike the postlesion fMRI digit maps, the postlesion optical imaging maps of digits exhibited close spatial correlations with the postlesion digit maps defined electrophysiologically (Fig. 13-5C). Electrophysiology and optical imaging maps of D3 and D4 were in close agreement (Fig. 13-5C). Portions of the D1 and D2 activations, as well as the second patch of D4 activation, were determined to be in area 3a, as indicated by the border between areas 3b and 3a (dotted lines in Fig. 13-5A–C). We do not know whether the responsive patches in areas 3a are expansions to area 3b digit territory or the newly acquired responsiveness of area 3a neurons to low-threshold tactile stimuli. Major findings about the spatial reorganization of the fMRI response after deafferentation are summarized in the schematic model (Fig. 13-7).

Comparison of spiking and LFP activity in input-intact and input-deprived (deafferentated) area 3b sites revealed stimulus frequency-dependent reductions in response strengths (Fig. 13-6). Deafferentation caused significant reduction in spiking rates, particularly to high-frequency stimuli, but not so in LFPs. This frequency-dependent reduction in spiking after disruption of dorsal column afferents indicates that functional changes occurring in the deafferentated cortex are functionally specific, such as the tactile frequency encoding in our experimental model.

To summarize, our studies showed that deafferentation alters several aspects of cortical processing. The weakened and diffused fMRI signal changes to stimuli likely compromise fMRI activation detection. This observation calls for more cautious interpretations about failed detection of pain-related activations in the S1 cortex, particularly in conditions where deafferentation is suspected. The finding of high frequency–dependent dissociation of LFP and spiking activity also indicates that the plastic changes occurring in the brain are developed in a functionally specific manner. Thus, to fully appreciate the role of the S1 cortex, particularly in chronic pain conditions, uses of appropriate forms of painful stimuli and paradigm are necessary.

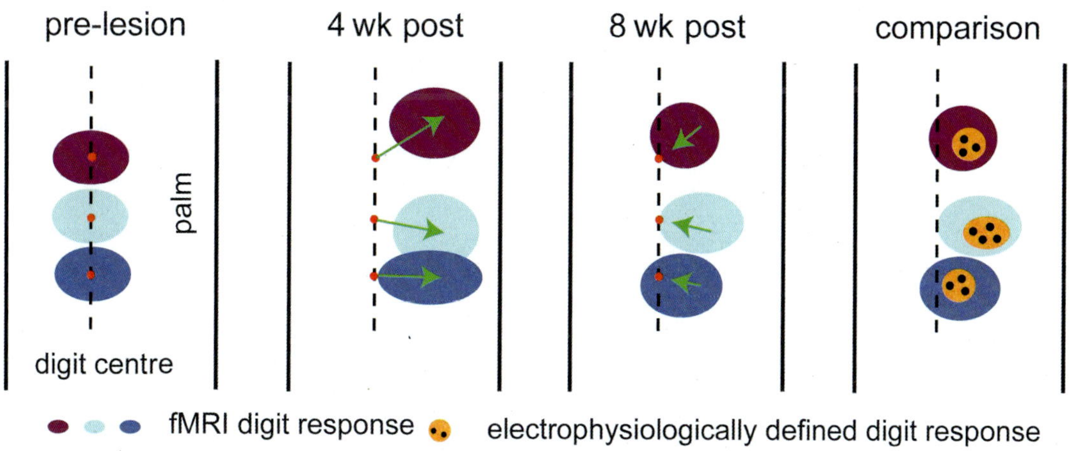

FIGURE 13-7 Spatial reorganization of the fMRI response relative to electrophysiologically determined response maps before and after deafferentation.

CONCLUSION

By taking advantage of submillimeter fMRI at high MRI field, we provided fMRI evidence supporting a differential engagement of areas 3a, 3b, and 1 of the S1 cortex in the processing of heat nociceptive versus tactile inputs. Analysis of resting-state fMRI signals revealed differential interareal functional connectivity among the subregions. We propose a separated interareal processing circuitry model for pain and touch within the S1 cortex. Our observations of the profound effects of deafferentation on fMRI signal, neuronal electrophysiological activity, and the relationships between the two types of signals highlight the importance of a better understanding of the neuronal basis for fMRI signal in general, and for nociceptive signal in particular. Our data demonstrated that we now have the tools necessary to start addressing those important questions.

ACKNOWLEDGEMENT

I am grateful for the helpful comments of Drs. Vania Apkarian and Robert Friedman on an earlier version of this chapter. I thank all the coauthors for their contributions to the original papers I mentioned in this chapter. I also thank Dr. John Gore for his financial support on resting-state fMRI projects, and Mrs. Chaohui Tang and Mr. Fuxue Xin for their assistance in data collection. The work presented in this chapter is supported by HIN grants (R21 DA024831 and R01 NS069909) and an imaging track grant from Dana Foundation.

REFERENCES

1. Ashaber M, Palfi E, Friedman RM, Palmer C, Jakli B, Chen LM, Kantor O, Roe AW, Negyessy L. Connectivity of somatosensory cortical area 1 form an anatomical substrate for the emergence of multifinger receptive fields and complex feature selectivity in the squirrel monkey (*Saimiri sciureus*). J Comp Neurol 2014;522(8):1769–85.
2. Biswal B, Yetkin FZ, Haughton VM, Hyde JS. Functional connectivity in the motor cortex of resting human brain using echo-planar MRI. Magn Reson Med 1995;34(4):537–41.
3. Blatow M, Nennig E, Durst A, Sartor K, Stippich C. fMRI reflects functional connectivity of human somatosensory cortex. Neuroimage 2007;37(3):927–36.
4. Bushnell MC, Duncan GH, Hofbauer RK, Ha B, Chen JI, Carrier B. Pain perception: is there a role for primary somatosensory cortex? Proc Natl Acad Sci USA 1999;96(14):7705–9.
5. Chen L, Mishra A, Newton AT, Morgan VL, Stringer EA, Rogers BP, Gore JC. Fine-scale functional connectivity in somatosensory cortex revealed by high-resolution fMRI. Magn Reson Imaging 2011;29(10):1330–7.
6. Chen L, Qi HX, Kaas JH. Dynamic reorganization of digit representations in somatosensory cortex of non-human primates after spinal cord injury. J Neurosci 2012;32(42)14649–63.
7. Chen LM, Dillenburger BC, Wang F, Friedman RM, Avison MJ. High-resolution functional magnetic resonance imaging mapping of noxious heat and tactile activations along the central sulcus in new world monkeys. Pain 2011;152(3):522–32.
8. Chen LM, Dillenburger BC, Wang F, Tang CH. Differential fMRI activation to noxious heat and tactile stimuli in parasylvian areas of new world monkeys. Pain 2012;153(1):158–69.
9. Chen LM, Friedman RM, Ramsden BM, LaMotte RH, Roe AW. Fine-scale organization of SI (area 3b) in the squirrel monkey revealed with intrinsic optical imaging. J Neurophysiol 2001;86(6):3011–29.
10. Chen LM, Friedman RM, Roe AW. Area-specific representation of mechanical nociceptive stimuli within SI cortex of squirrel monkeys. Pain 2009;141(3):258–68.
11. Chen LM, Qi HX, Kaas JH. Dynamic reorganization of digit representations in somatosensory cortex of nonhuman primates after spinal cord injury. J Neurosci 2012;32(42):14649–63.
12. Cheng H, Nair G, Walker TA, Kim MK, Pardue MT, Thule PM, Olson DE, Duong TQ. Structural and functional MRI reveals multiple retinal layers. Proc Natl Acad Sci USA 2006;103(46):17525–30.

13. Craig AD. Pain mechanisms: labeled lines versus convergence in central processing. Annu Rev Neurosci 2003;26:1–30.
14. Craig AD. Lamina I, but not lamina V, spinothalamic neurons exhibit responses that correspond with burning pain. J Neurophysiol 2004;92(4):2604–9.
15. Craig AD. Retrograde analyses of spinothalamic projections in the macaque monkey: input to ventral posterior nuclei. J Comp Neurol 2006;499(6):965–78.
16. Craig AD. Retrograde analyses of spinothalamic projections in the macaque monkey: input to the ventral lateral nucleus. J Comp Neurol 2008;508(2):315–28.
17. Davis KD. Neurophysiological and anatomical considerations in functional imaging of pain. Pain 2003;105 (1–2):1–3.
18. Dong WK, Chudler EH, Sugiyama K, Roberts VJ, Hayashi T. Somatosensory, multisensory, and task-related neurons in cortical area 7b (PF) of unanesthetized monkeys. J Neurophysiol 1994;72(2):542–64.
19. Dong WK, Salonen LD, Kawakami Y, Shiwaku T, Kaukoranta EM, Martin RF. Nociceptive responses of trigeminal neurons in SII-7b cortex of awake monkeys. Brain Res 1989;484(1–2):314–24.
20. Duong TQ, Kim DS, Ugurbil K, Kim SG. Spatiotemporal dynamics of the BOLD fMRI signals: toward mapping submillimeter cortical columns using the early negative response. Magn Reson Med 2000;44(2):231–42.
21. Favorov O, Li Y, Tommerdahl M, Whitsel B. Nociresponsive neurons in area 3a of squirrel monkeys. Soc Neurosci Abstr 2007;70:22.
22. Fukuda M, Moon CH, Wang P, Kim SG. Mapping iso-orientation columns by contrast agent-enhanced functional magnetic resonance imaging: reproducibility, specificity, and evaluation by optical imaging of intrinsic signal. J Neurosci 2006;26(46):11821–32.
23. Harel N. Ultra high resolution fMRI at ultra-high field. Neuroimage 2012;62(2):1024–8.
24. Harel N, Lin J, Moeller S, Ugurbil K, Yacoub E. Combined imaging-histological study of cortical laminar specificity of fMRI signals. Neuroimage 2006;29(3):879–87.
25. Harel N, Ugurbil K, Uludag K, Yacoub E. Frontiers of brain mapping using MRI. J Magn Reson Imaging 2006;23(6):945–57.
26. Kaas JH. What, if anything, is SI? Organization of first somatosensory area of cortex. Physiol Rev 1983;63(1):206–31.
27. Kaas JH. The functional organization of somatosensory cortex in primates. Ann Anat 1993;175(6):509–18.
28. Kaas JH. The evolution of the complex sensory and motor systems of the human brain. Brain Res Bull 2008;75(2–4):384–90.
29. Kaas JH, Garraghty PE. Hierarchical, parallel, and serial arrangements of sensory cortical areas: connection patterns and functional aspects. Curr Opin Neurobiol 1991;1(2):248–251.
30. Kenshalo DR. Pain and the primary somatosensory cortex is its role in pain overrated? Pain Forum 1996;5(3):181–3.
31. Kenshalo DR, Iwata K, Sholas M, Thomas DA. Response properties and organization of nociceptive neurons in area 1 of monkey primary somatosensory cortex. J Neurophysiol 2000;84(2):719–29.
32. Kenshalo DR Jr, Chudler EH, Anton F, Dubner R. SI nociceptive neurons participate in the encoding process by which monkeys perceive the intensity of noxious thermal stimulation. Brain Res 1988;454(1–2):378–82.
33. Kenshalo DR Jr, Isensee O. Responses of primate SI cortical neurons to noxious stimuli. J Neurophysiol 1983;50(6):1479–96.
34. Kim SG, Duong TQ. Mapping cortical columnar structures using fMRI. Physiol Behav 2002;77(4–5):641–4.
35. Kim SG, Fukuda M. Lessons from fMRI about mapping cortical columns. Neuroscientist 2008;14(3):287–99.
36. Logothetis NK, Pauls J, Augath M, Trinath T, Oeltermann A. Neurophysiological investigation of the basis of the fMRI signal. Nature 2001;412(6843):150–7.
37. Moayedi M, Davis KD. Theories of pain: from specificity to gate control. J Neurophysiol 2013;109(1):5–12.
38. Negyessy L, Palfi E, Ashaber M, Palmer C, Jakli B, Friedman RM, Chen LM, Roe AW. Intrinsic horizontal connections process global tactile features in the primary somatosensory cortex: neuroanatomical evidence. J Comp Neurol 2013;521(12):2798–817.
39. Op de Beeck HP, Haushofer J, Kanwisher NG. Interpreting fMRI data: maps, modules and dimensions. Nat Rev Neurosci 2008;9(2):123–35.
40. Orban GA. Functional MRI in the awake monkey: the missing link. J Cogn Neurosci 2002;14(6):965–969.
41. Qi HX, Chen LM, Kaas JH. Reorganization of somatosensory cortical areas 3b and 1 after unilateral section of dorsal columns of the spinal cord in squirrel monkeys. J Neurosci 2011;31(38):13662–75.
42. Robinson CJ, Burton H. Somatotopographic organization in the second somatosensory area of *M. fascicularis*. J Comp Neurol 1980;192(1):43–67.

43. Tommerdahl M, Delemos KA, Favorov OV, Metz CB, Vierck CJ Jr, Whitsel BL. Response of anterior parietal cortex to different modes of same-site skin stimulation. J Neurophysiol 1998;80(6):3272–83.
44. Tommerdahl M, Delemos KA, Vierck CJ Jr, Favorov OV, Whitsel BL. Anterior parietal cortical response to tactile and skin-heating stimuli applied to the same skin site. J Neurophysiol 1996;75(6):2662–70.
45. Treede RD, Apkarian AV, Bromm B, Greenspan JD, Lenz FA. Cortical representation of pain: functional characterization of nociceptive areas near the lateral sulcus. Pain 2000;87(2):113–9.
46. Vierck CJ, Whitsel BL, Favorov OV, Brown AW, Tommerdahl M. Role of primary somatosensory cortex in the coding of pain. Pain 2013;154(3):334–44.
47. Vierck CJ, Whitsel BL, Favorov OV, Tommerdahl M. Response to the letter to the editor of pain by *S. Canavero*. Pain 2013;154(7):1158–9.
48. Vincent JL, Patel GH, Fox MD, Snyder AZ, Baker JT, Van Essen DC, Zempel JM, Snyder LH, Corbetta M, Raichle ME. Intrinsic functional architecture in the anaesthetized monkey brain. Nature 2007;447(7140):83–6.
49. Wang Z, Chen LM, Negyessy L, Friedman RM, Mishra A, Gore JC, Roe AW. The relationship of anatomical and functional connectivity to resting-state connectivity in primate somatosensory cortex. Neuron 2013;78(6):1116–26.
50. Wang Z, Qi HX, Kaas JH, Roe AW, Chen LM. Functional signature of recovering cortex: Dissociation of local field potentials and spiking activity in somatosensory cortices of spinal cord injured monkeys. Exp Neurol 2013;249:132–43.
51. Whitsel BL, Petrucelli LM, Sapiro G. Modality representation in the lumbar and cervical fasciculus gracilis of squirrel monkeys. Brain Res 1969;15(1):67–78.
52. Yang PF, Chen LM. Functional MRI mapping of nociceptive cold and tactile activations in somatosensory areas in anesthetized monkeys[abstract 268.12]. Neuroscience 2013:9–13.

CHAPTER 14

phMRI Measures of Analgesics in Preclinical Studies

Lino Becerra and David Borsook

Whether analgesics affect the PNS or CNS, they affect brain processing in terms of brain alterations as a consequence of the underlying disease or in terms of pain relief. Chronic pain affects multiple brain processes, and most analgesics act on the CNS [3, 4]. However, the ability to evaluate pharmacological agent actions on the brain has been the purview of positron emission tomography that can evaluate drug–receptor interactions (if an appropriate radioactive ligand has been developed) [26]. Relatively recently, the use of functional MRI (fMRI) to evaluate the direct effects of a drug on brain networks has allowed for a new science of pharmacological MRI (phMRI) to evaluate whole brain network and brain subnetwork processing [25].

Preclinical studies of pharmacological analgesic agents involve behavioural testing to assess the degree of efficacy of a drug and/or its side effects [2]. The tests include reactive/reflexive probes such as mechanical (von Frey hairs), thermal, and chemical stimuli as well as operant-based ones in which the animal alters free-moving behaviour on the basis of the presence of a pharmacological agent or in pursuit of one. Inferences about drug effects/mechanisms are deduced on the basis of observed behaviour and the known or hypothesized mechanism of action of the drug. Such an approach has been the current standard, and it has been relatively unsuccessful for many disease models, including pain. In analgesic drug development for chronic pain, the disconnection between observed behaviour modulated by a drug and human trials is fairly high, questioning the validity of the method. Current approaches in animal behaviour have included place preference as an index of pain relief—thus conferring what is considered to be a measure of spontaneous or ongoing pain [23].

phMRI—THE METHOD

phMRI, in its simplest form, is a variant of common fMRI approaches: a drug is administered either acutely or chronically, and the corresponding change in brain activity is detected with fMRI techniques (such as BOLD or rCBV/rCBF changes) [1, 6, 20]. The challenging aspect of phMRI is that most drugs have a relatively slow dynamic change, and it is similar to those induced by physiology or the scanner itself [1]. Hence, careful attention has to be given to extract the phMRI response from background noise. Pharmacokinetic/Pharmacodynamic (PK/PD) models could help in selecting a model for the phMRI response [20]. Other exploratory approaches, such as independent component analysis, could be used to identify potential spatial patterns and time courses [10].

The presence of a pharmacological agent can induce changes in CNS as it can trigger a cascade of responses, including excitation/inhibition of neurons. These effects can be detected with imaging [1, 6, 20]. In addition, following administration of an analgesic (acutely or chronically), modulation of a pain stimulus can be assessed with imaging and its differential effects across the several pain networks (e.g., modulating more an affective response than a sensory one) can be defined. The presence of an anaesthetic agent to perform these experiments could alter the analgesic effect as well as the measured signal; anaesthetics modulate brain metabolism as well as neuronal firing [16, 22]. These effects are strongly dependent on the anaesthetic level. Hence, the use of awake imaging could reduce these effects since no anaesthetic is needed [16, 22].

This methodology also provides an opportunity to assess chronic dosing—administering a drug for a period of time and later observing associated changes either to an acute administration of a drug or in intrinsic brain networks.

phMRI is not the only tool available to assess brain changes induced by the administration of a drug. Recently, it has been determined that the brain has a collection of networks that remain active even during resting conditions [24]. In humans, the determination of these intrinsic networks in the healthy individuals and how they are modified in a disease condition has allowed a better characterization of the disease and provided new approaches for treatment [12]. Follow-up studies indicate whether the treatment has "normalized" brain function as it relates to behavioural outcomes. For chronic pain, this has opened the possibility to study spontaneous pain in these patients, which is actually the major complaint of their condition. Following the administration of an analgesic in a chronic pain patient, intrinsic brain networks are monitored to see whether the drug indicates a normalization of the networks or lack thereof. Of note is that imaging might detect brain changes before the patient experiences them. Functional imaging also provides a methodology (functional connectivity MRI, fcMRI) to specifically question whether a particular structure function (e.g., the periaqueductal grey area [PAG]) has reestablished normal function through its connectivity to other brain areas [18].

fMRI/phMRI EVALUATION OF DE NOVO PHARMACOLOGICAL EFFECTS

The development of a new analgesic is difficult, is costly, and takes time. Given that pain and pain relief are a brain process, one of the major hurdles is to better understand where drugs act in the CNS and how they may alter perturbed neural networks known to exist in chronic pain. While the development of most analgesics has focused on symptom relief, new approaches that take into consideration disease modification are now being addressed.

The study of acute drug effects on brain systems with fMRI has been coined "pharmacological MRI" or phMRI as it deals with the brain activation/deactivation patterns usually associated with the acute (typically a bolus injection) administration of the drug. Several known analgesic drugs have been studied in this fashion and include opioids (morphine [20], remifentanil [20], buprenorphine [1], heroin [27]), gabapentinoids (gabapentin) [13], NMDA antagonists (ketamine) [19], antidepressants (desipramine) [17], nicotinic receptor agents [9], cannabinoids [11], and membrane stabilizers (Lidocaine) [21] (Fig. 14-1).

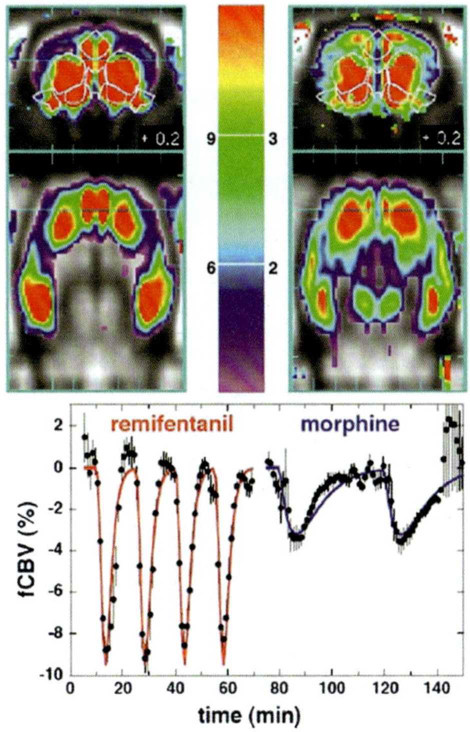

FIGURE 14-1 Patterns of brain activation following administration of remifentanil (**left images**) and morphine (**right images**). Below image shows the time course for infusion of both remifentanil and morphine. Activity was detected through changes in CBF as induced by the administration of a contrast agent [20]. The very different PK/PD of both drugs is evident from their time courses.

Within Class Evaluation: The Opioid Example

The study of morphine and remifentanil presents a unique opportunity to assess the pharmacodynamics of these different drugs [20]. Remifentanil is a fast-acting μ-opioid agonist that is metabolized within minutes of administration; morphine has extended effects lasting tens of minutes. In the study of Liu et al. [20], the drugs were administered at different doses. The resulting phMRI signal (measured as changes in cerebral blood volume) depicts a close relationship with the dosage. Analysis of the temporal dynamics of the response allowed them to define different aspects of the response and ascribe them to underlying neurobiological processes. The distribution of activity level across the brain indicates a good match of opioid receptor density distribution in the brain with structures such as the cingulate and the thalamus, displaying high levels of activity. In humans, a phMRI study of morphine indicated a similar response, with basal ganglia, thalamus, and other structures displaying a high level of activity.

Recently, we have published a study of the administration of buprenorphine in healthy humans and rodents [1]. The study involved the use of two doses, and their phMRI responses were measured. In both humans and rodents, we observed a similar pattern of activation, and, as with morphine and remifentanil, the areas of more activity matched the distribution of opioid receptors. The study also looked at dose effects in both species, and similar patterns of increased activity with dose were observed. This is one of the few studies in which effects of the same drugs across species have been reported (Fig. 14-2).

In an interesting study of heroin tolerance, Xi et al. [27] performed a phMRI study in heroin-naïve rats and rats that have self-administered (SA) heroin for 8–9 days. The phMRI response in the SA group, compared with the saline group, displayed an attenuated

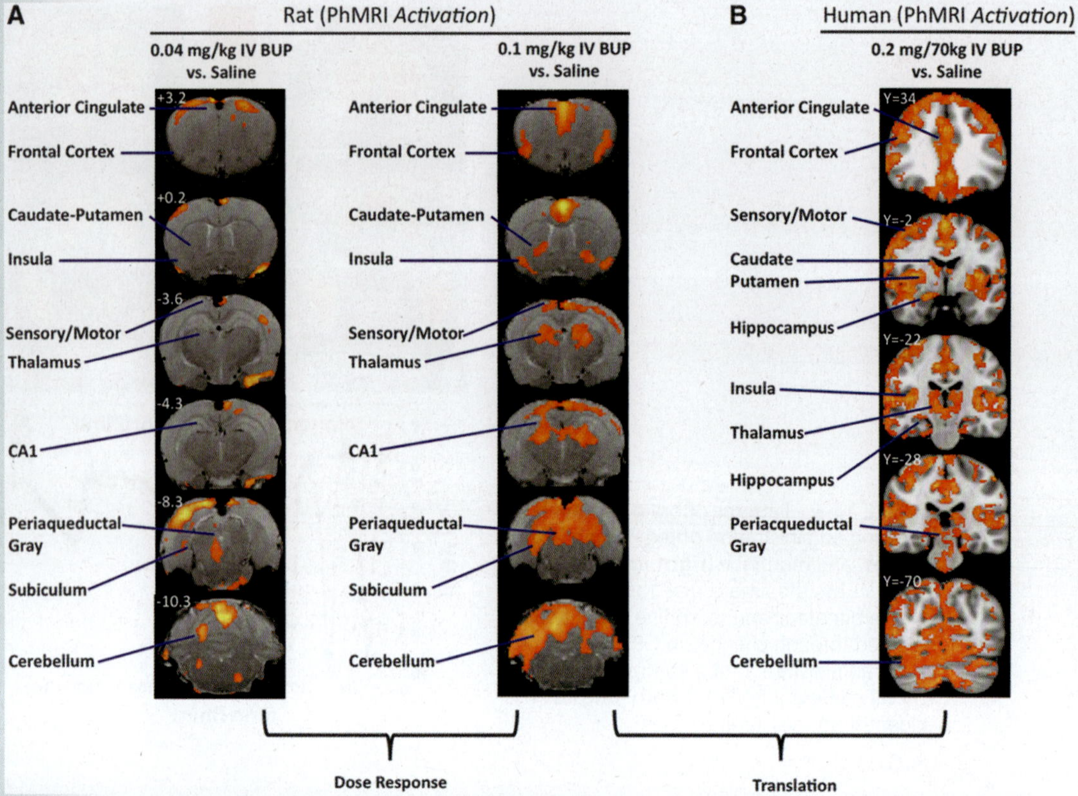

FIGURE 14-2 phMRI response to burprenorphine in **(A)** awake rodents and **(B)** humans. The activation maps following two doses of buprenorphine in humans and rats indicate the similarities and differences in activation across species. The differences in activation for different doses allow one to perform dose–response curves for different structures [1].

response in the prefrontal cortex and nucleus accumbens, suggesting that chronic exposure to heroin might increase the drug self-administration behaviour and intake (Fig. 14-3).

Preclinical phMRI Evaluation of Other Analgesics Used for Chronic Pain

Gabapentinoids

Gabapentin has a relatively long PK/PD process, and even with an intravenous (i.v.) injection, the temporal evolution of the signal is fairly long, as reported by Governo et al. [13]. Areas of deactivation, induced by inhibitory processes driven by gabapentin, were observed in the hippocampus and other structures; however, an increase in response was observed in the PAG. No human studies have been performed to assess the direct effect of gabapentin to compare with. More recently, another study has been reported in which the phMRI response in an animal model of neuropathic pain (SNL) was compared with naïve animals; they observed a stronger phMRI response in the hippocampus in the animal models compared with the control ones [15].

NMDA Antagonists

Ketamine is an NMDA antagonist that has found applications in chronic pain treatment. It has been studied separately in humans and rats: in humans, it has been shown to activate the cingulate, thalamus, insula, temporal lobes, and prefrontal areas, and there is a decrease

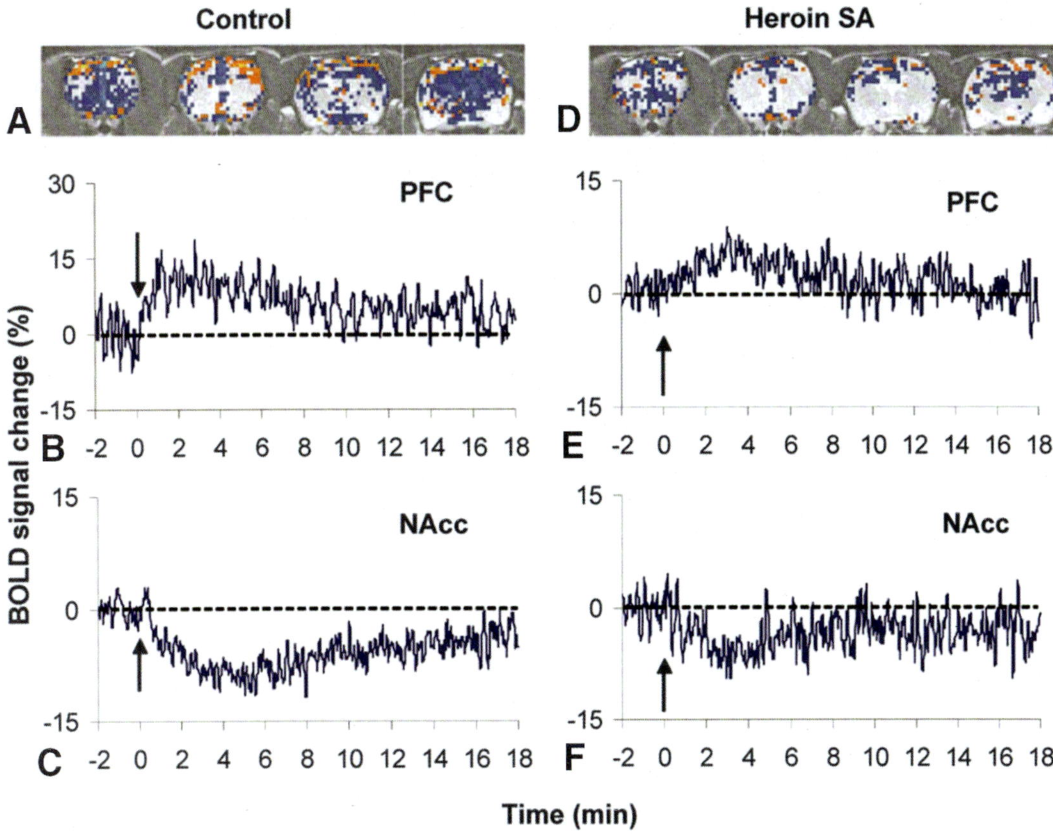

FIGURE 14-3 phMRI assessment of tolerance. In a study of self-administration of heroin, Xi et al. [27] demonstrated the attenuated response to an i.v. administration of heroin in rats that were allowed to self administer (SA) heroin for 2 weeks compared with naïve rats. Panels A and D display statistical maps of the response to a phMRI heroin challenge in naive **(A)** and SA rats **(D)**. Overall, there was reduced activity detected in SA animals compared to controls. The attenuated response in the frontal cortex (Panel **E**: SA animals vs. Panel **B**: Controls) and the accumbens (**F** vs **C**), indicate dampened responses in structures involved in reward processing and provide a measurement of the development of tolerance in SA animals.

in the subgenual cingulate cortex [19]. In rats under α chloralose [14], similar results were observed with prefrontal, limbic, association and sensorimotor cortices, and basal ganglia displaying increased activity. Of note is that this study also reports the effects of ketamine in the presence of isoflurane, and most of the results observed with α chloralose are reversed with isoflurane, suggesting a strong drug–anaesthesia interaction.

Cannabinoids

Activation of cannabinoid receptor CB1 and/or CB2 provides an analgesic effect [8]. phMRI results of a nonselective CB1/CB2 agonist indicate a good match of activation maps with autoradiographic CB1 receptor density binding maps. Interestingly, when rats were pretreated with a CB1 antagonist, the observed activation was eliminated, suggesting a phMRI activation driven by CB1 receptor activation.

Nicotinic Agonists

Nicotinic receptors are studied intensely for their potential therapeutic effects for drug abuse, neurocognitive disorders, and pain. Chin et al. [7] studied with awake phMRI the activation pattern of an $\alpha_4\beta_2$-nicotinic receptor agonist and found good matching with autoradiographic measures. They also observed differential dose effects of the activation patterns and that region-specific changes were associated with behavioural profiles of the drug. Interestingly, they performed the same experiments under α-chloralose anaesthesia, and observed that relationships were weak or nonexistent, suggesting a potential drug–anaesthesia interaction.

Antidepressants

Some antidepressants are used for the treatment of chronic neuropathic pain. In a study of SNL rats exposed chronically to desipramine, Jones et al. [17] found that SNL animals exposed had a larger phMRI response in sensorimotor and insular cortices and globus pallidus, whereas sham animals had larger activity in areas associated with learning and memory. These results suggest that alterations in brain function can be clearly defined in animal models of pain compared with sham controls and that, consequently, drug action is different.

Sodium Channel Modulators

The modulatory effects of Lidocaine were investigated with spinal cord fMRI [28] and with the measurement of blood volume changes in the presence of a contrast agent. They used transcutaneous electrical stimulation to observe activation in the spinal cord and its modulation with the application of Lidocaine administered locally or i.v. They observed a reduction of the activity in the spinal cord in the presence of Lidocaine irrespective of route of administration. Given that Lidocaine is thought to block damaged nerves peripherally, the fact that systemic administration also reduces pain transmission seems to indicate that it might block normal neural activity (Fig. 14-4).

CONCLUSIONS

Taking together, these results point to the utility of phMRI in assessing de novo effects as well as following chronic drug administration. The resemblance of some similarity of activity patterns (e.g., opioids) with human studies further supports the notion that phMRI studies in humans and rodents provide an opportunity to assess in an interactive mode analgesic effects and profiles across species.

As described previously, the use of phMRI or fMRI of evoked stimuli under an analgesic allows for the delineation of differential drug effects on the CNS; drugs that act on emotional pathways will probably offer important benefits compared with sensory modulation in chronic pain that affects emotional/motivation networks. This richness of information should help better understand drug mechanisms of action as well as define therapeutic effects (or lack thereof).

Future developments in understanding brain processing of pain and its modulation by analgesics should include the analysis of nonreflexive tests behaviourally and the results from nonevoked fMRI studies. In that regard, the advancement of our understanding of intrinsic brain networks in health and disease and in the presence of an analgesic will better help the interpretation of therapeutic effects and disease state/progression. In addition, the development of drugs that offer restorative processes (i.e., disease modification) will clearly be transformative.

Clearly, this is a field that is slowly evolving; the methodologies, from acquiring data to performing awake/anaesthetized studies, to the analysis pipelines, need to be standardized for proper comparisons across studies/institutions. Nevertheless, animal imaging holds tremendous potential as an avenue to provide insight into disease and therapeutic approaches.

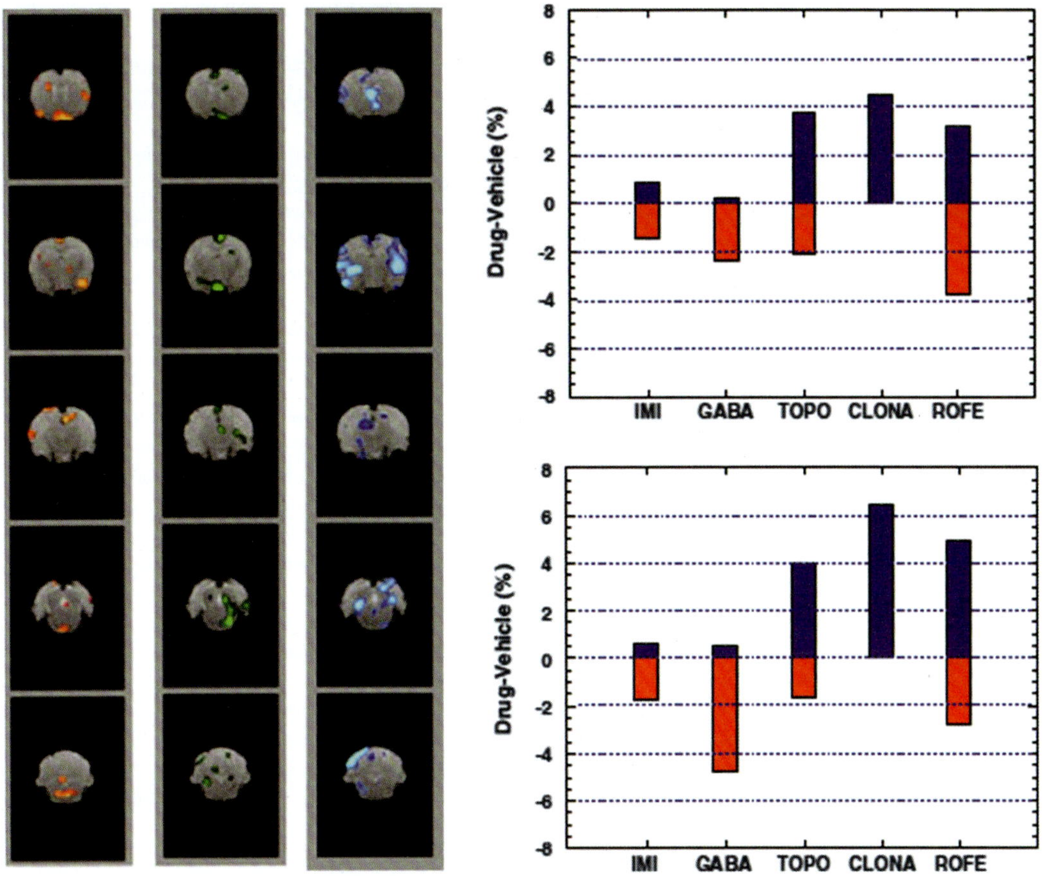

FIGURE 14-4 Drug modulation of pain response to noxious stimulus. As an example of differences in the modulation of an fMRI response to pain by drugs, a study of five drugs in awake rats indicated marked differences [5]. The brain slices indicate response to a saline injection (**middle column,** *green activation pattern*) following administration of imipramine (**left column,** *red-yellow activation pattern*) and following clonazepam (**right column,** *blue-light blue activation pattern*). Visually, imipramine produced reduced activation compared with saline, but clonazepam seems to produce the opposite effect. The bar graphs show quantification of volumes of activation comparing imipramine (IMI), gabapentin (GABA), clonazepam (CLONA), and rofecoxib (ROFE) with saline activation. "Desired effects" appear in red bars as reduction in activation, potentially indicating analgesic effects, whereas "undesired effects" appear in blue bars as presumably indicating potentiation of the noxious stimulus-induced brain activation [5].

REFERENCES

1. Becerra L, Upadhyay J, Chang PC, Bishop J, Anderson J, Baumgartner R, Schwarz AJ, Coimbra A, Wallin D, Nutile L, et al. Parallel buprenorphine phMRI responses in conscious rodents and healthy human subjects. J Pharmacol Exp Ther 2013;345(1):41–51.
2. Borsook D, Becerra L. CNS animal fMRI in pain and analgesia. Neurosci Biobehav Rev 2011;35(5):1125–43.
3. Borsook D, Becerra L, Hargreaves R. Biomarkers for chronic pain and analgesia, part 1: the need, reality, challenges, and solutions. Discov Med 2011;11(58):197–207.
4. Borsook D, Becerra L, Hargreaves R. Biomarkers for chronic pain and analgesia. part 2: how, where, and what to look for using functional imaging. Discov Med 2011;11(58):209–19.
5. Borsook D, Pendse G, Aiello-Lammens M, Glicksman M, Gostic J, Sherman S, Korn J, Shaw M, Stewart K, Gostic R, et al. CNS response to a thermal stressor in human volunteers and rats may predict the clinical utility of analgesics. Drug Dev Res 2007;68(1):23–41.
6. Chen YC, Choi JK, Andersen SL, Rosen BR, Jenkins BG. Mapping dopamine D_2/D_3 receptor function using pharmacological magnetic resonance imaging. Psychopharmacology (Berl) 2005;180(4):705–15.

7. Chin CL, Pauly JR, Surber BW, Skoubis PD, McGaraughty S, Hradil VP, Luo Y, Cox BF, Fox GB. Pharmacological MRI in awake rats predicts selective binding of alpha4beta2 nicotinic receptors. Synapse 2008;62(3):159–68.
8. Chin CL, Tovcimak AE, Hradil VP, Seifert TR, Hollingsworth PR, Chandran P, Zhu CZ, Gauvin D, Pai M, Wetter J, et al. Differential effects of cannabinoid receptor agonists on regional brain activity using pharmacological MRI. Br J Pharmacol 2008;153(2):367–79.
9. Choi JK, Mandeville JB, Chen YI, Kim YR, Jenkins BG. High resolution spatial mapping of nicotine action using pharmacologic magnetic resonance imaging. Synapse 2006;60(2):152–7.
10. Dieler AC, Samann PG, Leicht G, Eser D, Kirsch V, Baghai TC, Karch S, Schule C, Pogarell O, Czisch M, et al. Independent component analysis applied to pharmacological magnetic resonance imaging (phMRI): new insights into the functional networks underlying panic attacks as induced by CCK-4. Curr Pharm Des 2008; 14(33):3492–507.
11. Dodd GT, Stark JA, McKie S, Williams SR, Luckman SM. Central cannabinoid signaling mediating food intake: a pharmacological-challenge magnetic resonance imaging and functional histology study in rat. Neuroscience 2009;163(4):1192–200.
12. Fox MD, Greicius M. Clinical applications of resting state functional connectivity. Front Syst Neurosci 2010;4:19.
13. Governo RJ, Morris PG, Marsden CA, Chapman V. Gabapentin evoked changes in functional activity in nociceptive regions in the brain of the anaesthetized rat: an fMRI study. Br J Pharmacol 2008;153(7):1558–67.
14. Hodkinson DJ, de Groote C, McKie S, Deakin JF, Williams SR Differential effects of anaesthesia on the phMRI response to acute ketamine challenge. Br J Med Med Res 2012;2(3):373–85.
15. Hooker BA, Tobon G, Baker SJ, Zhu C, Hesterman J, Schmidt K, Rajagovindan R, Chandran P, Joshi SK, Bannon AW, et al. Gabapentin-induced pharmacodynamic effects in the spinal nerve ligation model of neuropathic pain. Eur J Pain 2014;18(2):223–37.
16. Hyder F, Rothman DL, Shulman RG. Total neuroenergetics support localized brain activity: implications for the interpretation of fMRI. Proc Natl Acad Sci USA 2002;99(16):10771–6.
17. Jones KL, Finn DP, Governo RJ, Prior MJ, Morris PG, Kendall DA, Marsden CA, Chapman V. Identification of discrete sites of action of chronic treatment with desipramine in a model of neuropathic pain. Neuropharmacology 2009;56(2):405–13.
18. Linnman C, Moulton EA, Barmettler G, Becerra L, Borsook D. Neuroimaging of the periaqueductal gray: state of the field. Neuroimage 2012;60(1):505–22.
19. Littlewood CL, Jones N, O'Neill MJ, Mitchell SN, Tricklebank M, Williams SC. Mapping the central effects of ketamine in the rat using pharmacological MRI. Psychopharmacology (Berl) 2006;186(1):64–81.
20. Liu CH, Greve DN, Dai G, Marota JJ, Mandeville JB. Remifentanil administration reveals biphasic phMRI temporal responses in rat consistent with dynamic receptor regulation. Neuroimage 2007;34(3):1042–53.
21. Luo Z, Yu M, Smith SD, Kritzer M, Du C, Ma Y, Volkow ND, Glass PS, Benveniste H. The effect of intravenous lidocaine on brain activation during non-noxious and acute noxious stimulation of the forepaw: a functional magnetic resonance imaging study in the rat. Anesth Analg 2009;108(1):334–44.
22. Martin C, Martindale J, Berwick J, Mayhew J. Investigating neural-hemodynamic coupling and the hemodynamic response function in the awake rat. Neuroimage 2006;32(1):33–48.
23. Navratilova E, Xie JY, King T, Porreca F. Evaluation of reward from pain relief. Ann N Y Acad Sci 2013;1282:1–11.
24. Pizoli CE, Shah MN, Snyder AZ, Shimony JS, Limbrick DD, Raichle ME, Schlaggar BL, Smyth MD. Resting-state activity in development and maintenance of normal brain function. Proc Natl Acad Sci USA 2011;108(28):11638–43.
25. Posner J, Hellerstein DJ, Gat I, Mechling A, Klahr K, Wang Z, McGrath PJ, Stewart JW, Peterson BS. Antidepressants normalize the default mode network in patients with dysthymia. JAMA Psychiatry 2013;70(4):373–82.
26. Sprenger T, Berthele A, Platzer S, Boecker H, Tolle TR What to learn from in vivo opioidergic brain imaging? Eur J Pain 2005;9(2):117–21.
27. Xi ZX, Wu G, Stein EA, Li SJ. Opiate tolerance by heroin self-administration: an fMRI study in rat. Magn Reson Med 2004;52(1):108–14.
28. Zhao F, Williams M, Welsh DC, Meng X, Ritter A, Abbadie C, Cook JJ, Reicin AS, Hargreaves R, Williams DS. fMRI investigation of the effect of local and systemic lidocaine on noxious electrical stimulation-induced activation in spinal cord. Pain 2009;145(1–2):110–9.

SECTION 4

Acute Pain

CHAPTER 15

Central Nervous System Mechanisms Supporting the Construction of an Experience of Pain Intensity

Robert C. Coghill

OVERVIEW

The process of building a subjectively available experience of pain and its intensity engages multiple levels of the CNS. For nociceptive pain, information related to noxious stimulus intensity is first transduced by multiple different types of primary afferent nociceptors. Primary afferent input derived from discrete body regions is integrated over multiple spinal levels and differing time frames. This afferent input is encoded by populations of wide dynamic range (WDR) and nociceptive specific (NS) neurons. These neurons transmit this processed information rostrally where it is elaborated into an individually unique subjective experience of pain magnitude by widely distributed supraspinal processes.

PSYCHOPHYSICS

In order to appreciate the neural mechanisms supporting the experience of pain intensity, it is critical to first develop an understanding of the relationship between stimulus intensity and perceived intensity as well as how pain intensity can be measured.

Classic work by Hardy et al. [11] in the 1940s and 1950s pioneered the psychophysical assessment of experimentally induced pain. They conducted an extensive series of studies using controlled noxious stimulation to assess both pain thresholds and suprathreshold sensations of pain. Using paradigms in which subjects detected differences between pairs of stimuli delivered with differing energies, they developed the "dol" scale based on just noticeable differences (i.e., the smallest detectable differences) between pairs of noxious stimuli.

During this time period, significant questions arose regarding the validity of psychophysical assessments based on just noticeable differences. The evolution of direct scaling techniques led to the development of scales of perceptual magnitude with ratio scale properties. Studies of multiple sensory modalities by Stevens [29] led to the observation that the relationship between perceived magnitude of a stimulus (Ψ) and the stimulus intensity (Φ) could be described by a power function in which $\Psi = k\Phi^{\beta}$. In this equation, β represents an exponent and k represents a proportionality constant. Early magnitude estimation studies indicated that perceived pain intensity generated by radiant heat from the Hardy–Wolff–Goodell dolorimeter could be fit to a power function in which the exponent β approximated 1 [1]. Consistent with information from other sensory modalities, β varies substantially from one noxious stimulus modality to another. For example, noxious heat delivered via a contact stimulus has an exponent of 3.5–3.8 [4], whereas cold pain has exponents of 2.2–3.0 [12]. Since exponents greater than 1 produce a positively accelerating curve, small changes in stimulus intensity at the upper end of the noxious range can produce profoundly large changes in perceived pain intensity.

Accurate assessment of pain magnitude depends critically upon the psychometric properties of the assessment instrument. In particular, ratio scale properties are heavily important for relating the magnitude of perceived pain to neural activity. For example, if one stimulus produces half as much perceived pain intensity than another, it should be associated with half as much neural activity. Fortunately, a number of well-validated ratio scales for pain magnitude exist. These range from verbal descriptor scales [13] to combined verbal/numerical scales [3] and visual analogue scales [24]. Such scales are employed in the imaging studies described subsequently. Surprisingly, the widely used 0–10 numerical rating scale does not exhibit ratio scale properties [22] and may potentially amplify sex differences [25].

ENCODING AND UTILIZATION OF INTENSITY-RELATED INFORMATION WITHIN THE SPINAL CORD

Noxious stimulus-related information is conveyed to the dorsal horn of the spinal cord by both Aδ and C nociceptors. This information is integrated in both the spatial and temporal domains by NS and WDR neurons [23]. NS neurons respond nearly exclusively to noxious stimuli, whereas WDR neurons respond robustly to both noxious and innocuous stimuli. Both NS and WDR neurons exhibit graded responses to progressive increases in noxious stimulus intensity. However, studies in awake, behaving monkeys indicate that WDR neurons can encode stimulus intensity with sufficient accuracy to support behavioural discrimination [17].

WDR neurons have a pronounced centre/surround receptive field organization. Both noxious and innocuous stimuli delivered to the central receptive field zone will produce excitatory activity, whereas only noxious stimuli will produce excitatory activity when delivered to the considerably larger surround zone. Accordingly, a single WDR neuron alone is unlikely to provide the CNS with sufficient information to encode a distinction between noxious and innocuous stimuli. However, given the substantial overlap of the surround excitatory receptive fields, a noxious stimulus will recruit larger numbers of WDR neurons than an innocuous stimulus, and thus, populations of WDR neurons can contribute to the encoding of distinctions between noxious and innocuous stimuli, as well as to intensity [23].

Consistent with the predictions based on receptive field organization, spinal cord imaging studies indicate that intensity-related information is encoded by progressive recruitment of neural populations, in addition to the increasing discharge frequencies of nociceptive neurons (Fig. 15-1) [6]. The rostro-caudal distribution of noxious stimulus-related activity increases in proportion to noxious stimulus intensity. At the high end of the noxious range, spinal cord regions contralateral to the stimulated body site are even recruited. This bilateral activation from a unilateral stimulus is a prominent feature of supraspinal processing.

This bilateral and multisegmental activation at the spinal level reflects the engagement of thousands of neurons during the processing of nociceptive information and represents substantial computational power. Classic studies by Sherrington indicate that, even at the spinal level, intensity-related information can be utilized by the CNS to guide behavioural responses. For example, spinal cord–transected dogs exhibit paw withdrawal responses that

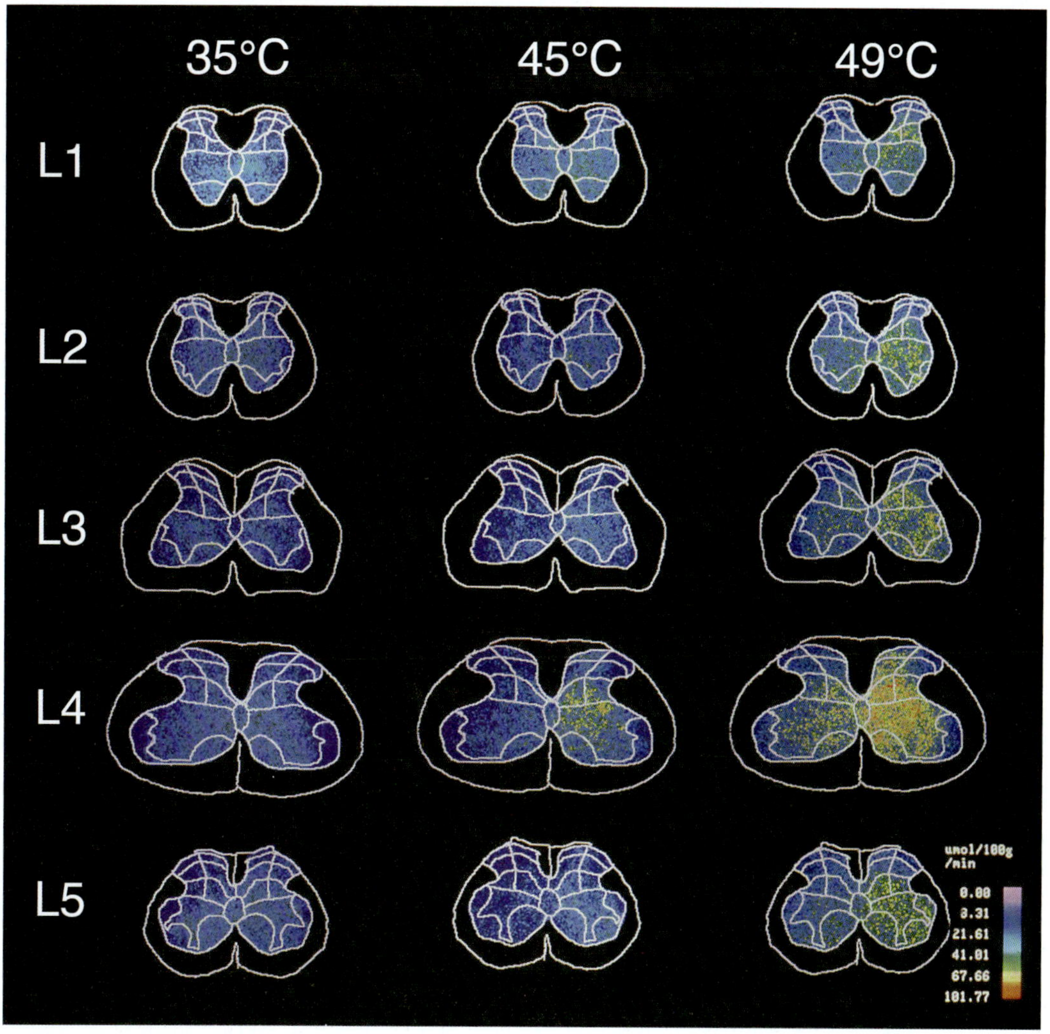

FIGURE 15-1 Spinal cord activation during graded noxious stimulation. Autoradiographic studies using ^{14}C-2-deoxyglucose to map activation of the rat spinal cord revealed that progressive increases in noxious stimulus intensity produced progressive recruitment of neural activity. Noxious thermal stimuli were applied to the hind paw of a spinal cord–transected unanaesthetized rat. In the low end of the noxious range (45°C), activation was largely restricted to the deep dorsal horn in spinal cord segment L4. When stimulus intensity was increased to 49°C, activation spread from L2 to L5 ipsilaterally, and also involved contralateral regions of L4. (Reproduced from Coghill et al. [6].)

are graded in clear proportion to stimulus intensity [26]. Moreover, reflexive responses to nociceptive information can be prioritized over postural reflexes [26]. Thus, even at this early level, the CNS makes "decisions" based on intensity-related information.

DISTRIBUTED PROCESSING OF INTENSITY-RELATED INFORMATION IN THE HUMAN BRAIN

Classic views by Melzack and Casey [18] postulated that sensory-discriminative components of pain are processed by a contralaterally directed flow of afferent information that involves thalamic regions such as the ventroposterior lateral nucleus and the S1 cortex.

They proposed that this system operated in parallel with affective-motivational components being processed by a medially directed system involving the medial thalamus and prefrontal cortex (PFC).

Early studies, in which brain regions exhibiting relationships with pain intensity were identified, revealed patterns of activation, which deviated substantially from these existing notions [7, 8, 21]. Although contralateral regions such as the S1 cortex were determined to be activated in an intensity-related manner in some studies [7], markedly different patterns of activation were detected in other brain regions (Fig. 15-2). First, in many areas, pain intensity–related activation was detected bilaterally despite the unilateral nature of the stimulus [7, 8]. Brain regions such as the thalamus, S2, anterior cingulate cortex (ACC), and insula all exhibited this pattern of activity, with more intense stimuli recruiting more ipsilateral activity. Second, brain regions thought to be important in the affective-motivational component of pain, such as the PFC and ACC, exhibited intensity-related activation [7, 8, 21]. Accordingly, intensity-related processing can be accomplished by a wide variety of brain regions, including those outside of regions traditionally thought of as somatosensory. Thus, the processing of intensity-related information is accomplished in a highly distributed fashion.

These imaging findings, when taken together with imaging and/or psychophysical studies of patients with brain lesions, further support the notion that intensity-related information processing can be accomplished in a distributed fashion. Psychophysical studies on a split-brain patient indicate that both cerebral cortical hemispheres receive sufficient input from subcortical sites to construct a subjectively available experience of pain intensity [28]. Importantly, the surgical destruction of the corpus callosum in this patient eliminates the possibility that direct cortico-cortical interhemispheric transfer of intensity-related information supported the capacity of the hemisphere ipsilateral to stimulation to construct and subsequently report an experience of pain intensity. Highly intense stimuli resulted in reports of pain intensity that were nearly equal between hemispheres, whereas weaker stimuli were more readily available to the contralateral hemisphere. This pattern of psychophysical reports mirrors bilateral activation patterns at spinal, thalamic, and cortical levels. That one hemisphere ipsilateral to stimulation is sufficient to support the generation of an experience of pain intensity is further confirmed by imaging studies of hemispherectomized patients [19]. These individuals exhibited activation of the insular cortex, S2, and the ACC when stimuli were delivered ipsilateral to the remaining cortical hemisphere.

BRAIN MECHANISMS ASSOCIATED WITH THE EVALUATION OF PAIN INTENSITY

Although many brain regions exhibit activation that is significantly related to pain intensity (Fig. 15-2), determining which regions contribute to evaluation and subjective awareness of intensity, as opposed to contributing to other intensity-driven processes such as affect, attention, or motor control, remains challenging. However, rating and discrimination paradigms can provide some insight into the neural mechanisms that support evaluation of pain intensity.

Following noxious stimulation, retrospective ratings of pain intensity with a combined numerical/verbal descriptor scale produce significant bilateral activation of the anterior insula, frontal operculum, and the ACC, among other regions [14]. This activation overlaps significantly with that evoked during noxious stimulation. Continuous ratings of thermal

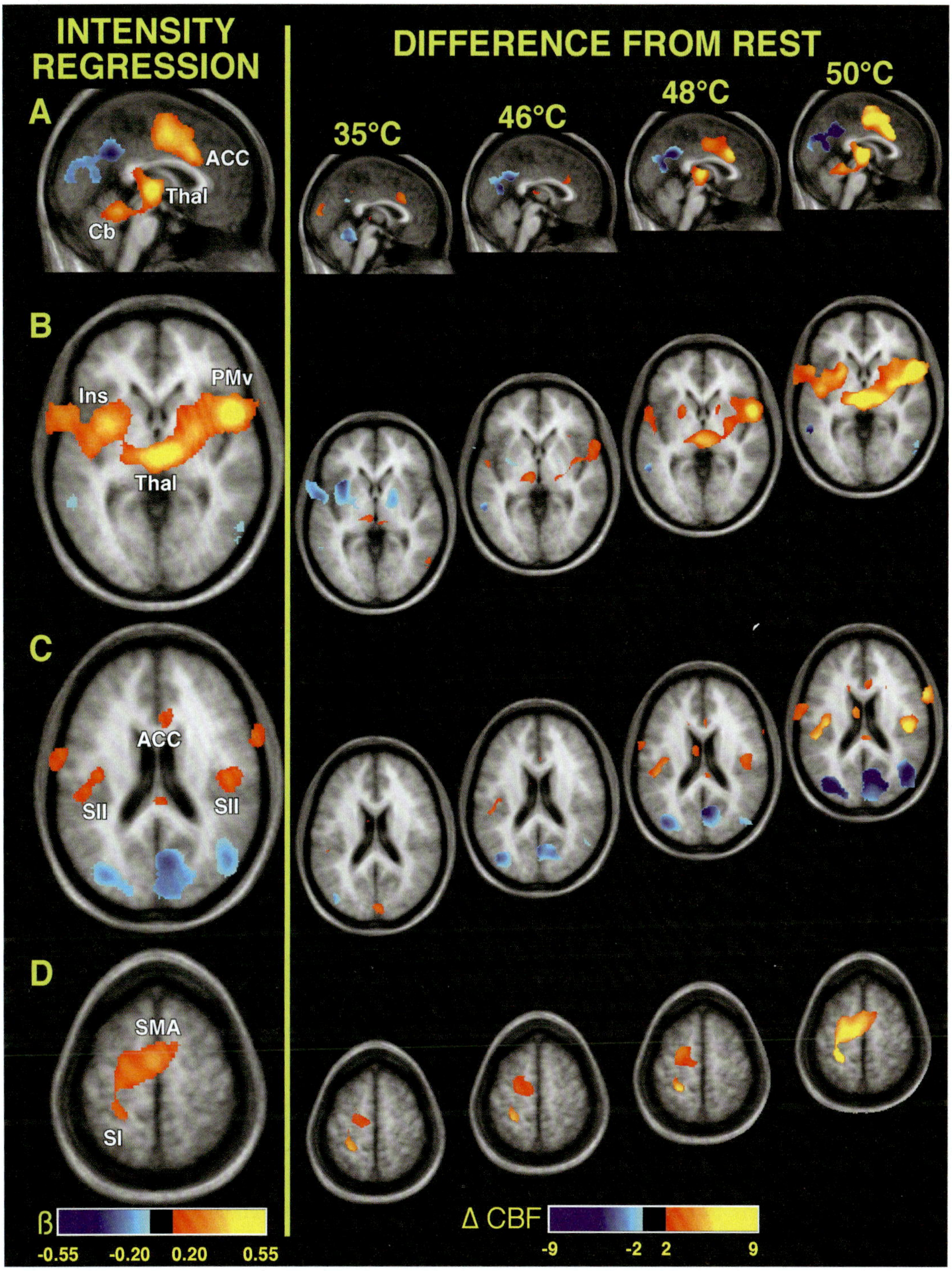

FIGURE 15-2 Brain activation during graded noxious stimulation. Positron emission tomography using $H_2{}^{15}O$ to map cerebral blood flow in healthy human volunteers revealed that progressive increases in noxious stimulus intensity produced progressive increases in neural activity. S1 cortex was one of the few brain regions to exhibit contralaterally focused increases in activity. The majority of other brain regions exhibited bilateral increases in activity. In many of these regions, ipsilateral activity was engaged only at the upper end of the noxious range, much like the pattern of activity seen at the spinal levels. Moreover, brain regions, such as the posterior cingulate cortex and precuneus, now known to be associated with the default-mode network, exhibited progressive decreases in activity as perceived pain intensity increased. (Reproduced from Coghill et al. [7].)

pain obtained via a finger span technique in healthy subjects similarly produce activation of the anterior insular cortex and ACC, indicating that this activity is not solely related to memory recall, but is importantly involved with the cognitive act of rating pain magnitude [2]. Visual stimuli delivered to the same subjects also produced activation of these regions, indicating that the mechanisms supporting the evaluation of pain magnitude are also related to the evaluation of intensity in other sensory modalities [2]. Thus, the insula has been proposed as a brain region that contributes to magnitude estimation [2, 20].

Brain mechanisms associated with pain intensity evaluation have also been assessed using a two-alternative, forced choice delayed-match-to-sample task [20]. In a way, this task harkens back to the early assessments of just noticeable differences by Hardy et al. [11]. In this task, subjects received two sequential stimuli (T1 and T2) separated by 30 seconds. T1 temperature was fixed at 48°C, and T2 was varied from 48° to 50°C. While T2 was still on, subjects were instructed to press a button to indicate that T2 was either the same as or different from T1. This task offers an advantage over continuous rating tasks in that interpretation of activation associated with the evaluation of pain intensity is complicated by neither dynamic changes in stimulus intensity nor movements and other outputs needed to make a rating. Moreover, since the evaluation period was defined by a window of time from T2 onset to slightly before the button push, brain activation during the comparison of incoming afferent information with previously experienced activation could be examined relatively selectively. Using this paradigm, the anterior insula, ACC, and regions of the PFC in the vicinity of the frontal pole were determined to be engaged in the evaluation of pain intensity [20].

It is important to consider that the act of discrimination in this delayed match-to-sample task involves a complex chain of events. Environmental/cognitive cues prime the somatosensory system for the acquisition of information in a selected domain by engaging attention. Information is acquired and retained within memory, and, finally, during the evaluation phase, incoming information is compared with previously experienced information in order to provide a context in which to formulate a response. Thus, activation during discrimination/intensity evaluation must necessarily involve multiple components. Lobanov et al. [16] separately examined these different phases of the discrimination task in both the intensity and spatial domains. During the period after presentation of the cue to attend to either the intensity or the location of a noxious stimulus, regions including the S1 cortex, the anterior insular cortex, and the PFC were activated during preparations to attend to intensity. During the acquisition period (T1) for intensity-related information, activation above and beyond that of pain itself was detected within the ACC. During the memory period, activation was again noted within the anterior insular cortex and ACC. Finally, during the intensity discrimination period, robust activation was noted in the anterior insula, PFC, and ACC. In this particular paradigm, many intensity components overlapped substantially with spatial components, suggesting that common processes were engaged despite the differing targets (intensity vs. spatial) of discrimination. Throughout all of these different paradigms, S1 and S2 cortices do not display consistent differential activation during discrimination, although they may exhibit attentional priming-related activation. Thus, these somatosensory regions may play a critical role in preprocessing afferent input and feeding information rostrally into the insular cortex [20].

The insula is anatomically situated in a manner to be a cortico-limbic pathway for somatosensory information [9]. The S1 cortex projects to S2 and the posterior parietal cortex (PPC); S2 and the PPC project to the posterior insula; the posterior insula projects to the anterior insula; and the anterior insula projects to the ACC, amygdala, PFC, and parahippocampal gyrus [9]. The majority of these connections are reciprocal, such that information can flow bidirectionally. Accordingly, this structure clearly has connectivity that supports a role in the evaluation of intensity information. The insula can link contextual information from memory, affect, and attention with somatosensory input. Furthermore, lesions of this structure may diminish the influence of contextual information on the construction of an experience of pain intensity [27]. Subjects with anterior insular lesions exhibit markedly higher ratings of pain intensity than age-matched control subjects, raising the possibility that prior information about the safety of the experimental stimulus could not be adequately utilized during the generation of an experience of pain intensity. In contrast, individuals with more posteriorly focused lesions of the insula have marked reduction of pain sensitivity, consistent with the idea that this region of the insula is more closely related to afferent processing [10].

INDIVIDUAL DIFFERENCES IN THE SUBJECTIVE EXPERIENCE OF PAIN

The experience of pain magnitude varies widely from one subject to the next, even when the nociceptive stimulus is held constant. Brain regions such as the S1 cortex, ACC, and PFC are all activated more frequently and to a greater magnitude in highly sensitive versus insensitive individuals (Fig. 15-3) [5]. Surprisingly, given the robustly detectable differences in the S1 cortex, ACC, and PFC, no differences were detected within the thalamus. This suggests that nociceptive input is elaborated into an individually unique subjective experience by mechanisms above the level of the thalamus. This pattern contrasts with that seen when stimulus–response relationships are examined within individuals [7]. In those experiments, the thalamus clearly responds in a highly graded fashion to monotonic increases in noxious stimulus intensity within individuals. This discordance highlights the distinction between nociceptive processing and the subjective experience of pain intensity.

Expectations and other forms of prior information clearly shape the experience of pain intensity [15]. Tremendous overlap between expectation-related activation and pain-related activation is noted within numerous regions within the cerebral cortex. Such regions include the anterior insula, ACC, and PFC, among other areas. Thus, this convergence of top-down activation with bottom-up activity is a critical determinant of the experience of pain intensity. As each individual is carrying his/her own unique past history, assessment of the present environment, and set of predicted future outcomes, it is not surprising that the construction of an experience of pain yields vast interindividual differences.

INDIVIDUALLY UNIQUE PATTERNS OF BRAIN ACTIVATION AND THE FEASIBILITY OF NEUROIMAGING BIOMARKERS FOR PAIN

As addressed in other chapters, substantial research effort is being devoted to the development of neuroimaging biomarkers for pain. The development of such biomarkers depends critically upon our ability to transition from group-based studies to studies with adequate sensitivity to detect pain-related activation within single individuals. Critical knowledge gaps remain that raise substantial questions about the feasibility of developing neuroimaging biomarkers for pain. For example, we have no idea whether different individuals instantiate an experience of pain using the same brain mechanisms. As already mentioned,

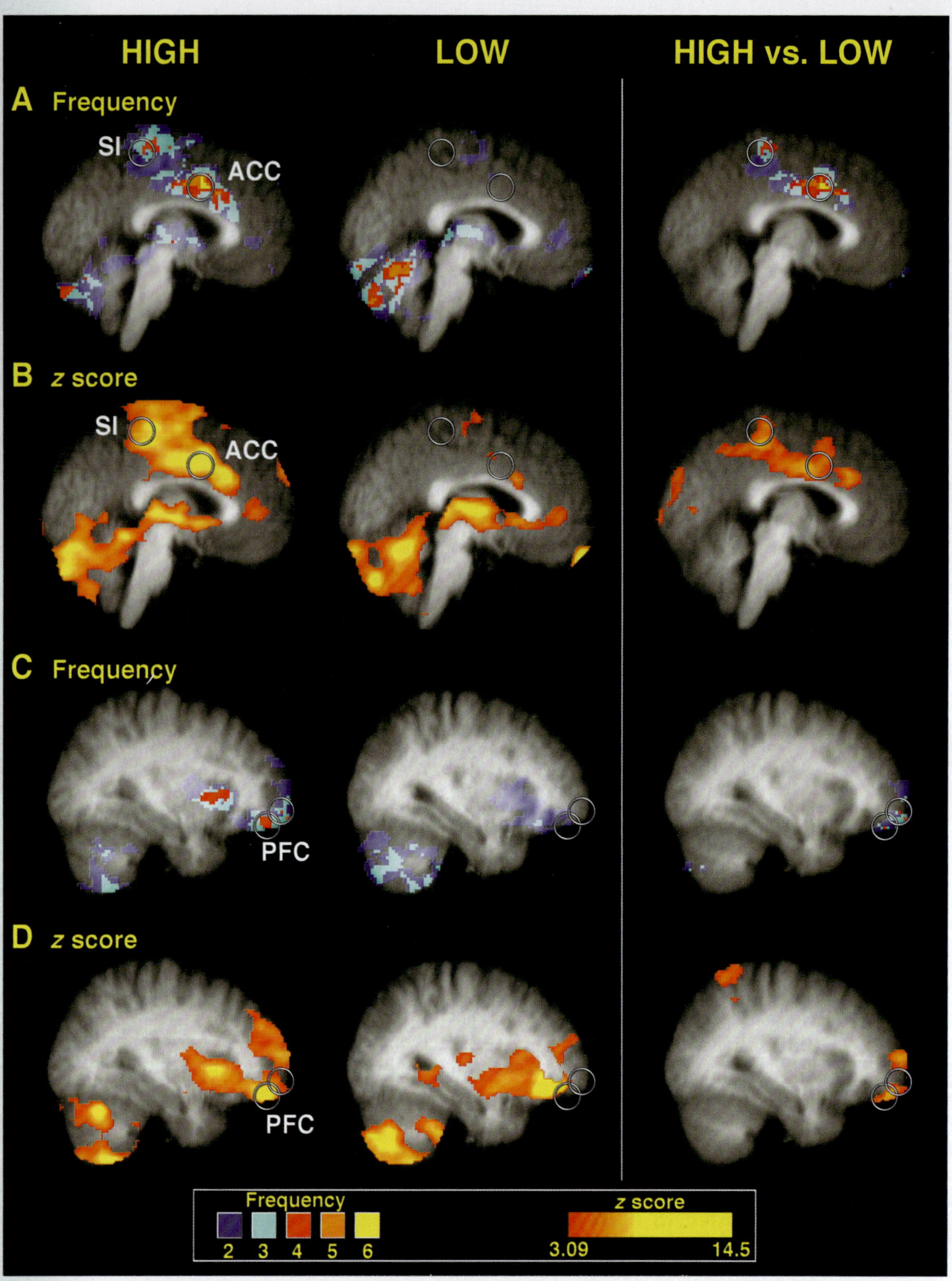

FIGURE 15-3 Highly sensitive individuals exhibit greater frequency and magnitude of pain-related brain activation than insensitive individuals. Functional MRI studies using the BOLD effect as an index of neural activity in healthy human volunteers revealed that highly sensitive individuals produced more frequent and greater magnitude of activation following 49°C stimulation than insensitive individuals. These differences were detected within the S1 cortex, ACC, and PFC. Surprisingly, such differences at the thalamic level were not evident, suggesting that the nociceptive input is elaborated into an individually unique experience of pain by suprathalamic mechanisms. (Reproduced from Coghill et al. [5] with permission.)

hemispherectomized subjects can generate a subjectively available experience of pain from stimuli applied contralateral to their missing hemisphere. Do healthy subjects generate an experience of pain using individually unique patterns of activity? If so, do we need to consider that there may be multiple biomarkers for pain?

Our experience of pain and its intensity is a truly individually unique experience, even when evoked by carefully defined experimental stimuli. Chronic pain by itself is hugely complex, with multiple different percepts arising from multiple distinct pathologies that may all be encompassed within one chronic pain syndrome. As neuroimaging moves from the laboratory to the clinic and then from the clinic to the courtroom, we need to ensure that we have the knowledge base to make accurate inferences about single individuals and their individually unique brain mechanisms that give rise to their subjective experience of pain.

ACKNOWLEDGEMENT

The author is supported by NIH grants R01NS039426 and R21AT007247.

REFERENCES

1. Adair ER, Stevens JC, Marks LE. Thermally induced pain, the Dol scale, and the psychophysical power law. Am J Psychol 1968;81(2):147–64.
2. Baliki MN, Geha PY, Apkarian AV. Parsing pain perception between nociceptive representation and magnitude estimation. J Neurophysiol 2009;101(2):875–87.
3. Coghill RC, Gracely RH. Validation of the combined numerical/verbal descriptor scale for pain. Am Pain Soc Abstr 1996;15:A86.
4. Coghill RC, Mayer DJ, Price DD. Wide dynamic range but not nociceptive specific neurons encode multidimensional features of prolonged repetitive heat pain. J Neurophysiol 1993;69:703–16.
5. Coghill RC, McHaffie JG, Yen YF. Neural correlates of interindividual differences in the subjective experience of pain. Proc Natl Acad Sci USA 2003;100(14):8538–42.
6. Coghill RC, Price DD, Hayes RL, Mayer DJ. Spatial distribution of nociceptive processing in the rat spinal cord. J Neurophysiol 1991;65:133–40.
7. Coghill RC, Sang CN, Maisog JM, Iadarola MJ. Pain intensity processing within the human brain: a bilateral, distributed mechanism. J Neurophysiol 1999;82:1934–43.
8. Derbyshire SW, Jones AK, Gyulai F, Clark S, Townsend D, Firestone LL. Pain processing during three levels of noxious stimulation produces differential patterns of central activity. Pain 1997;73:431–45.
9. Friedman DP, Murray EA, O'neil JB, Mishkin M. Cortical connections of the somatosensory fields of the lateral sulcus of macaques: evidence for a corticolimbic pathway for touch. J Comp Neurol 1986;252:323–47.
10. Greenspan JD, Lee RR, Lenz FA. Pain sensitivity alterations as a function of lesion location in the parasylvian cortex. Pain 1999;81(3):273–82.
11. Hardy JD, Wolff HG, Goodell H. Pain sensations and reactions. Baltimore, MD: Williams & Wilkins; 1952.
12. Harrison JL, Davis KD. Cold-evoked pain varies with skin type and cooling rate: a psychophysical study in humans. Pain 1999;83:123–35.
13. Heft MW, Gracely RH, Dubner R, McGrath PA. A validation model for verbal description scaling of human clinical pain. Pain 1980;9:363–73.
14. Kong J, White NS, Kwong KK, Vangel MG, Rosman IS, Gracely RH, Gollub RL. Using fMRI to dissociate sensory encoding from cognitive evaluation of heat pain intensity. Hum Brain Mapp 2006;27(9):715–21.
15. Koyama T, McHaffie JG, Laurienti PJ, Coghill RC. The subjective experience of pain: Where expectations become reality. Proc Natl Acad Sci USA 2005;102(36):12950–5.
16. Lobanov OV, Quevedo AS, Hadsel MS, Kraft RA, Coghill RC. Frontoparietal mechanisms supporting attention to location and intensity of painful stimuli. Pain 2013;154(9):1758–68.
17. Maixner W, Dubner R, Bushnell MC, Kenshalo DR, Oliveras J-L. Wide-dynamic-range dorsal horn neurons participate in the encoding process by which monkeys percieve the intensity of noxious heat stimuli. Brain Res 1986;374:385–8.

18. Melzack R, Casey KL. Sensory, motivational, and central control determinants of pain. In: DR Kenshalo, editor. The skin senses. Springfield, IL: Thomas; 1968. pp. 423–435.
19. Olausson H, Ha B, Duncan GH, Morin C, Ptito A, Ptito M, Marchand S, Bushnell MC. Cortical activation by tactile and painful stimuli in hemispherectomized patients. Brain 2001;124(Pt 5):916–27.
20. Oshiro Y, Quevedo AS, McHaffie JG, Kraft RA, Coghill RC. Brain mechanisms supporting discrimination of sensory features of pain: a new model. J Neurosci 2009;29(47):14924–31.
21. Porro CA, Cettolo V, Francescato MP, Baraldi P. Temporal and intensity coding of pain in human cortex. J Neurophysiol 1998;80(6):3312–20.
22. Price DD, Bush FM, Long S, Harkins SW. A comparison of pain measurement characteristics of mechanical visual analogue and simple numerical rating scales. Pain 1994;56(2):217–26.
23. Price DD, Hayes RL, Ruda M, Dubner R. Spatial and temporal transformations of input to spinothalamic tract neurons and their relation to somatic sensations. J Neurophysiol 1978;41:933–47.
24. Price DD, McGrath PA, Rafii A, Buckingham B. The validation of visual analogue scales as ratio scale measures for chronic and experimental pain. Pain 1983;17:45–56.
25. Price DD, Patel R, Robinson ME, Staud R. Characteristics of electronic visual analogue and numerical scales for ratings of experimental pain in healthy subjects and fibromyalgia patients. Pain 2008;140(1):158–66.
26. Sherrington CS. The integrative action of the nervous system. London, UK: Archibald Constable; 1908.
27. Starr CJ, Sawaki L, Wittenberg GF, Burdette JH, Oshiro Y, Quevedo AS, Coghill RC. Roles of the insular cortex in the modulation of pain: insights from brain lesions. J Neurosci 2009;29(9):2684–94.
28. Stein BE, Price DD, Gazzaniga MS. Pain perception in a man with total corpus callosum transection. Pain 1989;38:51–56.
29. Stevens SS. On the psychophysical law. Psychol Rev 1957;64(3):153–181.

CHAPTER 16

The "Pain Matrix": Myths and (Unpleasant) Truths

G. D. Iannetti and A. Mouraux

The ability to identify and react to impending threat is crucial for avoiding body damage and ensuring survival. In humans and non-human primates, the occurrence of potentially noxious events in the sensory environment is detected by all five senses. In particular, in the ever-changing sensory environment of modern life, the auditory, visual, and somatosensory systems rapidly encode information about threats and trigger cortical responses underlying appropriate behaviour. In the seemingly simple act of crossing a busy road in southern Italy, auditory and visual information allow choosing the movement repertoire to avoid, in most cases, being injured by the fast motorbike overtaking the car queuing at the red traffic light. In a similar way, transient noxious somatosensory stimuli are detected by the nociceptive system. The activation of the nociceptive system generates cortical responses that result in different physiological outcomes. One of these possible outcomes is the perception of pain. Other outcomes are, for example, autonomic responses, such as an increase in heart rate and blood pressure, or appropriate motor responses.

Many investigators have attempted to understand how the perception of pain emerges from nociception within the human brain, using noninvasive functional neuroimaging techniques such as electroencephalography (EEG), magnetoencephalography (MEG), positron emission tomography (PET), and functional magnetic resonance imaging (fMRI) [7, 19]. It is important to note that, with some interesting exceptions [3, 43, 49], the majority of these investigations have examined the cortical responses elicited by *transient* nociceptive stimuli. Such stimuli reveal activity within a wide array of brain regions, consistently including the S1 and S2 cortices, the insula, and the anterior cingulate cortex (ACC) [25]. When interpreting the functional significance of these brain responses, initial reports were extremely cautious, taking into consideration the notion that pain perception is only one of the possible outcomes of the cortical activation elicited by the incoming nociceptive input. For example, Carmon et al. [8] concluded that "it is possible that only the arousing and alerting effect of pain is responsible" for the elicited brain responses. Similarly, Chapman et al. [9, 10] stated that these responses "cannot be considered neurophysiological representations of pain sensations." However, as the number of studies focusing on these brain responses increased, investigators began interpreting them in a more pain-specific way, building the basis for the notion that they reflect "the activation of the neural circuit subserving the processing of the affective and motivational dimensions of pain" [11], or the activity of a cortical network "mediating pain experience itself" [46], that is, the so-called pain matrix [20]. Pushing their interpretations one step further, some investigators ascribed different parts of this "pain matrix" to different aspects of pain perception, a notion that is supported by equivocal experimental evidence that has, nevertheless, gained wide acceptance [7]. In particular, it was proposed that S1 and S2 would be specifically involved in encoding the sensory-discriminative aspects of pain perception (sometimes referred to as the "lateral pain system" or the "somatic node"), whereas the ACC would be specifically involved in the affective and cognitive aspects of pain perception (sometimes referred to as the "medial pain system" or the "affective node") [1, 4, 57]. Expectedly, the prospect of being able to measure noninvasively the neural activity underlying different aspects of pain perception has generated considerable enthusiasm in the field of pain neuroscience, by opening the possibility of using functional neuroimaging to understand how pain sensations are represented in the brain, and how this representation may be modulated by specific experimental factors. This has led not a few authors to propose that the "pain matrix" can be used, for example, as a specific biomarker for drug development [52], as "objective evidence of pain perception" in minimally conscious patients [6], or as an "objective measure of pain" that could even constitute medico-legal evidence when seeking compensation [38].

Three arguments are most often put forward to justify the notion that these brain responses are specific for pain: (1) these responses are consistently obtained by stimuli eliciting a sensation of pain, (2) their magnitude often correlates with the perceived intensity of pain, and (3) factors modulating pain can also modulate the magnitude of these brain responses.

In this chapter, we will take a radically different standpoint, and argue that the neural activity captured in the so-called pain matrix is likely to *largely* reflect cortical processes that are not at all specific for pain and, hence, that these brain responses cannot be easily used as a direct reflection of the cortical representation of pain in the human brain. Second, we will examine whether recently developed approaches such as time–frequency analysis of EEG signals or multivoxel pattern analysis (MVPA) of fMRI data could overcome some of the limitations of more conventional analyses and thereby be used to isolate cortical activity that is truly specific for nociception or pain.

THE "PAIN MATRIX": AN INVALID CONSTRUCT BASED ON REVERSE INFERENCE

The first and most fundamental argument put forward to claim that the "pain matrix" reflects the neural activity through which pain emerges from nociception within the human brain is that the different brain regions constituting this "pain matrix" are consistently activated by stimuli that elicit a perception of pain (for a review, see [7, 19]).[1] Such a conclusion is a typical example of *reverse inference*, in which a mental state is inferred from a pattern of neural activation. Poldrack [47] argued that the validity of a reverse inference must be treated probabilistically, with the likelihood of the inference being correct depending on the degree of exclusivity of the relationship between the cognitive state (in our case, the perception of pain) and the pattern of brain activation (in our case, the activity within the "pain matrix"). If the brain regions constituting the "pain matrix" are activated only when subjects experience pain, the reverse inference is likely to be correct. However, if the brain regions constituting the "pain matrix" are also activated in situations where no pain is present, the reverse inference is likely to be incorrect. As reviewed in the following paragraph, while the "pain matrix" is indeed activated in most situations where pain is perceived, it is also frequently activated in situations where pain is not present, suggesting that the reverse inference leading authors to conclude that pain emerges from activation of the "pain matrix" is not justified.

[1] The second argument commonly put forward to support this claim is discussed in the following section.

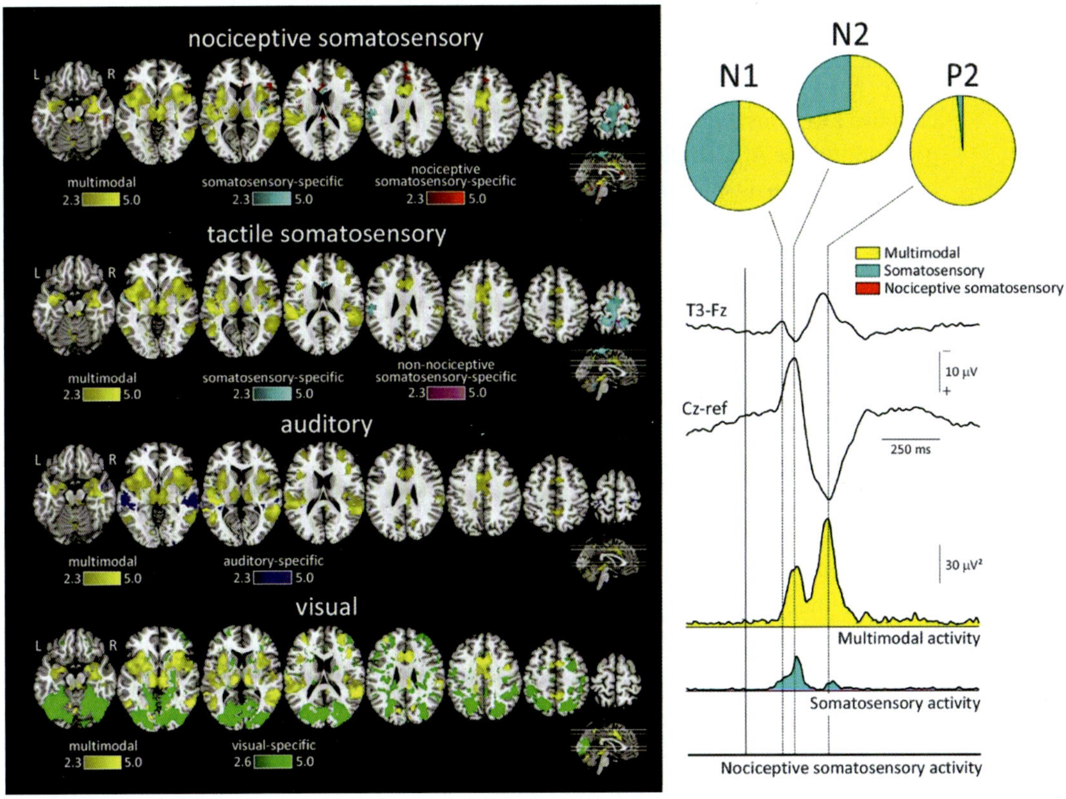

FIGURE 16-1 **Left panel:** conjunction analyses of the BOLD fMRI responses elicited by transient stimuli of four modalities (pain, touch, audition, and vision). Random-effect group analysis, voxel threshold $Z > 2.3$ and cluster threshold $P < 0.05$, corrected for multiple comparisons. Voxels responding to all four types of sensory stimuli are shown in yellow. Voxels uniquely responding to stimuli delivered to the body (either nociceptive or non-nociceptive) are shown in cyan. Nociceptive-specific voxels—voxels displaying significant activation only to nociceptive somatosensory stimuli—are shown in red. Note the large amount of spatial overlap between the responses elicited by all four modalities of sensory stimulation. **Right panel:** multimodal and somatosensory-specific activities contributing to nociceptive-evoked EEG responses (laser-evoked potentials, LEPs). The greater part of the LEP waveform is explained by multimodal brain activity (that is, activity also elicited by stimuli of other sensory modalities). The time course of this multimodal activity, expressed as global field power (μV^2), is shown in yellow. Note how multimodal activity explains the greater part of the N1 and N2 waves and almost all of the P2 wave. The contribution of somatosensory-specific brain activity (i.e., activity elicited by both nociceptive and non-nociceptive somatosensory stimuli), shown in light blue, is largely confined to the time interval corresponding to the N1 and N2 waves. Note also the lack of nociceptive-specific somatosensory activity contributing to the LEP. (Adapted from Iannetti and Mouraux [25].)

Indeed, several studies have highlighted that the EEG and fMRI responses elicited by nociceptive stimuli can be extremely similar to those elicited by non-nociceptive somatosensory stimuli [32, 36]. In two studies, we compared directly the brain responses elicited by nociceptive stimuli perceived as painful with the brain responses elicited by a range of salient but never painful tactile, auditory, and visual stimuli [39, 42] (Fig. 16-1). In both studies, stimuli were presented within a random sequence, using a large and unpredictable interstimulus interval (5–10 seconds), to maximize their saliency content. In the first study [42], we used a blind source separation technique (Probabilistic Independent Component Analysis, PICA [5]) to decompose the EEG responses elicited by nociceptive, tactile, auditory, and visual stimuli into a set of physiologically independent components. The results clearly demonstrated that the event-related potentials (ERPs) elicited by nociceptive stimuli can be entirely explained by a combination of multimodal neural activity (i.e., neural activity that is elicited by any sensory stimulus, independently of sensory modality) and somatosensory-specific (i.e., neural activity that is elicited by both nociceptive and tactile somatosensory stimuli), but not nociceptive-specific neural activity. Source analyses showed that the multimodal neural activity explaining the greater part of nociceptive ERPs was optimally modelled by generators located in bilateral operculo-insular regions and/or the ACC, indicating that the brain activity captured by the so-called pain matrix can also be elicited by non-nociceptive sensory stimuli that do not result in painful percepts. This finding led us to propose that the "pain matrix" is mainly the reflection of multimodal neural activity entirely unspecific for nociception and pain. Importantly, although the blind source separation algorithm succeeded in identifying modality-specific neural activity contributing uniquely to non-nociceptive auditory and visual ERPs—with a scalp topography compatible with sources located in primary auditory and visual areas—not a single component contributed uniquely to the nociceptive ERP.

In the second study [39], we compared the hemodynamic responses elicited by the same types of stimuli using fMRI. The fMRI data were analysed using mass-univariate analysis and general linear modelling [18], the most common approach to detect regional-average changes in brain activation. We found that nociceptive, tactile, auditory, and visual stimuli elicited spatially indistinguishable responses in the insula, in most of S2, as well as in the anterior cingulate. In addition to this multimodal activity, nociceptive and tactile somatosensory stimuli elicited an identical response in S1 and in a small region of S2. Strikingly, although auditory stimuli elicited a clear auditory-specific response in the primary auditory cortex, and visual stimuli elicited a clear visual-specific response in the primary visual cortex, there was no spatially segregated brain region that was exclusively activated by nociceptive stimuli.

Taken together, these observations suggest that the "pain matrix" identified using currently available functional neuroimaging techniques that sample neural activity at regional level [18] mainly reflects multimodal neural activity, that is, the activity of neurons that respond to a range of stimuli regardless of their sensory modality [39]. However, as detailed in the section "Novel Approaches to Characterize the Cortical Representation of Pain," the possibility that the activity of nociceptive-specific neurons does contribute to the responses recorded using these techniques, but that this activity cannot be isolated from the activity of spatially intermingled non-nociceptive-specific neurons, cannot be ruled out.

In any case, it is obvious that the so-called pain matrix is not exclusive to the processing of nociceptive input or the perception of pain. Therefore, the reverse inference that pain is experienced *because* the "pain matrix" is activated is not justified.

THE "PAIN MATRIX" CORRELATES WITH STIMULUS SALIENCY, NOT PAIN PERCEPTION

The second argument put forward in support of the view that the "pain matrix" constitutes the neural substrate for pain perception is the observation that the magnitude of the responses elicited in the "pain matrix" can predict the amount of subjective pain perception [13]. For these reasons, some investigators have suggested that one of the main functions of these brain responses is to specifically encode the intensity of pain perception [48, 40].

However, several EEG studies have shown that in many circumstances, the magnitude of the "pain matrix" response can be clearly dissociated from both the intensity of the nociceptive stimulus and the intensity of perceived pain [12, 14, 24, 33, 40, 44]. For example, in Iannetti et al. [24], we delivered trains of three identical nociceptive stimuli separated by a constant 1-second interstimulus interval, using four different stimulus intensities. Following the first stimulus, there was a strong correlation between the magnitude of the nociceptive ERP and the intensity of perceived pain. However, following the second and third stimuli of the train, this correlation was disrupted: the magnitude of the ERPs elicited by the second and third stimuli was markedly reduced and, most importantly, no longer reflected the intensity of perceived pain. A similar dissociation was reported by Clark et al. [12], in an experiment where nociceptive stimuli were preceded by a visual cue: when the duration of the delay between the visual cue and the nociceptive stimulus was unpredictable, the magnitude of the ERP elicited by the nociceptive stimulus was increased, whereas the intensity of pain perception was unaffected. An example of an opposite dissociation is sleep deprivation, which determines an increase of laser-evoked pain ratings, but a reduction of both parasylvian and vertex EEG responses [53]. Taken together, these different observations constitute evidence that the "pain matrix" is not *directly* involved in encoding pain intensity.

Also using EEG, it was shown that when a nociceptive stimulus is repeated at a short and constant interstimulus interval, it elicits an ERP of smaller magnitude [24, 55]. This effect of stimulus repetition is largely determined by the duration of the interstimulus interval: the shorter the interval, the more pronounced the response decrement [59]. Previous studies have demonstrated that the effect of stimulus repetition on the magnitude of nociceptive ERPs cannot be attributed to refractoriness of afferent nociceptive pathways or cortical generators. Indeed, both Mouraux et al. [40] and Wang et al. [59] showed that stimulus repetition affects the magnitude of nociceptive ERPs if the interstimulus interval remains constant from trial to trial, but not if the interstimulus interval is varied randomly from trial to trial. In other words, the effect of stimulus repetition appears to be strongly conditioned by the *context* within which the repetition occurs. The fact that stimulus repetition reduces the magnitude of nociceptive ERPs only when the interstimulus interval remains constant across trials could be related to the fact that, in these circumstances, stimulus repetition reduces the saliency of the repeated stimuli.

The influence of context on the magnitude of the "pain matrix" response has also been investigated directly in experiments examining the effect of introducing a change in a monotonous sequence of nociceptive stimuli—for example, changing the location, timing, or intensity of the stimulus [51, 54, 56] (Fig. 16-2). These different studies showed that introducing a change in one of the features defining the stimulus reverts, although to different degrees, the habituation of nociceptive ERPs. When the change consists in a difference in stimulus intensity, an interesting finding is observed. Dishabituation of the nociceptive ERP occurs only when the change entails an increase of stimulus intensity, but not when it entails a decrease of stimulus intensity [51]. This observation provides evidence that the cortical responses elicited by a salient sensory stimulus are not simply sensitive to novelty. Instead, it indicates that these responses are determined mainly by the saliency content of the eliciting stimulus.

The saliency of a given sensory stimulus is commonly defined as its ability to stand out relative to the background [27]. Therefore, the saliency of a stimulus is not defined by a particular physical dimension of the stimulus, but by how much the stimulus contrasts with its surrounding, along one or more physical dimensions. For example, a red flower is salient when it stands isolated in a green grass field, but not when it is surrounded by hundreds of other red poppies. Stimulus saliency is also defined by how much the stimulus contrasts with past experiences [45]. Similarly, the repeated ringing noise produced by a telephone will stand out more when it rings for the first time. It is generally recognized that the ability

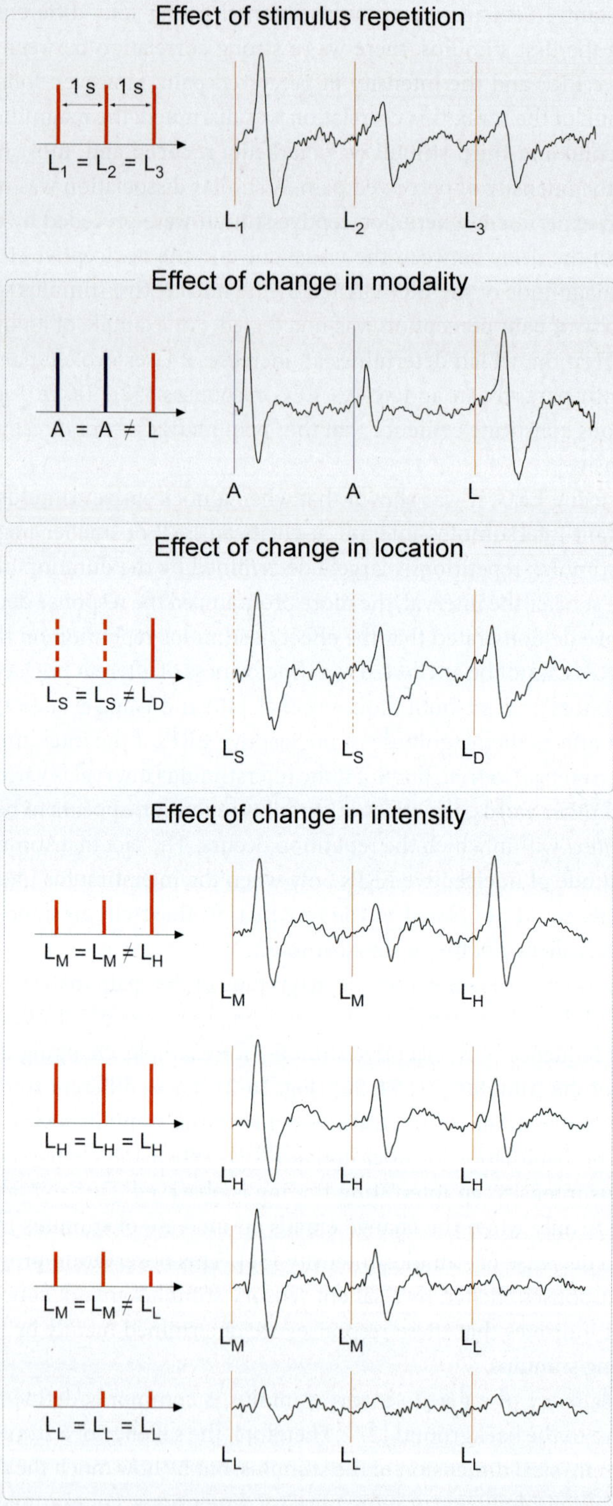

FIGURE 16-2 A summary of experiments exploring the habituation and dishabituation of LEPs. The repetition of identical laser stimuli at short and constant intervals of 1 second determines a clear habituation of the corresponding LEP response. By changing selectively the main features defining a sensory stimulus, we were able to identify those determining a significant response dishabituation. Changes of stimulus modality (as in [56]) and increases of stimulus intensity (as in [51]) were most effective at producing a dishabituation of the LEP response.

to detect, reorient attention, and prioritize the cortical processing of salient sensory input is crucial for survival. Indeed, this ability allows individuals to adapt swiftly and efficiently their behaviour to the changing environment. Because of their noxious nature, nociceptive stimuli have intrinsically high saliency content, and, for this reason, this ability to detect and react to salient sensory input is often considered as one of the most important functions of nociception.

Because the "pain matrix" does not appear to reflect activity that is specific for nociception or pain, and because the magnitude of the "pain matrix" response appears to be largely determined by factors that define saliency, we recently proposed that the "pain matrix" largely reflects the activity of a multimodal cortical network involved in the detection, orientation of attention, and reaction to salient sensory input, regardless of the sensory modality through which that input is conveyed. Importantly, this proposal agrees well with the results of other studies [15, 17] showing that the occurrence of a sudden change in the environment elicits activity within brain regions constituting most of the "pain matrix," regardless of the sensory modality conveying that change. More generally, it agrees with the notion of a "saliency network" subtending the detection of salient sensory input and prompting appropriate behavioural responses, including the insula and the anterior cingulate (i.e., key regions of the "pain matrix") [16].

Viewing the "pain matrix" as a multimodal network related to the detection of salient stimuli would account for a number of experimental observations. First, the fact that nociceptive stimuli consistently elicit activity within this network of brain areas: because of their homeostatic relevance, nociceptive stimuli often have inherently high saliency content. Also, graded nociceptive stimuli elicit graded responses in this network of brain areas, and such graded responses, albeit not being specific for pain *perception*, still allow achieving accurate prediction of the perceived pain across multiple subjects [58]. Second, it would account for the fact that, in most circumstances, the magnitude of the "pain matrix" response correlates with both the intensity of the stimulus and the intensity of pain: indeed, transient stimuli of greater energy, or stimuli perceived as more painful, are also more salient (i.e., they are more contrasted relative to the surrounding environment). Third, it would explain why watching a noxious stimulus being delivered to another individual (as in studies on empathy for pain) or why watching a menacing stimulus such as a needle approaching the hand [11] or experiencing social rejection [31] can elicit activity within the "pain matrix" [26]. Indeed, although none of these stimuli activate nociceptors, they all have a highly salient content.

In the classical hierarchical view of sensory processing, multimodal cortical activity mainly reflects higher order sensory and cognitive processes that occur after sensory information has undergone preliminary processing through modality-specific cortical structures [31, 38]. However, another possibility is that at least part of the multimodal cortical responses is consequent to the convergence, already at subcortical level, of various sources of sensory information belonging to different sensory modalities. We recently provided evidence supporting this hypothesis in Liang et al. [34, 35]. Using dynamic causal modelling of fMRI data combined with Bayesian Model Selection, we investigated the functional connectivity between the brain responses elicited by salient somatosensory, visual, and auditory stimuli in the thalamus; primary sensory cortices; and two core regions of the "pain matrix": the insula and the ACC. We observed that salient sensory input activates the insula and anterior cingulate mainly through direct connections from the thalamus, that is, without being first processed in primary and secondary sensory-specific areas.

Direct multimodal thalamo-cortical projections to these brain regions could originate from unspecific laminar thalamic nuclei, probably part of the "thalamic matrix," constituted by calbindin-positive cells that are present in all thalamic nuclei, and thus ignore the classical nuclear organization of the thalamus [28, 29]. The "thalamic matrix" cells project diffusely to virtually all sensory and motor cortices, and especially to the ACC, and could serve to trigger broad cortical activation following the detection of salient events. Thus, the thalamo-cortical projections from this parallel thalamic system could represent one of the neuroanatomical substrates for the multimodal cortical responses constituting the largest part of the "pain matrix" identified using conventional functional neuroimaging techniques.

In concluding this section, it is important to acknowledge that the interpretation we put forward—that the "pain matrix" reflects the detection of salient sensory events—is also based on reverse inference, and that other explanations are possible. Indeed, the occurrence of a salient stimulus triggers not only attentional mechanisms involved in the detection of salience, increase of arousal, and/or the reorientation of attention, but also emotions and autonomic responses such as changes in heart rate or arterial blood pressure. Hence, *rebus sic stantibus*, the repeated observations of a relationship between stimulus saliency and the magnitude of the "pain matrix" response do not allow us to conclude that this relationship is exclusive. Indeed, the validity of this reverse inference relies on the probability that the relationship between these responses and saliency detection is univocal. Future studies should thus attempt to disentangle experimentally saliency detection, emotion, and autonomic responses.

NOVEL APPROACHES TO CHARACTERIZE THE CORTICAL REPRESENTATION OF PAIN

The ease with which individuals can distinguish between the perception of painful and nonpainful sensations, even when their saliency content is similar, is in striking contrast to the similarity of the EEG and fMRI brain responses elicited by nociceptive and non-nociceptive stimuli [39, 42]. This observation raises an unavoidable question. Why have functional neuroimaging techniques such as EEG and fMRI largely failed to identify obvious differences between the patterns of brain activity elicited by these different stimuli? A first possible explanation is that the magnitude and spatial extent of the brain response elicited by transient nociceptive stimuli has hampered the identification of weaker, possibly nociceptive- or pain-specific sources of neural activity. A second possible explanation is that the widely used methods to analyse EEG and fMRI are based on the identification of regional changes in cortical activity, and have failed to isolate the activity of nociceptive-specific neurons because these neurons are not organized in spatially segregated cortical regions and, instead, are intermingled with neurons also responding to non-nociceptive sensory input. Indeed, in contrast to other main senses, there appears to be no cortical area devoted exclusively to the initial processing of thalamo-cortical nociceptive input (i.e., a primary nociceptive cortex). Recent results obtained using novel neuroimaging analysis techniques such as time–frequency decomposition of EEG/MEG data, and MVPA of fMRI data have provided evidence that both explanations could be true.

As detailed in the section "The "Pain Matrix" Correlates with Stimulus Saliency, Not Pain Perception," stimulus saliency is likely to be a main determinant of the magnitude of nociceptive ERPs, since their magnitude correlates with pain perception when nociceptive stimuli are presented in isolation, but not when their saliency is reduced by repetition at a short and constant interval [24, 51]. Recently, using a time–frequency decomposition of EEG and MEG data to identify non-phase-locked stimulus-evoked activity (i.e., stimulus-evoked activity that is cancelled out by conventional across-trial averaging in the time domain, see [41] for details), several studies have shown that nociceptive stimuli elicit a short lasting early-latency increase in signal power within the γ-band range of frequencies [21–23, 60]. This elusive feature of the EEG/MEG response to nociceptive stimulation has been proposed to originate in S1 and/or the primary motor cortex. Most importantly, Zhang et al. [60] showed that the magnitude of this response correlates with the intensity of pain perception even when the saliency of the stimulus is reduced by repetition, thereby providing evidence indicating that they reflect cortical processes more closely related to nociception and the intensity of pain perception (Fig. 16-3).

MVPA is a machine learning technique that can be used as a pattern classifier to identify the representational content of the fMRI responses elicited in different experimental

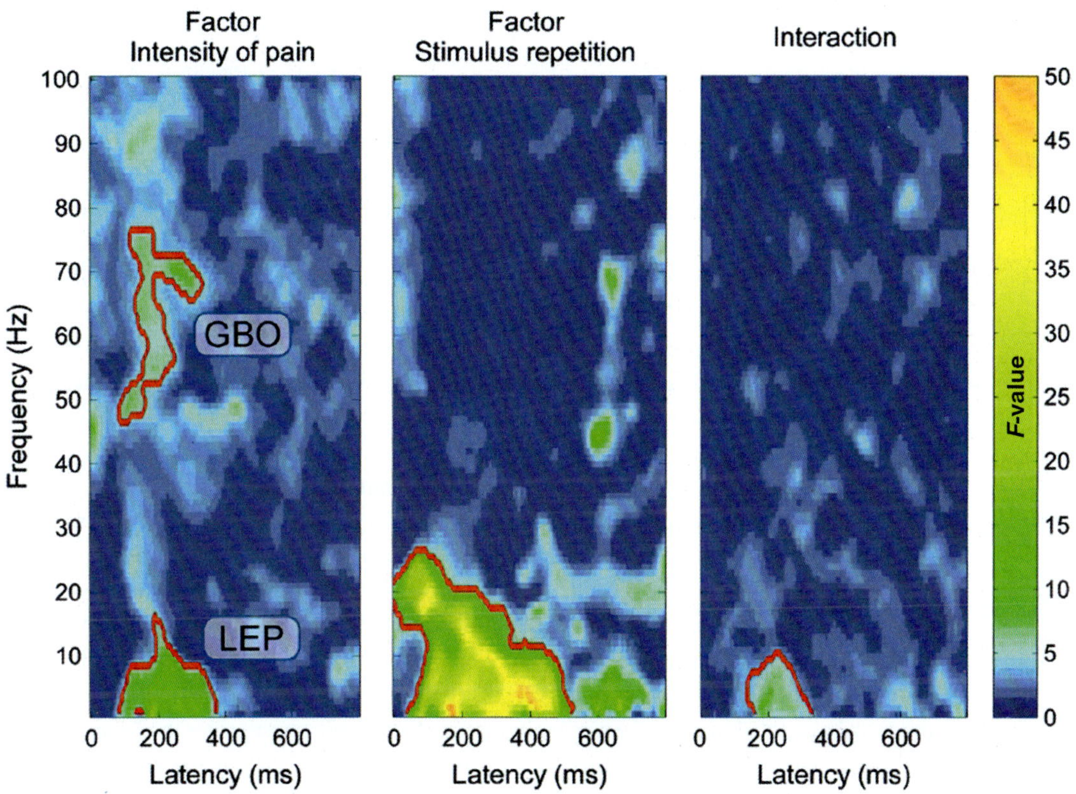

FIGURE 16-3 Effect of stimulus repetition and intensity of pain on the time–frequency representations of laser-induced EEG oscillations. A point-by-point two-way repeated-measures ANOVA was used to assess the effect of stimulus repetition and intensity of pain on the EEG responses elicited by nociceptive stimulation in the time–frequency domain. The time–frequency pixels significantly affected by each experimental factor (or their interaction) are outlined in red. The colour scale represents the *F*-values. Intensity of pain significantly modulated the time–frequency representations in two distinct regions *(in red)*: low-frequency cluster (LEP: 86–367 ms, 1–16 Hz) and high-frequency γ-band cluster (GBO: 86–328 ms, 47–76 Hz). The factor stimulus repetition significantly modulated the time–frequency representations in one low-frequency cluster (1–523 ms, 1–26 Hz), which was larger than the LEP cluster. In addition, there was a significant interaction between the two factors in a low-frequency cluster (141–328 ms, 1–10 Hz), indicating that the stimulus repetition reduced the strength of the relationship between intensity of perception and magnitude. (Adapted from Zhang et al. [60].)

conditions (e.g., by stimuli of different sensory modalities). Whereas conventional approaches to analyse fMRI signals—such as mass-univariate analyses using general linear modelling—detect regional-average changes in activation and consider one single voxel at a time within a given brain region, MVPA detects fine-grained patterns of activity across multiple voxels. Therefore, MVPA can be used to disclose, within a given brain region, fine-grained spatial differences in brain activity across experimental conditions even when the regional-average activity detected using conventional univariate analyses does not differ. MVPA often takes the form of solving a classification problem—for example, guessing whether an fMRI response is elicited by a nociceptive or a non-nociceptive stimulus. In *within-subject MVPA*, the fMRI dataset obtained from an experiment is divided into a training dataset (constituted by, e.g., three out of four fMRI runs) and a test dataset (constituted by, e.g., the fourth run). The training dataset, together with the known labels (identifying the different stimulus categories, e.g., "nociceptive" and "touch"), is used to train a classifier that learns the spatial pattern of responses to each stimulus category. This classifier is then applied to the test dataset to assess its ability to predict the category of the stimulus eliciting the responses of each sample. A good classification accuracy implies that the data (i.e., the spatial distribution of the blood oxygenation level–dependent [BOLD] signal within a given brain region) contain sufficient information to distinguish correctly the different stimulus categories or experimental conditions. A "leave-one-run-out" cross-validation approach is commonly employed, by repeating the procedure using each single run as test dataset and all other runs as the training dataset.

Recently, we performed within-subject MVPA on the fMRI responses elicited by brief and intense nociceptive, tactile, auditory, and visual stimuli. Importantly, these stimuli were matched in terms of saliency, thus reducing the confound represented by saliency-related differences [34]. We found that, although all four types of stimuli elicited spatially similar *regional* responses within the different brain regions constituting the "pain matrix" (as identified using conventional mass-univariate analysis and general linear modelling; [39]), MVPA was able to successfully distinguish the responses elicited by the different stimuli, indicating significant differences in the fine-grained spatial distribution of the activity within the tested brain regions (Fig. 16-4). Importantly, this was also the case when MVPA was performed using fMRI responses *normalized* across multiple voxels, demonstrating that the ability of MVPA to distinguish between the different types of stimuli was not due to mean differences in signal intensity. This demonstration of consistent differences in the spatial pattern of activation indicates that, within the "pain matrix," the neural activity elicited by stimuli perceived as painful can actually be distinguished from the neural activity elicited by other stimuli because each of the different stimuli does not activate the same neuronal populations. Interestingly, MVPA was able to effectively distinguish painful from nonpainful stimuli using the signals sampled in several other brain regions than those constituting the "pain matrix," including unexpected regions such as the primary visual or auditory cortex. This additional result raises the possibility that the quality of the perceptual outcome triggered by nociceptive stimuli does not only emerge from activity within the areas constituting the "pain matrix."

FUTURE DIRECTIONS

The large body of experimental evidence that the cortical responses elicited by transient nociceptive stimuli largely reflect the detection and reaction to potentially dangerous environmental changes implies that such responses are not necessarily adequate to explore

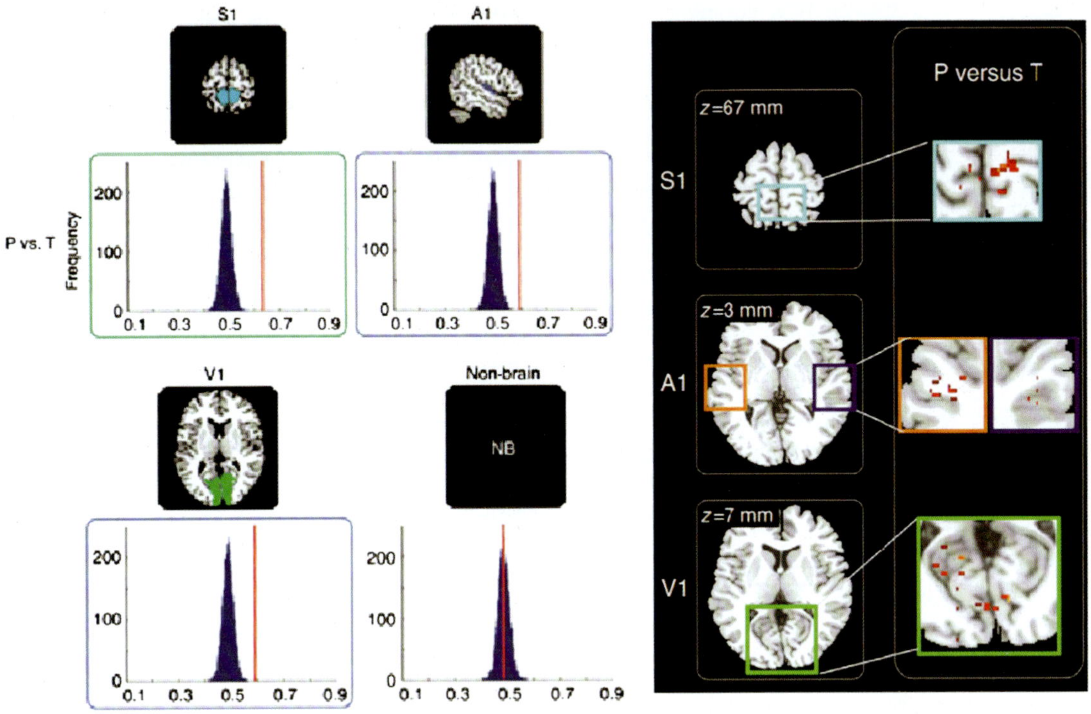

FIGURE 16-4 Accuracies and corresponding null distributions of classifications of BOLD fMRI responses elicited by nociceptive and tactile transient stimuli. Classification accuracies are indicated by vertical red lines, and compared with null distributions generated from 10,000 random permutations. fMRI signal is extracted from the primary somatosensory (S1), auditory (A1), and visual cortices (V1), and from a control, non-brain region (NB). The green frame highlights a pertinent classification (i.e., pain [P] vs. touch [T] in the primary somatosensory cortex). The blue frames highlight two non pertinent classifications (i.e., discrimination between pain and touch in A1 and V1). Permutation tests (*n* 1/4 10,000) show that all classification accuracies are significantly greater than chance level ($P < 0.0001$) except the accuracies from the non-brain control area. This finding indicates that primary sensory cortices contain fine-grained signature of stimuli belonging to different senses. (Adapted from Liang et al. [34].)

the neural activity underlying the actual emergence of pain. As discussed in the section "Novel Approaches to Characterize the Cortical Representation of Pain," the use of advanced analysis approaches might help in teasing out more pain-specific brain responses. Most importantly, experimental designs involving long-lasting nociceptive stimulation that results in tonic pain sensations constitute a promising strategy to enhance the likelihood of extracting neural activities more specifically related to the actual perception of pain and, possibly, more closely related to the pathophysiology of clinical pain conditions.

Finally, recent studies have shown that it is possible to isolate brain activity correlating with spontaneous fluctuations of ongoing pain in patients [2]. Future studies will allow the determination of whether these new approaches can be used to study directly the cortical mechanisms underlying sustained clinical pain.

REFERENCES

1. Albe-Fessard D, Berkley KJ, Kruger L, Ralston HJ III, Willis WD Jr. Diencephalic mechanisms of pain sensation. Brain Res 1985;356(3):217–96.
2. Apkarian AV, Baliki MN, Farmer MA. Predicting transition to chronic pain. Curr Opin Neurol 2013;26(4): 360–7.

3. Apkarian AV, Krauss BR, Fredrickson BE, Szeverenyi NM. Imaging the pain of low back pain: functional magnetic resonance imaging in combination with monitoring subjective pain perception allows the study of clinical pain states. Neurosci Lett 2001;299(1–2):57–60.
4. Avenanti A, Bueti D, Galati G, Aglioti SM. Transcranial magnetic stimulation highlights the sensorimotor side of empathy for pain. Nat Neurosci 2005;8(7):955–60.
5. Beckmann CF, Smith SM. Probabilistic independent component analysis for functional magnetic resonance imaging. IEEE Trans Med Imaging 2004;23(2):137–52.
6. Boly M, Faymonville ME, Schnakers C, Peigneux P, Lambermont B, Phillips C, Lancellotti P, Luxen A, Lamy M, Moonen G, et al. Perception of pain in the minimally conscious state with PET activation: an observational study. Lancet Neurol 2008;7(11):1013–20.
7. Bushnell MC, Apkarian AV. Representation of pain in the brain. In: McMahon S, M Koltzenburg M, editors. Textbook of pain, 5th edition. Churchill Livingstone; 2005. pp. 267–89.
8. Carmon A, Mor J, Goldberg J. Evoked cerebral responses to noxious thermal stimuli in humans. Exp Brain Res 1976;25(1):103–7.
9. Chapman CR, Chen AC, Colpitts YM, Martin RW. Sensory decision theory describes evoked potentials in pain discrimination. Psychophysiology 1981;18(2):114–20.
10. Chapman CR, Colpitts YH, Mayeno JK, Gagliardi GJ. Rate of stimulus repetition changes evoked potential amplitude: dental and auditory modalities compared. Exp Brain Res 1981;43(3–4):246–52.
11. Cheng Y, Lin CP, Liu HL, Hsu YY, Lim KE, Hung D, Decety J. Expertise modulates the perception of pain in others. Curr Biol 2007;17(19):1708–13.
12. Clark JA, Brown CA, Jones AK, El-Deredy W. Dissociating nociceptive modulation by the duration of pain anticipation from unpredictability in the timing of pain. Clin Neurophysiol 2008;119(12):2870–8.
13. Coghill RC, Sang CN, Maisog JM, Iadarola MJ. Pain intensity processing within the human brain: a bilateral, distributed mechanism. J Neurophysiol 1999;82(4):1934–43.
14. Dillmann J, Miltner WH, Weiss T. The influence of semantic priming on event-related potentials to painful laser-heat stimuli in humans. Neurosci Lett 2000;284(1–2):53–6.
15. Downar J, Crawley AP, Mikulis DJ, Davis KD. A multimodal cortical network for the detection of changes in the sensory environment. Nat Neurosci 2000;3(3):277–83.
16. Downar J, Crawley AP, Mikulis DJ, Davis KD. A cortical network sensitive to stimulus salience in a neutral behavioral context across multiple sensory modalities. J Neurophysiol 2002;87(1):615–20.
17. Downar J, Mikulis DJ, Davis KD. Neural correlates of the prolonged salience of painful stimulation. Neuroimage 2003;20(3):1540–51.
18. Friston KJ, Holmes AP, Poline JB, Grasby PJ, Williams SC, Frackowiak RS, Turner R. Analysis of fMRI time-series revisited. Neuroimage 1995;2(1):45–53.
19. Garcia-Larrea L, Frot M, Valeriani M. Brain generators of laser-evoked potentials: from dipoles to functional significance. Neurophysiol Clin 2003;33(6):279–92.
20. Garcia-Larrea L, Peyron R. Pain matrices and neuropathic pain: a review. Pain 2013;154(Suppl 1):S29–S43.
21. Gross J, Schnitzler A, Timmermann L, Ploner M. Gamma oscillations in human primary somatosensory cortex reflect pain perception. PLoS Biol 2007;5(5):e133.
22. Hauck M, Lorenz J, Zimmermann R, Debener S, Scharein E, Engel AK. Duration of the cue-to-pain delay increases pain intensity: a combined EEG and MEG study. Exp Brain Res 2007;180(2):205–15.
23. Hu L, Xiao P, Zhang ZG, Mouraux A, Iannetti GD. Single-trial time-frequency analysis of electrocortical signals: baseline correction and beyond. Neuroimage 2014;84:879–87.
24. Iannetti GD, Hughes NP, Lee MC, Mouraux A. Determinants of laser-evoked EEG responses: pain perception or stimulus saliency? J Neurophysiol 2008;100(2):815–28.
25. Iannetti GD, Mouraux A. From the neuromatrix to the pain matrix (and back). Exp Brain Res 2010;205(1):1–12.
26. Iannetti GD, Mouraux A. Can the functional MRI responses to physical pain really tell us why social rejection "hurts"? Proc Natl Acad Sci USA 2011;108(30):E343.
27. Itti L, Koch C. Computational modelling of visual attention. Nat Rev Neurosci 2001;2(3):194–203.
28. Jones EG. Viewpoint: the core and matrix of thalamic organization. Neuroscience 1998;85(2):331–45.
29. Jones EG. The thalamic matrix and thalamocortical synchrony. Trends Neurosci 2001;24(10):595–601.
30. Kaas JH, Collins CE. The organization of sensory cortex. Curr Opin Neurobiol 2001;11(4):498–504.
31. Kross E, Berman MG, Mischel W, Smith EE, Wager TD. Social rejection shares somatosensory representations with physical pain. Proc Natl Acad Sci USA 2011;108(15):6270–5.
32. Kunde V, Treede RD. Topography of middle-latency somatosensory evoked potentials following painful laser stimuli and non-painful electrical stimuli. Electroencephalogr Clin Neurophysiol 1993;88(4):280–9.

33. Lee MC, Mouraux A, Iannetti GD. Characterizing the cortical activity through which pain emerges from nociception. J Neurosci 2009;29(24):7909–16.
34. Liang M, Mouraux A, Hu L, Iannetti GD. Primary sensory cortices contain distinguishable spatial patterns of activity for each sense. Nat Commun. 2013;4:1979.
35. Liang M, Mouraux A, Iannetti GD. Bypassing primary sensory cortices—a direct thalamocortical pathway for transmitting salient sensory information. Cereb Cortex 2013;23(1):1–11.
36. Lui F, Duzzi D, Corradini M, Serafini M, Baraldi P, Porro CA. Touch or pain? Spatio-temporal patterns of cortical fMRI activity following brief mechanical stimuli. Pain 2008;138(2):362–74.
37. Mesulam MM. From sensation to cognition. Brain 1998;121 (Pt 6):1013–52.
38. Miller G. Neuroscience. Brain scans of pain raise questions for the law. Science 2009;323(5911):195.
39. Mouraux A, Diukova A, Lee MC, Wise RG, Iannetti GD. A multisensory investigation of the functional significance of the "pain matrix." Neuroimage 2011;54(3):2237–49.
40. Mouraux A, Guerit JM, Plaghki L. Refractoriness cannot explain why C-fiber laser-evoked brain potentials are recorded only if concomitant Aδ-fiber activation is avoided. Pain 2004;112(1–2):16–26.
41. Mouraux A, Iannetti GD. Across-trial averaging of event-related EEG responses and beyond. Magn Reson Imaging 2008;26(7):1041–54.
42. Mouraux A, Iannetti GD. Nociceptive laser-evoked brain potentials do not reflect nociceptive-specific neural activity. J Neurophysiol 2009;101(6):3258–69.
43. Mouraux A, Iannetti GD, Colon E, Nozaradan S, Legrain V, Plaghki L. Nociceptive steady-state evoked potentials elicited by rapid periodic thermal stimulation of cutaneous nociceptors. J Neurosci 2011;31(16):6079–87.
44. Mouraux A, Plaghki L. Cortical interactions and integration of nociceptive and non-nociceptive somatosensory inputs in humans. Neuroscience 2007;150(1):72–81.
45. Naatanen R, Paavilainen P, Rinne T, Alho K. The mismatch negativity (MMN) in basic research of central auditory processing: a review. Clin Neurophysiol 2007;118(12):2544–90.
46. Ploghaus A, Tracey I, Gati JS, Clare S, Menon RS, Matthews PM, Rawlins JN. Dissociating pain from its anticipation in the human brain. Science 1999;284(5422):1979–81.
47. Poldrack RA. Can cognitive processes be inferred from neuroimaging data? Trends Cogn Sci 2006;10(2): 59–63.
48. Porro CA. Functional imaging and pain: behavior, perception, and modulation. Neuroscientist 2003;9(5): 354–69.
49. Porro CA, Cettolo V, Francescato MP, Baraldi P. Temporal and intensity coding of pain in human cortex. J Neurophysiol 1998;80(6):3312–20.
50. Rainville P. Brain mechanisms of pain affect and pain modulation. Curr Opin Neurobiol 2002;12(2):195–204.
51. Ronga I, Valentini E, Mouraux A, Iannetti GD. Novelty is not enough: laser-evoked potentials are determined by stimulus saliency, not absolute novelty. J Neurophysiol 2013;109(3):692–701.
52. Schweinhardt P, Bountra C, Tracey I. Pharmacological FMRI in the development of new analgesic compounds. NMR Biomed 2006;19(6):702–711.
53. Tiede W, Magerl W, Baumgartner U, Durrer B, Ehlert U, Treede RD. Sleep restriction attenuates amplitudes and attentional modulation of pain-related evoked potentials, but augments pain ratings in healthy volunteers. Pain 2010;148(1):36–42.
54. Torta DM, Liang M, Valentini E, Mouraux A, Iannetti GD. Dishabituation of laser-evoked EEG responses: dissecting the effect of certain and uncertain changes in stimulus spatial location. Exp Brain Res 2012;218(3):361–372.
55. Treede RD, Lorenz J, Baumgartner U. Clinical usefulness of laser-evoked potentials. Neurophysiol Clin 2003;33(6):303–14.
56. Valentini E, Torta DM, Mouraux A, Iannetti GD. Dishabituation of laser-evoked EEG responses: dissecting the effect of certain and uncertain changes in stimulus modality. J Cogn Neurosci 2011;23(10):2822–37.
57. Valeriani M, Betti V, Le Pera D, De Armas L, Miliucci R, Restuccia D, Avenanti A, Aglioti SM. Seeing the pain of others while being in pain: a laser-evoked potentials study. Neuroimage 2008;40(3):1419–28.
58. Wager TD, Atlas LY, Lindquist MA, Roy M, Woo CW, Kross E. An fMRI-based neurologic signature of physical pain. N Engl J Med 2013;368(15):1388–97.
59. Wang AL, Mouraux A, Liang M, Iannetti GD. Stimulus novelty, and not neural refractoriness, explains the repetition suppression of laser-evoked potentials. J Neurophysiol 2010;104(4):2116–24.
60. Zhang ZG, Hu L, Hung YS, Mouraux A, Iannetti GD. Gamma-band oscillations in the primary somatosensory cortex—a direct and obligatory correlate of subjective pain intensity. J Neurosci 2012;32(22):7429–38.

CHAPTER 17

The Descending Pain Modulatory System in Humans

Irene Tracey and Melvin Mezue

Ever since Sherrington [56] noted increased nociceptive reflexes after rat spinal cord transection, it has been thought that descending spinal influences are involved in the processing of pain. However, investigation of the descending modulation of pain truly began following the seminal report showing that electrical stimulation of the midbrain periaqueductal grey matter (PAG) produced adequate analgesia in the rat to permit abdominal surgery without general anaesthetic [50]. Several preceding studies had already suggested the modulatory effects of supraspinal centres on nonspecific sensory inputs in the spinal cord [9, 19], and the gate control theory proposed by Melzack and Wall [38] proposed that supraspinal influences affected nociceptive spinal excitability. Such studies and the gate theory galvanized the concept that powerful descending influences on dorsal horn nociceptive processing occurred in everyday situations and opened the floodgates for further research.

In the decades following Reynolds' report, the PAG became an important region of study in the pain field. Soon, animal behaviour studies began to report that stimulation of the region produced selective loss of nocifensive behaviour without any changes in responses to other non-noxious stimuli or in general alertness and movement [36]. With the discovery of endogenous opioid activity sites, and the analgesic effect of microinjection of opioids into the PAG [76], it became clear that this region has a profound inhibitory role on the sensation of pain. Further, analgesia was produced with PAG stimulation in human chronic pain patients without any additional motor or sensory effects [7]. Research into the connections of the PAG identified other associated brainstem nuclei, which form a network that modulates nociceptive inputs at the spinal dorsal horn. Although early studies focused on the inhibitory effect of supraspinal modulation, it is now clear that this influence can be facilitatory as well as inhibitory. The dynamic balance between these two is altered in various psychological and pathological conditions, and disruption of this equilibrium may be key in the development of chronic pain states ([22] and references below). The PAG acts as a point of convergence between the cortical, forebrain, and spinal projections that combined are referred to as the descending pain modulatory system (DPMS). Although many of the structures that provide these inputs to the brainstem have been independently identified to have a role in pain modulation, the ultimate perception of pain involves a complex integration of these inputs, accounting for how variances in physical, emotional, and contextual factors influence pain experiences. This is supported by several studies using functional connectivity analyses where changes in coupling between cortical regions and the PAG produce analgesia in a range of contexts but perhaps most commonly illustrated during placebo analgesia and attentional modulation [13, 44, 62, 64]. More recently, aberrant functional coupling of the PAG to key subcortical and cortical brain regions during the interictal phase in migraine patients versus controls highlights further the PAG's role in clinical pain states [34]: an increasingly common finding across human clinical imaging studies and in altered hormonal states [3, 24, 31, 35, 37, 55, 67, 77].

THE DPMS: CORE AND ASSOCIATED BRAIN REGIONS

It should not be forgotten that important top-down cerebral influences result in pain modulation via changes in emotional and cognitive states from the limbic brain (Fig. 17-1). At this stage, it remains unclear in humans to what extent they mediate their influence on pain perception either in whole or in part via the DPMS.

In humans, the effects of attention, expectation, and other psychological variables on pain have been examined with the use of behavioural and functional imaging studies and support active engagement of the DPMS in most circumstances, but not all (reviewed in [60, 72]). Lately, evidence to support the DPMS acting at the level of the human dorsal horn by inhibiting nociceptive processing has come from spinal cord imaging during attentional modulation of pain perception [58]. In rodents, modulation of glutaminergic signalling in the anterior cingulate cortex and amygdala has been linked with the affective aspects of pain perception, supporting direct limbic involvement in the processing of the negative affective components of pain [11, 25]. Behaviourally, there is evidence that negative affect can increase or even decrease the perception of pain, with respect to the level of perceived threat—high threat can lead to stress-induced analgesia [73]. Furthermore, chronic pain patients often find their problems exacerbated by mood disorders, and there is a well-established link in chronic pain patients between depression and pain. Neuroimaging studies have allowed the investigation of the underlying neural correlates. The value of imaging for identifying the brain regions that are either part of or influence the DPMS is perhaps most striking in the various studies that have investigated the neural correlates of the placebo and nocebo effects. This has been shown to involve several opioid-rich limbic and brainstem structures [5, 13, 44, 69], and these regions alongside other regions we consider relevant are discussed in brief subsequently.

Prefrontal Cortex

The involvement of prefrontal structures in pain perception is complex and well documented. Involvement of the ventrolateral prefrontal cortex (VLPFC) during cognitive modulation may have a role in changing the emotional context and subsequent perception of pain—a process known as reappraisal [72, 60]. Activation in this region has been associated with voluntary attenuation of emotion [41, 45], perceived control over pain [51], belief-related pain modulation [72], and placebo analgesia [43]. The role of the VLPFC in emotional regulation may be mediated through its connectivity with the anterior insula cortex [39, 42, 65]. The orbitofrontal cortex (OFC) is also involved in emotional processing, but is associated with encoding of the reward value of stimuli and the anticipation of future outcome [27]. Recent findings have highlighted that information from the OFC (together with the PAG) prior to pain stimulation accurately predicts the trial-by-trial perception of pain [8]. Conversely, dorsolateral prefrontal cortex (DLPFC) activity has been shown to negatively correlate with perceived pain, in association with disruption of thalamic–midbrain coupling by the left DLPFC and increased

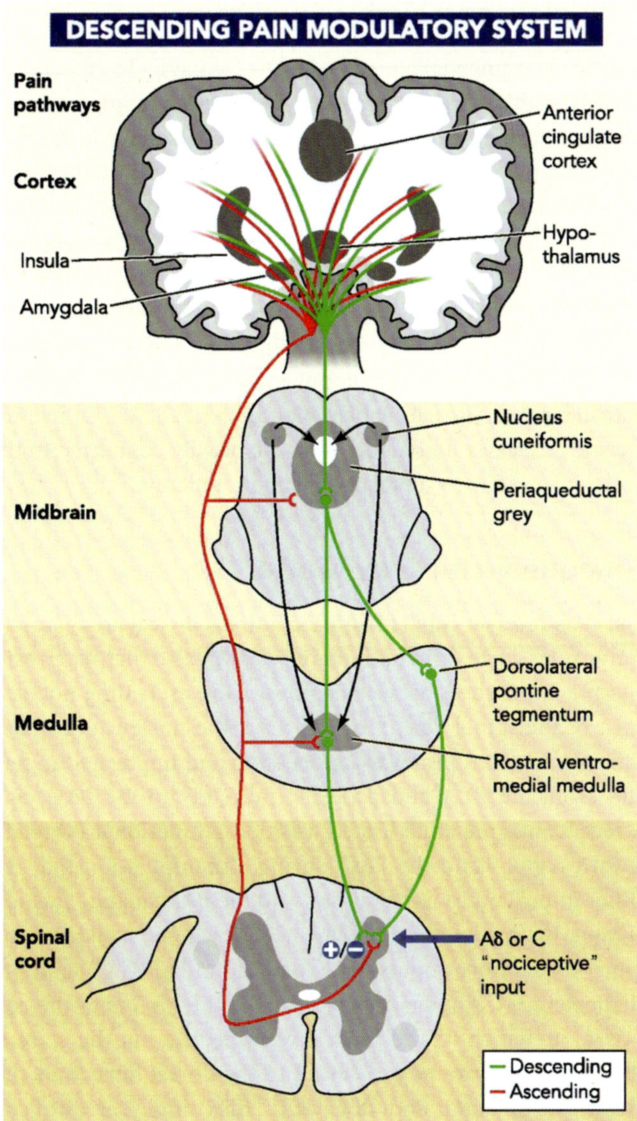

FIGURE 17-1 The descending pain modulatory system. (Schematic adapted from Bingel and Tracey [4].)

anterior insular connectivity with the right DLPFC [32]. The role of the DLPFC in top-down pain inhibition is further supported by evidence that direct current stimulation of this region has some efficacy against experimental pain [6].

Others have reported a role for the medial prefrontal cortex (MPFC) in predicting pharmacological antihyperalgesic responses in healthy volunteers [54], and pain chronification in back pain patients (via functional connections with the nucleus accumbens) [1]. Furthermore, these prefrontal regions have all been shown with white matter tract imaging to be structurally connected with midbrain structures important in descending pain modulation [18]. Alongside the dominant role of the rostral anterior cingulate cortex as a key part of the DPMS, these more recently identified roles of human prefrontal cortical regions in pain experiences and their anatomical connection to the brainstem provide a basis for direct cognitive and emotional modulation of pain perception via, in part or whole, the DPMS.

Amygdala and Limbic Forebrain

The two key amygdala nuclei relevant for pain and anxiety processing are the basolateral nucleus of the amygdala (BLA), which processes information from the cortical and forebrain limbic areas, and the central nucleus (CeA), which receives nociceptive specific inputs from the spino-parabrachial system [40, 46]. The BLA projects to the CeA, which in turn projects densely to the PAG. In rodents, morphine microinjection into the BLA has been shown to reduce glutaminergic excitation and so reduce nocifensive reflex behaviour in rats [11]. In humans, neuroimaging studies have reported both increases and decreases in amygdala activity in response to pain, with peak activity in clinical studies located in the BLA region (reviewed recently in [57]). The amygdala has also been shown to be involved in opioid and cannabinoid analgesia in healthy human pain models, illustrating its potential role in mediating pain modulation [28, 71]. Of relevance to this chapter's content, the amygdala and limbic forebrain are heavily connected to the PAG and other brainstem nuclei involved with supraspinal pain modulation.

Periaqueductal Grey Matter

The PAG receives inputs from the limbic cortical areas (rostral anterior cingulate cortex and insular cortex), hypothalamus, amygdala (that receives inputs from the hippocampus and neocortex), as well as inputs from ascending nociceptive fibres from the dorsal horn of the spinal cord [16]. Of note, the nucleus accumbens in the ventral striatum, which is involved in reward processing and implicated in pain modulation, receives inputs from the BLA and projects indirectly to the PAG via the lateral hypothalamus. A recent imaging study nicely verified a functional correlation and link between such reward regions and the PAG during a manipulation that rendered pain pleasant [30]. Other important brainstem inputs to the PAG include the pontomedullary reticular formation, the nucleus cuneiformis (NCF, which is adjacent to the PAG and also receives spinal dorsal horn inputs), the locus coeruleus (LC), and other brainstem noradrenergic nuclei [23]. The main projection of the PAG is to the rostral ventromedial medulla (RVM), to which it is reciprocally connected, but there are also projections to the noradrenergic cell groups projecting to the dorsal horn, and smaller rostral projections to the medial thalamus and OFC [16]. This complex array of connections allows top-down control of nociception as well as feedback modulation: without doubt, the PAG is in a pivotal position to influence pain perception. It is cytoarchitectonically heterogenous, with its ventrolateral and dorsolateral portions contributing differently to pain modulation. Importantly, the PAG (together with the anterior cingulate cortex, amygdala, and RVM) contains a high level of opioid receptors, and its involvement in endogenous pain modulation is directly linked to the opioid responsiveness of its cells, as shown by several neuroimaging studies [44, 71]. However, most imaging studies highlight its role in pain perception, sensitization, cognitive pain modulation, and placebo/nocebo responses (see reviews [31, 60, 61]). Imaging this region is not trivial due to its size and the inherent physiological noise in this brain region, and so special imaging requirements are needed and deployed in most studies to date. Going forward, imaging at ultrahigh field will undoubtedly bring added benefits, and this was illustrated recently in a 7-T study that allowed functional parcellation of the different divisions of the PAG affording us new and exciting research opportunities [53].

Rostral Ventromedial Medulla

The RVM is a functionally defined area in the midline pontomedullary reticular region of the brainstem—the main common output for descending pro- and antinociceptive signals. The RVM contains the midline serotonergic nucleus raphe magnus and is closely related to the adjacent ventrolateral reticular formation. Both medial and lateral parts of the RVM have to be blocked to completely stop descending inhibitory effects from PAG stimulation [52]. The RVM receives inputs from the PAG, NCF, adjacent reticular nuclei, A5 and A7 noradrenergic cell groups in the dorsolateral pons, and some ascending spinal nociceptive inputs (mainly via the NCF and adjacent reticular nuclei). It also receives direct projections from higher limbic cortical regions, including the CeA, hypothalamus, and prefrontal cortices. The RVM projects to deep and superficial layers of the dorsal horn and directly modulates the excitability of the nociceptive neurons. Although 5-HT spinal receptors may be either facilitatory or inhibitory to nociceptive signalling depending on receptor subtype [59, 61], the RVM's serotonergic projections likely affect 5-HT-1A spinal receptors, which are thought to be antinociceptive [66]. Microstimulation or opioid microinjection into the RVM produces profound and selective analgesia comparable to that seen in the PAG [76], confirmed recently in a human imaging study of opioid analgesia [71]. Conversely, anatomical lesions or pharmacological inactivation of the RVM abolishes the analgesic effect of PAG stimulation [15]. Such studies supported the role of the PAG–RVM system as an inhibitor of nociception and the RVM as the final supraspinal relay point. However, a series of reports from Zhuo and Gebhart [79–81] showed that low-intensity electrical stimulation of the RVM facilitates the tail-flick nocifensive reflex at the same sites where inhibition can also be produced. Furthermore, focal microinjection of the neuropeptide cholecystokinin (CCK) into the RVM has been shown to be pronociceptive and hyperalgesic [21]. Fitting with a pronociceptive role, the RVM has been shown to be important in hyperalgesia and maintenance of spontaneous pain in some neuropathic and inflammatory models [10, 22, 47, 70]. Neuroimaging of the brainstem in humans has revealed regions of the mesencephalic and pontine reticular formation to be important in postinjury pain sensitization and patients [17, 29, 77]. These studies combined confirm that descending control from the RVM in humans is facilitatory as well as inhibitory to nociception. The neural basis of this complex modulation is understood from an earlier key study by Fields et al. [14] that categorized two subsets of RVM neurons (ON = facilitation and OFF = inhibition cells) based on their state changes in association with nocifensive withdrawal. The neurobiology of these cell types is beyond the scope of this chapter and the resolution of neuroimaging—even at high field—but is of tremendous relevance and interest.

Dorsal Pontomesencephalic Formation and NCF

The dorsal pontomesencephalic formation includes the NCF and parabrachial nucleus (PBN). The NCF/PBN region receives major inputs from lamina I of spinal and trigeminal horns and smaller inputs from the deeper laminae of the spinal cord. Its projections are mainly to the RVM, creating a spinal–bulbar–spinal loop thought to mediate facilitation or inhibition at the dorsal horn [59]. The discovery of ON and OFF cells in a region of the NCF/PBN that was shown to suppress nocifensive behaviour in rats on microstimulation suggests that input into the RVM from this region may be important in pain modulation [20, 78]. Importantly, activity in this area has also been shown in a functional magnetic resonance imaging (fMRI) study to be correlated with RVM activity in visceral pain, which supports the view of a brainstem–spinal loop modulating nociceptive inputs in humans [12]. The NCF is ventrolateral to the PAG and has been identified as an important part of the pain modulation network, owing to its inputs from the prefrontal cortex, hypothalamus, and amygdala; strong association with the adjacent PAG; and projection to the nucleus raphe magnus of the RVM. These put the NCF in a prime position to receive autonomic, executive, and affective information, so it can bidirectionally modulate pain perception. In humans, an fMRI study by Zambreanu et al. [77] identified the NCF as a major region of brainstem activation in a healthy volunteer model of hyperalgesia subsequent to the development of central sensitization (CS).

LC and Noradrenergic Nuclei

The dorsolateral pontine tegmentum noradrenergic neurons are important contributors to the modulation of pain and include the LC and the A5 and A7 noradrenergic cell groups [16]. The LC is the most studied of this group and is principally a noradrenaline-producing nucleus having an important role in stress and anxiety behaviour modulation—mediating arousal via its widespread excitatory effects in the brain. Electrical or chemical stimulation of the LC produces descending antinociception by inhibiting nociceptive activity in the dorsal horn [26]. The LC receives major excitatory afferents from the ventrolateral medullary reticular formation and inhibitory afferents from the dorsomedial rostral medulla, as well as smaller inputs from the posterior hypothalamus, mesencephalic reticular formation, and some forebrain regions [33]. A projection from the central nucleus of the amygdala may be important in allowing emotional pain to trigger noradrenergic responses. The LC projects widely to the forebrain and sensory brainstem nuclei, and provides noradrenergic innervation to spinal cord neurons—mostly in the ventral horn but also in the dorsal horn [48]. The LC is also activated in experimentally induced inflammation, where it attenuates the development of hyperalgesia [63]. These observations suggest that noradrenergic neurons have important inhibitory effects, both as contributors to the PAG–RVM system and as an independent descending antinociceptive pathway, but to date there are no explicit neuroimaging reports of its role in human pain modulation. This is likely due to its small size and limitations on signal-to-noise producing sufficient measurable activity via commonly deployed neuroimaging tools. Hopefully, this will improve as more studies at ultrahigh field are performed.

Response to Injury—Peripheral and Central Sensitization: Role of the DPMS

A common feature of the nervous system is its ability to modify its properties in response to inputs—termed plasticity. In this vein, activity-dependent plasticity following noxious stimulation of nociceptors manifests in several forms [68, 75]. Of potentially far greater clinical import is CS, thought to be a major mechanism in the development of inflammatory and neuropathic pain conditions, supported by long-standing evidence of hyperalgesia and allodynia amongst certain patient groups [2, 49, 74].

Several preclinical and human studies have indicated that CS and spontaneous neuropathic pain are maintained by descending supraspinal facilitation, largely from the RVM and associated structures [10, 29, 44, 59, 70]. Such validation across species is reassuring, particularly because of our inability in human neuroimaging studies to distinguish ON from OFF cell activity, and therefore relies on careful paradigm design and concomitant behavioural measures to interpret likely descending facilitation from less descending inhibition (that would produce the same behavioural outcome).

CONCLUSION

The evidence outlined above suggests that active regulation by various excitatory and inhibitory CNS circuits, gated by brainstem structures, can decrease or increase pain perception, depending on several cognitive, mood, or contextual factors. Disruptions of these circuits at the supraspinal or spinal level can contribute to abnormal and pathological pain amplification.

REFERENCES

1. Baliki MN, Petre B, Torbey S, Herrmann KM, Huang L, Schnitzer TJ, Fields HL, Apkarian AV. Corticostriatal functional connectivity predicts transition to chronic back pain. Nat Neurosci 2012;15(8):1117–9.
2. Baron R. Mechanisms of disease: neuropathic pain—a clinical perspective. Nat Clin Pract Neurol 2006;2(2): 95–106.
3. Becerra L, Morris S, Bazes S, Gostic R, Sherman S, Gostic J, Pendse G, Moulton E, Scrivani S, Keith D, et al. Trigeminal neuropathic pain alters responses in CNS circuits to mechanical (brush) and thermal (cold and heat) stimuli. J Neurosci 2006;26(42):10646–57.
4. Bingel U, Tracey I. Imaging CNS modulation of pain in humans. Physiology (Bethesda) 2008;23:371–80.
5. Bingel U, Wanigasekera V, Wiech K, Ni Mhuircheartaigh R, Lee MC, Ploner M, Tracey I. The effect of treatment expectation on drug efficacy: imaging the analgesic benefit of the opioid remifentanil. Sci Transl Med 2011;3(70):70ra14.
6. Boggio PS, Zaghi S, Lopes M, Fregni F. Modulatory effects of anodal transcranial direct current stimulation on perception and pain thresholds in healthy volunteers. Eur J Neurol 2008;15(10):1124–30.
7. Boivie J, Meyerson BA. A correlative anatomical and clinical study of pain suppression by deep brain stimulation. Pain 1982;13(2):113–26.
8. Brodersen KH, Wiech K, Lomakina EI, Lin CS, Buhmann JM, Bingel U, Ploner M, Stephan KE, Tracey I. Decoding the perception of pain from fMRI using multivariate pattern analysis. NeuroImage 2012;63(3): 1162–70.
9. Carpenter D, Engberg I, Lundberg A. Differential supraspinal control of inhibitory and excitatory actions from the FRA to ascending spinal pathways. Acta Physiol Scand 1965;63:103–10.
10. De Felice M, Sanoja R, Wang R, Vera-Portocarrero L, Oyarzo J, King T, Ossipov MH, Vanderah TW, Lai J, Dussor GO, et al. Engagement of descending inhibition from the rostral ventromedial medulla protects against chronic neuropathic pain. Pain 2011;152(12):2701–9.
11. Deyama S, Nakagawa T, Kaneko S, Uehara T, Minami M. Involvement of the bed nucleus of the stria terminalis in the negative affective component of visceral and somatic pain in rats. Behav Brain Res 2007;176(2):367–71.
12. Dunckley P, Wise RG, Fairhurst M, Hobden P, Aziz Q, Chang L, Tracey I. A comparison of visceral and somatic pain processing in the human brainstem using functional magnetic resonance imaging. J Neurosci 2005;25(32):7333–41.
13. Eippert F, Bingel U, Schoell ED, Yacubian J, Klinger R, Lorenz J, Buchel C. Activation of the opioidergic descending pain control system underlies placebo analgesia. Neuron 2009;63(4):533–43.
14. Fields HL, Bry J, Hentall I, Zorman G. The activity of neurons in the rostral medulla of the rat during withdrawal from noxious heat. J Neurosci 1983;3(12):2545–52.
15. Fields HL, Heinricher MM, Mason P. Neurotransmitters in nociceptive modulatory circuits. Annu Rev Neurosci 1991;14:219–45.
16. Fields HW, Hessler C, Hibbits S, Jamerson PA, Mintun M. Develop a hospital-based nursing sabbatical program. Nurs Manage 2006;37(11):10–12.
17. Gwilym SE, Keltner JR, Warnaby CE, Carr AJ, Chizh B, Chessell I, Tracey I. Psychophysical and functional imaging evidence supporting the presence of central sensitization in a cohort of osteoarthritis patients. Arthritis Rheum 2009;61(9):1226–34.

18. Hadjipavlou G, Dunckley P, Behrens TE, Tracey I. Determining anatomical connectivities between cortical and brainstem pain processing regions in humans: a diffusion tensor imaging study in healthy controls. Pain 2006;123(1–2):169–78.
19. Hagbarth KE, Kerr DI. Central influences on spinal afferent conduction. J Neurophysiol 1954;17(3):295–307.
20. Haws CM, Williamson AM, Fields HL. Putative nociceptive modulatory neurons in the dorsolateral pontomesencephalic reticular formation. Brain Res 1989;483(2):272–82.
21. Heinricher MM, Neubert MJ. Neural basis for the hyperalgesic action of cholecystokinin in the rostral ventromedial medulla. J Neurophysiol 2004;92(4):1982–9.
22. Heinricher MM, Tavares I, Leith JL, Lumb BM. Descending control of nociception: specificity, recruitment and plasticity. Brain Res Rev 2009;60(1):214–25.
23. Herbert H, Saper CB. Organization of medullary adrenergic and noradrenergic projections to the periaqueductal gray matter in the rat. J Comp Neurol 1992;315(1):34–52.
24. Iannetti GD, Zambreanu L, Wise RG, Buchanan TJ, Huggins JP, Smart TS, Vennart W, Tracey I. Pharmacological modulation of pain-related brain activity during normal and central sensitization states in humans. Proc Natl Acad Sci USA 2005;102(50):18195–200.
25. Johansen JP, Fields HL. Glutamatergic activation of anterior cingulate cortex produces an aversive teaching signal. Nat Neurosci 2004;7(4):398–403.
26. Jones SL, Gebhart GF. Inhibition of spinal nociceptive transmission from the midbrain, pons and medulla in the rat: activation of descending inhibition by morphine, glutamate and electrical stimulation. Brain Res 1988;460(2):281–96.
27. Kahnt T, Heinzle J, Park SQ, Haynes JD. The neural code of reward anticipation in human orbitofrontal cortex. Proc Natl Acad Sci USA 2010;107(13):6010–5.
28. Lee MC, Ploner M, Wiech K, Bingel U, Wanigasekera V, Brooks J, Menon DK, Tracey I. Amygdala activity contributes to the dissociative effect of cannabis on pain perception. Pain 2013;154(1):124–34.
29. Lee MC, Zambreanu L, Menon DK, Tracey I. Identifying brain activity specifically related to the maintenance and perceptual consequence of central sensitization in humans. J Neurosci 2008;28(45):11642–9.
30. Leknes S, Berna C, Lee MC, Snyder GD, Biele G, Tracey I. The importance of context: when relative relief renders pain pleasant. Pain 2013;154(3):402–10.
31. Linnman C, Moulton EA, Barmettler G, Becerra L, Borsook D. Neuroimaging of the periaqueductal gray: state of the field. NeuroImage 2012;60(1):505–22.
32. Lorenz J, Minoshima S, Casey KL. Keeping pain out of mind: the role of the dorsolateral prefrontal cortex in pain modulation. Brain 2003;126(Pt 5):1079–91.
33. Luppi PH, Aston-Jones G, Akaoka H, Chouvet G, Jouvet M. Afferent projections to the rat locus coeruleus demonstrated by retrograde and anterograde tracing with cholera-toxin B subunit and *Phaseolus vulgaris* leucoagglutinin. Neuroscience 1995;65(1):119–60.
34. Mainero C, Boshyan J, Hadjikhani N. Altered functional magnetic resonance imaging resting-state connectivity in periaqueductal gray networks in migraine. Ann Neurol 2011;70(5):838–45.
35. Mainero C, Zhang WT, Kumar A, Rosen BR, Sorensen AG. Mapping the spinal and supraspinal pathways of dynamic mechanical allodynia in the human trigeminal system using cardiac-gated fMRI. NeuroImage 2007;35(3):1201–10.
36. Mayer DJ, Price DD. Central nervous system mechanisms of analgesia. Pain 1976;2(4):379–404.
37. Mayer EA, Berman S, Suyenobu B, Labus J, Mandelkern MA, Naliboff BD, Chang L. Differences in brain responses to visceral pain between patients with irritable bowel syndrome and ulcerative colitis. Pain 2005;115(3):398–409.
38. Melzack R, Wall PD. Pain mechanisms: a new theory. Science 1965;150(3699):971–9.
39. Mitchell DG. The nexus between decision making and emotion regulation: a review of convergent neurocognitive substrates. Behav Brain Res 2011;217(1):215–31.
40. Neugebauer V, Li W, Bird GC, Han JS. The amygdala and persistent pain. Neuroscientist 2004;10(3):221–34.
41. Ochsner KN, Ray RD, Cooper JC, Robertson ER, Chopra S, Gabrieli JD, Gross JJ. For better or for worse: neural systems supporting the cognitive down- and up-regulation of negative emotion. NeuroImage 2004;23(2):483–99.
42. Peltz E, Seifert F, DeCol R, Dorfler A, Schwab S, Maihofner C. Functional connectivity of the human insular cortex during noxious and innocuous thermal stimulation. NeuroImage 2011;54(2):1324–35.
43. Petrovic P, Kalso E, Petersson KM, Andersson J, Fransson P, Ingvar M. A prefrontal non-opioid mechanism in placebo analgesia. Pain 2010;150(1):59–65.

44. Petrovic P, Kalso E, Petersson KM, Ingvar M. Placebo and opioid analgesia—imaging a shared neuronal network. Science 2002;295(5560):1737–40.
45. Phan KL, Fitzgerald DA, Nathan PJ, Moore GJ, Uhde TW, Tancer ME. Neural substrates for voluntary suppression of negative affect: a functional magnetic resonance imaging study. Biol Psychiatry 2005;57(3):210–19.
46. Phelps EA, LeDoux JE. Contributions of the amygdala to emotion processing: from animal models to human behavior. Neuron 2005;48(2):175–87.
47. Porreca F, Ossipov MH, Gebhart GF. Chronic pain and medullary descending facilitation. Trends Neurosci 2002;25(6):319–25.
48. Proudfit HK, Clark FM. The projections of locus coeruleus neurons to the spinal cord. Prog Brain Res 1991;88:123–41.
49. Rasmussen PV, Sindrup SH, Jensen TS, Bach FW. Symptoms and signs in patients with suspected neuropathic pain. Pain 2004;110(1–2):461–9.
50. Reynolds DV. Surgery in the rat during electrical analgesia induced by focal brain stimulation. Science 1969;164(3878):444–5.
51. Salomons TV, Johnstone T, Backonja MM, Shackman AJ, Davidson RJ. Individual differences in the effects of perceived controllability on pain perception: critical role of the prefrontal cortex. J Cogn Neurosci 2007;19(6):993–1003.
52. Sandkuhler J, Gebhart GF. Relative contributions of the nucleus raphe magnus and adjacent medullary reticular formation to the inhibition by stimulation in the periaqueductal gray of a spinal nociceptive reflex in the pentobarbital-anesthetized rat. Brain Res 1984;305(1):77–87.
53. Satpute AB, Wager TD, Cohen-Adad J, Bianciardi M, Choi JK, Buhle JT, Wald LL, Barrett LF. Identification of discrete functional subregions of the human periaqueductal gray. Proc Natl Acad Sci USA 2013;110(42):17101–6.
54. Seifert F, Bschorer K, De Col R, Filitz J, Peltz E, Koppert W, Maihofner C. Medial prefrontal cortex activity is predictive for hyperalgesia and pharmacological antihyperalgesia. J Neurosci 2009;29(19):6167–75.
55. Seifert F, Maihofner C. Representation of cold allodynia in the human brain—a functional MRI study. NeuroImage 2007;35(3):1168–80.
56. Sherrington C. The integrative action of the nervous system. New Haven, CT: Yale University Press; 1906.
57. Simons LE, Moulton EA, Linnman C, Carpino E, Becerra L, Borsook D. The human amygdala and pain: evidence from neuroimaging. Hum Brain Mapp 2014;35(2):527–38.
58. Sprenger C, Eippert F, Finsterbusch J, Bingel U, Rose M, Buchel C. Attention modulates spinal cord responses to pain. Curr Biol 2012;22(11):1019–22.
59. Suzuki R, Rygh LJ, Dickenson AH. Bad news from the brain: descending 5-HT pathways that control spinal pain processing. Trends Pharmacol Sci 2004;25(12):613–7.
60. Tracey I. Getting the pain you expect: mechanisms of placebo, nocebo and reappraisal effects in humans. Nat Med 2010;16(11):1277–83.
61. Tracey I, Dickenson A. SnapShot: pain perception. Cell 2012;148(6):1308–1308.e2.
62. Tracey I, Ploghaus A, Gati JS, Clare S, Smith S, Menon RS, Matthews PM. Imaging attentional modulation of pain in the periaqueductal gray in humans. J Neurosci 2002;22(7):2748–52.
63. Tsuruoka M, Willis WD Jr. Bilateral lesions in the area of the nucleus locus coeruleus affect the development of hyperalgesia during carrageenan-induced inflammation. Brain Res 1996;726(1–2):233–6.
64. Valet M, Sprenger T, Boecker H, Willoch F, Rummeny E, Conrad B, Erhard P, Tolle TR. Distraction modulates connectivity of the cingulo-frontal cortex and the midbrain during pain—an fMRI analysis. Pain 2004;109(3):399–408.
65. Veit R, Singh V, Sitaram R, Caria A, Rauss K, Birbaumer N. Using real-time fMRI to learn voluntary regulation of the anterior insula in the presence of threat-related stimuli. Soc Cogn Affect Neurosci 2012;7(6):623–34.
66. Viisanen H, Pertovaara A. Roles of the rostroventromedial medulla and the spinal 5-HT(1A) receptor in descending antinociception induced by motor cortex stimulation in the neuropathic rat. Neurosci Lett 2010;476(3):133–7.
67. Vincent K, Warnaby C, Stagg CJ, Moore J, Kennedy S, Tracey I. Brain imaging reveals that engagement of descending inhibitory pain pathways in healthy women in a low endogenous estradiol state varies with testosterone. Pain 2013;154(4):515–24.
68. von Hehn CA, Baron R, Woolf CJ. Deconstructing the neuropathic pain phenotype to reveal neural mechanisms. Neuron 2012;73(4):638–52.

69. Wager TD, Rilling JK, Smith EE, Sokolik A, Casey KL, Davidson RJ, Kosslyn SM, Rose RM, Cohen JD. Placebo-induced changes in fMRI in the anticipation and experience of pain. Science 2004;303(5661):1162–7.
70. Wang R, King T, De Felice M, Guo W, Ossipov MH, Porreca F. Descending facilitation maintains long-term spontaneous neuropathic pain. J Pain 2013;14(8):845–53.
71. Wanigasekera V, Lee MC, Rogers R, Kong Y, Leknes S, Andersson J, Tracey I. Baseline reward circuitry activity and trait reward responsiveness predict expression of opioid analgesia in healthy subjects. Proc Natl Acad Sci USA 2012;109(43):17705–10.
72. Wiech K, Ploner M, Tracey I. Neurocognitive aspects of pain perception. Trends Cogn Sci 2008;12(8):306–13.
73. Wiech K, Tracey I. The influence of negative emotions on pain: behavioral effects and neural mechanisms. NeuroImage 2009;47(3):987–94.
74. Woolf CJ. Central sensitization: implications for the diagnosis and treatment of pain. Pain 2011;152 (3 Suppl):S2–15.
75. Woolf CJ, Salter MW. Neuronal plasticity: increasing the gain in pain. Science 2000;288(5472):1765–9.
76. Yaksh TL, Rudy TA. Narcotic analgesics: CNS sites and mechanisms of action as revealed by intracerebral injection techniques. Pain 1978;4(4):299–359.
77. Zambreanu L, Wise RG, Brooks JC, Iannetti GD, Tracey I. A role for the brainstem in central sensitisation in humans: evidence from functional magnetic resonance imaging. Pain 2005;114(3):397–407.
78. Zemlan FP, Behbehani MM. Nucleus cuneiformis and pain modulation: anatomy and behavioral pharmacology. Brain Res 1988;453(1–2):89–102.
79. Zhuo M, Gebhart GF. Characterization of descending inhibition and facilitation from the nuclei reticularis gigantocellularis and gigantocellularis pars alpha in the rat. Pain 1990;42(3):337–50.
80. Zhuo M, Gebhart GF. Characterization of descending facilitation and inhibition of spinal nociceptive transmission from the nuclei reticularis gigantocellularis and gigantocellularis pars alpha in the rat. J Neurophysiol 1992;67(6):1599–614.
81. Zhuo M, Gebhart GF. Biphasic modulation of spinal nociceptive transmission from the medullary raphe nuclei in the rat. J Neurophysiol 1997;78(2):746–58.

CHAPTER 18

Evoked Potentials in Relation to Pain Perception

A. Mouraux, G. D. Iannetti, Ulf Baumgärtner, and Rolf-Detlef Treede

The ongoing electrical activity of the human brain can be directly and noninvasively sampled through the skull, using electroencephalography (EEG) [66]. Recording the EEG thus constitutes a unique means to study brain function in humans. Compared with other noninvasive methods to sample human brain activity such as functional magnetic resonance imaging (fMRI) or positron emission tomography (PET), one important advantage of EEG (and its magnetic counterpart, magnetoencephalography, MEG) is its high temporal resolution. This makes it possible to distinguish neural events occurring close in time and, thereby, to study the detailed chronometry of the different brain responses elicited by a sensory stimulus. Indeed, the scalp potentials composing the EEG are related *directly* to the underlying neural activity, whereas fMRI and PET rely on the increase in blood flow related to the haemodynamic response following neural activity, and thus measure neural activity *indirectly* [47].

However, when interpreting EEG signals, it is important to consider the following two points. First, that EEG signals primarily reflect the synchronized occurrence of slow post-synaptic potentials occurring within a population of similarly oriented cortical pyramidal neurons and, hence, that the EEG reflects only a fraction of the electrical activity of the human brain [56]. Second, that EEG measures a spatially blurred mixture of a series of neural activities. Because of the distance between the neurons generating the activity and the electrodes recording that activity, and the conductance of the interposed anatomical structures, the changes in scalp potential induced by the activity occurring within a given neuronal population are spread over a large area of the scalp. Consequently, EEG has a relatively low spatial resolution, that is, the ability of EEG to resolve two neural events in space is relatively low.

An interesting application of EEG is the recording of event-related potentials (ERPs) [66]. The delivery of a brief stimulus belonging to virtually any sensory modality elicits transient changes of EEG potentials, which appear as mono- or polyphasic deflections embedded in the background EEG, and reflect the fact that the event triggers synchronized neural activity within different brain regions. For example, the transient activation of somatosensory afferents elicited by transcutaneous median nerve stimulation elicits a succession of positive and negative deflections in the EEG signal, corresponding to (a) subcortical activity within the dorsal column nuclei, medial lemniscus, and thalamus, followed by (b) cortical activity within the primary somatosensory cortex (S1), and (c) later responses occurring in other cortical areas (such as the secondary somatosensory cortex) thought to reflect higher order processing stages [17]. Therefore, the recording of ERPs has been widely used to study the neural activity involved in a given brain function, in particular, the cortical activity involved in processing sensory input of a given sensory modality. Furthermore, stimulus-evoked sensory ERPs are widely used in clinical practice as a proxy for the state of the afferent pathways activated by the sensory stimulus. For example, a dysfunction of somatosensory pathways can be demonstrated by the observation of a significant increase in latency or reduction of amplitude of the ERPs elicited by somatosensory stimulation [17].

In 1976, Carmon et al. [11] introduced the use of laser stimulators to selectively and transiently activate heat-sensitive nociceptive afferents, and thereby record ERPs reflecting the neural responses elicited by synchronized nociceptive somatosensory input [6]. The technique is now widely used both in basic research, to study the neural processes elicited by a sudden nociceptive input, and in a clinical setting, to assess the function of nociceptive pathways in patients [20, 76].

Here, we will (a) critically review the functional significance of the EEG responses that are commonly measured in response to transient nociceptive stimulation (e.g., laser-evoked potentials [LEPs]), (b) present some novel approaches to measure neural activities that could be more specific for nociception such as the recording of γ-band oscillations and steady-state evoked potentials, and (c) discuss the clinical usefulness of recording ERPs elicited by nociceptive stimuli, to assess pain pathways in humans.

In this context, it is important to distinguish between pain and nociception [46]. Pain, as defined by the IASP, is a *subjective* experience that may be induced by a nociceptive stimulus but may also occur without any noticeable stimulus. Nociception is the encoding of nociceptive stimuli by peripheral nociceptive nerve endings and the processing of the resulting afferent activity in higher order neurons of the so-called nociceptive system. Nociceptive signal processing can thus be explored experimentally using electrophysiological or functional neuroimaging techniques that sample this neural activity. However, and although several authors refer to these responses as "pain-evoked" [80, 86], this does not imply that they reflect neural activity directly responsible for pain perception. Hence, increases or decreases in the magnitude of these responses should not be taken as *objective* evidence for changes in pain perception.

EEG RESPONSES ELICITED BY A TRANSIENT NOCICEPTIVE STIMULUS

Selective Activation of Nociceptive Free Nerve Endings

The study of any sensory system requires the availability of a quantifiable stimulus that activates selectively the sensory system under investigation. The issue of the selectivity of sensory stimuli is especially relevant in the study of nociception as, within the skin, nociceptive free nerve endings are in the close vicinity of non-nociceptive mechanoreceptors conveying vibrotactile sensations and, within peripheral nerves, nociceptive and non-nociceptive axons are intermingled. Therefore, characterizing the brain responses to nociceptive input requires a stimulus that is able to activate nociceptive afferents without concurrently activating nearby non-nociceptive somatosensory afferents. Furthermore, it is important to highlight that some free nerve endings respond selectively to gentle warm or cool stimuli and, hence, are not considered as nociceptors (although the neural encoding and processing of these inputs appear to be largely similar to that of nociceptive input, i.e., thermonociception) [4, 29, 40]. Differential sensitivity to different stimulus modalities

TABLE 18-1 Innervation of the Skin by Nociceptive and Non-Nociceptive Sensory Afferents

Fibre Class	Receptor	Function	Location
Aβ	Merkel	SA1 (touch)	Dermal–epidermal junction
	Meissner	RA (brush)	Dermal–epidermal junction
	Ruffini	SA2 (stretch)	Dermis
	Pacini	PC (vibration)	Subcutis
Aδ	Free ending	Innocuous cold	Epidermis?
	Free ending	Polymodal nociceptors	Superficial epidermis
	Free ending	Mechano-nociceptors	Superficial epidermis
C	?	Dynamic light touch	–
	Free ending	Innocuous warm	Epidermis?
	Free ending	Nociceptors	Superficial epidermis

(electrical, mechanical, thermal) and differences in location of nerve terminals in different skin layers have been exploited for this purpose. Table 18-1 summarizes these properties of cutaneous afferents.

Several methods can be used to transiently activate nociceptors: direct electrical stimulation, punctate mechanical stimulation, and thermal stimulation.

Direct electrical stimulation. Transcutaneous electrical stimuli delivered over a peripheral nerve are easy to control, and activate peripheral afferents in a highly synchronous manner. However, the electrical activation threshold of large-diameter non-nociceptive Aδ afferents conveying vibrotactile sensations is lower than that of small-diameter nociceptive Aδ and C afferents [75], because of the large diameter and higher density of voltage-gated sodium channels of Aδ axons. Thus, when the intensity of electrical stimulation is sufficient to activate nociceptive afferents, coactivation of non-nociceptive somatosensory afferents is unavoidable. Because, as detailed in the section "Functional Significance," it is difficult to isolate ERPs elicited by the simultaneous activation of nociceptive and non-nociceptive afferents, transcutaneous electrical stimulation cannot be used to reliably study the brain responses elicited by nociceptive input.

Intraepidermal and epicutaneous electrical stimulation. It has been proposed that very focal electrical stimuli delivered to the epidermis (e.g., intraepidermal electrical stimulation using a very short-needle electrode or epicutaneous electrical stimulation using a punctate electrode applied against the skin surface) can be used to activate superficial epidermal free nerve endings without concomitantly activating non-nociceptive mechanoreceptors located more deeply in the skin [41], because current density declines rapidly with distance from the stimulating electrodes and tactile receptors are located deeper in the skin than nociceptors (Table 18-1). Converging evidence indicates that provided that low intensities of stimulation are used, intraepidermal electrical stimulation can selectively activate skin nociceptors [55]. However, the selectivity of this approach is greatly dependent on the intensity of the stimulus [44]. Thus, the elicited responses are usually of very small amplitude (because of the small number of activated afferents), and lose their selectivity as soon as the intensity is increased. Some authors have suggested improving the reliability of the elicited responses by increasing the strength of the stimulus-evoked afferent volley through temporal summation (by delivering short trains of stimuli instead of a single pulse) and/or spatial summation (by using multiple electrode contacts instead of a single contact) [38, 39].

Mechanical pinprick stimulation. Recently, it has been suggested that punctate mechanical stimulation could be used to elicit ERPs related to the preferential activation of mechanosensitive nociceptive afferents [32]. Although such stimuli may also activate low-threshold mechanoreceptors of the lemniscal pathway, low forces applied to small areas are relatively selective for superficial epidermal nerve endings, that is, mechanosensitive nociceptors [26]. The finding that the ERPs elicited by punctate mechanical stimulation were (a) increased during central sensitization and (b) reduced in a patient with a lesion disrupting the spinothalamic tract contralateral to the clinically affected skin site suggests that these responses predominantly reflect activity conveyed through nociceptive afferent pathways.

Thermal stimulation. It is currently considered as the most appropriate method to activate the thermonociceptive system selectively [63]. C-fibre nociceptors are more sensitive to heat than Aδ-fibre nociceptors, and Aβ-fibre mechanoreceptors do not respond to heat [4]. Heat stimuli can also activate low-threshold thermosensitive free nerve endings conveying innocuous warm sensations (i.e., warm fibres) [29]. Indeed, noxious heat stimuli activate a molecular transduction mechanism that is specific for heat-sensitive free nerve endings, involving heat-sensitive TRP channels [63]. Because some of these heat-sensitive channels are also expressed in keratinocytes, some authors have proposed that these cells could also contribute to the neural responses to heat [49]. Reliably recording time-locked responses such as ERPs requires the synchronous and reproducible activation of a population of heat-sensitive afferents, and this can be achieved only if the stimulus is able to bring the skin above thermal activation threshold within a very short time. This constitutes the main advantage of laser stimulators compared with other thermal stimulators such as contact heat thermodes and conventional sources of radiant heat [62]. Indeed, lasers can generate stimuli with very high power density and, hence, can achieve very steep skin heating ramps, crossing the thermal activation threshold of nociceptors in only a few milliseconds [27].

Although currently recognized as the most reliable method to elicit nociceptive ERPs [20], laser stimulation does have its limitations. First, long interstimulus intervals (ISIs) must separate two stimuli applied at the same location, to avoid skin overheating, nociceptor habituation, and/or sensitization, which is a limitation for all natural stimuli that activate nociceptors. The length of the ISI (usually between 3 and 30 seconds) depends on the wavelength of the laser source (shorter wavelength lasers require a longer ISI as they heat a larger volume of skin, and more time is needed for this irradiated volume to release heat and reach the baseline temperature [43]). Second, unless sophisticated feedback-controlled laser stimulators are used [13], baseline skin temperature has to be carefully monitored throughout the ERP recording, as the skin temperature following the delivery of a laser pulse of fixed energy is dependent on the baseline temperature. Hence, variations in baseline skin temperature will inevitably lead to variations in the strength of the nociceptive input.

Fast-rising contact heat stimulators have been proposed as an alternative [1]. Similarly to feedback-controlled laser stimulators, these devices solve the issue of baseline temperature, which is monitored through thermocouples embedded in the surface of the contact heat stimulator. However, the heating ramps achieved by contact heat stimulators remain far less steep than those achieved by laser stimulators, thereby reducing the synchronicity of the afferent input. Second, the increase of temperature can be monitored at the surface of the skin, but not at a depth where nociceptive free nerve endings are located. Third, heat transfer to the skin depends on the actual contact of the flat surface of the thermode and the surface of the skin.

Notably, it has been recently suggested that contact thermodes may be used to deliver transient cooling stimuli. Such stimuli could constitute an interesting alternative to study the neural responses elicited by the activation of free nerve endings responding to decreases in skin temperature [2, 4]. Using thermodes originally designed to deliver heat stimuli that were reprogrammed to deliver decreasing temperature ramps, it was demonstrated that evoked potentials can be elicited by small temperature steps of −1.5° to −5.0°C [2]. The stimuli elicit a vivid cooling sensation which is reliably detected by healthy subjects. When interpreting the functional significance of these responses, it is important to take into consideration the fact that this technique does not allow studying the function of cold *nociceptors* (many cold-sensitive nociceptors have thresholds as low as 0°C [69]), as the elicited responses are predominantly related to the activation of cool receptors responding to the dynamic innocuous cooling of the skin. Also, further work is needed to validate the technique of cool-evoked potentials.

Scalp Distribution and Latency

Brief laser pulses selectively excite Aδ and C-fibre free nerve endings located in the superficial layers of the skin [7], and elicit a number of brain responses that can be detected in the EEG and MEG, both in the time domain (e.g., laser-evoked potentials and magnetic fields; LEPs and LEFs) [25] and in the time–frequency domain (laser-induced oscillations) [28, 50, 64] (Fig. 18-1). LEPs comprise a number of waves that are time-locked to the onset of the stimulus.

The largest wave is a negative–positive complex (called N2–P2, peaking at 200–350 ms when stimulating the hand dorsum), maximal at the scalp vertex. This N2–P2 complex is preceded by a smaller negative wave (N1) that overlaps in time and space with the larger subsequent N2 wave, and has a maximal distribution over the temporal-central region contralateral to the stimulated hand (Fig. 18-2). Using source modelling, the N1 was initially proposed to derive from S1 [73]. Later, it was proposed to have predominant generator sources in S2 bilaterally [70, 71]. Activation of these regions at the latency of the N1 wave has been confirmed by subdural [3, 58, 83] and stereotactic [22, 23] EEG recordings in epilepsy surgery patients (Fig. 18-2). Recently, the contribution of S1 to the N1 wave has been reemphasized in a study showing that the N1 wave is clearly identified as a lateralized peak when stimulating the hand but not as clearly when stimulating the foot [70, 81]. This difference in scalp topography is explained by the fact that, in S1, the representation of the hand is more lateralized than the representation of the foot. Bilateral operculo-insular (S2 and the insula) activation is thought to predominantly contribute to the N2 wave, whereas the midcingulate cortex would contribute to both the N2 and the P2 waves [25]. Recently, it was suggested that the contralateral S1 also contributes to the very final part of the LEP response (i.e., the return to baseline following the P2 wave) [30].

Importantly, the latency of the N1, N2, and P2 waves is compatible with the conduction velocity of Aδ fibres, but not with the slower conduction velocity of unmyelinated C fibres. Furthermore, teased-fibre studies in monkeys have shown that brief laser stimuli activate only heat-sensitive afferents responding in a phasic manner to transient increases in skin temperature (type II A fibre mechano-heat nociceptors [AMH-II] [75]). Therefore, it is generally considered that LEPs reflect cortical activity exclusively related to the arrival of nociceptive input transmitted by peripheral AMH-II.

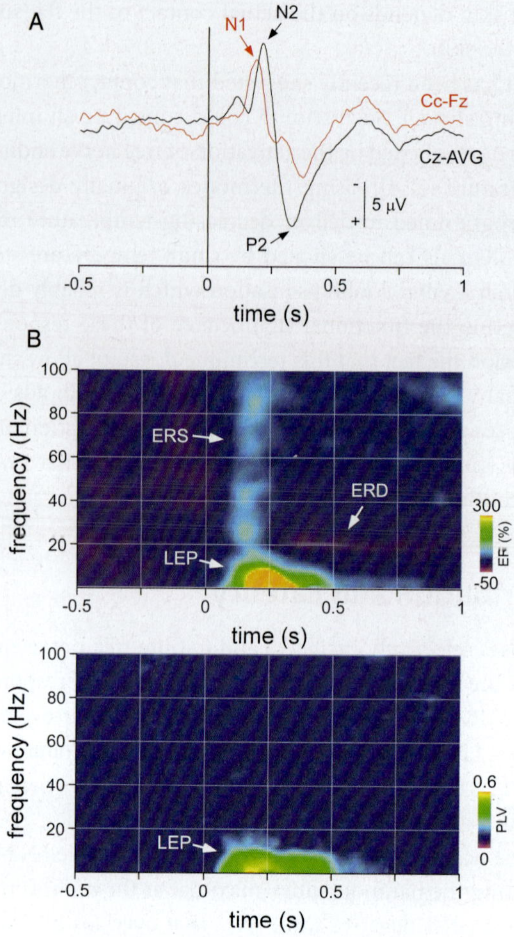

FIGURE 18-1 EEG responses elicited by a transient nociceptive stimulus.
A: Nociceptive event-related potentials (ERPs) elicited by a brief (40 ms) CO_2 laser stimulus delivered to the hand dorsum (group-level average of the ERP waveforms obtained in 17 healthy participants following 40 stimuli delivered to the left and right hand dorsum, respectively). The black waveform shows the laser-evoked potential (LEP) recorded from the scalp vertex (Cz, average reference). Note the large negative–positive complex consisting of a negative wave (N2) peaking 200–250 ms after stimulus onset, followed by a positive wave (P2) peaking 300–400 ms after stimulus onset. The red waveform shows the LEP recorded from the contralateral central electrode (left hand: C4; right hand: C3) referenced to the frontal electrode Fz. Note the earlier negative wave (N1) peaking approximately 150–200 ms after stimulus onset. **B:** Group-level average time–frequency representation of phase-locked and non-phase-locked EEG responses elicited by brief (4 ms) Nd:Yap laser stimuli delivered to the left and right hand dorsum (signals recorded from the central electrode C3/C4 contralateral to the stimulated hand; adapted from Zhang et al. [87]). The upper graph shows the average changes in oscillation amplitude as a function of time and frequency (increases and decreases relative to baseline are shown in yellow and purple, respectively). The lower graph shows the average phase-locking value (PLV) [42], a measure of phase-locking across trials (phase-locked and non-phase-locked responses appear in *yellow and red/blue*, respectively). Note that in addition to the phase-locked LEP, the stimulus also elicits a transient and early non-phase-locked enhancement of oscillations in the α, β, and γ bands (ERS, event-related synchronization). Also note that the stimulus induces a long-lasting reduction of power in the α band (ERD, event-related desynchronization).

Several methods have been proposed to activate heat-sensitive C-fibre afferents without concomitantly activating Aδ-fibre afferents (reviewed in [61]). Unlike the concomitant activation of Aδ and C fibres, the isolated activation of C fibres elicits an N2–P2 complex at latencies compatible with the conduction velocity of C fibres. The morphology and scalp topography of this "ultra-late" N2–P2 complex is highly similar to the morphology and scalp topography of the N2–P2 complex related to the activation of Aδ fibres [59, 60].

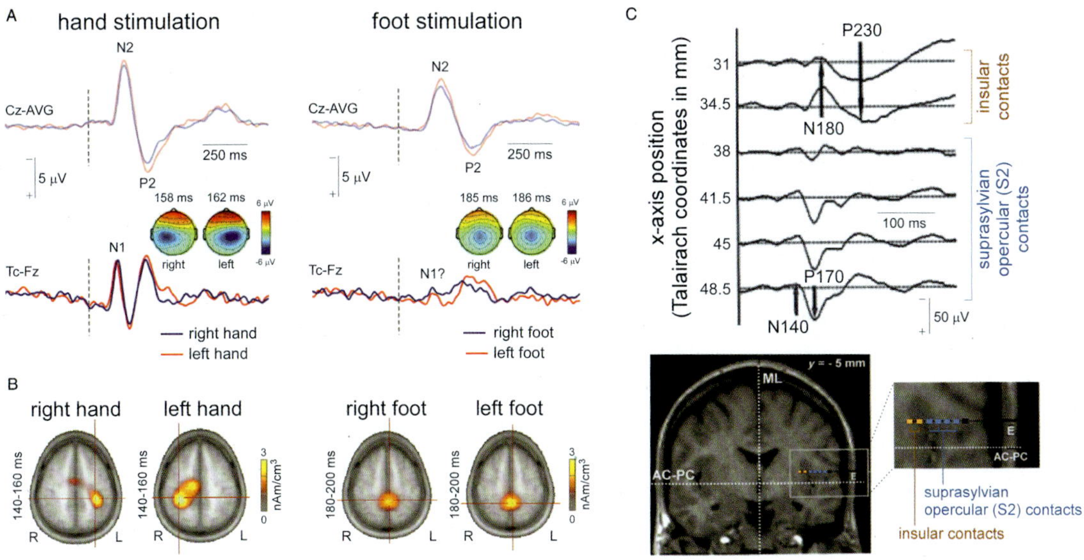

FIGURE 18-2 Scalp topography and possible sources of the N1 wave of laser-evoked brain potentials. **A:** The N1 wave is the earliest event-related potential (ERP) recorded following laser stimulation of the hand and foot dorsum. Following stimulation of the hand dorsum, the N1 wave appears as a clear negative peak maximal at the central and/or temporal electrode contralateral to the stimulated hand. In contrast, the N1 wave cannot always be detected following stimulation of the foot dorsum. The signals recorded following stimulation of the right and left sides are shown in blue and red (contralateral temporal electrode Tc referenced to the frontal electrode Fz). The signals recorded from the vertex (Cz) are shown in pale blue and red for comparison. **B:** Distributed source analysis of the early activity of laser-evoked potentials performed using CLARA. Note that the locations of the sources of the earliest part of the LEP waveform elicited by the stimulation of the hand and of the foot are compatible only with the corresponding hand and foot areas in the primary somatosensory cortex (S1). **C:** Stereotactic recording of laser-evoked potentials elicited by stimulation of the left hand dorsum using a depth electrode implanted in the right operculo-insular cortex of a patient undergoing a presurgical evaluation of intractable epilepsy. Note the early-latency response (N140–P170) recorded at electrode contacts in the secondary somatosensory cortex (S2), indicating that this brain structure could contribute to the N1 wave recorded from the scalp. Also note the later response (N180–P230) recorded at electrode contacts located in the insula, indicating that this brain structure could contribute to the later N2 wave. (Adapted from Frot and Mauguiere [24] and Valentini et al. [81].)

However, it is worth noting that the recording of C-fibre LEPs is not straightforward when stimuli are directed to body extremities (e.g., the hand dorsum and foot), possibly because variability in conduction velocity desynchronizes the C-fibre afferent volley when conduction distance is large. Indeed, C-fibre LEPs are more easily recorded when stimuli are delivered to proximal body territories such as the innervation territory of the trigeminal nerve [19], and the skin overlying the vertebral spinous processes [35].

Functional Significance

Typically, the ERPs elicited by a non-nociceptive somatosensory, auditory, or visual stimulus can be summarized as a succession of ERPs within which early-latency cortical components reflect low-level processing occurring in primary sensory cortices and late-latency components reflect higher order processing steps occurring in secondary sensory and multimodal cortical areas [66]. For example, the earliest cortical response to non-nociceptive transcutaneous electrical stimulation of the median nerve consists of a succession of early-latency ERPs (N20, P27, and P45) hypothesized to reflect cortical activity elicited in S1 contralateral to the stimulated hand. These early-latency components are followed by later components hypothesized to reflect higher order processing within other S1 subareas, secondary somatosensory and/or multimodal cortices. Early ERP components are often called "exogenous" because they are mostly influenced by the physical properties of the stimulus, whereas late ERP components are called "endogenous" because they are thought to primarily reflect stimulus-evoked cognitive processes such as the orientation of attention or target detection. Importantly, both "exogenous" and "endogenous" ERPs can be influenced by the cognitive state. For example, both can be modulated by the focus of selective attention, through a top-down effect on the responsiveness of the neuronal populations responding to the attended stimulus or stimulus feature.

Given that nociceptive ERPs are usually obtained by delivering only a small number of stimuli using a large ISI, an important question that must be addressed is whether the N1, N2, and P2 waves should be considered as early-latency nociceptive-specific "exogenous" responses, late multimodal "endogenous" responses, or a mixture of the two.

As discussed in the previous section, the N1 wave of LEPs is generated by overlapping activity in S1, S2, and parts of the insula. However, unlike the earliest components of non-nociceptive somatosensory ERPs, the amplitude of the N1 wave is significantly reduced by stimulation if repeated a small number of times [33, 67], and could even disappear when the stimulus is repeated a large number of times. These observations, combined with the fact that stimulus repetition does not similarly affect the sensation elicited by the stimulus [33], suggest that the N1 wave cannot be considered as a strictly "exogenous" component whose magnitude is determined solely by the physical properties of the stimulus (e.g., stimulus intensity). Lastly, blind source separation of nociceptive and non-nociceptive somatosensory ERPs failed to isolate a spatially distinguishable response to nociceptive stimulation [53], suggesting that the N1 wave may reflect either the activity of S1 nociceptive-specific neurons that are very close in space to S1 touch-specific neurons, or the activity of wide–dynamic range neurons responding to both nociceptive and non-nociceptive somatosensory inputs.

Several investigators have highlighted the similarity between the morphology and scalp topography of the N2 and P2 waves of nociceptive ERPs and that of the so-called vertex potentials, which can be elicited by any sensory stimulus provided that the stimuli are delivered using relatively large ISIs (reviewed in [34]) (Fig. 18-3). Comparing directly the scalp topographies of the ERPs elicited by nociceptive laser stimuli and non-nociceptive transcutaneous electrical stimuli, Treede et al. [73] found that the P2 wave of LEPs exhibited a more posterior scalp topography than the P2 wave elicited by electrical stimulation. This difference could suggest that LEPs and "vertex potentials" at least partly reflect distinct cortical processes. However, it could also be explained by differences in stimulus saliency leading to a stronger or weaker engagement of attentional processes such as those underlying the late cognitive P3 wave [45]. Using similarly salient laser, electrical, auditory, and visual stimuli combined with a joint blind source separation of the elicited ERPs, Mouraux et al. [53] found that the N2–P2 wave of LEPs could be explained entirely by multimodal neural activity also contributing to the "vertex potentials" elicited by non-nociceptive stimuli, possibly originating from anterior cingulate and/or bilateral operculo-insular regions.

Another important point to consider when interpreting the functional significance of nociceptive ERPs is the fact that their magnitude is strongly dependent on the context within which the eliciting stimulus is delivered. In other words, and unlike early-latency "exogenous" ERPs elicited by non-nociceptive somatosensory, auditory, or visual stimuli, the magnitude of nociceptive ERPs is not simply determined by the physical features of the eliciting stimulus, in particular, its intensity. A large number of studies have shown that the magnitude of nociceptive ERPs often correlates extremely well with the energy of the

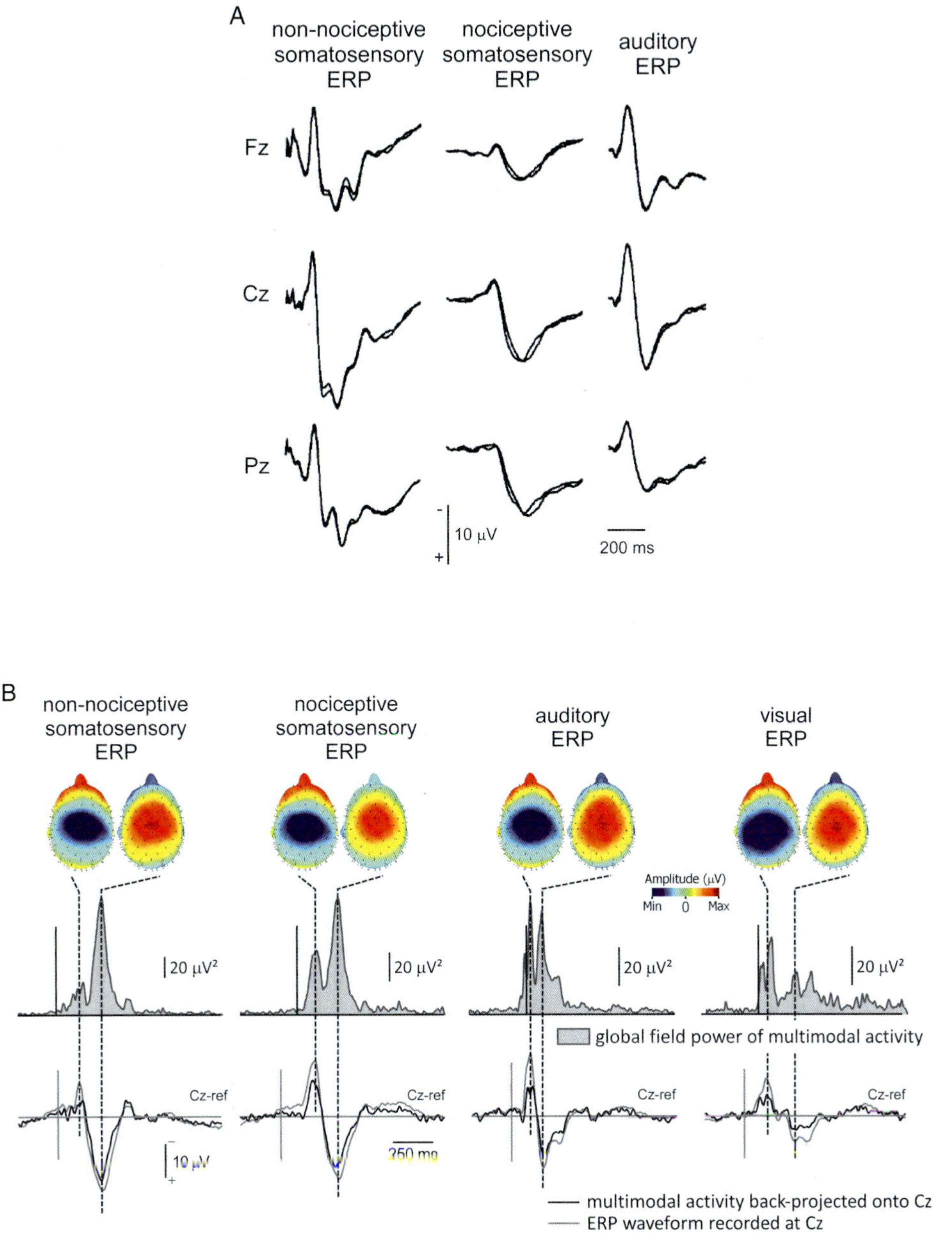

FIGURE 18-3 Comparison of nociceptive somatosensory ERPs and late components of non-nociceptive sensory ERPs. A: Non-nociceptive somatosensory (electrical stimulation of the median nerve), nociceptive (laser stimulation of the hand dorsum), and auditory (brief tone) ERPs recorded at frontal, central, and parietal electrodes Fz, Cz, and Pz (group-level average of 24 subjects; 80 stimulus repetitions). Note the similarity of the negative–positive complex elicited by nociceptive stimulation and the late negative–positive complex elicited by non-nociceptive somatosensory and auditory stimulation. Also note the more posterior scalp topography of the positive wave elicited by nociceptive stimulation. (Adapted from Treede et al. [73].) **B:** Blind source separation of nociceptive (laser stimulation of the hand dorsum), non-nociceptive somatosensory (electrical stimulation of the superficial radial nerve), auditory (brief tone), and visual (brief flash) ERPs performed using a Probabilistic Independent Component Analysis. The middle graphs show the time course of independent components contributing to all four ERP waveforms and probably reflecting multimodal activity. The lower graphs show the respective contribution of this multimodal activity to the ERP waveforms recorded at electrode Cz. Note that most of the nociceptive ERP and most of the late components of non-nociceptive ERPs can be explained by this source of multimodal activity. The upper graphs show the scalp maps of the negative and positive peaks of this activity. (Adapted from Mouraux and Iannetti [53].)

applied stimulus [51, 57]. Some studies have shown an even stronger relationship with the perceived intensity of pain [5, 10, 36, 72], to an extent allowing accurate predictions of perceived pain intensity [31]. However, several studies have shown that, in several circumstances, this relationship can be clearly disrupted [12, 14, 21, 33]. These exceptions are important as they show that the correlation between magnitude of the nociceptive ERP and pain is not obligatory. For example, when a nociceptive stimulus is repeated at a short and constant ISI (e.g., a constant 1-second ISI), it elicits an ERP of smaller magnitude, while the intensity of perceived pain is entirely unaltered [33] (see also Fig. 16-2). This effect of stimulus repetition is largely determined by the duration of the ISI: the shorter the interval, the more pronounced the response decrement [8, 65, 78]. Previous studies have convincingly shown that such effects of stimulus repetition on the magnitude of nociceptive ERPs cannot be explained by refractoriness of the afferent neural pathways or of the underlying cortical generators. Indeed, stimulus repetition affects the magnitude of nociceptive ERPs if the ISI remains constant from trial to trial, but it does not if the ISI is varied randomly from trial to trial [52] (Fig. 18-4). In other words, the effect of stimulus repetition appears to be strongly conditioned by the *context* within which the repetition occurs.

Importantly, many studies have shown that the magnitude of the "vertex potentials" elicited by non-nociceptive somatosensory, auditory, and visual stimuli is strongly reduced when stimuli are repeated using a constant ISI, but not when they are repeated using a varying ISI [9, 48, 84]. This further suggests that nociceptive N2–P2 and "vertex potentials" reflect similar brain processes, which are largely independent of the activated sensory channel and strongly dependent on the context in which the stimuli are presented.

Taken together, these findings indicate that the magnitude of nociceptive ERPs is strongly determined by the saliency of the eliciting stimulus and, hence, that these responses are very indirectly related to the intensity of the stimulus and/or of the elicited pain percept. Furthermore, this suggests that nociceptive ERPs may predominantly reflect the activity of a multimodal cortical network involved in the detection and reaction to salient sensory input, regardless of the sensory channel through which that input is conveyed. This interpretation is fully consistent with the data from dipole source analyses and direct intracranial recordings showing that the anterior midcingulate cortex contributes strongly to the N2–P2, as this region is thought to be strongly involved in orienting responses.

NOCICEPTIVE γ-BAND OSCILLATIONS AND STEADY-STATE EVOKED POTENTIALS

Nociceptive laser pulses also elicit non-phase-locked EEG responses [50, 58, 64, 87]. These can be summarized as (a) a short-lasting enhancement of signal power at frequencies around 10 Hz, starting approximately 160 ms after stimulus onset when stimulating the hand dorsum, followed by (b) a long-lasting reduction of signal power within the same frequency band, starting approximately 500 ms after stimulus onset. These responses are maximally observed at the scalp vertex. However, the neural generators and the functional significance of these two non-phase-locked responses remain largely unknown. More recently, it has been described that nociceptive laser pulses also elicit a short-lasting enhancement of γ-band oscillation (GBO, 40–100 Hz), which predominates over the central region contralateral to the stimulated hand, suggesting that it is generated in the contralateral S1 [28]. In striking contrast to nociceptive ERPs detected in the time domain, it was recently

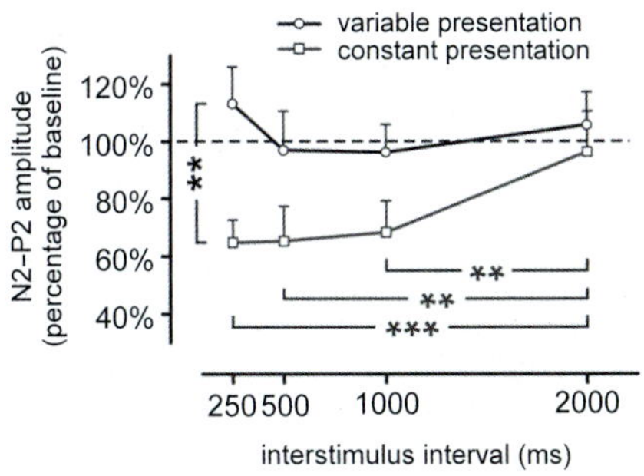

FIGURE 18-4 Effect of stimulus repetition on the magnitude of nociceptive ERPs using constant or variable presentation rates. Brief pairs of laser stimuli were delivered to the hand dorsum using an ISI ranging from 250 to 2000 ms. In the constant presentation condition, the ISI was identical across all trials of each block. In the variable presentation condition, the ISI was varied randomly across trials. Therefore, the time of occurrence of the second stimulus was both less novel and more predictable in the variable condition compared with the constant condition. Note that in the constant condition, stimulus repetition induced a marked reduction of the magnitude of the N2–P2 wave. In contrast, there was no habituation of the nociceptive ERP in the variable condition. (Adapted from Wang et al. [85].)
Note: ** $P<.01$; *** $P<.001$

shown that these GBOs correlate with the intensity of pain perception regardless of stimulus repetition, thus suggesting that this EEG response could reflect cortical activity more directly related to pain perception [87]. Therefore, GBOs elicited by nociceptive stimuli could constitute a unique means to study the cortical activity related to the perception of pain in humans. Further data are required to determine whether these responses can be assessed reliably at single-subject level, to confirm that they truly originate from S1 (some studies have suggested that they could also originate from the primary motor cortex, M1 [68]), and to characterize the temporal relationship between these responses and perception.

When repeated periodically, a sensory stimulus can elicit a sustained EEG response, referred to as a steady-state evoked potential (SS-EP) [82]. SS-EPs are fundamentally different from ERPs elicited by isolated transient sensory stimuli, because they result from the entrainment at the frequency of stimulation of a population of neurons responding to the periodically applied stimulus. This approach is interesting, as it could be used as a means to study the cortical activity related to the processing of sustained nociceptive input in humans, reducing the confound of novelty-related neural activities that are known to contribute largely to nociceptive ERPs (reviewed in [15]).

The recording of nociceptive SS-EPs is technically challenging because of the need to deliver nociceptive stimuli in very rapid succession (e.g., 7 Hz or above). Nevertheless, it was recently shown that nociceptive SS-EPs can be recorded using both laser stimulation (trains of laser stimuli delivered at a 7-Hz repetition rate [54]) and intraepidermal electrical stimulation (10-second trains of electrical stimuli delivered using a range of frequencies between 7 and 43 Hz [16]). Direct comparison of these nociceptive SS-EPs with the SS-EPs elicited by non-nociceptive somatosensory stimulation (transcutaneous radial nerve stimulation; mechanical vibrotactile stimulation) showed that nociceptive and non-nociceptive somatosensory SS-EPs exhibit remarkably different scalp distributions, indicating that they reflect the entrainment of distinct neuronal populations (Fig. 18-5). Furthermore, nociceptive SS-EPs reflect cortical activity that is sustained during the whole stimulation period, indicating that, unlike nociceptive ERPs, they reflect cortical processes that do not habituate over time.

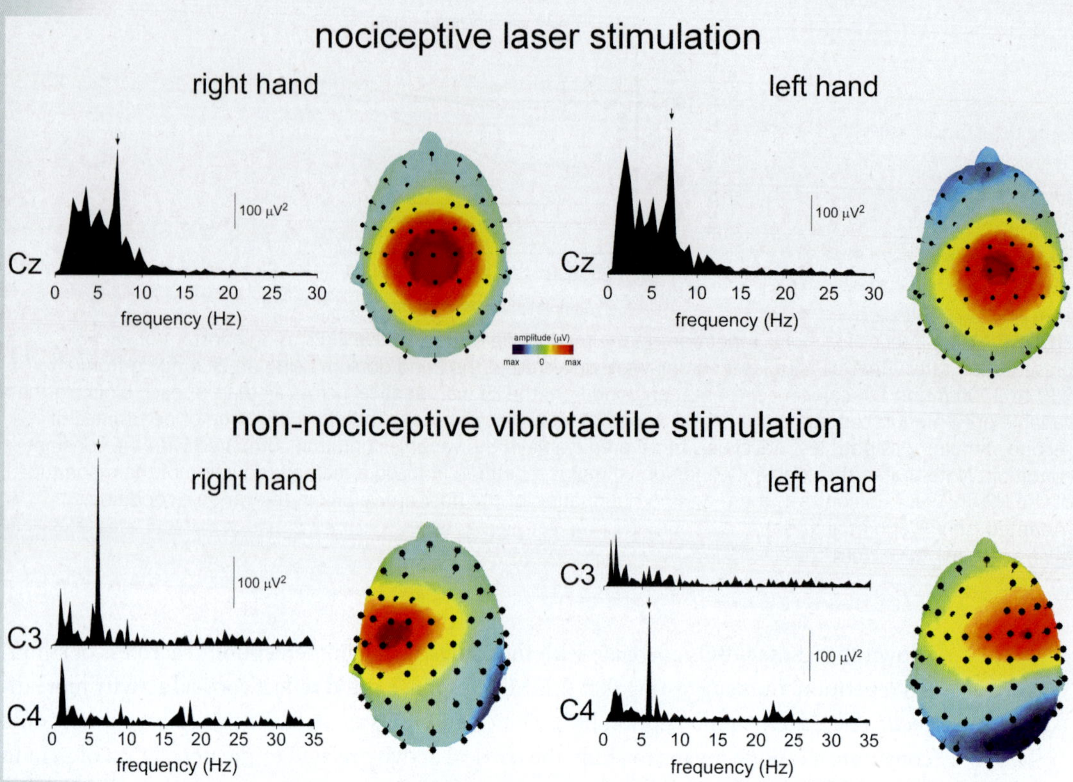

FIGURE 18-5 Nociceptive and non-nociceptive steady-state evoked potentials (SS-EPs). Nociceptive SS-EPs were elicited using 2.3-second trains of CO_2 laser stimuli delivered to the left- and right-hand dorsum at a frequency of 7 Hz. To avoid skin overheating, the target of the stimulus was displaced between each stimulus of the train using a computer-controlled mirror. Note the significant peak of EEG power at 7 Hz, corresponding to the stimulation frequency. Also note the symmetrical scalp topography of the elicited SS-EPs, maximal at the scalp vertex. Non-nociceptive somatosensory SS-EPs were elicited using 3-second trains of transcutaneous electrical stimuli delivered to the left and right superficial radial nerves at a modulation frequency of 6 Hz. Note the significant peak of EEG power at 6 Hz, visible on the central electrode contralateral to the stimulated hand (C3/C4). Also note the clearly lateralized scalp topography of the elicited SS-EPs, maximal over the parietal region contralateral to the stimulated hand. (Adapted from Mouraux et al. [54].)

CLINICAL USEFULNESS OF NOCICEPTIVE ERPs

LEPs have been demonstrated to be related to the activation of AMH-II [74, 75, 79]. Because of this specificity, LEPs are useful to document dysfunctions of small-fibre primary sensory afferents, the spinothalamic tract, brainstem, and thalamocortical projections conveying thermonociceptive signals to the brain. Their clinical usefulness is increased by the ability of laser pulses to elicit cortical responses when applied to virtually all skin territories, including the glabrous skin [37, 77]. For these reasons, LEPs have been recommended as the easiest and most reliable neurophysiological method to assess the function of nociceptive pathways and diagnose clinical pain of neuropathic origin [18, 20]. Indeed, even if LEPs reflect cortical activities that are not entirely specific for the nociceptive system, their generation still relies on the functional state of the nociceptive system, at both peripheral and central levels.

REFERENCES

1. Arendt-Nielsen L, Chen ACN. Lasers and other thermal stimulators for activation of skin nociceptors in humans. Neurophysiol Clin 2003;33(6):259–68.
2. Baumgärtner U, Greffrath W, Treede RD. Contact heat and cold, mechanical, electrical and chemical stimuli to elicit small fiber-evoked potentials: merits and limitations for basic science and clinical use. Neurophysiol Clin 2012;42(5):267–80.
3. Baumgärtner U, Vogel H, Ohara S, Treede RD, Lenz F. Dipole source analyses of laser evoked potentials obtained from subdural grid recordings from primary somatic sensory cortex. J Neurophysiol 2011;106(2):722–30.
4. Belmonte C, Viana F. Molecular and cellular limits to somatosensory specificity. Mol Pain 2008;4:14.
5. Beydoun A, Morrow TJ, Shen JF, Casey KL. Variability of laser-evoked potentials: attention, arousal and lateralized differences. Electroencephalogr Clin Neurophysiol 1993;88(3):173–81.
6. Bromm B, Jahnke MT, Treede RD. Responses of human cutaneous afferents to CO_2 laser stimuli causing pain. Exp Brain Res 1984;55(1):158–66.
7. Bromm B, Treede RD. Nerve fibre discharges, cerebral potentials and sensations induced by CO_2 laser stimulation. Hum Neurobiol 1984;3(1):33–40.
8. Bromm B, Treede RD. Human cerebral potentials evoked by CO_2 laser stimuli causing pain. Exp Brain Res 1987;67(1):153–62.
9. Budd TW, Michie PT. Facilitation of the N1 peak of the auditory ERP at short stimulus intervals. Neuroreport 1994;5(18):2513–6.
10. Carmon A, Dotan Y, Sarne Y. Correlation of subjective pain experience with cerebral evoked responses to noxious thermal stimulations. Exp Brain Res 1978;33(3–4):445–53.
11. Carmon A, Mor J, Goldberg J. Evoked cerebral responses to noxious thermal stimuli in humans. Exp Brain Res 1976;25(1):103–7.
12. Chapman CR, Chen AC, Colpitts YM, Martin RW. Sensory decision theory describes evoked potentials in pain discrimination. Psychophysiology 1981;18(2):114–20.
13. Churyukanov M, Plaghki L, Legrain V, Mouraux A. Thermal detection thresholds of Aδ- and C-fibre afferents activated by brief CO_2 laser pulses applied onto the human hairy skin. PloS one 2012;7(4):e35817.
14. Clark JA, Brown CA, Jones AK, El-Deredy W. Dissociating nociceptive modulation by the duration of pain anticipation from unpredictability in the timing of pain. Clin Neurophysiol 2008;119(12):2870–8.
15. Colon E, Legrain V, Mouraux A. Steady-state evoked potentials to study the processing of tactile and nociceptive somatosensory input in the human brain. Neurophysiol Clin 2012;42(5):315–23.
16. Colon E, Nozaradan S, Legrain V, Mouraux A. Steady-state evoked potentials to tag specific components of nociceptive cortical processing. NeuroImage 2012;60(1):571–81.
17. Cruccu G, Aminoff MJ, Curio G, Guerit JM, Kakigi R, Mauguiere F, Rossini PM, Treede RD, Garcia-Larrea L. Recommendations for the clinical use of somatosensory-evoked potentials. Clin Neurophysiol 2008;119(8):1705–19.
18. Cruccu G, Anand P, Attal N, Garcia-Larrea L, Haanpaa M, Jorum E, Serra J, Jensen TS. EFNS guidelines on neuropathic pain assessment. Eur J Neurol 2004;11(3):153–62.
19. Cruccu G, Pennisi E, Truini A, Iannetti GD, Romaniello A, Le Pera D, De Armas L, Leandri M, Manfredi M, Valeriani M. Unmyelinated trigeminal pathways as assessed by laser stimuli in humans. Brain 2003; 126(Pt 10):2246–56.
20. Cruccu G, Sommer C, Anand P, Attal N, Baron R, Garcia-Larrea L, Haanpaa M, Jensen TS, Serra J, Treede RD. EFNS guidelines on neuropathic pain assessment: revised 2009. Eur J Neurol 2010;17(8):1010–18.
21. Dillmann J, Miltner WH, Weiss T. The influence of semantic priming on event-related potentials to painful laser-heat stimuli in humans. Neurosci Lett 2000;284(1–2):53–6.
22. Frot M, Garcia-Larrea L, Guenot M, Mauguiere F. Responses of the supra-sylvian (SII) cortex in humans to painful and innocuous stimuli: a study using intra-cerebral recordings. Pain 2001;94(1):65–73.
23. Frot M, Mauguiere F. Timing and spatial distribution of somatosensory responses recorded in the upper bank of the sylvian fissure (SII area) in humans. Cereb Cortex 1999;9(8):854–63.
24. Frot M, Mauguiere F. Dual representation of pain in the operculo-insular cortex in humans. Brain 2003; 126(Pt 2):438–50.
25. Garcia-Larrea L, Frot M, Valeriani M. Brain generators of laser-evoked potentials: from dipoles to functional significance. Neurophysiol Clin 2003;33(6):279–92.
26. Garnsworthy RK, Gully RL, Kenins P, Mayfield RJ, Westerman RA. Identification of the physical stimulus and the neural basis of fabric-evoked prickle. J Neurophysiol 1988;59(4):1083–97.

27. Greffrath W, Nemenov MI, Schwarz S, Baumgärtner U, Vogel H, Arendt-Nielsen L, Treede RD. Inward currents in primary nociceptive neurons of the rat and pain sensations in humans elicited by infrared diode laser pulses. Pain 2002;99(1–2):145–55.
28. Gross J, Schnitzler A, Timmermann L, Ploner M. Gamma oscillations in human primary somatosensory cortex reflect pain perception. PLoS Biol 2007;5(5):e133.
29. Hallin RG, Torebjork HE, Wiesenfeld Z. Nociceptors and warm receptors innervated by C fibres in human skin. J Neurol Neurosurg Psychiatry 1982;45(4):313–9.
30. Hu L, Valentini E, Zhang ZG, Liang M, Iannetti GD. The primary somatosensory cortex contributes to the latest part of the cortical response elicited by nociceptive somatosensory stimuli in humans. Neuroimage 2014;84:383–93.
31. Huang G, Xiao P, Hung YS, Iannetti GD, Zhang ZG, Hu L. A novel approach to predict subjective pain perception from single-trial laser-evoked potentials. Neuroimage 2013;81:283–93.
32. Iannetti GD, Baumgärtner U, Tracey I, Treede RD, Magerl W. Pinprick-evoked brain potentials: a novel tool to assess central sensitization of nociceptive pathways in humans. J Neurophysiol 2013;110(5):1107–16.
33. Iannetti GD, Hughes NP, Lee MC, Mouraux A. Determinants of laser-evoked EEG responses: pain perception or stimulus saliency? J Neurophysiol 2008;100(2):815–28.
34. Iannetti GD, Mouraux A. From the neuromatrix to the pain matrix (and back). Exp Brain Res 2010;205(1): 1–12.
35. Iannetti GD, Truini A, Romaniello A, Galeotti F, Rizzo C, Manfredi M, Cruccu G. Evidence of a specific spinal pathway for the sense of warmth in humans. J Neurophysiol 2003;89(1):562–70.
36. Iannetti GD, Zambreanu L, Cruccu G, Tracey I. Operculoinsular cortex encodes pain intensity at the earliest stages of cortical processing as indicated by amplitude of laser-evoked potentials in humans. Neuroscience 2005;131(1):199–208.
37. Iannetti GD, Zambreanu L, Tracey I. Similar nociceptive afferents mediate psychophysical and electrophysiological responses to heat stimulation of glabrous and hairy skin in humans. J Physiol 2006;577(Pt 1):235–48.
38. Inui K, Tsuji T, Kakigi R. Temporal analysis of cortical mechanisms for pain relief by tactile stimuli in humans. Cereb Cortex 2006;16(3):355–65.
39. Inui K, Wang X, Qiu Y, Tsuji T, Nakata H, Kakigi R. Cortical processing of noxious information in humans: a magnetoencephalographic study. Suppl Clin Neurophysiol 2006;59:127–33.
40. Jankovski A, Plaghki L, Mouraux A. Reliable EEG responses to the selective activation of C-fibre afferents using a temperature-controlled infrared laser stimulator in conjunction with an adaptive staircase algorithm. Pain 2013;154(9):1578–87.
41. Klein T, Magerl W, Hopf HC, Sandkuhler J, Treede RD. Perceptual correlates of nociceptive long-term potentiation and long-term depression in humans. J Neurosci 2004;24(4):964–71.
42. Lachaux JP, Rodriguez E, Martinerie J, Varela FJ. Measuring phase synchrony in brain signals. Hum Brain Mapp 1999;8(4):194–208.
43. Leandri M, Saturno M, Spadavecchia L, Iannetti GD, Cruccu G, Truini A. Measurement of skin temperature after infrared laser stimulation. Neurophysiol Clin 2006;36(4):207–18.
44. Legrain V, Mouraux A. Activating selectively and reliably nociceptive afferents with concentric electrode stimulation: yes we can! Provided that low stimulus intensities are used! Clin Neurophysiol 2013;124(2):424.
45. Linden DE. The p300: where in the brain is it produced and what does it tell us? Neuroscientist 2005;11(6): 563–76.
46. Loeser JD, Treede RD. The Kyoto protocol of IASP basic pain terminology. Pain 2008;137(3):473–7.
47. Logothetis NK, Pauls J, Augath M, Trinath T, Oeltermann A. Neurophysiological investigation of the basis of the fMRI signal. Nature 2001;412(6843):150–7.
48. Loveless N, Hari R, Hamalainen M, Tiihonen J. Evoked responses of human auditory cortex may be enhanced by preceding stimuli. Electroencephalogr Clin Neurophysiol 1989;74(3):217–27.
49. Lumpkin EA, Caterina MJ. Mechanisms of sensory transduction in the skin. Nature 2007;445(7130):858–65.
50. Mouraux A, Guerit JM, Plaghki L. Non-phase locked electroencephalogram (EEG) responses to CO_2 laser skin stimulations may reflect central interactions between A partial partial differential- and C-fibre afferent volleys. Clin Neurophysiol 2003;114(4):710–22.
51. Mouraux A, Guerit JM, Plaghki L. Non-phase locked electroencephalogram (EEG) responses to CO_2 laser skin stimulations may reflect central interactions between Aδ- and C-fibre afferent volleys. Clin Neurophysiol 2003;114(4):710–22.
52. Mouraux A, Guerit JM, Plaghki L. Refractoriness cannot explain why C-fiber laser-evoked brain potentials are recorded only if concomitant Aδ-fiber activation is avoided. Pain 2004;112(1–2):16–26.

53. Mouraux A, Iannetti GD. Nociceptive laser-evoked brain potentials do not reflect nociceptive-specific neural activity. J Neurophysiol 2009;101(6):3258–69.
54. Mouraux A, Iannetti GD, Colon E, Nozaradan S, Legrain V, Plaghki L. Nociceptive steady-state evoked potentials elicited by rapid periodic thermal stimulation of cutaneous nociceptors. J Neurosci 2011;31(16):6079–87.
55. Mouraux A, Iannetti GD, Plaghki L. Low intensity intra-epidermal electrical stimulation can activate Aδ-nociceptors selectively. Pain 2010;150(1):199–207.
56. Nunez PL, Srinivasan R. Electric fields of the brain: the neurophysics of EEG. New York, NY: Oxford University Press; 2006.
57. Ohara S, Crone NE, Weiss N, Treede RD, Lenz FA. Amplitudes of laser evoked potential recorded from primary somatosensory, parasylvian and medial frontal cortex are graded with stimulus intensity. Pain 2004;110 (1–2):318–28.
58. Ohara S, Crone NE, Weiss N, Treede RD, Lenz FA. Cutaneous painful laser stimuli evoke responses recorded directly from primary somatosensory cortex in awake humans. J Neurophysiol 2004;91(6):2734–46.
59. Opsommer E, Weiss T, Miltner WH, Plaghki L. Scalp topography of ultralate (C-fibres) evoked potentials following thulium YAG laser stimuli to tiny skin surface areas in humans. Clin Neurophysiol 2001;112(10): 1868–74.
60. Opsommer E, Weiss T, Plaghki L, Miltner WH. Dipole analysis of ultralate (C-fibres) evoked potentials after laser stimulation of tiny cutaneous surface areas in humans. Neurosci Lett 2001;298(1):41–4.
61. Plaghki L, Mouraux A. Brain responses to signals ascending through C-fibers. In: Hirata K, editor. International congress series, Vol. 1232. Amsterdam, The Netherlands: Elsevier; 2002. pp. 181–92.
62. Plaghki L, Mouraux A. How do we selectively activate skin nociceptors with a high power infrared laser? Physiology and biophysics of laser stimulation. Neurophysiol Clin 2003;33(6):269–77.
63. Plaghki L, Mouraux A. EEG and laser stimulation as tools for pain research. Curr Opin Investig Drugs 2005;6(1):58–64.
64. Ploner M, Gross J, Timmermann L, Pollok B, Schnitzler A. Pain suppresses spontaneous brain rhythms. Cerebral cortex 2006;16(4):537–40.
65. Raij TT, Vartiainen NV, Jousmaki V, Hari R. Effects of interstimulus interval on cortical responses to painful laser stimulation. J Clin Neurophysiol 2003;20(1):73–9.
66. Regan D. Human brain electrophysiology: evoked potentials and evoked magnetic fields in science and medicine. New York, NY: Elsevier; 1989.
67. Ronga I, Valentini E, Mouraux A, Iannetti GD. Novelty is not enough: laser-evoked potentials are determined by stimulus saliency, not absolute novelty. J Neurophysiol 2013;109(3):692–701.
68. Schulz E, Tiemann L, Witkovsky V, Schmidt P, Ploner M. Gamma oscillations are involved in the sensorimotor transformation of pain. J Neurophysiol 2012;108(4):1025–31.
69. Simone DA, Kajander KC. Excitation of rat cutaneous nociceptors by noxious cold. Neurosci Lett 1996;213(1):53–6.
70. Spiegel J, Hansen C, Treede RD. Laser-evoked potentials after painful hand and foot stimulation in humans: evidence for generation of the middle-latency component in the secondary somatosensory cortex. Neurosci Lett 1996;216(3):179–82.
71. Tarkka IM, Treede RD. Equivalent electrical source analysis of pain-related somatosensory evoked potentials elicited by a CO_2 laser. J Clin Neurophysiol 1993;10(4):513–9.
72. Timmermann L, Ploner M, Haucke K, Schmitz F, Baltissen R, Schnitzler A. Differential coding of pain intensity in the human primary and secondary somatosensory cortex. J Neurophysiol 2001;86(3):1499–503.
73. Treede RD, Kief S, Holzer T, Bromm B. Late somatosensory evoked cerebral potentials in response to cutaneous heat stimuli. Electroencephalogr Clin Neurophysiol 1988;70(5):429–41.
74. Treede RD, Lankers J, Frieling A, Zangemeister WH, Kunze K, Bromm B. Cerebral potentials evoked by painful, laser stimuli in patients with syringomyelia. Brain 1991;114 (Pt 4):1595–607.
75. Treede RD, Meyer RA, Campbell JN. Myelinated mechanically insensitive afferents from monkey hairy skin: heat-response properties. J Neurophysiol 1998;80(3):1082–93.
76. Truini A, Galeotti F, Romaniello A, Virtuoso M, Iannetti GD, Cruccu G. Laser-evoked potentials: normative values. Clini Neurophysiol 2005;116(4):821–6.
77. Truini A, Haanpaa M, Zucchi R, Galeotti F, Iannetti GD, Romaniello A, Cruccu G. Laser-evoked potentials in post-herpetic neuralgia. Clin Neurophysiol 2003;114(4):702–9.
78. Truini A, Rossi P, Galeotti F, Romaniello A, Virtuoso M, De Lena C, Leandri M, Cruccu G. Excitability of the Adelta nociceptive pathways as assessed by the recovery cycle of laser evoked potentials in humans. Exp Brain Res 2004;155(1):120–3.

79. Tsuji T, Inui K, Kojima S, Kakigi R. Multiple pathways for noxious information in the human spinal cord. Pain 2006;123(3):322–31.
80. Untergehrer G, Jordan D, Eyl S, Schneider G. Effects of propofol, sevoflurane, remifentanil, and (S)-ketamine in subanesthetic concentrations on visceral and somatosensory pain-evoked potentials. Anesthesiology 2013;118(2):308–17.
81. Valentini E, Hu L, Chakrabarti B, Hu Y, Aglioti SM, Iannetti GD. The primary somatosensory cortex largely contributes to the early part of the cortical response elicited by nociceptive stimuli. NeuroImage 2012;59(2):1571–81.
82. Vialatte FB, Maurice M, Dauwels J, Cichocki A. Steady-state visually evoked potentials: focus on essential paradigms and future perspectives. Prog Neurobiol 2010;90(4):418–38.
83. Vogel H, Port JD, Lenz FA, Solaiyappan M, Krauss G, Treede RD. Dipole source analysis of laser-evoked subdural potentials recorded from parasylvian cortex in humans. J Neurophysiol 2003;89(6):3051–60.
84. Wang AL, Mouraux A, Liang M, Iannetti GD. The enhancement of the N1 wave elicited by sensory stimuli presented at very short inter-stimulus intervals is a general feature across sensory systems. PloS One 2008;3(12):e3929.
85. Wang AL, Mouraux A, Liang M, Iannetti GD. Stimulus novelty, and not neural refractoriness, explains the repetition suppression of laser-evoked potentials. J Neurophysiol 2010;104(4):2116–24.
86. Zaslansky R, Sprecher E, Katz Y, Rozenberg B, Hemli JA, Yarnitsky D. Pain-evoked potentials: what do they really measure? Electroencephalogr Clin Neurophysiol 1996;100(5):384–91.
87. Zhang ZG, Hu L, Hung YS, Mouraux A, Iannetti GD. Gamma-band oscillations in the primary somatosensory cortex—a direct and obligatory correlate of subjective pain intensity J Neurosci 2012;32(22):7429–38.

CHAPTER 19

Placebo and Activity in the Central Nervous System

Christian Sprenger, Tor D. Wager, and Christian Büchel

The perception of pain is a complex multidimensional event, and is sensitive to various mental processes such as feelings, expectancies, and beliefs. It is therefore not a simple reflection of nociceptive activity, but rather the complex interplay of pro- and antinociceptive mechanisms in the human organism. Placebo analgesia represents one of the best studied examples of endogenous pain modulation. Although it was once considered as a kind of "response bias," placebo effects are now recognized as a class of genuine psychobiological effects in which pain reduction occurs after application of medication without an active agent, after sham procedures, or through symbols associated with treatment. Because, by definition, the observed pain reduction does not arise from the intervention, placebo effects are seen as effects of the higher level representation of the therapeutic procedure such as the meaning of a therapeutic measure to the patient and expectations regarding the therapeutic outcome. Consequently, it has been suggested that the term "placebo effect" be replaced by "meaning response" [41].

There is now extensive evidence from numerous clinical and experimental studies that placebo analgesia represents a real psychobiological phenomenon, and multiple meta-analyses have affirmed their effects on pain reports [30, 55] and brain systems involved in the processing of nociceptive input and the construction of pain [4, 38, 59]. However, it is important to strictly separate placebo effects from improvements in the placebo arm of a randomized clinical trial, because the latter might occur due to a variety of other mechanisms such as spontaneous improvement, natural symptom fluctuations, or regression to the mean. Experimental studies that compare a placebo with a no-placebo control treatment (which might differ only in instructions to participants or other contextual variables) are appropriate for isolating the effects of the treatment context itself.

Two psychological factors are frequently considered as key mediators in placebo analgesia: expectation and experience (i.e., learning processes), although additional factors such as a reduction of negative emotions might play a role [22]. On the basis of positive instructions related to treatment (e.g., drug) or certain contextual cues, the expectation of the patient regarding the therapeutic outcome might be manipulated, and this might lead to the occurrence of placebo effects [3, 7, 42]. However, many placebo effects can also be explained within the concept of classical conditioning. According to classical conditioning, the repeated association of a neutral stimulus (e.g., the colour or shape of a tablet) with the pharmacological action of the drug (pain relief, unconditioned response) leads to a conditioned response even if the active agent is subsequently removed and only the conditioned stimulus is presented [56, 57, 62]. Early theory [62] and more recent data [13] suggest that placebo responses are stronger when reinforced with conditioning procedures. However, the weight of evidence suggests that many forms of "conditioned" responses, including conditioned placebo responses, work mainly by affecting expectancies [32, 51].

In this respect, it is interesting to note that the concept of conditioned analgesia is related to the conditioning aspect of placebo analgesia. It has been shown in rodents [18] and humans [14] that conditioned analgesia is mediated by the release of endogenous opioids. Furthermore, the rostral anterior cingulate cortex (rACC) and the amygdala play a role in both placebo analgesia [11, 15, 44] and conditioned analgesia [14].

OPIOIDS

In 1978, Levine et al. [36] made the groundbreaking observation that the opioid antagonist naloxone can reduce the placebo analgesic effect in postoperative pain. As a consequence, the endogenous opioid system has attracted a high level of attention, and it became clear that this system is an integral component of the descending antinociceptive system, which plays a crucial role in pain modulation [1, 5, 20]. Since the initial observation by Levine et al. [36], several studies were able to replicate the observation that placebo analgesia is significantly reduced after the administration of the opioid antagonist naloxone [3, 6, 15]. In addition, more recent studies showed that placebo treatment (compared with control conditions identical except the instructions to participants) increases μ-opioid activity in the opioid-rich periaqueductal grey (PAG) [48, 61], medial prefrontal cortex, and other structures.

DOPAMINE

However, the endogenous opioid system appears not to be the only neurotransmitter system involved in placebo analgesia. A possible role of dopamine in the context of placebo effects was postulated following observations in patients suffering from Parkinson disease, where dorsal striatal dopaminergic effects were related to improvements in the patient's motor control, while effects in the ventral striatum (nucleus accumbens) were associated with expectations of improvement [23, 24]. The latter observation suggesting that the endogenous release of dopamine in the nucleus accumbens is related to the expectation of reward [21, 25] has led to the placebo-reward hypothesis, where the expectation of clinical benefit represents an anticipated reward. Both "reward"- and punishment-related dopamine activity has been strongly associated with motivated responses [19, 45], and midbrain and striatal dopamine interacts with opioids during multiple forms of behavioural analgesia in animals [2]. Thus, it is also meaningful that nucleus accumbens dopamine release has been observed to be involved in placebo analgesia [47, 48].

OTHER NEUROTRANSMITTERS

Besides opioids and dopamine, additional neurotransmitters seem to be involved in the neuronal mechanisms underlying placebo analgesia. Amanzio and Benedetti [3] observed that placebo analgesia after conditioning with the nonsteroidal anti-inflammatory drug ketorolac could not be reversed with the opioid antagonist naloxone but with the CB1 cannabinoid receptor antagonist rimonabant [8], revealing the involvement of the endocannabinoid system in placebo analgesia. Recently, it has also been shown that the hypothalamic–pituitary hormone oxytocin may enhance placebo analgesia [31]. Oxytocin has been previously associated with processes such as empathy, trust, and social learning [39]. Therefore, oxytocin might enhance placebo analgesia by reinforcing those key aspects of the physician–patient relationship.

IMAGING STUDIES

An early seminal study on the CNS mechanisms underlying placebo analgesia was conducted by Petrovic et al. [44] showing commonalities between opioid-induced and placebo-induced analgesia, employing $H_2[^{15}O]$ positron emission tomography (PET). Healthy participants were stimulated with painful thermal stimuli and received either the rapidly acting opioid remifentanil or a placebo (i.e., an intravenous saline solution with the instruction it would be a potent painkiller). Interestingly, both conditions exhibited increased activity in the rACC and an increased coupling between the rACC and the PAG. Hence, this study reported, for the first time, shared neuronal mechanisms of placebo analgesia and pharmacologically induced opioid analgesia. In addition, this and numerous subsequent studies demonstrated that pain relief during placebo analgesia is accompanied by decreased cerebral responses to pain in typical intensity encoding brain areas such as ACC, S2, insula, and thalamus [17, 59], demonstrating that the placebo effect actually alters the sensory, affective, and/or motivational processes associated with noxious stimuli and does not merely affect compliance with the investigator.

In analogy to studies investigating the role of opioids in sustained pain [64], the effect of endogenous opioids in placebo analgesia has been studied with $[^{11}C]$carfentanil–PET. This technique allows assessment of opioid ligand displacement ($[^{11}C]$carfentanil) by endogenous opioids and thus, indirectly, measurement of the release of endogenous opioids. These studies were able to reveal altered opioid receptor availability during placebo analgesia in several brain regions, including the rACC, lateral frontal regions, and in subcortical structures such as the PAG [61]. In addition, the aforementioned enhanced coupling between the rACC and the PAG during placebo analgesia was observed [61].

CONNECTIVITY

The involvement of the rACC and an enhanced functional coupling with brainstem structures such as the PAG is an observation that functional imaging studies investigating placebo analgesia have repeatedly made [11, 15, 60] and that not only pertains to placebo analgesia evoked by the administration of an intravenous injection but that has also been demonstrated in the context of locally induced placebo analgesia [15, 34, 60]. However, the involvement of this network is not specific to placebo analgesia; it is equally involved in other types of placebo effects—for example, on anxiety-related processes [43]—and even in different types of pain modulation [54].

DORSOLATERAL PREFRONTAL CORTEX

There is evidence showing that the dorsolateral prefrontal cortex (DLPFC) plays a crucial role in the generation of placebo analgesia. The DLPFC has been associated with the generation and manipulation of cognitive representations and also with the modulation of pain, consistent with an important role in expectancy-related pain modulation. Several studies have consistently shown an increase of neuronal activity within the DLPFC, particularly during the anticipation of pain. This increase correlated positively with the subsequent pain reduction and also with pain-related activity in brainstem regions such as the PAG. These studies therefore suggest a neuronal representation of positive treatment expectation by the placebo instruction within the DLPFC, which subsequently recruits a top-down pain modulatory network comprising the rACC and subcortical regions [15, 60]. In the first analysis using unbiased methods to predict the magnitude of placebo analgesia using multivariate patterns of brain activity, Wager et al. [58] found that anticipatory activity in the DLPFC was a crucial part of a predictive model that explained up to 40% of the variance in placebo responses. In addition, anticipatory activity was more strongly related to placebo response strength than activity during pain.

The essential relevance of the DLPFC in mediating placebo analgesia is supported by other experimental approaches and also clinical observations. In a heat-pain paradigm, a transient disruption of the DLPFC function by low-frequency repetitive transcranial magnetic stimulation (rTMS) completely blocked placebo analgesia, whereas the heat-pain perception itself was not affected [35]. Similarly, during the pharmacological manipulation of placebo analgesia by the opiate antagonist naloxone, the DLPFC activation in the anticipation phase is significantly reduced and the top-down recruitment of the rACC and subcortical brain regions is impaired, which is paralleled by a reduction of the individual placebo analgesic effect [15]. The important contribution of frontal brain regions to expectancy-related pain reduction is also supported by studies in patients with neurodegenerative diseases affecting frontal lobe function. Benedetti et al. [9] assessed the placebo response in patients suffering from Alzheimer disease and correlated the individual placebo response with both cognitive status using neuropsychological measures and functional connectivity among different brain regions using EEG. Their data showed a reduction of expectancy-induced analgesia in Alzheimer disease patients that correlated with neuropsychological measures of frontal lobe function and the connectivity of prefrontal regions with other brain regions. These results highlight that the functional and structural integrity of frontal brain networks subserving treatment expectancy is crucial for placebo analgesia. This is further supported by the observation that white matter integrity assessed by fractional anisotropy in the DLPFC and the rACC using diffusion tensor imaging is positively correlated with the individual placebo analgesic response [50].

BRAINSTEM

There is strong evidence from animal research that brainstem areas have a strong influence on the processing of afferent nociceptive stimuli via thoroughly characterized anatomical networks [5, 20]. Functional magnetic resonance imaging (fMRI) studies investigating placebo analgesia were able to demonstrate the involvement of brainstem regions during placebo analgesia that belong to the descending pain modulatory network. The PAG is a key element of the brainstem descending modulatory control systems that have been repeatedly shown to be associated with the analgesic response after a placebo [11, 15, 44, 60]. Interestingly, these studies also observed a placebo-specific increase in the correlation of activity between the rACC and the PAG, establishing a tight functional relationship. In a similar way, fMRI studies manipulating the expectation regarding pain without giving a placebo revealed the importance of brainstem centres in the expectancy-related modulation of pain [17].

However, it has been shown that brainstem regions can also be involved in other types of pain modulation [52, 53, 63], and are elicited by multiple types of affective events [33], including emotionally evocative pictures [10, 46]. It is thus possible that the brainstem participates in multiple top-down processes and has the ability to modulate afferent nociceptive information at multiple levels of processing, including potentially early nociceptive responses.

Neurophysiological studies have provided sophisticated insights into how brainstem regions are able to modulate the processing of afferent nociceptive information at the dorsal horn of the spinal cord. The PAG–rostral ventromedial medulla (RVM) axis seems to be especially important, and mediates multiple types of behavioural and stimulation-evoked analgesia [20, 28, 40]. It is important to note that this descending influence on the spinal cord dorsal horn is complex and that most brainstem regions display state-dependent facilitative as well as inhibitory properties. Therefore, in the healthy organism, brainstem control over nociceptive processing appears to be a dynamically balanced system adapted to actual external and internal requirements. Given the fact that the descending pain modulatory system is a highly conserved feature across different species and considering evidence that this system exists in humans [20, 29], a large interest emerged to investigate whether placebo analgesia already acts at the spinal level in humans.

SPINAL CORD

The first evidence for spinal modulation by placebo treatment came from a study showing a reduced area of secondary hyperalgesia due to placebo administration [37], a phenomenon most parsimoniously explained by spinal involvement. Subsequently, technical advances in spinal cord fMRI allowed measuring blood oxygenation level–dependent (BOLD) responses to thermal stimulation in the dorsal horn during placebo analgesia and revealed an inhibition of neuronal activity in the dorsal horn of the corresponding spinal segment [16]. This observation highlights the ability of the mechanisms involved in placebo analgesia to profoundly alter pain processing, namely, already at the level of the first synapse in the pain pathway. Together with further studies [26, 49], it became apparent that cognitive factors have the capacity to act on spinal pain processing. This is in agreement with previous observations [53] showing a similar recruitment of brainstem areas for various pain modulatory effects. Clinically, these mechanisms might turn out to be highly relevant, as the spinal cord is a main site for pain amplification and pain chronification processes, and cognitive factors have been shown to be important predictors in the chronification of pain [12, 27].

REFERENCES

1. Akil H, Watson SJ, Young E, Lewis ME, Khachaturian H, Walker JM. Endogenous opioids: biology and function. Annu Rev Neurosci 1984;7:223–55.
2. Altier N, Stewart J. The role of dopamine in the nucleus accumbens in analgesia. Life Sci 1999;65:2269–87.
3. Amanzio M, Benedetti F. Neuropharmacological dissection of placebo analgesia: expectation-activated opioid systems versus conditioning-activated specific subsystems. J Neurosci 1999;19:484–94.
4. Amanzio M, Benedetti F, Porro CA, Palermo S, Cauda F. Activation likelihood estimation meta-analysis of brain correlates of placebo analgesia in human experimental pain. Hum Brain Mapp 2013;34:738–52.
5. Basbaum AI, Fields HL. Endogenous pain control systems: brainstem spinal pathways and endorphin circuitry. Annu Rev Neurosci 1984;7:309–38.
6. Benedetti F. The opposite effects of the opiate antagonist naloxone and the cholecystokinin antagonist proglumide on placebo analgesia. Pain 1996;64:535–43.

7. Benedetti F, Amanzio M, Baldi S, Casadio C, Maggi G. Inducing placebo respiratory depressant responses in humans via opioid receptors. Eur J Neurosci 1999;11:625–31.
8. Benedetti F, Amanzio M, Rosato R, Blanchard C. Nonopioid placebo analgesia is mediated by CB_1 cannabinoid receptors. Nat Med 2011;17:1228–30.
9. Benedetti F, Arduino C, Costa S, Vighetti S, Tarenzi L, Rainero I, Asteggiano G. Loss of expectation-related mechanisms in Alzheimer's disease makes analgesic therapies less effective. Pain 2006;121:133–44.
10. Buhle JT, Kober H, Ochsner KN, Mende-Siedlecki P, Weber J, Hughes BL, Kross E, Atlas LY, McRae K, Wager TD. Common representation of pain and negative emotion in the midbrain periaqueductal gray. Soc Cogn Affect Neurosci 2013;8:609–16.
11. Bingel U, Lorenz J, Schoell E, Weiller C, Büchel C. Mechanisms of placebo analgesia: rACC recruitment of a subcortical antinociceptive network. Pain 2006;120:8–15.
12. Chou R, Shekelle P. Will this patient develop persistent disabling low back pain? JAMA 2010;303:1295–302.
13. Colloca L, Petrovic P, Wager TD, Ingvar M, Benedetti F. How the number of learning trials affects placebo and nocebo responses. Pain 2010;151:430–9.
14. Eippert F, Bingel U, Schoell E, Yacubian J, Büchel C. Blockade of endogenous opioid neurotransmission enhances acquisition of conditioned fear in humans. J. Neurosci 2008;28:5465–72.
15. Eippert F, Bingel U, Schoell ED, Yacubian J, Klinger R, Lorenz J, Buchel C. Activation of the opioidergic descending pain control system underlies placebo analgesia. Neuron 2009;63:533–43.
16. Eippert F, Finsterbusch J, Bingel U, Buchel C. Direct evidence for spinal cord involvement in placebo analgesia. Science 2009;326:404.
17. Fairhurst M, Wiech K, Dunckley P, Tracey I. Anticipatory brainstem activity predicts neural processing of pain in humans. Pain 2007;128:101–10.
18. Fanselow MS. Conditioned fear-induced opiate analgesia: a competing motivational state theory of stress analgesia. Ann N Y Acad Sci 1986;467:40–54.
19. Faure A, Reynolds SM, Richard JM, Berridge KC. Mesolimbic dopamine in desire and dread: enabling motivation to be generated by localized glutamate disruptions in nucleus accumbens. J Neurosci 2008;28: 7184–92.
20. Fields H. State-dependent opioid control of pain. Nat Rev Neurosci 2004;5:565–75.
21. Fiorillo CD, Tobler PN, Schultz W. Discrete coding of reward probability and uncertainty by dopamine neurons. Science 2003;299:1898–902.
22. Flaten MA, Aslaksen PM, Lyby PS, Bjørkedal E. The relation of emotions to placebo responses. Philos Trans R Soc Lond B Biol Sci 2011;366:1818–27.
23. De la Fuente-Fernandez R, Phillips AG, Zamburlini M, Sossi V, Calne DB, Ruth TJ, Stoessl AJ. Dopamine release in human ventral striatum and expectation of reward. Behav Brain Res 2002;136:359–63.
24. De la Fuente-Fernandez R, Ruth TJ, Sossi V, Schulzer M, Calne DB, Stoessl AJ. Expectation and dopamine release: mechanism of the placebo effect in Parkinson's disease. Science 2001;293:1164–6.
25. Garris PA, Kilpatrick M, Bunin MA, Michael D, Walker QD, Wightman RM. Dissociation of dopamine release in the nucleus accumbens from intracranial self-stimulation. Nature 1999;398:67–9.
26. Geuter S, Büchel C. Facilitation of pain in the human spinal cord by nocebo treatment. J Neurosci 2013;33:13784–90.
27. Hasenbring M. Predictors of efficacy in treatment of chronic low back pain. Curr Opin Anesthesiol 1998;11:553.
28. Heinricher MM, Tavares I, Leith JL, Lumb BM. Descending control of nociception: specificity, recruitment and plasticity. Brain Res Rev 2009;60:214–25.
29. Hosobuchi Y, Adams JE, Linchitz R. Pain relief by electrical stimulation of the central gray matter in humans and its reversal by naloxone. Science 1977;197:183–6.
30. Hrobjartsson A, Gotzsche PC. Is the placebo powerless? Update of a systematic review with 52 new randomized trials comparing placebo with no treatment. J Intern Med 2004;256:91–100.
31. Kessner S, Sprenger C, Wrobel N, Wiech K, Bingel U. Effect of oxytocin on placebo analgesia: a randomized study. JAMA 2013;310:1733–5.
32. Kirsch I. Conditioning, expectancy, and the placebo effect: comment on Stewart-Williams and Podd (2004). Psychol Bull 2004;130:341–3; discussion 344–5.
33. Kober H, Barrett LF, Joseph J, Bliss-Moreau E, Lindquist K, Wager TD. Functional grouping and cortical-subcortical interactions in emotion: a meta-analysis of neuroimaging studies. NeuroImage 2008;42:998–1031.
34. Kong J, Gollub RL, Rosman IS, Webb JM, Vangel MG, Kirsch I, Kaptchuk TJ. Brain activity associated with expectancy-enhanced placebo analgesia as measured by functional magnetic resonance imaging. J Neurosci 2006;26:381–8.

35. Krummenacher P, Candia V, Folkers G, Schedlowski M, Schonbachler G. Prefrontal cortex modulates placebo analgesia. Pain 2009;148:368–74.
36. Levine JD, Gordon NC, Fields HL. The mechanism of placebo analgesia. Lancet 1978;2:654–7.
37. Matre D, Casey KL, Knardahl S. Placebo-induced changes in spinal cord pain processing. J Neurosci 2006;26:559–63.
38. Meissner K, Bingel U, Colloca L, Wager TD, Watson A, Flaten MA. The placebo effect: advances from different methodological approaches. J Neurosci 2011;31:16117–24.
39. Meyer-Lindenberg A, Domes G, Kirsch P, Heinrichs M. Oxytocin and vasopressin in the human brain: social neuropeptides for translational medicine. Nat Rev Neurosci 2011;12:524–38.
40. Millan MJ. Descending control of pain. Prog Neurobiol 2002;66:355–474.
41. Moerman DE, Jonas WB. Deconstructing the placebo effect and finding the meaning response. Ann Intern Med 2002;136:471–6.
42. Montgomery GH, Kirsch I. Classical conditioning and the placebo effect. Pain 1997;72:107–13.
43. Petrovic P, Dietrich T, Fransson P, Andersson J, Carlsson K, Ingvar M. Placebo in emotional processing—induced expectations of anxiety relief activate a generalized modulatory network. Neuron 2005;46:957–69.
44. Petrovic P, Kalso E, Petersson KM, Ingvar M. Placebo and opioid analgesia—imaging a shared neuronal network. Science 2002;295:1737–40.
45. Salamone JD, Correa M, Mingote SM, Weber SM. Beyond the reward hypothesis: alternative functions of nucleus accumbens dopamine. Curr Opin Pharmacol 2005;5:34–41.
46. Satpute AB, Wager TD, Cohen-Adad J, Bianciardi M, Choi J-K, Buhle JT, Wald LL, Barrett LF. Identification of discrete functional subregions of the human periaqueductal gray. Proc Natl Acad Sci. USA 2013;110:17101–6.
47. Scott DJ, Stohler CS, Egnatuk CM, Wang H, Koeppe RA, Zubieta JK. Individual differences in reward responding explain placebo-induced expectations and effects. Neuron 2007;55:325–36.
48. Scott DJ, Stohler CS, Egnatuk CM, Wang H, Koeppe RA, Zubieta J-K. Placebo and nocebo effects are defined by opposite opioid and dopaminergic responses. Arch Gen Psychiatry 2008;65:220–31.
49. Sprenger C, Eippert F, Finsterbusch J, Bingel U, Rose M, Büchel C. Attention modulates spinal cord responses to pain. Curr Biol 2012;22:1–4.
50. Stein N, Sprenger C, Scholz J, Wiech K, Bingel U. White matter integrity of the descending pain modulatory system is associated with interindividual differences in placebo analgesia. Pain 2012;153:2210–7.
51. Stewart-Williams S, Podd J. The placebo effect: dissolving the expectancy versus conditioning debate. Psychol Bull 2004;130:324–40.
52. Tracey I. Getting the pain you expect: mechanisms of placebo, nocebo and reappraisal effects in humans. Nat Med 2010;16:1277–83.
53. Tracey I, Mantyh PW. The cerebral signature for pain perception and its modulation. Neuron 2007;55:377–91.
54. Valet M, Sprenger T, Boecker H, Willoch F, Rummeny E, Conrad B, Erhard P, Tolle TR. Distraction modulates connectivity of the cingulo-frontal cortex and the midbrain during pain: an fMRI analysis. Pain 2004;109: 399–408.
55. Vase L, Petersen GL, Riley JL, Price DD. Factors contributing to large analgesic effects in placebo mechanism studies conducted between 2002 and 2007. Pain 2009;145:36–44.
56. Voudouris NJ, Peck CL, Coleman G. Conditioned placebo responses. J Pers Soc Psychol [illegible]53.
57. Voudouris NJ, Peck CL, Coleman G. The role of conditioning and verbal expectancy in the placebo response. Pain 1990;43:121–8.
58. Wager TD, Atlas LY, Leotti LA, Rilling JK. Predicting individual differences in placebo analgesia: contributions of brain activity during anticipation and pain experience. J Neurosci 2011;31:439–52.
59. Wager TD, Fields H. Placebo analgesia. In: Wall PD, Melzack R, editors. Textbook of pain. Philadelphia, PA: Elsevier Churchill Livingstone; 2013. pp. 362–73.
60. Wager TD, Rilling JK, Smith EE, Sokolik A, Casey KL, Davidson RJ, Kosslyn SM, Rose RM, Cohen JD. Placebo-induced changes in FMRI in the anticipation and experience of pain. Science 2004;303:1162.
61. Wager TD, Scott DJ, Zubieta JK. Placebo effects on human mu-opioid activity during pain. Proc Natl Acad Sci USA 2007;104:11056–61.
62. Wickramasekera I. A conditioned response model of the placebo effect predictions from the model. Biofeedback Self Regul 1980;5:5–18.
63. Wiech K, Ploner M, Tracey I. Neurocognitive aspects of pain perception. Trends Cogn Sci 2008;12:306–13.
64. Zubieta JK, Smith YR, Bueller JA, Xu Y, Kilbourn MR, Jewett DM, Meyer CR, Koeppe RA, Stohler CS. Regional mu opioid receptor regulation of sensory and affective dimensions of pain. Science 2001;293:311.

SECTION 5

Neuroplasticity and Chronic Pain

CHAPTER 20

Functional Reorganization of the Brain with Chronic Pain

A. Vania Apkarian and Herta Flor

The chapter briefly reviews the accumulated evidence that the functional representation for perception of pain is modified in different types of clinical chronic pain conditions, in comparison with acute pain, and in relation to duration of persistence of chronic pain. We provide mechanistic explanations for this plasticity within the context of the classical electrophysiological studies performed in the late 20th century in monkey and rodent cortex, and in relation to more recent theories regarding the interaction between pain and brain learning circuitry. Moreover, we discuss clinical consequences of these results and some examples of practical applications that have already ensued.

Until the early 1970s, concepts regarding brain plasticity were limited to the early developmental stages, and it was commonly assumed that after a critical developmental period, brain anatomical properties become fixed and that further learning and experience would be reflected on physiological reorganizations grounded upon a fixed anatomical architecture. Two seminal observations revolutionized these concepts. The first was the demonstration of long-term potentiation (LTP), which soon afterwards was shown to be accompanied by structural changes [14]. The second was the determination that topographic cortical maps underlying body and auditory representations undergo injury- and experience-dependent plastic changes even in adulthood [63, 70], implying that synaptic circuitry is under dynamic control. Given the large scale of the observed changes, it was concluded that physiological changes are also accompanied by reorganization of the anatomy of synaptic inputs. There is now incontrovertible evidence that experience in the adult organism carves novel patterns of dendrites and spines, and perhaps axonal terminations, at the cellular level. Perhaps the best examples are morphological studies in rodents exposed to cocaine addiction and also rodents studied within an enriched environment [44, 78].

Pain research in the latter half of the 20th century was dominated by anatomical studies based on retrograde and anterograde tracer techniques and extracellular sharp electrode electrophysiological techniques. Both aimed at elucidating the presence and properties of nociceptors, and the projection pathways transmitting such information from the periphery to the spinal and to supraspinal targets [38, 49, 82]. Within the context of this 20th-century viewpoint and with the assumption that the adult nervous system is anatomically constant, the overriding assumption regarding chronic pain was simply that these nociceptors should be more activated for longer periods of time. Therefore, even the discovery that afferent fibre properties and spinal cord circuit properties are labile and undergo specific reorganization with inflammatory and neuropathic injuries was a surprise, and established an attempt of capturing the details (anatomical, physiological, and molecular) of these changes that continues unabated until today. The fact that supraspinal brain circuitry undergoes reorganization with pain was not seriously contemplated until the advent of modern noninvasive brain imaging technology, and even with this technology, such ideas were not pursued in detail until the clinical chronic pain condition became a scientific entity in need of being studied in and of itself.

Perhaps the first inkling that the brain in chronic pain was not fitting within the conceptual construct of late 20th-century notions was based on observing brain activity for acute painful stimuli when applied to patients with persistent or chronic pain [4]. The logic of performing such experiments was clear: If the brain circuitry involved in pain perception is preoccupied with a persistent pain state, then the superposition of an additional painful stimulus would identify which of the components of the system are preoccupied and thus unable to process the new incoming information. One of the few consistent observations that such experiments identified was decreased thalamic activity, see [4], coupled with the observation that most cortical regions observed to be activated in healthy subjects seemed to still be essentially showing a similar pattern of activity. As the thalamus is the primary relay for nociceptive information flow to the cortex, it was difficult to come up with adequate explanations/theories for the observation, especially if anatomical constancy was to be assumed. Thus, in the 1990s, there was a burgeoning of studies reporting some type of distortion of brain activity for acute painful stimuli, whether studied by positron emission tomography (PET) or functional magnetic resonance imaging (fMRI), in clinical pain patients, but the results were not uniform. This pushed many laboratories away from studying pain patients and towards further examination of the brain properties of pain encoding in the healthy subject and/or to attempt to design surrogate experimental models in healthy subjects hoping to identify characteristics that might apply to chronic pain.

It seemed that many of the human brain imaging studies were attempts to replicate the electrophysiology of the 1970s that used to be done in anaesthetized animals and now was being conducted in awake humans. Moreover, the realization was coupled with the sense that the methodologies available were simply not sufficient for specifically doing the science of chronic pain and that new approaches were called for to seriously advance the field.

FUNCTIONAL REORGANIZATION OF SENSORY AND MOTOR AREAS OF THE BRAIN

A series of magnetoencephalographic and electroencephalographic studies, soon followed by fMRI, showed that in patients with amputations, the map in primary somatosensory cortex changes in a manner that input from neighbouring areas occupies the region that formerly received input from the now amputated limb [19, 26, 54, 85]. These changes were mirrored in motor cortex [48, 53]. Interestingly, reorganizational changes were found only in amputees with phantom limb pain after amputation but not in amputees without pain. This suggests that pain may contribute to the changes observed and that the persisting pain might also be a consequence of the plastic changes that occur. In several studies in human upper extremity amputees, displacement of the lip representation in the primary motor and somatosensory cortex was positively correlated with the intensity of phantom limb pain, and was not present in pain-free amputees or healthy controls. Also, in the patients with phantom limb pain, but not the pain-free amputees, imagined movement of the phantom hand activated the neighbouring face area [53]. The coactivation occurs probably due to the high overlap of the hand, arm, and mouth representations. However, input from the residual limb may also contribute to postamputation changes [60].

Similar observations were made in patients with complex regional pain syndrome. In these patients, the representation of the affected hand tended to be smaller compared with that of the unaffected hand, and the individual digit representations had moved closer together [45, 56, 57, 68, 76]. The extent of the pathological changes in the cortical representations not only correlated with the intensity of pain [59, 68] but was also related to a degradation of sensibility in the affected hand.

Not only nerve lesion but also increased behaviourally relevant input related to musculoskeletal pain leads to changes in the cortical map [23, 34, 35]. For example, Flor et al. [23] reported a close association between pain chronicity and enhanced excitability and map expansion of the back representation in primary somatosensory cortex. The back representation had expanded and shifted towards the leg representation the longer the pain had persisted. Similar changes were reported by Giesecke et al. [34] using fMRI. Greatly enhanced representations of painful stimulation were also found in patients with fibromyalgia who showed more areas of the brain responding to painful stimulation of a standard value and also higher activation intensities [35].

Moreover, it was also shown that when the pain could be relieved by training or pharmacological interventions, the reorganization would also be reduced and this change was significantly correlated with pain reduction [24, 42, 58]. In some sense, these results were the human equivalent of the classic studies done by Merzenich and Kaas [46] years earlier, where careful sharp electrode mappings had demonstrated the fragility of the somatotopic maps [15]. However, these noninvasive mapping results were the first evidence of cortical electrical properties (meaning that the signals were direct measures of neuronal activity) in humans undergoing large-scale (cm) changes in their body maps related to the presence of unremitting pain. A main worry at the time, and that remains incompletely resolved, was the issue of the observed reorganization being some complex combination of secondary somatic and motor adaptations due to living with the discomfort of the persisting pain. That one observes at least partial recovery of maps towards the healthy control with pain relief was good evidence that the presence of the pain itself may be involved in the observed reorganization [25, 60]. Importantly, these studies for the first time also linked, at least indirectly, brain learning mechanisms (that must be involved in remappings; either through local LTP-type mechanisms or driven by the more global learning processes of the mesocorticolimbic circuitry) with chronic pain. Although these were exciting results, they were readily acceptable and were deemed to fit the classical view of distortions of cortical representation of pain, as the reorganization appeared to be localized to the sensorimotor cortex, a structure that is part of the classical concept for encoding nociceptive information through the spinothalamic pathway. However, it soon became clear that other areas are involved in these reorganizational processes that also involve large-scale increases in brain excitability (see below).

STRUCTURAL BRAIN CHANGES IN CHRONIC PAIN

A separate line of study examined brain chemistry, using magnetic resonance spectroscopy (MRS), and showed that specific cortical regions display abnormal chemical composition in chronic back pain patients as well as patients with complex regional pain syndrome [36, 37]. The chemical abnormality was outside of the somatosensory cortex, localized to the dorsolateral prefrontal cortex (DLPFC). In patients with fibromyalgia, as noted above, additional limbic areas were found to be altered, and MRS also revealed changes in the insula in these patients that were reversed with successful treatment [39]. One of the first studies examining the influence of a chronic pain state might have on cortical grey matter volume was done by Apkarian et al. [5]. Chronic back pain patients showed a decrease in grey matter volume in the DLPFC and the right thalamus compared with a matched group of healthy subjects. Although the authors were not able to show a causal link, they did show a correlation between the grey matter volume loss and pain duration. A later study by Schmidt-Wilcke et al. [73] also showed a correlation between duration of the chronic back pain and decreased grey matter volume, however, only within the primary somatosensory cortex and the brain stem. Increased grey matter volume was found in the bilateral striatum and the left thalamus.

The first studies to examine grey matter volume changes in fibromyalgia found not only a significantly reduced total volume of grey matter in patients compared with controls but also a correlation between disease duration and grey matter loss. Additionally, patients showed significantly reduced grey matter in the parahippocampal and cingulate gyrus, the insula, as well as the median frontal cortex [50]. It has been debated to what extent other factors than pain, for example, depression, might contribute to these changes [11, 71].

CHANGES IN LIMBIC AND FRONTAL CIRCUITRY

Although the initial studies, which focused on EEG and MEG recordings, showed mainly reorganizational changes in primary somatosensory and motor areas, it is clear that reorganization also affects areas involved in emotional and motivational processing and memory processes. For example, Witting et al. [84] examined the brain correlates of allodynia in patients with allodynia related to neuropathic pain. In this PET study, the authors observed that allodynia was related to enhanced ipsilateral insular and more orbitofrontal activation as well as a lack of contralateral S1 activation, which the authors explained in terms of a stronger emotional load and higher computational demands in the processing of a mixed sensation of brush and pain. The orbitofrontal activation is probably related to the mechanisms of descending pain modulation, but it might also be involved in anticipatory anxiety related to pain. Similarly, in trigeminal neuralgia, allodynia activated not only areas in the primary sensory pathway but also areas in the basal ganglia and frontal cortex [11]. Schweinhardt et al. [75] also observed a relationship of allodynia and caudal insular activity in pain patients. In complex regional pain syndrome (CRPS) patients, hyperalgesia was associated with enhanced activation in all pain-relevant areas, including S1 and S2.

In amputees, Willoch et al. [83] used hypnosis to induce painful phantom sensations and reported activation in areas such as the insula and the anterior cingulate cortex, regions that have been identified as important in the processing of affective pain components. However, the influence of the effort to create the specific sensation in the hypnotic condition cannot be controlled in this type of study. In a study that varied both acute and chronic pain intensity simultaneously, it was observed that chronic pain intensity changes covaried with prefrontal activation, whereas acute pain intensity changes covaried with insular activation, suggesting different processing modes for acute and chronic pain [6, 8]. A number of additional cross-sectional fMRI studies indicate preferential involvement of brain emotional and limbic circuitry in encoding fluctuations of ongoing pain for various chronic pain conditions [20, 31, 32, 40, 67].

Almost all studies on brain imaging show that there is a certain set of brain regions that usually show a deactivation during task performance compared with a rest condition.

This has led to the proposal of a "default-mode network" (DMN) of brain function [69]. Baliki et al. [7] suggested that long-term pain alters the functional connectivity of the cortical regions of the DMN. They studied chronic back pain patients and healthy controls and presented them with a simple visual attention task while measuring the blood oxygenation level–dependent (BOLD) response. They found no difference in task performance of both groups, but reduced brain deactivation in the medial prefrontal cortex, the amygdala, and the posterior cingulate cortex. The authors concluded that chronic pain alters several key DMN brain regions in the chronic back pain patients and that the disruption of the DMN may underlie many of the cognitive and behavioural impairments accompanying chronic pain (i.e., depression, anxiety, sleep disturbance, or decision-making abnormalities).

Most of the above-described research has been carried out in chronic pain patients either by administering nociceptive stimuli that mimic patients' chronic pain or by applying stimuli that challenge the nociceptive system. Thus, what we know so far is a momentary picture of cortical changes in chronic pain. Longitudinal studies that examine the transition from acute to chronic pain have only recently been reported. Baliki et al. [9, 10] investigated patients with a first occurrence of chronic back pain and reinvestigated them over a period of 1 year. They found a clear differentiation between patients in whom pain persisted over the period of this year and those in whom the pain decreased. In terms of pain intensity ratings, the persistent pain group rated their chronic back pain at about 60 (on a visual analogue scale from 0 [no pain] to 100 [worst pain imaginable]) on all the four visits throughout the year. The patients who were classified as recovering back pain patients showed decreased pain ratings: initially, they reported the same pain intensity rating as the persistent pain group, but dropped to about 20 at the end of the year. It is noteworthy that the recovering group did not report a complete amelioration of pain, but rather a decrease. Classification of the two groups (persistent versus recovering) was done at the end of the year based on the pain intensity ratings. The authors then looked for differences in functional connectivity between the two groups on the first visit. Initial greater functional connectivity between the nucleus accumbens and the prefrontal cortex predicted pain persistence. It seems that the connectivity between prefrontal regions and the nucleus accumbens, which is implicated in reward learning, is crucial for the transition from acute to chronic pain. In a separate but related article, Mansour et al. [61] investigated white matter structural changes between the two groups. Here, they found decreases in integrity of white matter tracts for the patients with persistent chronic back pain. Since most of the variance in white matter differences is explained by genetic factors, the differences observed might be a predisposition to pain chronicity. Investigating differences between patients with persistent and recovering back pain after 1 year, Mutso et al. [66] found decreased functional connectivity of the hippocampus and medial prefrontal cortex for patients with persistent pain. Especially the involvement of the hippocampus points towards dysfunctional learning processes.

To further elucidate brain processes involved in pain chronicity, Hashmi et al. [40] investigated a group of subacute patients in a very early phase of back pain (~2 months) and patients who had lived with their chronic pain for over 10 years. They found a shift of pain-related brain activation from regions involved in pain processing for the subacute patients towards regions implicated in emotions and reward processing for the chronic group. In a longitudinal design, they found that patients with persisting chronic back pain also showed a gradually diminishing response of regions encoding pain intensity over the course of 1 year. Using an automated meta-analysis of brain imaging, they could replicate this result. They found that acute and subacute pain engaged pain and reward circuits, whereas chronic back pain and persisting back pain showed a shift away from networks involved in acute pain processing towards networks involved in emotion and reward processing. In line with this, Kamping et al. [47] found that the pain perception and processing in fibromyalgia patients is not deficient per se, as they did not find any group differences between patients and healthy controls when using painful laser stimulation. However, when adding additional input, for example, pictures with emotional content, patients showed a deficient modulation of pain by positive mood. These results suggest that fibromyalgia patients are less efficient in modulating pain by positive affect and may benefit less from appetitive events than healthy control subjects and may thus have altered reward processing capacities. In line with the results given by Baliki et al. [47], these patients had a disturbed processing of rewards in the nucleus accumbens.

LEARNING, MEMORY, AND CHRONIC PAIN

As noted above, plastic changes in the CNS and specifically the brain can be viewed as indicative of learning processes that affect brain structure and function. Already in the 1960s and 1970s, operant and respondent learning as well as social observation were considered important factors in pain chronicity [17, 30, 33, 52]. For example, Fordyce's [30] description of the role of operant factors in chronic pain suggests that when an individual is exposed to a stimulus, which causes tissue damage, the immediate response is withdrawal and attempts to escape from noxious sensations. This may be accomplished by avoidance of activity believed to cause or exacerbate pain, help seeking to reduce symptoms, and so forth. These behaviours are observable and, consequently, subject to the principles of operant conditioning, that is, they respond to contingencies of reward and punishment. The operant view proposes that acute "pain behaviour" such as limping to protect a wounded limb from producing additional nociceptive input may come under the control of external contingencies of reinforcement and thus develop into a chronic pain problem. Pain behaviour (e.g., complaining, inactivity) may be positively reinforced directly, for example, by attention from a spouse or health care provider. Pain behaviour may also be maintained by the escape from noxious stimulation by the use of drugs or rest, or the avoidance of undesirable activities such as work (negative reinforcement). In addition, "well behaviour" (e.g., activity, working) may not be sufficiently reinforcing, and the more rewarding pain behaviours may, therefore, be maintained (lack of reinforcement of healthy behaviours). The pain behaviour originally elicited by organic factors may come to occur, totally or in part, in response to reinforcing environmental events. Because of the consequences of specific behavioural responses, it is proposed that pain behaviours may persist long after the initial cause of the pain is resolved or greatly reduced. The operant conditioning model considers pain as an internal subjective experience that may be maintained even after an initial physical basis of pain has resolved. Operant conditioning can lead to increased inactivity and invalidity and also plays an important role in the increase of medication levels since the intake of medication—especially on a *prn* basis when there are high pain levels—may be viewed as a consequence of a negative reinforcement process (a negative consequence, the pain, is removed by medication intake). Not only observable pain behaviours but also verbal expressions of pain and physiological variables may come under the control of the contingencies of reinforcement. For example, Flor et al. [27] showed that monetary and social reinforcement of acute pain ratings can lead to an increase or reduction of self-reported pain levels, depending on the direction of the reinforced response. This response was equally well acquired by chronic pain patients and healthy controls and did not yield any differences in central brain responses (somatosensory evoked potentials of the electroencephalogram, EEG). However, when reinforcement was withdrawn, only the healthy controls downregulated their pain ratings and their brain response (following the normal habituation curves). The chronic pain patients, however, maintained elevated pain responses during extinction, and this was also reflected in elevated brain potentials. The patients were unaware of this altered pain processing and lack of extinction. Becker et al. [12] showed recently that this implicit operant learning can also take place when the behaviour-contingent reduction or increase of pain is used as a reinforcing stimulus and behavioural adjustments of pain perception rather than verbal ratings or EEG measures are used.

Since the experience of pain is a very important biological stimulus, it is immediately evident that respondent (Pavlovian) emotional conditioning might also play an important role when pain is repeatedly experienced as it is the case in the transition from acute to chronic pain [52]. In the typical aversive classical conditioning paradigm, a previously neutral variable (later the conditioned stimulus, CS), when paired with a biologically significant aversive stimulus (unconditioned stimulus, US) comes to elicit a conditioned response (CR) that often, but not always, resembles the response to the unconditioned stimulus, the unconditioned response (UR). For example, if a certain movement has been associated with pain, just thinking about the movement may already elicit fear and muscle tension (previously elicited by pain) and may then motivate avoidance behaviours, and this also forms a central memory trace. Once an acute pain problem exists, fear of motor activities that the patient expects to result in pain may develop and motivate avoidance of activity. Nonoccurrence of pain is a powerful reinforcer for reduction of activity, and thus the original respondent conditioning may be followed by an operant learning process whereby the nociceptive stimuli and the associated responses need no longer be present for the avoidance behaviour to occur. In acute pain states, it may be useful to reduce movement, consequently avoiding pain, to accelerate the healing process. Pain related to sustained muscle contractions might, however, also be conceptualized as an unconditioned stimulus in the case where no acute injury was present and sympathetic activation and tension increases might be viewed as URs that may elicit more pain, and conditioning might proceed in the same fashion as outlined above. Thus, although the original association between pain and pain-related stimuli results in anxiety regarding these stimuli, with time the expectation of pain related to activity may lead to avoidance of adaptive behaviours even if the nociceptive stimuli and the related sympathetic activation are no longer present. Fear of pain and activity may become conditioned to an expanding number of situations. Avoided activities may involve simple motor behaviours, but also work, leisure, and sexual activity. In addition to the avoidance learning, pain may be exacerbated and maintained in these encounters with potentially pain-increasing situations due to the anxiety-related sympathetic activation and muscle tension increases that may occur in anticipation of pain and also as a consequence of pain. Thus, psychological factors may directly affect nociceptive stimulation and need not be viewed as only reactions to pain, and they also induce plastic changes in the brain. Vlaeyen and Linton [81] have documented that fear avoidance is a major predictor of chronic pain and disability.

Aversive emotional conditioning with painful stimuli as US has been shown to be exaggerated in chronic pain patients, specifically in the muscle that is relevant for the specific type of pain [74]. This site specificity of peripheral changes associated with pain-related memory traces is important because this may be a local aggravating factor that is, however, triggered by central changes. Craig [17] has shown and emphasized that viewing pain in others and responding to it is a major learning factor related to pain, and confirmed the role of social learning for pain processing, a factor that has so far received insufficient attention. Empathy for pain [77] is a prerequisite for social learning, but social learning goes beyond emotional involvement in others' pain.

Although the important role of these learning processes for chronic pain has already been formulated in the 1970s and 1980s, research in the neurosciences focused on the mechanisms of these learning processes only recently, and, specifically, the advent of neuroimaging has thus made the study of their central mechanisms feasible also in humans [2, 3, 22, 28].

As noted above, the neural signature of pain can also be altered by learning and memory processes. For example, Albanese et al. [1] showed that learning and memory tasks related to discrimination of stimuli alter the somatosensory and insular cortex, and Diesch and Flor [18] documented similar changes in primary somatosensory cortex as a consequence of Pavlovian conditioning. Furthermore, Schneider et al. [74] showed that Pavlovian conditioning is enhanced in chronic pain patients and both peripheral and brain responses to painful stimulation are enhanced and resistant to extinction. Most of these memory and learning processes are implicit and change the way pain is processed, without necessarily forming an explicit memory trace. This makes it difficult to change these pain-related learning processes, which increasingly involve emotional and motivational circuits, in treatment.

TREATMENTS BASED ON BRAIN CHANGES AND LEARNING

If ongoing pain is associated with abnormal cross talk from other brain regions such as those involved in emotion and motivation, then alterations of the respective brain region should alter the brain map and also pain [21, 65]. The prevention of somatosensory and emotional pain memories would be an important task in pain management, and there are at least four possible targets: (a) chronic pain must be prevented as early as possible by pharmacological and psychological interventions to keep pain memories from being established; (b) cortical reorganization related to injury or stimulation could further be prevented by using pharmacological agents that are known to impair cortical reorganization; (c) chronic states of pain could be reversed by using training procedures that are known to influence cortical reorganization and emotional learning; (d) pharmacological changes that are important for reorganization could be counteracted by using antagonists; and (e) stimulation methods such as transcranial magnetic stimulation or transcranial direct current stimulation or neurofeedback that can alter cortical excitation and inhibition and affect brain circuits might also be beneficial.

The prevention of chronic pain might be possible by using pharmacological agents that are known to also prevent or reverse cortical reorganization. Among these substances, GABA agonists, NMDA receptor antagonists, and anticholinergic substances seem to be the most promising. A double-blind placebo-controlled study that used the NMDA receptor antagonist memantine in the perioperative phase in acute amputations reported a decrease in the incidence of phantom limb pain from 72% to 20% 1 year after the amputation [72].

In chronic amputees, stimulation-related procedures were found to be effective. Intense input to the cortical amputation zone, such as by the use of a myoelectric prosthesis, was found to reduce both cortical reorganization and phantom limb pain [54]. Thus, extensive training with a myoelectric or sensorimotor prosthesis would seem useful in reducing phantom limb pain. In patients in whom the use of a prosthesis is not possible, sensory discrimination training might be beneficial. In one study, electrodes are closely spaced over the amputation stump in a region where their activity excites the nerve that supplied the amputated arm portion. Patients then had to discriminate the frequency and the location of the stimulation in an extended training that encompassed 90 minutes per day over a 2-week period. Substantial improvements in both two-point discrimination and phantom limb pain were found in the trained patients. These improvements were accompanied by changes in cortical reorganization indicating a normalization of the shifted mouth representation [24]. These findings are in line with other evidence suggesting that behavioural training can have massive effects on cortical representations. Direct modification of cortical activity by a biofeedback application might target slow cortical potentials, somatosensory evoked potentials or fields or EEG rhythms, or blood flow changes related to the experience of heightened pain.

Birbaumer et al. [13] used regional anaesthesia in upper limb amputees to treat phantom limb pain and observed a very rapid reversal of the somatosensory cortical reorganization in those who experienced substantial pain relief but not in those whose pain remained unchanged. More recently, noninvasive techniques such as transcranial magnetic stimulation (TMS) and transcranial direct current stimulation (tDCS) were proposed. Both techniques have been applied in several hundred subjects (patients and healthy volunteers) worldwide, and no significant side effects have been reported to date [43, 51].

Moseley [64] used a tripartite program for patients with CRPS. This program contained a hand laterality recognition task (recognizing a pictured hand to be left or right), imagined movements of the affected hand, and mirror therapy (adoption of the hand posture shown in a picture with both hands in a mirror box while watching the reflection of the unaffected hand). After a 2-week treatment, pain scores were significantly reduced. McCabe et al. [62] also found a reduction in pain ratings during and after mirrored visual feedback of movement of the unaffected limb in CRPS. In phantom limb pain, both imagery [55] and mirror treatment [16] were found to be effective, and changes in pain were closely matched by reversed cortical reorganization [29]. These studies suggest that modification of input into the affected brain region may alter pain sensation in chronic pain.

Patients who show high levels of pain behaviours and are very incapacitated by their pain should profit from operant behavioural treatment. The goals of this treatment are the decrease of pain behaviours in an effort to extinguish pain; the increase of activity levels and healthy behaviours related to work, leisure time, and the family; as well as medication reduction and management and the change of the behaviour of significant others [28]. The overall goal is to reduce disability by reducing pain and increasing healthy behaviours. Medication is switched from a *prn* basis to a fixed time schedule, where medication is given at certain times of the day to avoid negative reinforcement learning from occurring. Similar principles are applied to the enhancement of activity and the reduction of inactivity and invalidity. This approach has been found to be effective in patients with chronic back pain as well as other pain syndromes [79]. The cognitive-behavioural model of chronic pain emphasizes the role of cognitive, affective, and behavioural factors in the development and maintenance of chronic pain. The central tenet of cognitive-behavioural treatment is to reduce feelings of helplessness and uncontrollability and to establish a sense of control over pain in the patients. This is achieved by the modification of pain-eliciting and maintaining behaviours, cognitions, and emotions. The cognitive-behavioural approach teaches patients various techniques to deal effectively with episodes of pain. Pain-related cognitions are changed by cognitive restructuring and pain coping strategies such as attention diversion and use of imagery or relaxation that increases self-efficacy. Several studies have examined the efficacy of cognitive-behavioural pain management, which must be considered as a very effective treatment of chronic pain [79]. Both operant- and cognitive-behavioural therapies lead to a significant reduction in pain intensity. In addition, the cognitive therapy improves cognitive and affective variables, whereas the operant therapy showed significant improvements in physical functioning and behavioural variables and maintained at both the 6- and 12-month follow-ups [80].

Behavioural treatments that focus on the extinction of pain behaviours and the acquisition of healthy behaviours can also alter brain processes related to pain. Since pain seems to generally increase excitability, substances that decrease excitation such as gabapentin or pregabalin would also seem to be indicated as enhancers of extinction. Since extinction is context-specific, training as many varied behaviours as possible, training in many different environments, and the use of stress and pain episodes to train relapse prevention are important parts of this training. In addition, cognitive and emotional aspects of pain need to be targeted as outlined above.

CONCLUSION

Although recent neuroscientific evidence has shown that chronic pain leads to changes in many brain regions, this responsiveness of pain to plastic changes also opens the door to new intervention methods relying on stimulation, behavioural training, or pharmacological substances that prevent maladaptive memory formation or enhance extinction. For our understanding of chronic pain, it is essential to understand that the brain circuits that are involved in acute pain differ from those involved in chronic pain, where emotional and motivational components become more important than nociception.

REFERENCES

1. Albanese MC, Duerden EG, Rainville P, Duncan GH. Memory traces of pain in human cortex. J Neurosci 2007;27(17):4612–20.
2. Apkarian AV. Pain perception in relation to emotional learning. Curr Opin Neurobiol 2008;18(4):464–8.
3. Apkarian AV, Baliki MN, Geha PY. Towards a theory of chronic pain. Prog Neurobiol 2009;87(2):81–97.
4. Apkarian AV, Bushnell MC, Treede RD, Zubieta JK. Human brain mechanisms of pain perception and regulation in health and disease. Eur J Pain 2005;9(4):463–84.
5. Apkarian AV, Sosa Y, Sonty S, Levy RM, Harden RN, Parrish TB, Gitelman DR. Chronic back pain is associated with decreased prefrontal and thalamic gray matter density. J Neurosci 2004;24(46):10410–5.
6. Baliki MN, Chialvo DR, Geha PY, Levy RM, Harden RN, Parrish TB, Apkarian AV. Chronic pain and the emotional brain: specific brain activity associated with spontaneous fluctuations of intensity of chronic back pain. J Neurosci 2006;26(47):12165–73.
7. Baliki MN, Geha PY, Apkarian AV, Chialvo DR. Beyond feeling: chronic pain hurts the brain, disrupting the default-mode network dynamics. J Neurosci 2008;28(6):1398–1403.
8. Baliki MN, Geha PY, Fields HL, Apkarian AV. Predicting value of pain and analgesia: nucleus accumbens response to noxious stimuli changes in the presence of chronic pain. Neuron 2010;66(1):149–60.
9. Baliki MN, Petre B, Torbey S, Herrmann KM, Huang L, Schnitzer TJ, Fields HL, Apkarian AV. Corticostriatal functional connectivity predicts transition to chronic back pain. Nat Neurosci 2012;15(8):1117–9.
10. Baliki MN, Schnitzer TJ, Bauer WR, Apkarian AV. Brain morphological signatures for chronic pain. PLoS One 2011;6(10):e26010.
11. Becerra L, Morris S, Bazes S, Gostic R, Sherman S, Gostic J, Pendse G, Moulton E, Scrivani S, Keith D, et al. Trigeminal neuropathic pain alters responses in CNS circuits to mechanical (brush) and thermal (cold and heat) stimuli. J Neurosci 2006;26(42):10646–57.

12. Becker S, Kleinböhl D, Klossika I, Hölzl R. Operant conditioning of enhanced pain sensitivity by heat-pain titration. Pain 2008;140(1):104–14.
13. Birbaumer N, Lutzenberger W, Montoya P, Larbig W, Unertl K, Topfner S, Grodd W, Taub E, Flor H. Effects of regional anesthesia on phantom limb pain are mirrored in changes in cortical reorganization. J Neurosci 1997;17(14):5503–8.
14. Bliss TV, Lomo T. Long-lasting potentiation of synaptic transmission in the dentate area of the anaesthetized rabbit following stimulation of the perforant path. J Physiol 1973;232(2):331–56.
15. Buonomano DV, Merzenich MM. Cortical plasticity: from synapses to maps. Annu Rev Neurosci 1998;21: 149–86.
16. Chan BL, Witt R, Charrow A, Howard R, Magee A, Pasquina PF, Heilman KM, Tsao JW. A randomized trial of mirror therapy for lower limb phantom pain. Ann Neurol 2007;62:S32, S33.
17. Craig KD. Social modeling influences on pain. In: Sternbach RA, editor. The psychology of pain. New York, NY: Raven Press; 1978. pp. 73–110.
18. Diesch E, Flor H. Alteration in the response properties of primary somatosensory cortex related to differential aversive Pavlovian conditioning. Pain 2007;131(1–2):171–80.
19. Elbert T, Flor H, Birbaumer N, Knecht S, Hampson S, Larbig W, Taub E. Extensive reorganization of the somatosensory cortex in adult humans after nervous system injury. Neuroreport 1994;5(18):2593–7.
20. Farmer MA, Chanda ML, Parks EL, Baliki MN, Apkarian AV, Schaeffer AJ. Brain functional and anatomical changes in chronic prostatitis/chronic pelvic pain syndrome. J Urol 2011;186(1):117–24.
21. Flor H. New developments in the understanding and management of persistent pain. Curr Opin Psychiatry 2012;25(2):109–13.
22. Flor H. Psychological pain interventions and neurophysiology: implications for a mechanism-based approach. Am Psychol 2014;69(2):188–96.
23. Flor H, Braun C, Elbert T, Birbaumer N. Extensive reorganization of primary somatosensory cortex in chronic back pain patients. Neurosci Lett 1997;224(1):5–8.
24. Flor H, Denke C, Schaefer M, Grüsser S. Effect of sensory discrimination training on cortical reorganisation and phantom limb pain. Lancet 2001;357(9270):1763–4.
25. Flor H, Diers M, Andoh J. The neural basis of phantom limb pain. Trends Cogn Sci 2013;17(7):307–8.
26. Flor H, Elbert T, Knecht S, Wienbruch C, Pantev C, Birbaumer N, Larbig W, Taub E. Phantom-limb pain as a perceptual correlate of cortical reorganization following arm amputation. Nature 1995;375(6531):482–4.
27. Flor H, Knost B, Birbaumer N. The role of operant conditioning in chronic pain: an experimental investigation. Pain 2002;95(1–2):111–8.
28. Flor H, Turk DC. Chronic pain: an integrated biobehavioral approach. Seattle, WA: IASP Press; 2011.
29. Foell J, Bekrater-Bodmann R, Diers M, Flor H. Mirror therapy for phantom limb pain: brain changes and the role of body representation. Eur J Pain 2014;18(5):729–39.
30. Fordyce WE. Behavioral methods for chronic pain and illness. St. Louis, MO: Mosby; 1976.
31. Geha PY, Baliki MN, Chialvo DR, Harden RN, Paice JA, Apkarian AV. Brain activity for spontaneous pain of postherpetic neuralgia and its modulation by lidocaine patch therapy. Pain 2007;128(1–2):88–100.
32. Geha PY, Baliki MN, Harden RN, Bauer WR, Parrish TB, Apkarian AV. The brain in chronic CRPS pain: abnormal gray-white matter interactions in emotional and autonomic regions. Neuron 2008;60(4):570–81.
33. Gentry WD, Bernal GAA. Chronic pain. In: Williams RB, Gentry WD, editors. Behavioral approaches to medicine treatment. New York, NY: Ballinger; 1977. pp. 173–181.
34. Giesecke T, Gracely RH, Grant MA, Nachemson A, Petzke F, Williams DA, Clauw DJ. Evidence of augmented central pain processing in idiopathic chronic low back pain. Arthritis Rheum 2004;50(2):613–23.
35. Gracely RH, Petzke F, Wolf JM, Clauw DJ. Functional magnetic resonance imaging evidence of augmented pain processing in fibromyalgia. Arthritis Rheum 2002;46(5):1333–43.
36. Grachev ID, Fredrickson BE, Apkarian AV. Abnormal brain chemistry in chronic back pain: an in vivo proton magnetic resonance spectroscopy study. Pain 2000;89(1):7–18.
37. Grachev ID, Thomas PS, Ramachandran TS. Decreased levels of *N*-acetyl aspartate in dorsolateral prefrontal cortex in a case of intractable severe sympathetically mediated chronic pain (complex regional pain syndrome, type I). Brain Cogn 2002;49(1):102–13.
38. Haber LH, Moore BD, Willis WD. Electrophysiological response properties of spinoreticular neurons in the monkey. J Comp Neurol 1982;207(1):75–84.
39. Harris RE, Sundgren PC, Pang Y, Hsu M, Petrou M, Kim SH, McLean SA, Gracely RH, Clauw DJ. Dynamic levels of glutamate within the insula are associated with improvements in multiple pain domains in fibromyalgia. Arthritis Rheum 2008;58(3):903–7.

40. Hashmi JA, Baliki MN, Huang L, Baria AT, Torbey S, Hermann KM, Schnitzer TJ, Apkarian AV. Shape shifting pain: chronification of back pain shifts brain representation from nociceptive to emotional circuits. Brain 2013;136(Pt 9):2751–68.
41. Hsu MC, Harris RE, Sundgren PC, Welsh RC, Fernandes CR, Clauw DJ, Williams DA. No consistent difference in gray matter volume between individuals with fibromyalgia and age-matched healthy subjects when controlling for affective disorder. Pain 2009;143(3):262–7.
42. Huse E, Preissl H, Larbig W, Birbaumer N. Phantom limb pain. Lancet 2001;358(9286):1015.
43. Jensen MP, Day MA, Miro J. Neuromodulatory treatments for chronic pain: efficacy and mechanisms. Nat Rev Neurol 2014;10(3):167–78.
44. Jung CK, Herms J. Structural dynamics of dendritic spines are influenced by an environmental enrichment: an in vivo imaging study. Cereb Cortex 2014;24(2):377–84.
45. Juottonen K, Gockel M, Silen T, Hurri H, Hari R, Forss N. Altered central sensorimotor processing in patients with complex regional pain syndrome. Pain 2002;98(3):315–23.
46. Kaas JH. Plasticity of sensory and motor maps in adult mammals. Annu Rev Neurosci 1991;14:137–67.
47. Kamping S, Bomba IC, Kanske P, Diesch E, Flor H. Deficient modulation of pain by a positive emotional context in fibromyalgia patients. Pain 2013;154(9):1846–55.
48. Karl A, Birbaumer N, Lutzenberger W, Cohen LG, Flor H. Reorganization of motor and somatosensory cortex in upper extremity amputees with phantom limb pain. J Neurosci 2001;21(10):3609–18.
49. Kenshalo DR Jr, Giesler GJ Jr, Leonard RB, Willis WD. Responses of neurons in primate ventral posterior lateral nucleus to noxious stimuli. J Neurophysiol 1980;43(6):1594–614.
50. Kuchinad A, Schweinhardt P, Seminowicz DA, Wood PB, Chizh BA, Bushnell MC. Accelerated brain gray matter loss in fibromyalgia patients: premature aging of the brain? J Neurosci 2007;27(15):4004–7.
51. Lefaucheur JP. Use of repetitive transcranial magnetic stimulation in pain relief. Expert Rev Neurother 2008;8:799–808.
52. Linton SJ, Melin L, Götestam KG. Behavioral analysis of chronic pain and its management. In: Hersen M, Bellack A, Eisler M, editors. Progress in behavior modification. New York, NY: Academic Press; 1985. pp. 1–42.
53. Lotze M, Flor H, Grodd W, Larbig W, Birbaumer N. Phantom movements and pain: an fMRI study in upper limb amputees. Brain 2001;124(Pt 11):2268–77.
54. Lotze M, Laubis-Herrmann U, Topka H, Erb M, Grodd W. Reorganization in the primary motor cortex after spinal cord injury—a functional magnetic resonance (fMRI) study. Restor Neurol Neurosci 1999;14(2–3): 183–7.
55. MacIver K, Lloyd DM, Kelly S, Roberts N, Nurmikko T. Phantom limb pain, cortical reorganization and the therapeutic effect of mental imagery. Brain 2008;131(Pt 8):2181–91.
56. Maihofner C, Handwerker HO, Birklein F. Functional imaging of allodynia in complex regional pain syndrome. Neurology 2006;66(5):711–7.
57. Maihofner C, Handwerker HO, Neundorfer B, Birklein F. Patterns of cortical reorganization in complex regional pain syndrome. Neurology 2003;61(12):1707–15.
58. Maihofner C, Handwerker HO, Neundorfer B, Birklein F. Cortical reorganization during recovery from complex regional pain syndrome. Neurology 2004;63(4):693–701.
59. Maihöfner C, Schmelz M, Forster C, Neundorfer B, Handwerker HO. Neural activation during experimental allodynia: a functional magnetic resonance imaging study. Eur J Neurosci 2004;19(12):3211–8.
60. Makin TR, Scholz J, Filippini N, Henderson Slater D, Tracey I, Johansen-Berg H. Phantom pain is associated with preserved structure and function in the former hand area. Nat Comm 2013;4:1570.
61. Mansour AR, Baliki MN, Huang L, Torbey S, Herrmann KM, Schnitzer TJ, Apkarian AV. Brain white matter structural properties predict transition to chronic pain. Pain 2013;154(10):2160–8.
62. McCabe CS, Haigh RC, Ring EF, Halligan PW, Wall PD, Blake DR. A controlled pilot study of the utility of mirror visual feedback in the treatment of complex regional pain syndrome (type 1). Rheumatology 2003;42(1):97–101.
63. Merzenich MM, Nelson RJ, Stryker MP, Cynader MS, Schoppmann A, Zook JM. Somatosensory cortical map changes following digit amputation in adult monkeys. J Comp Neurol 1984;224(4):591–605.
64. Moseley GL. Why do people with complex regional pain syndrome take longer to recognize their affected hand? Neurology 2004;62(12):2182–6.
65. Moseley GL, Flor H. Targeting cortical representations in the treatment of chronic pain: a review. Neurorehabil Neural Repair 2012;26(6):646–52.
66. Mutso AA, Petre B, Huang L, Baliki MN, Torbey S, Herrmann K, Schnitzer TJ, Apkarian AV. Reorganization of hippocampal functional connectivity with transition to chronic back pain. J Neurophysiol 2014;111(5): 1065–76.

67. Parks EL, Geha PY, Baliki MN, Katz J, Schnitzer TJ, Apkarian AV. Brain activity for chronic knee osteoarthritis: dissociating evoked pain from spontaneous pain. Eur J Pain 2011;15(8):843.e1– e14.
68. Pleger B, Tegenthoff M, Ragert P, Forster AF, Dinse HR, Schwenkreis P, Nicolas V, Maier C. Sensorimotor retuning [corrected] in complex regional pain syndrome parallels pain reduction. Ann Neurol 2005;57(3): 425–9.
69. Raichle ME, MacLeod AM, Snyder AZ, Powers WJ, Gusnard DA, Shulman GL. A default mode of brain function. Proc Natl Acad Sci USA 2001;98(2):676–82.
70. Recanzone GH, Schreiner CE, Merzenich MM. Plasticity in the frequency representation of primary auditory cortex following discrimination training in adult owl monkeys. J Neurosci 1993;13(1):87–103.
71. Robinson ME, Craggs JG, Price DD, Perlstein WM, Staud R. Gray matter volumes of pain-related brain areas are decreased in fibromyalgia syndrome. J Pain 2011;12(4):436–43.
72. Schley M, Topfner S, Wiech K, Schaller HE, Konrad CJ, Schmelz M, Birbaumer N. Continuous brachial plexus blockade in combination with the NMDA receptor antagonist memantine prevents phantom pain in acute traumatic upper limb amputees. Eur J Pain 2007;11(3):299–308.
73. Schmidt-Wilcke T, Leinisch E, Ganssbauer S, Draganski B, Bogdahn U, Altmeppen J, May A. Affective components and intensity of pain correlate with structural differences in gray matter in chronic back pain patients. Pain 2006;125(1–2):89–97.
74. Schneider C, Palomba D, Flor H. Pavlovian conditioning of muscular responses in chronic pain patients: central and peripheral correlates. Pain 2004;112(3):239–47.
75. Schweinhardt P, Glynn C, Brooks J, McQuay H, Jack T, Chessell I, Bountra C, Tracey I. An fMRI study of cerebral processing of brush-evoked allodynia in neuropathic pain patients. NeuroImage 2006;32(1):256–65.
76. Schwenkreis P, Pleger B, Cornelius B, Weyen U, Dertwinkel R, Zenz M, Malin JP, Tegenthoff M. Reorganization in the ipsilateral motor cortex of patients with lower limb amputation. Neurosci Lett 2003;349(3):187–90.
77. Singer T, Seymour B, O'Doherty J, Kaube H, Dolan RJ, Frith CD. Empathy for pain involves the affective but not sensory components of pain. Science 2004;303(5661):1157–62.
78. Strickland TL, Miller BL, Kowell A, Stein R. Neurobiology of cocaine-induced organic brain impairment: contributions from functional neuroimaging. Neuropsychol Rev 1998;8(1):1–9.
79. Thieme K, Flor H, Turk DC. Psychological pain treatment in fibromyalgia syndrome: efficacy of operant behavioural and cognitive behavioural treatments. Arthritis Res Ther 2006;8(4):R121.
80. Thieme K, Turk DC, Flor H. Responder criteria for operant and cognitive-behavioral treatment of fibromyalgia syndrome. Arthritis Rheum 2007;57(5):830–6.
81. Vlaeyen JW, Linton SJ. Fear-avoidance and its consequences in chronic musculoskeletal pain: a state of the art. Pain 2000;85(3):317–32.
82. Willis WD, Coggeshall RE. Sensory mechanisms of the spinal cord. New York, NY: Plenum press; 1978.
83. Willoch F, Rosen G, Tolle TR, Oye I, Wester HJ, Berner N, Schwaiger M, Bartenstein P. Phantom limb pain in the human brain: unraveling neural circuitries of phantom limb sensations using positron emission tomography. Ann Neurol 2000;48(6):842–9.
84. Witting N, Kupers RC, Svensson P, Jensen TS. A PET activation study of brush-evoked allodynia in patients with nerve injury pain. Pain 2006;120(1–2):145–54.
85. Yang TT, Gallen CC, Ramachandran VS, Cobb S, Schwartz BJ, Bloom FE. Noninvasive detection of cerebral plasticity in adult human somatosensory cortex. Neuroreport 1994;5(6):701–4.

CHAPTER 21

Anatomical Reorganization of the Brain with Chronic Pain

Tobias Schmidt-Wilcke and Arne May

STRUCTURAL BRAIN IMAGING IN PAIN

In recent years, structural imaging methods have been applied to assess regional brain morphology in chronic pain patients. As with functional brain imaging, modern brain morphometry is essentially a statistical approach that compares specified parameters between two or more groups, for example, a group of patients and a group of healthy controls, which typically assumes that characteristics that distinguish these groups are associated with the disorder in question. Such parameters may include global measures (e.g., whole-brain volume, whole grey or white matter volume), regional measures (e.g., volume of a certain structure), as well as voxel/vertex based parameters including cortical thickness, voxel-based grey or white matter values (interpreted as regional grey or white matter density or volume), gyrification index, sulcal depth, and fractional anisotropy (in case of diffusion tensor imaging). Magnetic resonance–based morphometry is based on the approach of warping individual brains into a common space [3], placing the same anatomical structures across individuals into the same stereotactic positions, thereby making regional units accessible to statistical analysis. Structural brain imaging has been applied to many neurological and psychiatric diseases [8, 24, 40]. Only more recently has altered brain morphology also been described in various chronic pain conditions. The outcome parameters that have been investigated most frequently in chronic pain conditions are regional grey matter (GM) density and volume using voxel-based morphometry (VBM) [3] and cortical thickness [28]. Importantly, VBM and cortical thickness analysis, although both used to assess cortical GM, do not tap on the same constructs and thus do not yield interchangeable results [25, 26]. Diffusion tensor imaging (DTI), which provides measures of water diffusion, such as fractional anisotropy (FA) and mean diffusivity (MD), is regarded as a marker of white matter integrity.

SUMMARY OF IMPORTANT FINDINGS

Structural alterations of the brain in people with chronic pain have now been reported in a wide range of chronic pain conditions such as headaches [37, 41, 44] and facial pains [42, 55], back pain [1, 6, 29, 43], chronic widespread pain [7, 26, 30, 45], chronic neuropathic pain [20, 54], as well as chronic visceral pain [2, 31, 47]. The first studies applying VBM to detect alterations in regional brain morphology in chronic pain patients reported an increase in GM in the hypothalamus in cluster headache patients; a decrease in GM in the thalamus and dorsolateral prefrontal cortex (DLPFC) in chronic back pain patients; and a decrease in GM in the anterior cingulate cortex (ACC), midcingulate cortex (MCC), and posterior cingulate cortex, the insular cortex bilaterally, the mesial temporal lobe, and the brainstem in patients suffering from chronic tension-type headache. Since then, a number of studies have identified GM decreases in various pain syndromes, mostly in structures related to pain perception and modulation (e.g., DLPFC) and antinociception (e.g., pregenual/subgenual ACC [42, 47]). Some studies also reported increases in GM in the basal ganglia (globus pallidus/putamen) in chronic back pain patients [43], fibromyalgia patients [7, 45], vulvodynia patients [46], and patients suffering from temporomandibular disorder [55]. A recently published meta-analysis based on 23 VBM studies investigated various chronic pain conditions and described reductions in GM volume/density in several areas, including the insular cortex bilaterally, the ACC, the supplementary motor area, the thalamus, and the prefrontal cortex (the left inferior frontal gyrus and right medial frontal gyrus). The one region with higher GM volume was identified in the right medial temporal lobe.

Cortical thickness analyses have also been applied to investigate chronic pain states. Decreases in cortical thickness have been described in a number of studies, such as in the cingulate cortex of patients suffering from trigeminal neuropathic pain [9], fibromyalgia [26], and irritable bowel syndrome [11, 27]. Increases in cortical thickness, on the other hand, have been reported in the somatosensory cortices of migraine patients [10], patients with chronic low back pain [29], and female patients suffering from an irritable bowel syndrome [27].

Overall, the alterations seen in chronic pain syndromes seem to fall into one of two patterns. Most of the studies report a decrease in GM density/volume or a decrease in cortical thickness in structures known to be part of the salience network or regions involved in antinociception, or cognitive pain modulation (i.e., the dorsal ACC and MCC, the insular cortex, the pregenual ACC, and the DLPFC). Increases in regional GM, on the other hand, have been described in the basal ganglia [37, 43, 45, 46, 55], whereas cortical thickness increases were mainly found in the primary sensory cortex [10, 31]. Importantly, apart from pain *per se,* some of these findings might also be related to age and gender effects.

DTI has been applied less frequently to investigate chronic pain conditions [18, 32]. One of the first studies applying DTI described local alterations in MD and FA, indicating diminished white matter integrity in the thalamus, thalamocortical tracts, and subinsular regions of fibromyalgia patients [32]. Another study applying DTI and tractography in a patient population suffering from a complex regional pain syndrome found a decrease in FA in the left cingulum–callosal bundle, as well as altered white matter connectivity between the ventromedial prefrontal cortex and the insula (increased connectivity) and between the ventromedial prefrontal cortex and the basal ganglia (decreased connectivity) [18]. Also using tractography, higher degrees of structural connectivity between the thalamus, the prefrontal cortex, and the ACC, as well as decreased connectivity between the thalamus and the basal ganglia, have been reported in patients with irritable bowel syndrome compared with a control group [13]. Another study investigating patients with temporomandibular disorder identified the corpus callosum as having higher connectivity with the frontal pole, and lower connectivity to the DLPFC [36]. These studies underline the importance of considering alterations in network characteristics, especially of the pain system and salience network when describing altered brain structure in chronic pain patients.

LONGITUDINAL STUDIES AND TRANSIENT CHANGES

Only more recently, dynamic changes in chronic pain syndromes undergoing therapy or spontaneous remission have been described. The first study to demonstrate changes in brain morphology associated with pain investigated patients that developed a posttraumatic headache after a head injury. Initial decreases were observed in the ACC and DLPFC [37]. These changes resolved after 1 year, but only in those who became pain free; patients who continued to have pain additionally showed increases in GM in antinociceptive brainstem regions, in the thalamus, as well as the cerebellum. One study followed patients with a medication overuse headache (MOH), showing that patients with significant clinical improvement upon medication withdrawal showed a significant decrease of previously increased GM in the midbrain regions including periaqueductal grey and the nucleus cuneiformis [39]. MOH patients without improvement did not show this change; interestingly, these patients had less GM in the orbitofrontal cortex, a finding that had previously been described in MOH patients [44].

Another study investigated changes in regional brain morphology in patients suffering from painful hip arthritis. The thalamus in osteoarthritis patients exhibited a reduction in GM, preoperatively in comparison with healthy controls [21]. This reduction in GM volume could not be detected anymore 9 months after surgery (arthroplasty), indicating that a prolonged nociceptive input may induce changes in GM that are reversible after removal of the nociceptive source.

An 11-week cognitive behavioural therapy intervention for coping with chronic pain was associated with an increase in GM volume in prefrontal and somatosensory brain regions in patients suffering from chronic low back pain, suggesting that nonpharmacological treatment may act via a structural reorganization of pain modulatory regions like the DLPFC [48].

One study looked at changes of cortical thickness in chronic pain patients. Chronic low back pain patients showed a thinner cortex (decreased cortical thickness) in the DLPFC at baseline compared with healthy controls. Treatment was associated with an increase in cortical thickness in the DLPFC, which also correlated with reduction of pain and physical disability [49].

These studies suggest that structural changes in various brain regions can occur over time and are likely to be related to pain reduction or treatment via nociceptive source removal or even psychological treatment.

ALTERED BRAIN STRUCTURE—INTERPRETATIONS AND IMPLICATIONS

The neurobiological correlates of changes in regional brain morphology associated with chronic pain, in terms of tissue composition, are still not fully elucidated. To our knowledge, there is no study that has cross-correlated MRI and postmortem findings in humans. As such, our interpretations with respect to histological/cellular correlates of VBM/cortical thickness findings are dependent on animal studies in the framework of peripherally driven pain models, for example, induced by nerve or muscle damage [35].

GM decreases are likely to reflect tissue shrinkage, affecting neural tissue (neurons and glia), vasculature, and extracellular volume. In the light of spectroscopy findings, we have suggested that GM changes (decreases) might result from neurodegenerative processes that affect size or number of neurons and/or neuroglia [19]. This notion, however, has been challenged by several VBM studies that describe a reversibility of GM decreases either spontaneously [37] or after surgical intervention to treat a peripheral, nociceptive source (see above).

On the spinal level, animal studies have revealed neuronal apoptosis, with a predominant impact on GABAergic interneurons following prolonged nociceptive input [53]. We suggested that some chronic pain conditions are associated with decreased GABA levels (measured in supraspinal structures, e.g., insular cortex) [16, 38]. If neuronal loss preferentially affected inhibitory interneurons, it is conceivable that increased (spontaneous) activity in areas known to be involved in pain processing might influence subsequent pain perception and contribute to spontaneous pain, at the same time leading to GM decreases as revealed by structural brain imaging [20]. Astrocytes, as another subtype of neuroglia, are critically involved in potassium homeostasis and glutamate reuptake, thereby having a direct influence on neuronal activity and metabolism [23]. Given the literature suggesting increased glutamate/glutamine (GLX) levels in chronic pain states [24, 38] (e.g., fibromyalgia, diabetic neuropathy), another link to VBM findings could be the neurotoxic effect of excessive GLX levels, corroborating an overall decrease in neural tissue. However, to our knowledge, no clear association between GLX levels and GM density/volume has been established.

In recent years, changes in brain function and brain morphology have increasingly been interpreted in the light of the broader concept of neuroplasticity, which refers to the ability of brain tissue to reorganize itself and thereby change its function and morphology. This is especially relevant when considering the dynamic aspects of changes in brain morphology associated with chronic pain and pain chronification. Neural reorganization can range from synaptic plasticity to changes in complex neural circuitry (e.g., LTP, long-term depression, synaptic sprouting, neurogenesis [5], and glial reorganization). Neuroplasticity is thought to take place physiologically in response to new environmental demands, thereby improving the individual's goal-directed performance. Interestingly, it could be demonstrated that repeated painful stimulation resulted in a substantial increase of GM in classical somatosensory areas, including the MCC and somatosensory cortex [50]. These data are in line with most morphometric studies investigating structural brain plasticity as a result of exercise and learning [12, 17, 34]. In this context, we have proposed that a prolonged nociceptive input or a decrease in physiological sensory input may serve as a trigger for *maladaptive* neuroplasticity, which then serves as the actual basis of chronic pain (no longer—or only marginally—dependent upon the initial peripheral input).

Most of the studies investigating regional GM or cortical thickness in chronic pain patients are cross-sectional studies, inferring that differences between groups are based on dynamic changes that previously occurred in the pain patients. Indeed, it is highly likely that for most chronic pain conditions, GM changes are dynamic and take place over time, contributing to pain chronification. As outlined previously, some recent longitudinal studies demonstrated that GM changes can be induced by repeated experimental pain [50], and that changes associated with clinical pain can reverse spontaneously [37] and/or after therapy [22, 49], which underlines the structural dynamics of the system. However, brain morphology in certain brain regions correlates with experimental pain thresholds in healthy subjects [14, 15], indicating that brain structure and pain perception also interact in the nonchronic pain state. Thus, morphological changes in these brain regions might reflect pain sensitivity, or possibly even a certain vulnerability to develop a chronic pain condition.

Given that the larger part of changes in regional brain morphology do develop over time, we and others have proposed that the initial "reaction" of the brain is a GM increase in certain pain-transmitting areas [2, 7], such as the MCC, the somatosensory cortex, and the basal ganglia [50–52]. This initial increase in GM might at first be an adaptive mechanism. However, a transition to a chronic pain state might then take place in some patients, depending on the duration and persistence of the nociceptive input, local characteristics of the neural tissue, as well as other factors such as capacity/effectiveness of antinociceptive systems (for a conceptual approach, see Fig. 21-3). This transition is marked by a decrease in regional GM in the pain system. These changes, once they occur, are likely to contribute to an ongoing pain perception, even after the initial nociceptive source has been eliminated. These changes in GM vary between pain states and brain structures involved, and each alteration is likely to depend further on pain duration, pain occurrence (intermittent vs. persistent), and other factors influencing pain perception, such as personality traits and medication—all factors contributing to the high variability of VBM and cortical thickness findings across pain conditions and studies. Importantly, it is also conceivable that patients do not run through these phases successively, but react differently right from the beginning of the pain chronification process. We propose that these two phases/types could be descriptively referred to as an *atrophy* and a *hypertrophy phase/type* (see Figs. 21-1 and 21-2), characterized by reductions or higher levels in regional GM, as determined by structural brain imaging. Importantly, these terms, as suggested here, are used rather metaphorically and are not meant to make any assumptions on cellular/histological correlates, which remain to be determined.

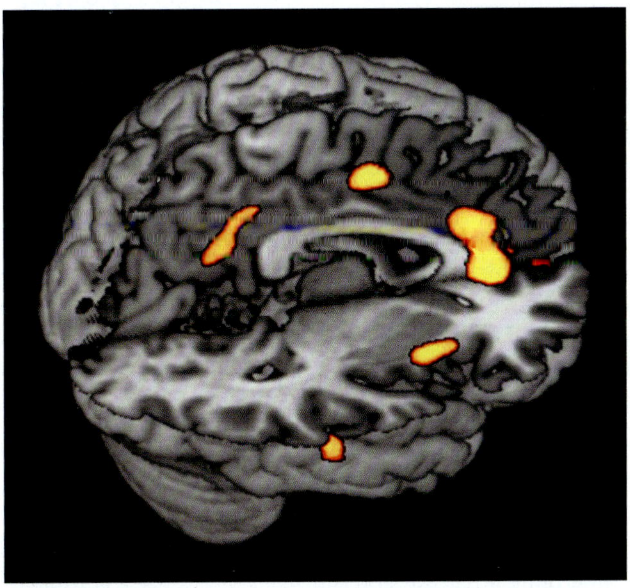

FIGURE 21-1 Anatomical reorganization of the brain with chronic pain. Chronic pain syndrome—chronic tension-type headache—associated with grey matter reductions in the cingulate cortex, the insular cortex, and the superior/middle temporal gyrus (reported in Schmidt-Wilcke et al. [44]).

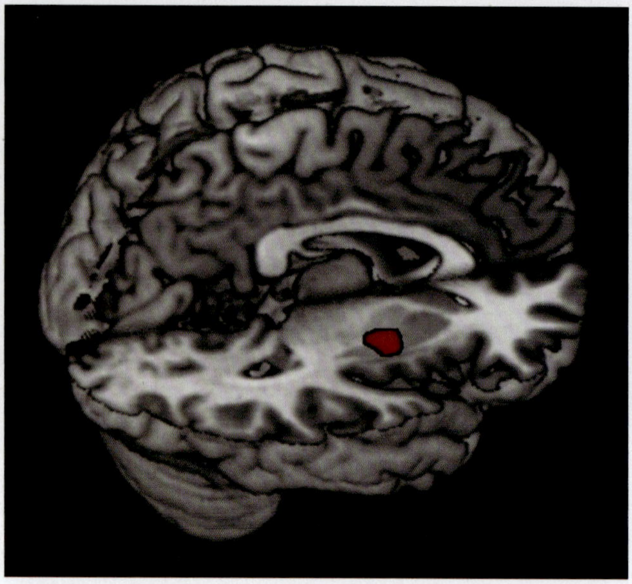

FIGURE 21-2 Structural alterations in chronic pain—hypertrophy type. Chronic pain syndrome—fibromyalgia—associated with higher levels of GM in the basal ganglia (putamen, reported in Schmidt-Wilcke et al. [45]).

LIMITATION AND CRITICISM

Apart from the ill-defined histological/cellular interpretation of VBM findings, discussed previously, there is quite a variability in reported findings, which is related to relatively small sample sizes, poor control for pain duration and comorbidities (e.g., depression and anxiety, medication intake), as well as differences in image preprocessing. Only in a few cases could study results be reproduced by another group. Structural brain imaging in fibromyalgia, for example, revealed conflicting results with one study reporting only decreases in the cingulum and in the medial temporal lobe, one study reporting decreases in the thalamus and superior temporal gyrus, but increases in the basal ganglia, and one study reporting decreases in the left insula, which disappeared after correcting for depression scores. A recently published study that looked more specifically at age effects reported an increase in GM in the basal ganglia in the under 50 group, whereas the older group showed a pattern of GM atrophy in various parts of the pain system, such as the cingulum. Apart from age, disease state, and comorbidities, which all need to be accounted for in a more systematic way, there is only seemingly a clear definition for chronic pain and pain chronification. As such, the term chronic pain only refers to the minimum amount of time for which the patient has had pain. Otherwise, it is rather uninformative on the pain days per month, the actual time of pain during the day, and the occurrence pattern (i.e., continuous vs. intermittent). In a patient suffering from intermittent pelvic pain, a proprioceptive input from a filling bladder might stimulate a hypersensitive pain system associated with an increase in GM in the somatosensory system. In turn, the proprioceptive signal may be interpreted as intermittent pain several times per day, while a chronic tension-type headache patient, associated with decrease in the cingulum and the insular cortices, might suffer from continuous pain, completely independent from any peripherally generated nociceptive or proprioceptive input. Although both pain states would be considered chronic, given that they occur for more than 3 months, the underlying mechanisms and the role of the brain (and

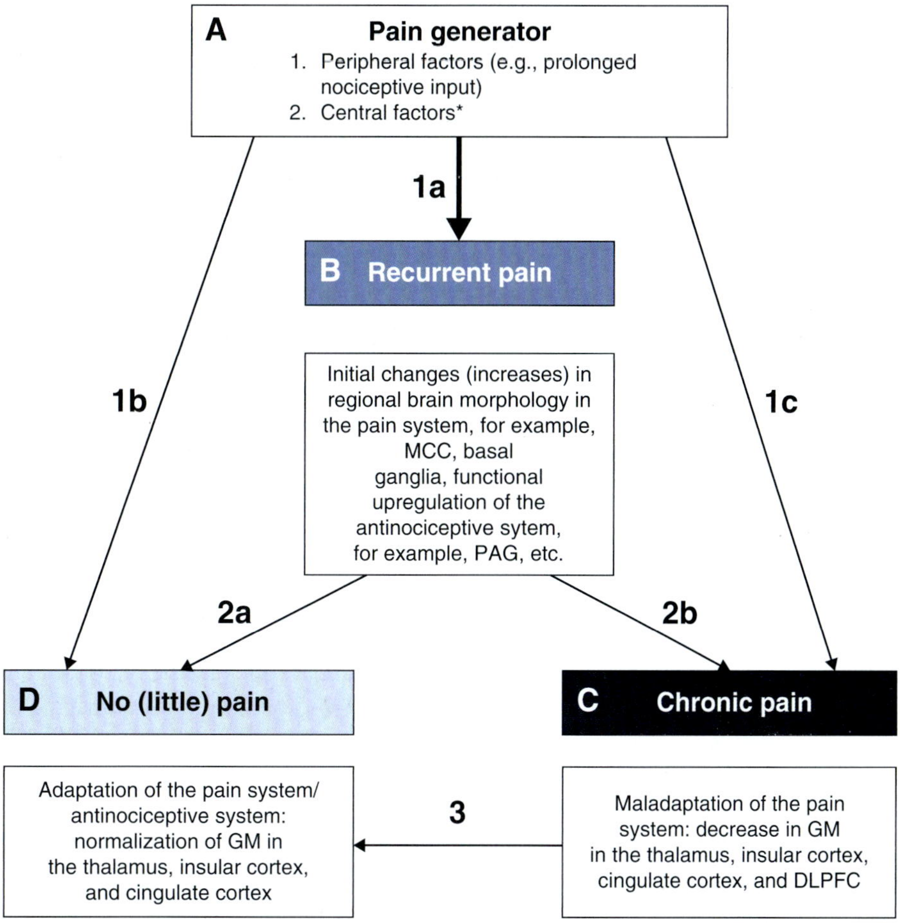

FIGURE 21-3 Structural changes in chronic pain—a conceptual approach. Possible mechanisms of pain chronification. **Box A:** Initially, a nociceptive source serves as a "pain generator," inducing recurrent pain associated with changes in regional brain morphology and metabolism. *Central factors such as anxiety and catastrophizing may increase vulnerability, sensitizing the brain to nociceptive neural input. Patients who progress to chronic pain show maladaptive changes in the pain system. Less commonly, this may occur without a preceding phase of recurrent/frequent pain (*arrow* 1c). **Box D:** Those patients who experience resolution of their intermittent (*arrow* 2a) or chronic pain (*arrow* 3), and those who do not experience pain despite having a peripheral pain generator (1b) show a "normalization" of or no change in GM in the pain system.

its structure) might be quite different. This kind of information is of essential importance in determining where in the structural reorganization process the patient might be and to launch imaging studies, which in that respect rely on more homogeneous study samples.

CONCLUSION AND OUTLOOK

The findings put forth by structural brain imaging have contributed substantially to the notion that chronic pain cannot be thought of as just an endless string of nociceptive signals being processed by an otherwise healthy/normal central pain system. Chronic pain has to be interpreted, at least in parts, as a result of neural reorganization of the CNS, associated with changes in regional brain structure. With respect to the variability of imaging findings, obstructing a clear picture of the interaction of pain and brain structure, we have proposed a biphasic model suggesting that a prolonged nociceptive input leads to an initial increase, mainly in the basal ganglia and primary sensory cortex, followed by a decrease in various parts of the pain system, particularly the cingulate and insular cortices. Arguably, the structural differences seen, especially those in dysfunctional pain syndromes, might not reflect a maladaptive process to a prolonged nociceptive input, but rather might be preexisting, leading to an increased vulnerability to the development of chronic pain via disturbed proprioception. Given that the large portion of pain syndromes where either no clear-cut nociceptive source can be identified or the degree of peripheral pathology does not correlate with the degree of pain or suffering, structural brain imaging has explicitly pointed to central mechanisms that are likely to play a critical role in the maintenance of chronic pain.

In addition to the need to fully elucidate the neural correlates of VBM, cortical thickness, and DTI findings, further improvement of structural brain imaging as research tools will not only depend on methodological improvements (higher magnetic field strength, optimized preprocessing protocols, etc.) but also heavily rely on the clinical information that is fed into the analyses. In this regard, statistical brain imaging is only as good as its clinical information; these techniques also have the capability to unravel differences in pathological mechanisms in clinically similar pain conditions.

New developments, such as structural network analysis [4, 31], multimodal imaging, that is, the combination of VBM/cortical thickness with other imaging methods, such as resting-state fMRI [26], and multivariate analyses are now being established and applied to unravel more complex features of structural changes seen in chronic pain patients. Multivariate analyses can be used to build classifiers, and thus have the potential to find clinical applications, such as helping to determine a certain chronification stage and/or the likelihood of subacute pain transitioning into a chronic pain condition [33]. In this regard, the development of structural brain imaging in the years to come will be quite exciting.

ACKNOWLEDGEMENT

We would like to thank Lauren Haag for very valuable discussion.

REFERENCES

1. Apkarian AV, Sosa Y, Sonty S, Levy RM, Harden RN, Parrish TB, Gitelman DR. Chronic back pain is associated with decreased prefrontal and thalamic gray matter density. J Neurosci 2004;24(46):10410–5.
2. As-Sanie S, Harris RE, Napadow V, Kim J, Neshewat G, Kairys A, Williams D, Clauw DJ, Schmidt-Wilcke T. Changes in regional gray matter volume in women with chronic pelvic pain: a voxel-based morphometry study. Pain 2012;153(5):1006–14.
3. Ashburner J, Friston KJ. Voxel-based morphometry—the methods. NeuroImage 2000;11(6 Pt 1):805–21.
4. Baliki MN, Schnitzer TJ, Bauer WR, Apkarian AV. Brain morphological signatures for chronic pain. PloS One 2011;6(10):e26010.
5. Bruel-Jungerman E, Davis S, Laroche S. Brain plasticity mechanisms and memory: a party of four. Neuroscientist 2007;13(5):492–505.
6. Buckalew N, Haut MW, Morrow L, Weiner D. Chronic pain is associated with brain volume loss in older adults: preliminary evidence. Pain Med 2008;9(2):240–8.
7. Ceko M, Bushnell MC, Fitzcharles MA, Schweinhardt P. Fibromyalgia interacts with age to change the brain. Neuroimage Clin 2013;3:249–60.

8. Chetelat G, Desgranges B, de la Sayette V, Viader F, Berkouk K, Landeau B, Lalevee C, Le Doze F, Dupuy B, Hannequin D, et al. Dissociating atrophy and hypometabolism impact on episodic memory in mild cognitive impairment. Brain 2003;126(Pt 9):1955–67.
9. DaSilva AF, Becerra L, Pendse G, Chizh B, Tully S, Borsook D. Colocalized structural and functional changes in the cortex of patients with trigeminal neuropathic pain. PloS One 2008;3(10):e3396.
10. DaSilva AF, Granziera C, Snyder J, Hadjikhani N. Thickening in the somatosensory cortex of patients with migraine. Neurology 2007;69(21):1990–5.
11. Davis KD, Pope G, Chen J, Kwan CL, Crawley AP, Diamant NE. Cortical thinning in IBS: implications for homeostatic, attention, and pain processing. Neurology 2008;70(2):153–4.
12. Draganski B, Gaser C, Busch V, Schuierer G, Bogdahn U, May A. Neuroplasticity: changes in grey matter induced by training. Nature 2004;427(6972):311–2.
13. Ellingson BM, Mayer E, Harris RJ, Ashe-McNally C, Naliboff BD, Labus JS, Tillisch K. Diffusion tensor imaging detects microstructural reorganization in the brain associated with chronic irritable bowel syndrome. Pain 2013;154(9):1528–41.
14. Elsenbruch S, Schmid J, Kullmann JS, Kattoor J, Theysohn N, Forsting M, Kotsis V. Visceral sensitivity correlates with decreased regional gray matter volume in healthy volunteers: a voxel-based morphometry study. Pain 2014;155(2):244–9.
15. Erpelding N, Moayedi M, Davis KD. Cortical thickness correlates of pain and temperature sensitivity. Pain 2012;153(8):1602–9.
16. Foerster BR, Petrou M, Edden RA, Sundgren PC, Schmidt-Wilcke T, Lowe SE, Harte SE, Clauw DJ, Harris RE. Reduced insular gamma-aminobutyric acid in fibromyalgia. Arthritis Rheum 2012;64(2):579–83.
17. Gaser C, Schlaug G. Brain structures differ between musicians and non-musicians. J Neurosci 2003;23(27): 9240–5.
18. Geha PY, Baliki MN, Harden RN, Bauer WR, Parrish TB, Apkarian AV. The brain in chronic CRPS pain: abnormal gray-white matter interactions in emotional and autonomic regions. Neuron 2008;60(4):570–81.
19. Grachev ID, Fredrickson BE, Apkarian AV. Abnormal brain chemistry in chronic back pain: an in vivo proton magnetic resonance spectroscopy study. Pain 2000;89(1):7–18.
20. Gustin SM, Peck CC, Wilcox SL, Nash PG, Murray GM, Henderson LA. Different pain, different brain: thalamic anatomy in neuropathic and non-neuropathic chronic pain syndromes. J Neurosci 2011;31(16):5956–64.
21. Gwilym SE, Filippini N, Douaud G, Carr AJ, Tracey I. Thalamic atrophy associated with painful osteoarthritis of the hip is reversible after arthroplasty: a longitudinal voxel-based morphometric study. Arthritis Rheum 2010;62(10):2930–40.
22. Hansson E, Ronnback L. Altered neuronal-glial signaling in glutamatergic transmission as a unifying mechanism in chronic pain and mental fatigue. Neurochem Res 2004;29(5):989–96.
23. Harris RE. Elevated excitatory neurotransmitter levels in the fibromyalgia brain. Arthritis Res Ther 2010;12(5):141.
24. Hazlett-Stevens H, Craske MG, Mayer EA, Chang L, Naliboff BD. Prevalence of irritable bowel syndrome among university students: the roles of worry, neuroticism, anxiety sensitivity and visceral anxiety. J Psychosom Res 2003;55(6):501–5.
25. Hutton C, Draganski B, Ashburner J, Weiskopf N. A comparison between voxel based cortical thickness and voxel-based morphometry in normal aging. NeuroImage 2009;48(2):371–80.
26. Jensen KB, Srinivasan P, Spaeth R, Tan Y, Kosek E, Petzke F, Carville S, Fransson P, Marcus H, Williams SC, et al. Overlapping structural and functional brain changes in patients with long-term exposure to fibromyalgia pain. Arthritis Rheum 2013;65(12):3293–303.
27. Jiang Z, Dinov ID, Labus J, Shi Y, Zamanyan A, Gupta A, Ashe-McNalley C, Hong JY, Tillisch K, Toga AW, Mayer EA. Sex-related differences of cortical thickness in patients with chronic abdominal pain. PloS One 2013;8(9):e73932.
28. Jones SE, Buchbinder BR, Aharon I. Three-dimensional mapping of cortical thickness using Laplace's equation. Hum Brain Mapp 2000;11(1):12–32.
29. Kong J, Spaeth RB, Wey HY, Cheetham A, Cook AH, Jensen K, Tan Y, Liu H, Wang D, Loggia ML, et al. S1 is associated with chronic low back pain: a functional and structural MRI study. Mol Pain 2013;9(1):43.
30. Kuchinad A, Schweinhardt P, Seminowicz DA, Wood PB, Chizh BA, Bushnell MC. Accelerated brain gray matter loss in fibromyalgia patients: premature aging of the brain? J Neurosci 2007;27(15):4004–7.
31. Labus JS, Dinov ID, Jiang Z, Ashe-McNalley C, Zamanyan A, Shi Y, Hong JY, Gupta A, Tillisch K, Ebrat B, et al. Irritable bowel syndrome in female patients is associated with alterations in structural brain networks. Pain 2014;155(1):137–79.

32. Lutz J, Jager L, de Quervain D, Krauseneck T, Padberg F, Wichnalek M, Beyer A, Stahl R, Zirngibl B, Morhard D, et al. White and gray matter abnormalities in the brain of patients with fibromyalgia: a diffusion-tensor and volumetric imaging study. Arthritis Rheum 2008;58(12):3960–9.
33. Mansour AR, Baliki MN, Huang L, Torbey S, Herrmann KM, Schnitzer TJ, Apkarian AV. Brain white matter structural properties predict transition to chronic pain. Pain 2013;154(10):2160–8.
34. May A, Hajak G, Ganssbauer S, Steffens T, Langguth B, Kleinjung T, Eichhammer P. Structural brain alterations following 5 days of intervention: dynamic aspects of neuroplasticity. Cereb Cortex 2007;17(1):205–10.
35. Metz AE, Yau HJ, Centeno MV, Apkarian AV, Martina M. Morphological and functional reorganization of rat medial prefrontal cortex in neuropathic pain. Proc Natl Acad Sci USA 2009;106(7):2423–8.
36. Moayedi M, Weissman-Fogel I, Salomons TV, Crawley AP, Goldberg MB, Freeman BV, Tenenbaum HC, Davis KD. White matter brain and trigeminal nerve abnormalities in temporomandibular disorder. Pain 2012;153(7):1467–77.
37. Obermann M, Nebel K, Schumann C, Holle D, Gizewski ER, Maschke M, Goadsby PJ, Diener HC, Katsarava Z. Gray matter changes related to chronic posttraumatic headache. Neurology 2009;73(12):978–83.
38. Petrou M, Pop-Busui R, Foerster BR, Edden RA, Callaghan BC, Harte SE, Harris RE, Clauw DJ, Feldman EL. Altered excitation-inhibition balance in the brain of patients with diabetic neuropathy. Acad Radiol 2012;19(5):607–12.
39. Riederer F, Gantenbein AR, Marti M, Luechinger R, Kollias S, Sandor PS. Decrease of gray matter volume in the midbrain is associated with treatment response in medication-overuse headache: possible influence of orbitofrontal cortex. J Neuroscience 2013;33(39):15343–9.
40. Sastre-Garriga J, Ingle GT, Chard DT, Cercignani M, Ramio-Torrenta L, Miller DH, Thompson AJ. Grey and white matter volume changes in early primary progressive multiple sclerosis: a longitudinal study. Brain 2005;128(Pt 6):1454–60.
41. Schmidt-Wilcke T, Ganssbauer S, Neuner T, Bogdahn U, May A. Subtle grey matter changes between migraine patients and healthy controls. Cephalalgia 2008;28(1):1–4.
42. Schmidt-Wilcke T, Hierlmeier S, Leinisch E. Altered regional brain morphology in patients with chronic facial pain. Headache 2010;50(8):1278–85.
43. Schmidt-Wilcke T, Leinisch E, Ganssbauer S, Draganski B, Bogdahn U, Altmeppen J, May A. Affective components and intensity of pain correlate with structural differences in gray matter in chronic back pain patients. Pain 2006;125(1–5)89–97.
44. Schmidt-Wilcke T, Leinisch E, Straube A, Kampfe N, Draganski B, Diener HC, Bogdahn U, May A. Gray matter decrease in patients with chronic tension type headache. Neurology 2005;65(9):1483–6.
45. Schmidt-Wilcke T, Luerding R, Weigand T, Jurgens T, Schuierer G, Leinisch E, Bogdahn U. Striatal grey matter increase in patients suffering from fibromyalgia—a voxel-based morphometry study. Pain 2007;132(Suppl 1):S109–16.
46. Schweinhardt P, Kuchinad A, Pukall CF, Bushnell MC. Increased gray matter density in young women with chronic vulvar pain. Pain 2008;140(3):411–9.
47. Seminowicz DA, Labus JS, Bueller JA, Tillisch K, Naliboff BD, Bushnell MC, Mayer EA. Regional gray matter density changes in brains of patients with irritable bowel syndrome. Gastroenterology 2010;139(1):48–57.e42.
48. Seminowicz DA, Shpaner M, Keaser ML, Krauthamer GM, Mantegna J, Dumas JA, Newhouse PA, Filippi CG, Keefe FJ, Naylor MR. Cognitive-behavioral therapy increases prefrontal cortex gray matter in patients with chronic pain. J Pain 2013;14(12):1573–84.
49. Seminowicz DA, Wideman TH, Naso L, Hatami-Khoroushahi Z, Fallatah S, Ware MA, Jarzem P, Bushnell MC, Shir Y, Ouellet JA, et al. Effective treatment of chronic low back pain in humans reverses abnormal brain anatomy and function. J Neurosci 2011;31(20):7540–50.
50. Teutsch S, Herken W, Bingel U, Schoell E, May A. Changes in brain gray matter due to repetitive painful stimulation. NeuroImage 2008;42(2):845–9.
51. Tu CH, Niddam DM, Chao HT, Chen LF, Chen YS, Wu YT, Yeh TC, Lirng JF, Hsieh JC. Brain morphological changes associated with cyclic menstrual pain. Pain 2010;150(3):462–8.
52. Tu CH, Niddam DM, Chao HT, Liu RS, Hwang RJ, Yeh TC, Hsieh JC. Abnormal cerebral metabolism during menstrual pain in primary dysmenorrhea. NeuroImage 2009;47(1):28–35.
53. Whiteside GT, Munglani R. Cell death in the superficial dorsal horn in a model of neuropathic pain. J Neurosci Res 2001;64(2):168–73.
54. Yoon EJ, Kim YK, Shin HI, Lee Y, Kim SE. Cortical and white matter alterations in patients with neuropathic pain after spinal cord injury. Brain Res 2013;1540:64–73.
55. Younger JW, Shen YF, Goddard G, Mackey SC. Chronic myofascial temporomandibular pain is associated with neural abnormalities in the trigeminal and limbic systems. Pain 2010;149(2):222–8.

CHAPTER 22

Resting-State Alterations in Chronic Pain

Diana M. Torta, Franco Cauda, Vitaly Napadow, and Marwan N. Baliki

RESTING STATE

Early histological studies of brain tissue showed that neuronal elements of the brain construct a complicated structural network. During the past two decades, advances in brain imaging techniques, namely functional magnetic resonance imaging (fMRI), have shown that human brains exhibit modular and hierarchical attributes in common with other complex systems. In this respect, brain functions can be described as global integration of information across different modules or networks. Such networks are thought to provide the physiological basis for information processing and mental representations, and to reflect the cumulative effect of learned experiences throughout lifetime.

Brain functional organization is generally inferred from the correlation between nodal activities (comprising individual voxels or groups of voxels or regions) on the basis of blood oxygenation level–dependent (BOLD) fMRI or coherence in electro- or magnetoencephalogram (EEG/MEG) signals acquired during task or rest. Resting-state fMRI (rs-fMRI), in particular, has become an important basis for studying the functional network properties of the brain. Usually, rs-fMRI focuses on the analysis of spontaneous fluctuations in the BOLD signal [21]. During rs-fMRI, participants are required to relax and not think of anything in particular; the cofluctuation of the BOLD signal across distinct brain regions is thought to reflect functional connectivity (FC) between brain areas. That is, areas that fluctuate together are probably functionally wired together. Typically, these fluctuations are evaluated in very low-frequency ranges (~0.008–0.25 Hz). Importantly, rs-fMRI per se is unable to provide a measure of causality (e.g., activity in one brain area causing activity in another area), indeed, the only inference that can be extracted from this analysis remains correlative. The most popular techniques for performing rs-fMRI analysis include (1) independent component analysis (ICA), (2) seed-based correlation, and (3) graph theoretical approaches (Fig. 22-1), with ICA and seed-based correlation being the most commonly used. In seed-based correlation, the signal is extracted from a specific region of interest (ROI) and its temporal profile correlated with that of all other brain voxels [8, 21]. Alternatively, ICA is a data-driven approach that considers all activated voxels and groups them into clusters that are correlated with their spontaneous fluctuations [11].

RESTING STATE AND CHRONIC PAIN

Rs-fMRI techniques offer the unique opportunity of studying brain activity without the administration of a task. They have been widely exploited to characterize the "rest" activity of the brain in several pathological conditions, such as depression, schizophrenia, dementia,

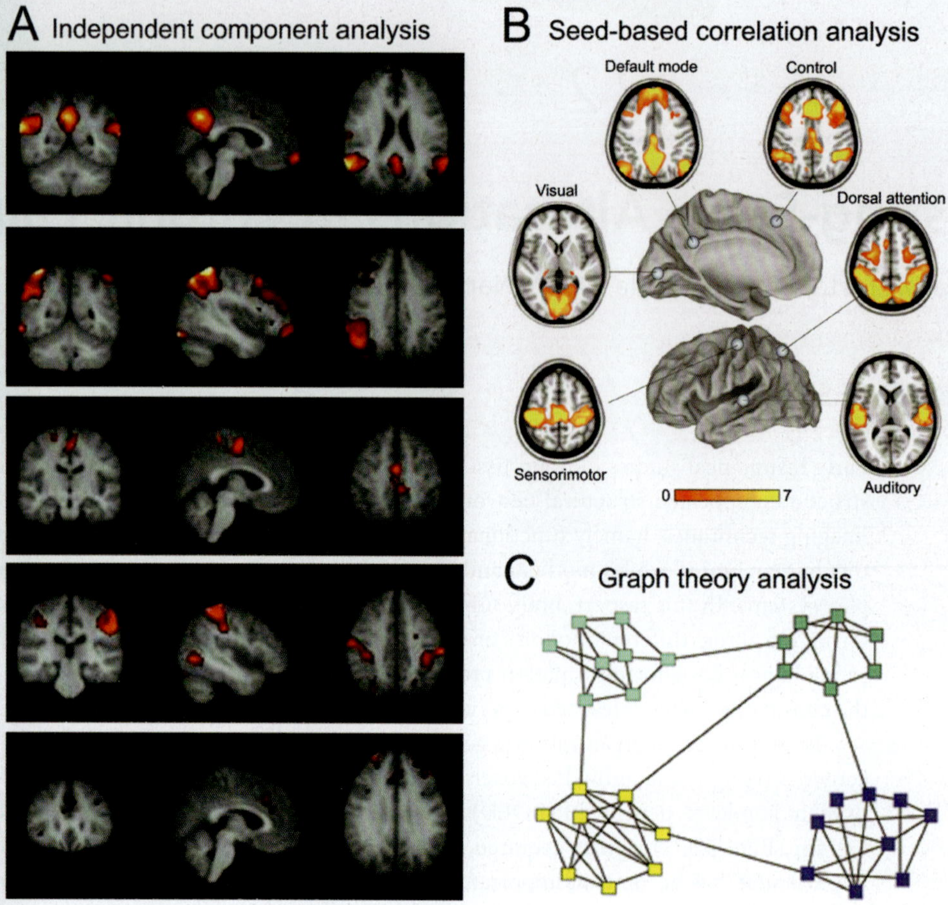

FIGURE 22-1 Methods for analyzing the brain as a network. A: Independent component analysis (ICA) shows that the resting state has consistent spatial temporal patterns. (Adapted from Damoiseaux et al. [18].) **B:** Same networks can be inferred from seed-based correlation analysis (Zhang and Raichle [49]). **C:** Diagram showing the modular properties of brain networks. Each colour represents a separate functional unit. Graph measurements can be used to identify topological properties.

and chronic pain (see [20] for a critical discussion). Chronic pain is a condition in which pain persists beyond the healing phase. Chronic pain states are usually divided into neuropathic and inflammatory, depending on the underlying etiology [1] (see also [44]). The site of pain is also considered when describing the pain syndrome. Research is now attempting to ascertain whether, at a cortical level, specific signatures can be identified for each chronic pain state, in terms of both anatomical and functional peculiarities [19]. To date, multiple brain functional and anatomical studies show that various chronic pain conditions are associated with metabolic and anatomical changes within large-scale distributed networks underlying various physiological processes, including autonomic, sensorimotor, cognitive, and emotional processes. Such outcomes emphasize the divergence in brain representation of chronic and acute pain, which negate the notion that brain activity associated with chronic pain is localized to a definitive neural substrate, reflecting peripheral and spinal changes following injury.

Within this framework, the application of rs-fMRI to the study of chronic pain has, at least, two advantages. First, since pain is a complex experience, emerging from the integration of information between multiple brain regions [2, 16, 32], rs-fMRI is able to picture brain activity in terms of networks and not of single areas. Second, chronic pain states are characterized by a fluctuation of the ongoing pain. In this sense, rs-fMRI offers the unique chance of detailing the natural state of chronic pain, correlating spontaneous BOLD fluctuations with concomitant changes in pain perception. The number of studies characterizing rs-fMRI connectivity in chronic pain is increasing, as outlined in Table 22-1.

Chronic back pain, fibromyalgia (FM), and migraine remain the most explored, but insights have also been provided for postherpetic neuralgia and diabetic pain, temporomandibular disorder, complex regional pain syndrome (CRPS), and irritable bowel syndrome (IBS).

Chronic Back Pain

The first evidence of the impact of chronic pain on functional brain networks was reported in chronic back pain patients [6]. The authors observed that patients, compared with controls, had lower deactivations of the default-mode network (DMN) during the performance of a simple visual task. The DMN is a commonly observed brain network comprising the ventromedial prefrontal cortex (PFC), the posterior cingulate cortex (PCC), the precuneus, the medial temporal gyri, and the inferior parietal cortices. It is thought to be implicated in self-referential cognitive processing, self-awareness, and self-monitoring. The involvement of the medial prefrontal cortex (MPFC) in online monitoring of pain fluctuations has been confirmed by subsequent studies. For instance, Baliki and colleagues [5] demonstrated that increased fluctuation power in this region was synchronous with spontaneous pain changes. BOLD oscillations in the MPFC of back pain patients were also characterized by an aberrant high-frequency (0.12–0.20 Hz) power. Adding to this, Tagliazucchi et al. [43] observed that the middle frontal gyrus showed increased FC with the bilateral insula in these patients. A recent study also found that DMN–insula connectivity was associated with clinical pain at the time of the scan, and that increases in pain following physical manoeuvres in these patients were correlated with increased DMN–insula connectivity, specifically linking this potential neuroimaging biomarker with clinical pain [29].

Another fruitful approach to the study of network dynamics is given by the application of graph theories [10]. Balenzuela and colleagues [4] applied graph theoretical analysis to the resting-state BOLD time series of healthy controls and chronic back pain patients. They first calculated the mutual coactivity of 90 brain regions, selected on an anatomical basis, and then constructed network modules. Network modules were defined in terms of density of the nodes by which they are constructed: nodes of a module should be similar among one another and different with respect to nodes of other modules. Network modules were then portioned to obtain communities, modules having a similar temporal profile. Interestingly, the authors observed that healthy controls and chronic low back pain (cLBP) patients did not differ in the number of identified communities. Instead, the two groups differed for memberships, meaning that brain regions were not grouped in the same way. This suggests that the FC of some regions is altered. In detail, patients showed increased functional correlation in regions such as the orbitofrontal cortex, the insula, and the anterior cingulate cortex (ACC).

Altogether, these findings suggest that chronic back pain is associated with abnormal high-frequency activity in the prefrontal regions, accompanied by increased FC between these areas, the insula, and the ACC.

A divergent result was obtained by Kornelsen and colleagues [28]. They used ICA to compare the DMN of failed back surgery patients with that of healthy volunteers. These authors concluded that healthy controls showed significantly larger and more active clusters

TABLE 22-1 **Summary of Studies Characterizing Resting-State Functional Connectivity in Chronic Pain**

Study	Chronic Pain State	Resting-State Method	Affected Areas or Networks	Main Findings (Patients Compared with Controls)	Control Group	Relation with Clinical Characteristics
Balenzuela et al. [10]	Back pain	Whole-brain network topology (mutual partial correlation)	Frontal lobes, anterior cingulate, insula, basal ganglia, somatosensory cortices, parietotemporal, sensorimotor, frontomedial communities	Same number of communities, different memberships. Different FC between frontal lobes and anterior cingulate	Healthy volunteers	Not explored
Baliki et al. [5]	Back pain	Power spectral analysis (0.01–0.20 Hz)	Medial PFC and DMN	Increased power of high-frequency oscillations (0.12–0.20) in medial PFC	Healthy volunteers	Increased fluctuations were synchronous to spontaneous pain changes
Tagliazucchi et al. [43]	Back pain	Seed-based correlation analysis	Middle frontal gyrus, right and left angular gyri	Increased correlation between middle frontal gyrus, angular gyrus, and right and left insula	Healthy volunteers	
Loggia et al. [29]	Back pain	ICA	DMN, pregenual ACC, left inferior parietal lobule, rINS, and clinical pain	Stronger DMN connectivity to the pgACC, left inferior parietal lobule, and rINS in patients		Positive correlation between patients' baseline clinical pain and strength between the DMN and rINS (DMN–rINS connectivity) Changes in DMN–insula connectivity related to manoeuvres used to exacerbate pain
Napadow et al. [34]	FM	ICA	DMN, EAN, MVN	Greater connectivity within DMN and EAN	Healthy volunteers	Spontaneous pain correlated with greater intrinsic connectivity between insula and both DMN and rEAN
Cifre et al. [17]	FM	Seed-based	Insula, ACC, basal ganglia	Increased FC between insula and ACC and basal ganglia; between S2 and the amygdala; the MPFC with PCC. Reduced connectivity between insula and PAG.		Negative correlations between depression

Study	Chronic Pain State	Resting-State Method	Affected Areas or Networks	Main Findings (Patients Compared with Controls)	Control Group	Relation with Clinical Characteristics
Kim et al. [25]	FM	PSD (0.01–0.25 Hz)	S1 SMA, DLPFC, amygdala	Increased PSD in S1, SMA, DLPFC, and amygdala	Healthy female volunteers	No association with depression or anxiety
Schwedt et al. [38]	Migraine	Seed-based correlation analysis	Anterior insula, amygdala, pulvinar, mediodorsal thalamus, middle temporal cortex, PAG	Lack of correlation between left anterior insula and precuneus and right anterior insula and pulvinar in patients. Positive correlation between left insula and left middle temporal cortex in patients (negative correlation in controls).		Connectivity of insula–mediodorsal thalamus and insula–PAG correlated with duration of pain
Xue et al. [47]	Migraine without aura	ICA	DMN, CEN, SN	Aberrant intrinsic connectivity between the CEN and SN; greater connectivity between the DMN and the insula and the CEN and the insula	Healthy controls	Greater connectivity of the DMN and rCEN correlated with the duration of the migraine
Xue et al. [46]	Migraine without aura	ALFF and ROI-based seed voxel correlational analysis (0.01–0.08 Hz)	rACC, thalamus, insula, bilateral PFC, DMN, executive network	(1) Reduced power in left rACC and bilateral PFC; increased power in thalamus. (2) A general increase in FC.		
Hadjikhani et al. [22]	Migraine with and without aura	Seed voxel correlation	Amygdala, thalamus, anterior insula, S2	Increased connectivity between the amygdala and insula, S2/parietal operculum, thalamus, temporal pole, Heschl gyrus		
Yuan et al., [48]	Migraine without aura	Seed voxel correlation	Basal ganglia, somatosensory regions	Increased FC between basal ganglia and somatosensory regions	Healthy controls	Correlation between monthly rate of attacks and increased FC between the bilateral caudate and the insula. Correlation between disease duration and increased FC between the right nucleus accumbens and the bilateral ACC.

TABLE 22-1 (Continued)

Study	Chronic Pain State	Resting-State Method	Affected Areas or Networks	Main Findings (Patients Compared with Controls)	Control Group	Relation with Clinical Characteristics
Mainero et al. [30]	Migraine	Seed-based		Greater connectivity from PAG to thalamus, S1, M1, posterior parietal cortex, S2		Increased number of monthly attacks correlates with reduced connectivity between PAG and PFC, ACC, amygdala, and medial thalamus
Otti et al. [35]	Chronic pain disorder	ICA, power density frequency spectra (0–0.24 Hz)	Insula, cingulate cortex, middle frontal gyrus (anterior DMN [aDMN], FIN)	Higher PSD in aDMN and FIN		No correlation
Malinen et al. [31]	Various pain states	Spectral power density (0.12–0.25) and seed-based		Increased PD in insula and ACC. Lack of functional connection between the insula and ACC.		
Ichesco et al. [24]	Temporo-man-dibular disorder	Seed-based	Insula, ACC	Increased FC between the left anterior insula and pregenual ACC		Negative correlation between insular cortex and ACC connectivity, and clinical pain
Kornelsen et al. [28]	Back pain (failed back surgery)	ICA		Reduction of FC in DMN. Increased FC in the left angular gyrus, the right middle and inferior frontal gyrus, and the left cingulate.		
Hong et al. [23]	IBS	Power spectrum magnitude (0.01–0.16)	Insula, amygdala, somato-sensory cortices	No overall disease effects. Gender effect on changes in power spectrum distribution.		Correlation between skewedness of the distribution and discomfort in women

Study	Chronic Pain State	Resting-State Method	Affected Areas or Networks	Main Findings (Patients Compared with Controls)	Control Group	Relation with Clinical Characteristics
Cauda et al. [14]	Diabetic neuropathic pain	ICA, power spectra	Fusiform and lingual gyri, inferior temporal gyrus, dorsal ACC, postcentral gyrus, precuneus, DLPFC, frontopolar cortex, right superior and left inferior frontal gyri, both thalami, both insulae, inferior parietal lobuli, right mammillary body	Dorsal ACC bilaterally, but also the pre- and postcentral gyri (S1/M1). Greater connectivity between precuneus, DLPFC, and frontopolar cortex is seen in patients. Higher frequency in patients	Healthy controls	
Cauda et al. [15]	Diabetic neuropathic pain	Seed voxel	Primary somatosensory cortex, ventral posterior lateral thalamic nucleus, medial dorsal thalamic nucleus	Reduced thalamic–cortical connectivity		
Cauda et al. [12]	Diabetic neuropathic pain	Seed voxel	Parietal, frontal, and cingulate cortices	Reduced connectivity in attentional networks		

Abbreviations: PFC, prefrontal cortex; DMN, default-mode network; ICA, independent component analysis; rINS, right insula; pgACC, pregenual anterior cingulate cortex; EAN, executive attentional network; MVN, medial visual network; rEAN, right EAN; ACC, anterior cingulate cortex; MPFC, medial prefrontal cortex; PCC, posterior cingulate cortex; PAG, periaqueductal grey; IBS, irritable bowel syndrome; FC, functional connectivity; PSD, power spectral density; SMA, supplementary motor area; DLPFC, dorsolateral prefrontal cortex; SN, saliency network; ALFF, amplitude of low-frequency fluctuation; ROI, region of interest; rACC, rostral ACC; FIN, frontoinsular network; CEN, central executive network.

in the medial frontal gyrus, right precuneus, and left supramarginal parietal gyrus. However, they also reported greater FC in the left angular gyrus, the right middle and inferior frontal gyri, and the dorsolateral prefrontal cortex (DLPFC) in patients. Greater FC was observed, in chronic back pain, between the insula, the midcingulate cortex, and somatomotor regions.

Fibromyalgia

FM is characterized by widespread pain that varies in location and intensity [45]. Although psychogenic origins of this disturbance have been put forward, evidence exists that FM patients show altered brain activity in response to experimental painful stimuli [25, 41]. Napadow and colleagues [34] explored rs-fMRI in FM, focusing on the DMN and attentional networks, such as the executive attentional network (EAN, also known as the frontoparietal control network). Key nodes of the EAN comprise the DLPFC and the posterior parietal cortex [39, 40]. Contrary to the DMN, which is involved in internal monitoring, the EAN appears to contribute to external monitoring, executive decision making, and working memory. The authors highlighted greater connectivity within the DMN and the right EAN in patients. Increased FC was also observed between the two networks and the insula. Moreover, the medial visual network (MVN), which was used as a control, did not show functional differences between patients and controls. Importantly, spontaneous clinical pain, which was rated by patients at the time of the scan, correlated positively with increased FC between the insula and the two networks, suggesting a close linkage, as also noted by Loggia et al. for cLBP patients (mentioned previously).

In a subsequent study, Napadow and colleagues [33] demonstrated that FC between the DMN and insula may serve as a possible surrogate biomarker for pain reduction in FM. The authors reexamined FM patients after 4 weeks of successful (analgesic) nonpharmacological treatment and reported concomitant significantly decreased DMN–insula connectivity posttreatment.

Cifre and colleagues [17] showed a pattern of increased/decreased FC in FM patients, with increased FC occurring mainly at the level of MPFC, PCC, ACC, and the insula. Decreased FC was instead observed between the thalamus, insula, and periaqueductal grey (PAG).

Kim and coworkers [27], by applying power spectrum density transformation to BOLD fluctuations, observed increased frequency power in the primary somatosensory cortex (S1), the supplementary motor area (SMA), the DLPFC, and the amygdalae. As already observed by Napadow and colleagues [33], occipital and temporal sites did not show differences between groups, suggesting that only somatosensory and prefrontal regions were characterized by increased power spectral density in FM.

Migraine

Rs-fMRI studies in migraine patients have so far focused mainly on chronic migraine without aura, leaving yet unexplored other forms of headache. Xue and colleagues [47] used ICA to explore the FC of the DMN and the central executive and salience networks (CEN and SN) in a cohort of migraine patients without aura. They observed an aberrant intrinsic connectivity within the bilateral CEN and SN. In addition, they found increased FC between the DMN and the rCEN and the insula. In a second study, Xue and colleagues [46] explored both the power spectrum density and the ROI-based FC in patients with migraine without aura. Their results showed that the power of the fluctuations was decreased in the rostral ACC (rACC) and in the bilateral PFC of the patients. Conversely, increased power was reported in the thalamus. A second, ROI-based analysis on the regions showing abnormal power spectrum amplitude revealed increased FC between the left rACC, bilateral frontal lobe, and the parietal lobe, and between the left PFC, right precuneus, and bilateral parietal lobe.

Another ROI-based study conducted on interictal migraineurs [38] has suggested that altered FC in migraineurs includes the anterior insula to the pulvinar, middle temporal cortex, mediodorsal thalamus, precuneus, and PAG. Migraineurs showed, on average, a greater strength of FC between the anterior insula and the thalami, and the anterior insula and the PAG. Patients were also characterized by a reduced strength between the anterior insula, cingulate cortex, and the precuneus. In patients, stronger functional connections were observed between the amygdalae and the superior frontal gyrus. A stronger FC between the PAG and prefrontal regions, anterior cingulate, and amygdalae was also reported by Mainero and colleagues [30]. Specifically, these authors reported a positive correlation between the number of migraine attacks per month and the FC within somatosensory regions. Concomitantly, the frequency of attacks was negatively correlated with FC between the PAG and prefrontal regions. Mainero and colleagues also showed that patients with a history of allodynia exhibited significantly reduced connectivity between the PAG and prefrontal regions compared with migraineurs without allodynia.

The role of subcortical structures in migraineurs has been further pointed out by two recent studies by Yuan and colleagues [48], and Hadjikhani and colleagues [22]. Yuan and colleagues explored the FC of the basal ganglia and several somatosensory regions. Their results revealed, in line with previous evidence, that FC between these structures was increased, with an augmented number of monthly attacks correlating positively with the FC between the bilateral caudate and the insula. Longer disease duration was correlated with increased FC between the right nucleus accumbens and the bilateral ACC. In the Hadjikhani and colleagues' study [22], resting-state FC between the amygdalae and the cortex in migraineurs with or without aura was compared with that of other chronic pain states, such as trigeminal neuralgia and carpal tunnel syndrome. Their findings suggested that only migraine (both with and without aura) was related to increased connectivity between the amygdalae and the insula. Their results are interesting, as, by comparing different chronic pain conditions, they could pinpoint putative pathology-specific changes.

Diabetic Neuropathic Pain

Three studies conducted by Cauda and colleagues [12–15] explored the FC of different brain networks in diabetic neuropathic pain. The authors focused their investigation both on DMN and attentional and thalamocortical networks. Their findings showed that patients (1) were characterized by reduced DMN connectivity, but increased frontal, insular, and thalamic connectivity and had a power spectrum changing to higher frequencies; (2) had alterations in both ventral and dorsal attentional networks; and (3) presented reduced FC between the ventral posterior lateral nucleus of the thalamus, the insula, and the middle frontal gyrus. Altogether, these results evidenced that functional alterations and power spectrum frequency shifts modify thalamocortical connectivity, occurring for all neural networks that participate in elaborating nociceptive, painful stimuli, and salient events.

Other Pain Conditions

Reports of altered rs-FC in other pain conditions have been documented for CRPS, temporomandibular disorder (TMD), and IBS. Bolwerk and colleagues [9] showed that, compared with healthy controls, CRPS patients exhibited reduced connectivity within the DMN but increased connectivity between somatomotor regions and the cingulate cortex, the precuneus, the thalamus, and the PFC. A similar FC increase was observed between the intraparietal sulcus and the aforementioned areas.

Ichesco and colleagues [24] confined their interest to the cinguloinsular FC in patients suffering from TMD. They observed increased FC between the left anterior insular cortex and pregenual anterior cingulate, both in resting state and during the administration of pain stimuli. The connectivity between the insula and the cingulate cortex was negatively correlated with clinical pain intensity.

In a study conducted on IBS, Hong and colleagues [23] showed that differences in frequency power of brain oscillations also have a gender component. The authors found that brain oscillations of greater magnitude were more frequent in women, and also in those not affected by IBS. This increase was more prominent in the amygdala and in the hippocampus. Female IBS also exhibited greater power in the insula, compared with male IBS, and a power distribution more skewed towards lower frequencies in somatosensory regions. These results are important, as they suggest that some functional characteristics usually attributed to chronic pain may also be partly accounted for by gender. Indeed, certain chronic pain states are characterized by a greater female prevalence.

Interestingly, chronic pain conditions usually considered of somatoform origin, such as the chronic pain disorder, also present some FC alterations. Otti and colleagues' [35] results of an investigation carried out on patients diagnosed with chronic pain disorders indicated that the frontoinsular salience networks and the anterior DMN oscillated at higher frequencies in patients. These results raise the question of the role of emotional homeostasis and introspection in FC modifications.

SIMILARITIES AND DIFFERENCES AMONG CONDITIONS, AND INTERPRETATION OF THE FINDINGS

Regardless of the underlying chronic pain state, a common finding, first evidenced by Cauda and colleagues, is that patients show a power of brain spectrum skewed towards high frequencies. Areas showing increased power spectra also have altered FC; this suggests a common functional mechanism underlying plastic changes. Malinen and colleagues [31], by exploring temporal and spatial brain activity during rest in patients suffering from a wide range of pain conditions (CRPS type II, phantom limb pain, lumbar spine degeneration, cervical spine degeneration, postsurgical pain), showed stronger spectral power in the insula, and to a weaker extent in the cingulate cortex. The FC of the two sites was also altered. These data pinpointed aberrant high-frequency activity in selective brain regions as a common feature of chronic pain. Although no definitive conclusion should be drawn, such alterations are likely to be tightly pain-related and, thus, maladaptive. Studies conducted by Baliki and colleagues [5] have indicated that these functional changes correlate with ongoing fluctuations of chronic pain and are not related to attentional demands alone [6].

In addition, the few longitudinal available studies [33] suggest that increased FC in patients can be significantly reduced by effective pain therapies.

There are, however, at least two open questions in this kind of research. First, why do these studies observe similar changes despite very different underlying etiologies in chronic pain states? EEG studies have suggested, by observing increased levels of power spectrum in various pain states [36, 37, 42], that chronic pain is associated with altered brain oscillations possibly related to dysfunctional thalamocortical loops. It may be proposed that the mere fact of having pain modifies brain functions and that this occurs similarly across pain states. However, morphometric studies have revealed peculiar white matter alterations in different pain states [3]. These pathology-specific modifications thus open the possibility that different chronic pain states have peculiar "signatures." The same hypothesis can be put forward for functional alternations. In this view, a parsimonious explanation for the present findings is that studies have so far focused on a limited number of brain networks, leaving unexplored functional alterations in others. It may be that some brain networks, such as the DMN, are indeed always affected in a similar fashion in chronic pain conditions (Fig. 22-2). As the DMN is crucial in internal self-monitoring, aberrant activity can be interpreted as failure in disengaging attentional focus from the internal states. It remains to be elucidated whether similar DMN alterations observed in other pathological states, such as Alzheimer disease and schizophrenia, reflect the same functional imbalance or, rather, other pathophysiological mechanisms.

Second, it should be explored whether altered functional circuits constitute a signature for pain states, or precede the process of chronification. The transition from acute to chronic pain, typical of certain pain conditions, occurs only in a portion of patients and, presently, seems to be associated with functional characteristics present prior to the chronification phase [7].

The role of comorbidities is yet to be fully understood, for what concerns both its role in pain chronification and its effect on FC. Commonly, patients suffering from chronic pain also report high levels of comorbidities such as anxiety and depression, which, as primary pathologies, associated with altered rs-fMRI connectivity. Most rs-fMRI studies control for these comorbidities when examining brain activity at rest, but find a correlation between FC and psychiatric comorbidities only rarely [17]. Conversely, correlations between spontaneous pain and brain fluctuations are sometimes directly reported [29, 33, 34], and pain report at the time of the scan is important for attributing specificity to the rs-fMRI marker.

Finally, rs-fMRI connectivity is not devoid of possible confounds. Motion and cardiovascular artefacts can affect the results significantly. Indeed, head motion can reduce spectral power at 0.007–0.05 Hz and increase it at 0.12–0.167 Hz. Importantly, the effect of motion confounds is greater in association networks such as the DMN and frontoparietal control network [26]. Therefore, further steps in rs-fMRI research should be undertaken to disentangle possible biomarkers of chronic pain from biological noise, which can be more evident in patients than controls.

In conclusion, rs-fMRI analysis has been used to uncover significantly altered functional brain connectivity in different chronic pain populations. As this analysis approach is relatively new and methods for performing rs-fMRI analyses are still evolving, future studies are likely to better delineate just how altered rs-fMRI reflects and even maintains persistent pain in chronic pain populations.

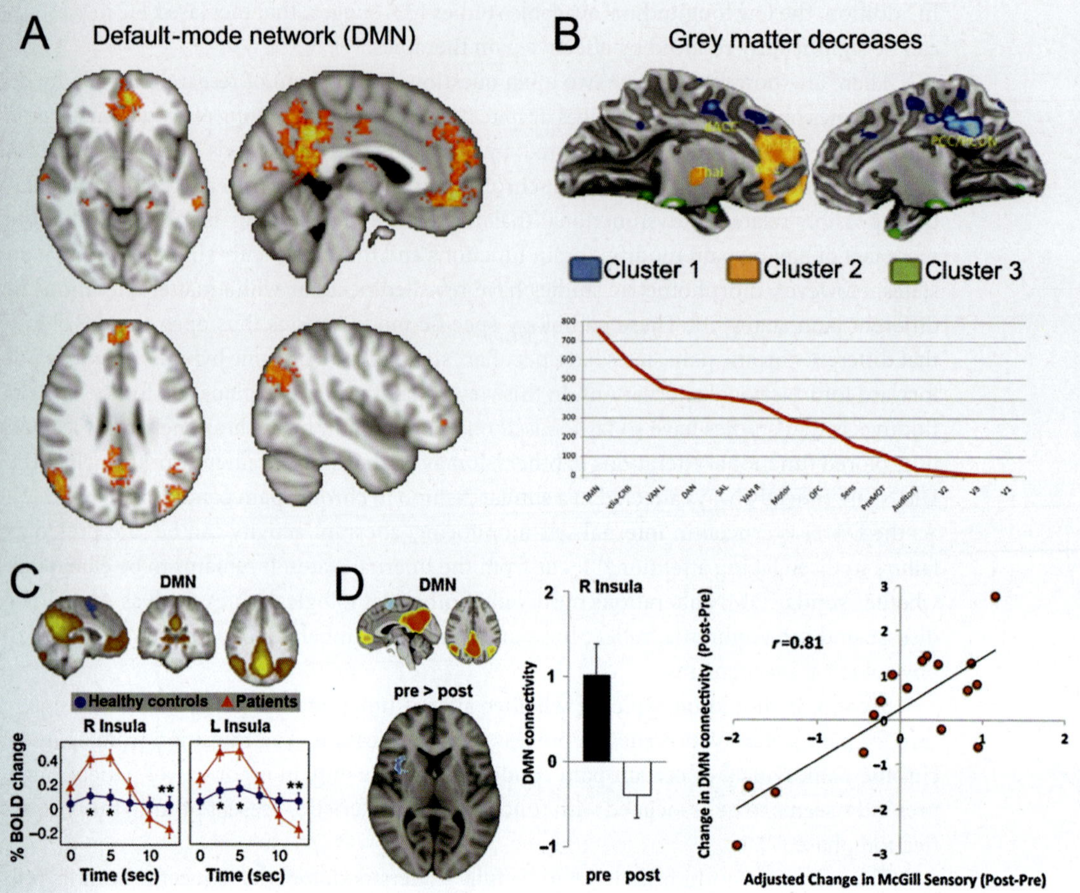

FIGURE 22-2 The role of the DMN in chronic pain. A: Default mode representation from automated meta-analysis of 117 studies in *Neurosynth*. **B:** Brain images represent the results of the model-based clustering of grey matter decreases across chronic pain conditions (32 studies). Lower panel shows the global involvement of each large-scale brain network in the pain-related grey matter alterations. (The results from all the pathologies are placed here together, and the values are expressed in mm^3 of altered brain volume.) All the networks except auditory, V1, V2, and V3 are significantly different from zero, with the DMN showing the most changes. (Adapted from Cauda et al. [13].) **C:** Functional connectivity changes between DMN and insula. Tagliazucchi et al. found that the insula is more likely to show increased activity immediately following MPFC activity, only in pain patients but not healthy controls. **D:** Napadow et al. showed that the correlation between DMN and insula activity reduces following treatment in fibromyalgia patients. In addition to these changes, this coupling was related to a change in pain parameters. These results collectively suggest that the DMN shows increased coupling with pain-related regions, indicating that chronic pain alters brain dynamics at rest. $*p < 0.05$, $**p < 0.001$

REFERENCES

1. Apkarian AV, Baliki MN, Geha PY. Towards a theory of chronic pain. Prog Neurobio 2009;87(2):81–97.
2. Apkarian AV, Hashmi JA, Baliki MN. Pain and the brain: specificity and plasticity of the brain in clinical chronic pain. Pain 2011;152(3 Suppl):S49–64.
3. Apkarian AV, Sosa Y, Sonty S, Levy RM, Harden RN, Parrish TB, Gitelman DR. Chronic back pain is associated with decreased prefrontal and thalamic gray matter density. J Neurosci 2004;24(46):10410–5.
4. Balenzuela P, Chernomoretz A, Fraiman D, Cifre I, Sitges C, Montoya P, Chialvo DR. Modular organization of brain resting state networks in chronic back pain patients. Front Neuroinform 2010;4:116.
5. Baliki MN, Baria AT, Apkarian AV. The cortical rhythms of chronic back pain. J Neurosci 2011;31(39): 13981–90.
6. Baliki MN, Geha PY, Apkarian AV, Chialvo DR. Beyond feeling: chronic pain hurts the brain, disrupting the default-mode network dynamics. J Neurosci 2008;28(6):1398–403.

7. Baliki MN, Petre B, Torbey S, Herrmann KM, Huang L, Schnitzer TJ, Fields HL, Apkarian AV. Corticostriatal functional connectivity predicts transition to chronic back pain. Nat Neurosci 2012;15(8):1117–9.
8. Biswal B, Zerrin Yetkin F, Haughton VM, Hyde JS. Functional connectivity in the motor cortex of resting human brain using echo-planar MRI. Magn Reson Med 1995;34(4):537–41.
9. Bolwerk A, Seifert F, Maihöfner C. Altered resting-state functional connectivity in complex regional pain syndrome. J Pain 2013;14(10):1107–15.
10. Bullmore E, Sporns O. Complex brain networks: graph theoretical analysis of structural and functional systems. Nat Rev Neurosci 2009;10(3):186–98.
11. Calhoun VD, Adali T. Multisubject independent component analysis of fMRI: a decade of intrinsic networks, default mode, and neurodiagnostic discovery. IEEE Rev Biomed Eng 2012;5:60–73.
12. Cauda F, D'Agata F, Sacco K, Duca S, Cocito D, Paolasso I, Isoardo G, Geminiani G. Altered resting state attentional networks in diabetic neuropathic pain. J Neurol Neurosurg Psychiatry 2010;81(7):806–11.
13. Cauda F, Palermo S, Costa T, Torta R, Duca S, Vercelli U, Geminiani G, Torta DM. Gray matter alterations in chronic pain: A network-oriented meta-analytic approach. Neuroimage Clin. 2014;4:676–86.
14. Cauda F, Sacco K, D'Agata F, Duca S, Cocito D, Geminiani G, Migliorati F, Isoardo G. Low-frequency BOLD fluctuations demonstrate altered thalamocortical connectivity in diabetic neuropathic pain. BMC Neurosci 2009;10:138.
15. Cauda F, Sacco K, Duca S, Cocito D, D'Agata F, Geminiani GC, Canavero S. Altered resting state in diabetic neuropathic pain. PLoS One 2009;4(2):e4542.
16. Cauda F, Torta DM, Sacco K, Geda E, D'Agata F, Costa T, Duca S, Geminiani G, Amanzio M. Shared "core" areas between the pain and other task-related networks. PLoS One 2012;7(8):e41929.
17. Cifre I, Sitges C, Fraiman D, Munoz MA, Balenzuela P, Gonzalez-Roldan A, Martinez-Jauand M, Birbaumer N, Chialvo DR, Montoya P. Disrupted functional connectivity of the pain network in fibromyalgia. Psychosom Med 2012;74(1):55–62.
18. Damoiseaux JS, Rombouts SA, Barkhof F, Scheltens P, Stam CJ, Smith SM, Beckmann CF. Consistent resting state networks across healthy subjects. Proc Natl Acad Sci U S A. 2006;103(37):13848–53.
19. Farmer MA, Baliki MN, Apkarian AV. A dynamic network perspective of chronic pain. Neurosci Lett 2012;520(2):194–203.
20. Fox MD, Greicius M. Clinical applications of resting state functional connectivity. Front Syst Neurosci 2010;4:19.
21. Fox MD, Raichle ME. Spontaneous fluctuations in brain activity observed with functional magnetic resonance imaging. Nat Rev Neurosci 2007;8(9):700–11.
22. Hadjikhani N, Ward N, Boshyan J, Napadow V, Maeda Y, Truini A, Caramia F, Tinelli E, Mainero C. The missing link: enhanced functional connectivity between amygdala and visceroceptive cortex in migraine. Cephalalgia 2013;33(15):1264–8.
23. Hong JY, Kilpatrick LA, Labus J, Gupta A, Jiang Z, Ashe-McNalley C, Stains J, Heendeniya N, Ebrat B, Smith S, et al. Patients with chronic visceral pain show sex-related alterations in intrinsic oscillations of the resting brain. J Neurosci 2013;33(29):11994–2002.
24. Ichesco E, Quintero A, Clauw DJ, Peltier S, Sundgren PM, Gerstner GE, Schmidt-Wilcke T. Altered functional connectivity between the insula and the cingulate cortex in patients with temporomandibular disorder: a pilot study. Headache 2012;52(3):441–54.
25. Jorge LL, Amaro E Jr. Brain imaging in fibromyalgia. Curr Pain Headache Rep 2012;16(5):388–98.
26. Kim J, Van Dijk K, Libby A, Napadow V. Frequency-dependent relationship between resting state fMRI signal power and head motion is localized within distributed association networks. Brain Connect 2014;4(1):30–9.
27. Kim JY, Kim SH, Seo J, Han SW, Nam EJ, Kim SK, Lee HJ, Lee SJ, Kim YT, Chang Y. Increased power spectral density in resting-state pain-related brain networks in fibromyalgia. Pain 2013;154(9):1792–7.
28. Kornelsen J, Sboto-Frankenstein U, McIver T, Gervai P, Wacnik P, Berrington N, Tomanek B. Default mode network functional connectivity altered in failed back surgery syndrome. J Pain 2013;14(5):483–91.
29. Loggia ML, Kim J, Gollub RL, Vangel MG, Kirsch I, Kong J, Wasan AD, Napadow V. Default mode network connectivity encodes clinical pain: an arterial spin labeling study. Pain 2013;154(1):24–33.
30. Mainero C, Boshyan J, Hadjikhani N. Altered functional magnetic resonance imaging resting-state connectivity in periaqueductal gray networks in migraine. Ann Neurol 2011;70(5):838–45.
31. Malinen S, Vartiainen N, Hlushchuk Y, Koskinen M, Ramkumar P, Forss N, Kalso E, Hari R. Aberrant temporal and spatial brain activity during rest in patients with chronic pain. Proc Natl Acad Sci USA 2010;107(14): 6493–7.

32. Moulton EA, Pendse G, Becerra LR, Borsook D. BOLD responses in somatosensory cortices better reflect heat sensation than pain. J Neurosci 2012;32(17):6024–31.
33. Napadow V, Kim J, Clauw DJ, Harris RE. Decreased intrinsic brain connectivity is associated with reduced clinical pain in fibromyalgia. Arthritis Rheum 2012;64(7):2398–403.
34. Napadow V, LaCount L, Park K, As-Sanie S, Clauw DJ, Harris RE. Intrinsic brain connectivity in fibromyalgia is associated with chronic pain intensity. Arthritis Rheum 2010;62(8):2545–55.
35. Otti A, Guendel H, Wohlschlager A, Zimmer C, Noll-Hussong M. Frequency shifts in the anterior default mode network and the salience network in chronic pain disorder. BMC Psychiatry 2013;13:84.
36. Saab CY. Pain-related changes in the brain: diagnostic and therapeutic potentials. Trends Neurosci 2012;35(10):629–37.
37. Sarnthein J, Stern J, Aufenberg C, Rousson V, Jeanmonod D. Increased EEG power and slowed dominant frequency in patients with neurogenic pain. Brain 2006;129(Pt 1):55–64.
38. Schwedt TJ, Schlaggar BL, Mar S, Nolan T, Coalson RS, Nardos B, Benzinger T, Larson-Prior LJ. Atypical resting-state functional connectivity of affective pain regions in chronic migraine. Headache 2013;53(5):737–51.
39. Seeley WW, Menon V, Schatzberg AF, Keller J, Glover GH, Kenna H, Reiss AL, Greicius MD. Dissociable intrinsic connectivity networks for salience processing and executive control. J Neurosci 2007;27(9):2349–56.
40. Sridharan D, Levitin DJ, Menon V. A critical role for the right fronto-insular cortex in switching between central-executive and default-mode networks. Proc Natl Acad Sci USA 2008;105(34):12569–74.
41. Staud R. Brain imaging in fibromyalgia syndrome. Clin Exp Rheumatol 2011;29(6 Suppl 69):S109–17.
42. Stern J, Jeanmonod D, Sarnthein J. Persistent EEG overactivation in the cortical pain matrix of neurogenic pain patients. NeuroImage 2006;31(2):721–31.
43. Tagliazucchi E, Balenzuela P, Fraiman D, Chialvo DR. Brain resting state is disrupted in chronic back pain patients. Neurosci Lett 2010;485(1):26–31.
44. Treede RD, Jensen TS, Campbell JN, Cruccu G, Dostrovsky JO, Griffin JW, Hansson P, Hughes R, Nurmikko T, Serra J. Neuropathic pain: redefinition and a grading system for clinical and research purposes. Neurology 2008;70(18):1630–5.
45. Wolfe F. New American College of Rheumatology criteria for fibromyalgia: a twenty-year journey. Arthritis Care Res (Hoboken) 2010;62(5):583–4.
46. Xue T, Yuan K, Cheng P, Zhao L, Yu D, Dong T, von Deneen KM, Gong Q, Qin W, Tian J. Alterations of regional spontaneous neuronal activity and corresponding brain circuit changes during resting state in migraine without aura. NMR Biomed 2013;26(9):1051–8.
47. Xue T, Yuan K, Zhao L, Yu D, Dong T, Cheng P, von Deneen KM, Qin W, Tian J. Intrinsic brain network abnormalities in migraines without aura revealed in resting-state fMRI. PLoS One 2012;7(12):e52927.
48. Yuan K, Zhao L, Cheng P, Yu D, Dong T, Xing L, Bi Y, Yang X, von Deneen KM, Liang F, et al. Altered structure and resting-state functional connectivity of the basal ganglia in migraine patients without aura. J Pain 2013;14(8):836–44.
49. Zhang D, Raichle ME. Disease and the brain's dark energy. Nat Rev Neurol. 2010;6(1):15–28.

CHAPTER 23

Understanding Pain Mechanisms Using Rodent Brain Imaging: Opportunities and Pitfalls

David A. Seminowicz, Catherine S. Hubbard, and Radi Masri

ADVANTAGES AND LIMITATIONS OF RODENT fMRI

Neuroimaging gives us the ability to noninvasively explore activity in the human brain and determine brain regional activity correlated with action, thought, language, and perception, in health and disease. Why then would we want to perform imaging on nonhuman species when we can do all those things in people? In this chapter, we focus on the potential use of rodent structural and functional MRI to bolster our understanding of chronic and acute pain mechanisms. Although other neuroimaging techniques such as positron emission tomography (PET) and electroencephalography (EEG) have been used in rodents, by far the most common imaging technique has been MRI, and we suspect its use will increase in the future.

The major advantages of neuroimaging studies in rodents over humans come from the possibilities of running longitudinal studies in which invasive manipulations can be applied and genetic and environmental (diet, enrichment, social) factors can be controlled. We can scan animals before and after induction of a model of chronic pain, and we can use invasive or noninvasive manipulations to test a putative intervention and the brain mechanisms associated with its effects. Examples of invasive interventions include motor cortex stimulation, deep brain stimulation [37, 55], pharmacological interventions, including delivery by topical application [25], systemic injection [20, 24], intracerebroventricular infusion [29], brain lesions, and optogenetics [1, 43]. Upon completion of the imaging study, we can harvest the rodents' CNS or other tissue of interest to further examine mechanisms and link changes in MRI with genetic, protein, or morphological aspects of the tissue. Altogether, these advantages could lead to the rapid identification of brain targets that can then be tested in humans, completing the cycle from reverse to forward translation.

We note up front that a major limitation of rodent neuroimaging is that we ultimately seek to understand pain in humans, and rodents do not have human brains or experience pain in a human way. Moreover, rodents do not express many aspects of chronic pain; absent are many psychosocial factors of the human disease. Thus, we approach studies attempting to make a link between rodent and human pain with great caution. Crucial to successful translation of rodent to human models is the development of experiments built on straightforward hypotheses. In the next section, we outline the major imaging techniques applied to rodent imaging in pain and other fields, and in the following section, we give two examples of experiments that we believe made important contributions to the pain field by following the guidelines described above, including using longitudinal designs and testing simple hypotheses.

RODENT IMAGING

Anatomical Imaging

In humans, MRI-based assessment of brain anatomy is used extensively as a diagnostic tool to assess brain injury. It is also used as a research tool to study pathological conditions where brain injury is pronounced, such as traumatic brain injury (TBI), stroke, cancer, and neurodegenerative diseases such as Alzheimer's. Similar to humans, advanced methods that examine changes in brain morphometry have been described in rodents. These methods include deformation-based morphometry (DBM) [39, 40], voxel-based morphometry (VBM) [65], and cortical thickness analysis (CTA) [41]. Anatomical imaging in rodents can also be used to investigate changes in white matter [75] via anatomical connectivity using diffusion tensor imaging (DTI) and newer techniques like diffusion kurtosis imaging [79]. DTI-based white matter tract atlases are currently available for mice [32], making comparisons with normal reference anatomy possible. Morphometric changes in rodents can be induced with learning [42], similar to what has been shown in humans [18].

Functional "Pain" Imaging in Rodents

Thompson and Bushnell [71] have reviewed papers on rodent imaging with noxious stimulation up to early 2012. Of the more than 30 fMRI and PET studies included, the following general trends were evident: most studies involved anaesthesia (usually α-chloralose or isoflurane), the most commonly used noxious stimulus was electrical, followed by formalin injection into the paw, and the most commonly reported regional activations were in the primary somatosensory and motor cortices (S1/M1), thalamus, anterior cingulate cortex (ACC), and prefrontal cortex (PFC), with less consistent reports of activation in the insula, secondary somatosensory cortex (S2), caudate–putamen, hypothalamus, periaqueductal grey (PAG), hippocampus, and amygdala. Compare that with the activations reported across over 100 fMRI studies employing painful stimulation in humans, where the strongest activations were in thalamus, ACC, anterior and posterior insula, S2, PFC (inferior, middle, superior, and medial frontal gyri), with less frequent reports of activation in inferior parietal, putamen, cerebellum, posterior cingulate cortex (PCC), S1, and M1 [19].

Although the overlap between regions activated in humans and rodents is obvious, we must be cautious of overextending the similarities as they might relate to behaviour. The thalamus, S1, and ACC reliably show blood oxygenation level–dependent (BOLD) responses via activation of the spinothalamic tract, but activation of other regions might be more difficult to compare between species. Moreover, the prefrontal and posterior parietal lobes in rodents make up a tiny fraction of the rodent brain, whereas in humans, these regions are substantial. PFC activation in the rat might reflect a response related to decision-making, reward, or motivation [14, 23, 31, 54, 56, 57], but is unlikely to be comparable to the thoughts, feelings, inhibitions, and motivational goals represented in the PFC of humans undergoing a painful experience. Furthermore, because rodents are usually anaesthetized, the stimulus is not experienced as painful (see section below on anaesthesia). Therefore, it is important to keep in mind the limitations of rodent models and to cautiously draw links to the human case.

Resting-State Functional Connectivity

In human brain imaging research, one of the fastest expanding areas is resting-state connectivity [62, 68]. In the rat, resting-state fMRI has recently begun to appear and will surely soon dominate the rodent fMRI literature. Resting-state fMRI allows one to interrogate functional brain networks without imposing a task, thus allowing a researcher to test the connectivity of several networks in a single dataset. Several studies have indicated abnormal resting-state activity in humans suffering from chronic pain [3, 11–13]. However, there are still limited data on how rodent resting-state networks (RSNs) are affected in models of chronic pain.

Assuming that RSNs reflect relatively static circuit connectivity, resting-state fMRI is much less dependent on current behavioural state and thus less susceptible to problems related to anaesthesia. Reliable RSNs involving S1, thalamus, and caudate–putamen have been demonstrated in rats under medetomidine anaesthesia [58,77]. Several other resting-state fMRI studies have been performed in rats under anaesthesia [9, 30, 49, 59] as well as in awake rats [27, 34, 44, 45, 76]. Becerra and colleagues [8] reported that seven RSNs could be robustly identified in awake rats. These included cerebellar, "default mode" (DMN), basal ganglia–hypothalamus, basal ganglia–thalamus–hippocampus, autonomic, somatosensory, and interoceptive networks. Liang et al. [44] reported three major brain modules in awake rat resting-state fMRI, all of which involved the PFC: one module in which PFC was connected with somatosensory, thalamus, and hippocampus; a second module in which PFC was connected with amygdala, insula, and hypothalamus, likely related to emotional and autonomic function; and a third module in which PFC was connected with most of the cortical mantle.

EXAMPLES OF SUCCESSFUL RODENT MRI STUDIES

In the first example, we test the hypothesis that brain morphometric changes—usually grey matter volume decreases—repeatedly reported in people with chronic pain [15] were the effect of long-term pain or disease, rather than a neuroanatomical predisposition to develop chronic pain. Since studies in humans up to that point were cross-sectional, the latter explanation could not be excluded. To address this problem, rats were scanned before and at multiple time points after spared nerve injury (SNI), a model of peripheral neuropathic pain [67]. Behavioural assessments were also made at approximately the same time points. The major findings of the study were that PFC showed decreased volume, but only at the later (4- and 5-month) time points (Fig. 23-1A). The decrease in prefrontal volume coincided with the presence of anxiety-like behaviour (Fig. 23-1B and C). A second finding was that decreased volume in sensory areas including S1 and the ACC correlated with mechanical hyperalgesia (Fig. 23-2). Together, these results strongly suggest that cortical grey matter decreases are an effect of long-term pain and related to disease severity.

The second example of successful use of rodent neuroimaging to address a specific hypothesis comes from our work in a model of central neuropathic pain [66]. We examined resting-state functional connectivity in a well-characterized rat model of spinal cord injury (SCI) [16, 51, 73] to test the hypothesis that central pain is associated with

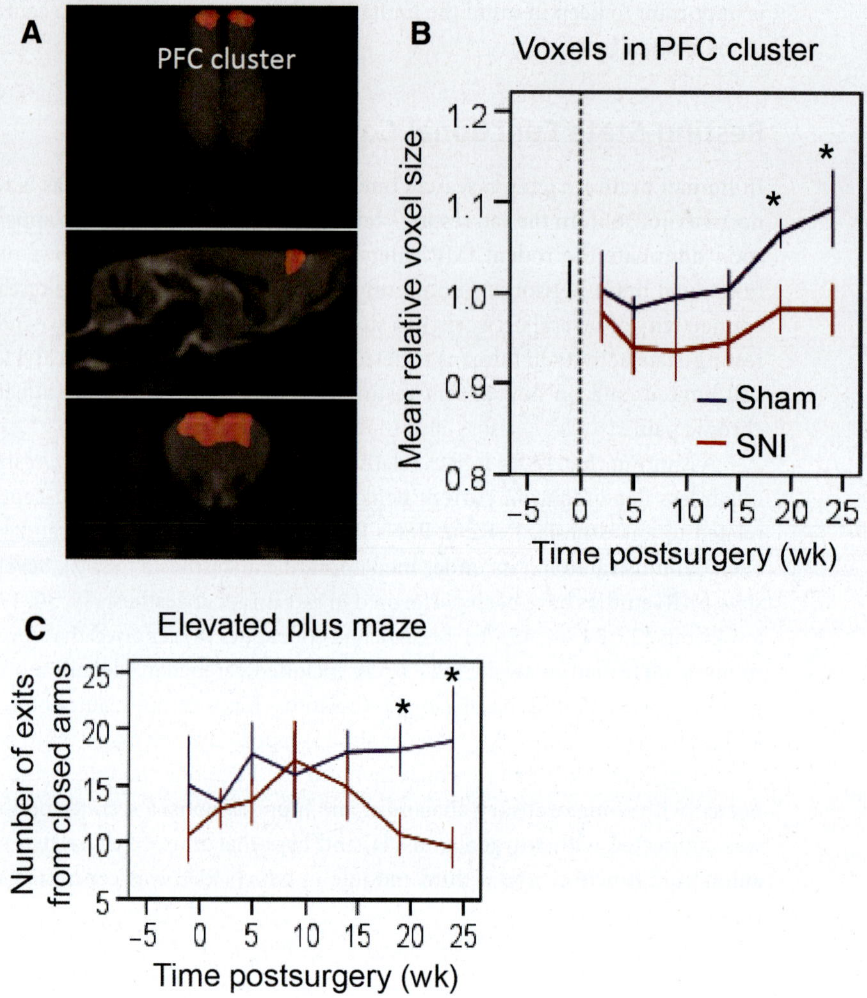

FIGURE 23-1 **A:** Deformation-based morphometry: linear mixed-effects model results for one significant cluster from the whole-brain analysis, PFC, which includes secondary motor cortex (M2), ACC area 24, and ACC area 32. **B:** PFC volume was significantly lower in SNI than sham rats at time points 19 and 24 weeks postsurgery, but not at earlier time points. $^*P < 0.05$ simple effects tests. Error bars represent 1 SEM. The vertical dashed line indicates the approximate time the surgeries were performed. **C:** SNI rats also began to display anxiety-like behaviours several months after injury, demonstrated here as decreased exits from the closed arms of the elevated plus maze. $^*P < 0.05$ simple effects tests. All brain images are shown in neurological convention: left side of the image is left side of the brain. (Adapted from Seminowicz et al. [67], with permission from Elsevier.)

corticothalamic asynchrony, as proposed previously [72]. After demonstrating that RSNs could be reliably identified in our sample (Fig. 23-3), we showed that thalamocortical asynchrony was present in spinal cord–injured rats 7 days postinjury, consistent with the finding of enhanced pain-like behaviour at this time point (Fig. 23-4). Having multiple time points in that experiment was crucial, since the thalamocortical asynchrony had a greatly reduced effect 14 days postinjury and might have been overlooked if only that time point was examined. Furthermore, to perform a similar experiment in humans would be extremely difficult considering the variability in SCI, and the use of a prospective design would be impractical.

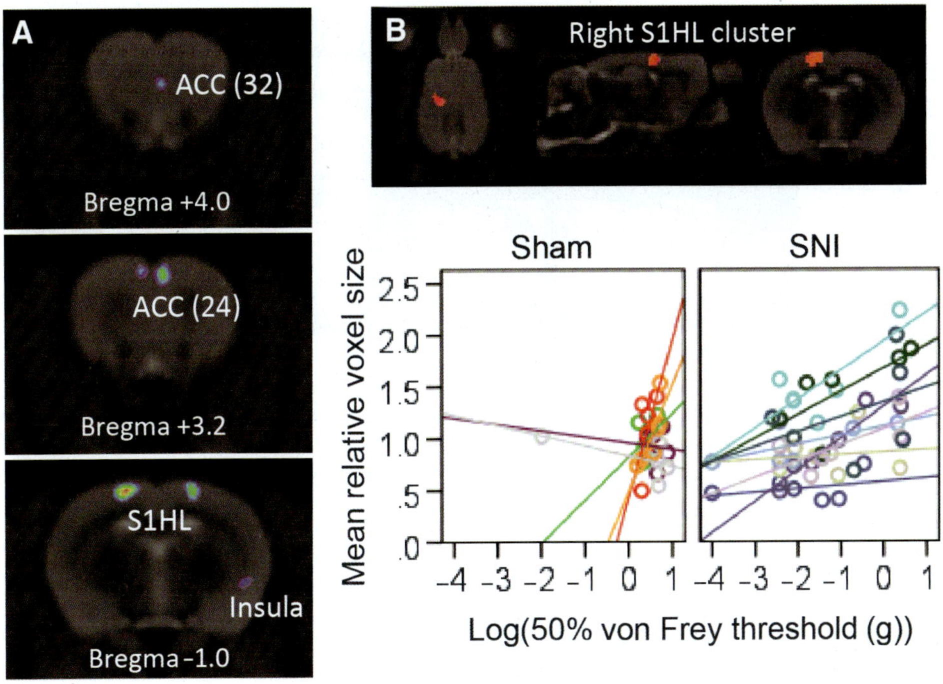

FIGURE 23-2 Results from the von Frey (mechanical hyperalgesia) analysis, showing **A:** significant clusters where increasing mechanical hypersensitivity predicted decreased volume in rats with SNI. Six significant clusters were identified in the analysis and are shown in the figure. **B:** The scatter plot for one region (right S1HL) is shown (mean relative voxel sizes, or the Jacobian determinant mean values, indicate an expansion (>1) or compression (<1) relative to the reference space), and a regression line is added for each rat. The von Frey scores for all time points postsurgery are included. (Reprinted from Seminowicz et al. [67], with permission from Elsevier.)

CONSIDERATIONS, LIMITATIONS, AND FUTURE APPLICATIONS FOR RODENT NEUROIMAGING

Cellular Correlates

Intuitively, one would expect morphometric changes to correlate with a reduction or shrinkage of neuronal or glial cells, reduced dendritic branching, or a reduction of extracellular water content. An early study reported diffusion-weighted imaging (DWI) could predict postmortem histopathology in a rodent model of TBI [2]. However, currently, there is no definitive link between MRI-based morphometric brain changes and neuronal pathology. Furthermore, the cellular mechanisms of morphometric changes are likely to differ between neurodegenerative (e.g., Alzheimer's disease), chronic illness (e.g., chronic pain, depression), and neurodevelopmental (e.g., schizophrenia, autism) conditions, making the search for cellular mechanisms very difficult and perhaps irrelevant. Related to our findings in the rat model described above, the morphometric changes we reported—decreased PFC volume 4–5 months after nerve injury [67]—could be related to early increases in basal dendrites (increased branching and spine density) and in *N*-methyl-D-aspartate (NMDA) currents [52] in the same region, leading to excitotoxicity and cell degeneration in the long term. Our own histological data suggested proliferation of astrocytes in the region of volume decrease [53], but this finding needs replication.

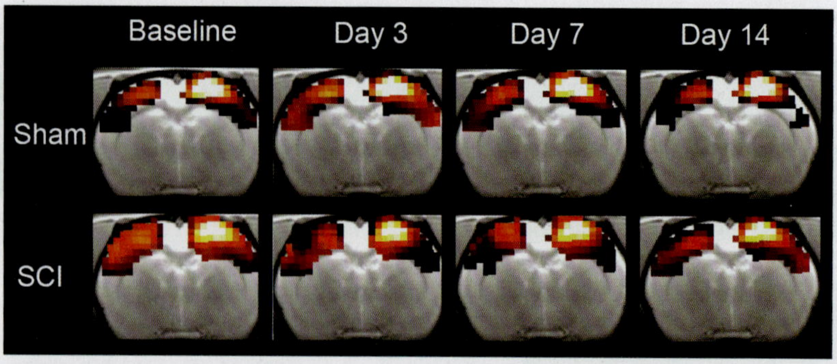

FIGURE 23-3 Reliability of functional connectivity in SCI and sham-operated animals. The right hindpaw representation in the primary somatosensory cortex (S1HL) seed network is shown for each group (top row = sham, bottom row = SCI) before surgery (baseline) and 3, 7, and 14 days after surgery. Images were thresholded at a *T*-value of 3 to highlight the extent of the network, and masked by the combined baseline scans for both groups. (Adapted from Seminowicz et al. [66], with permission.)

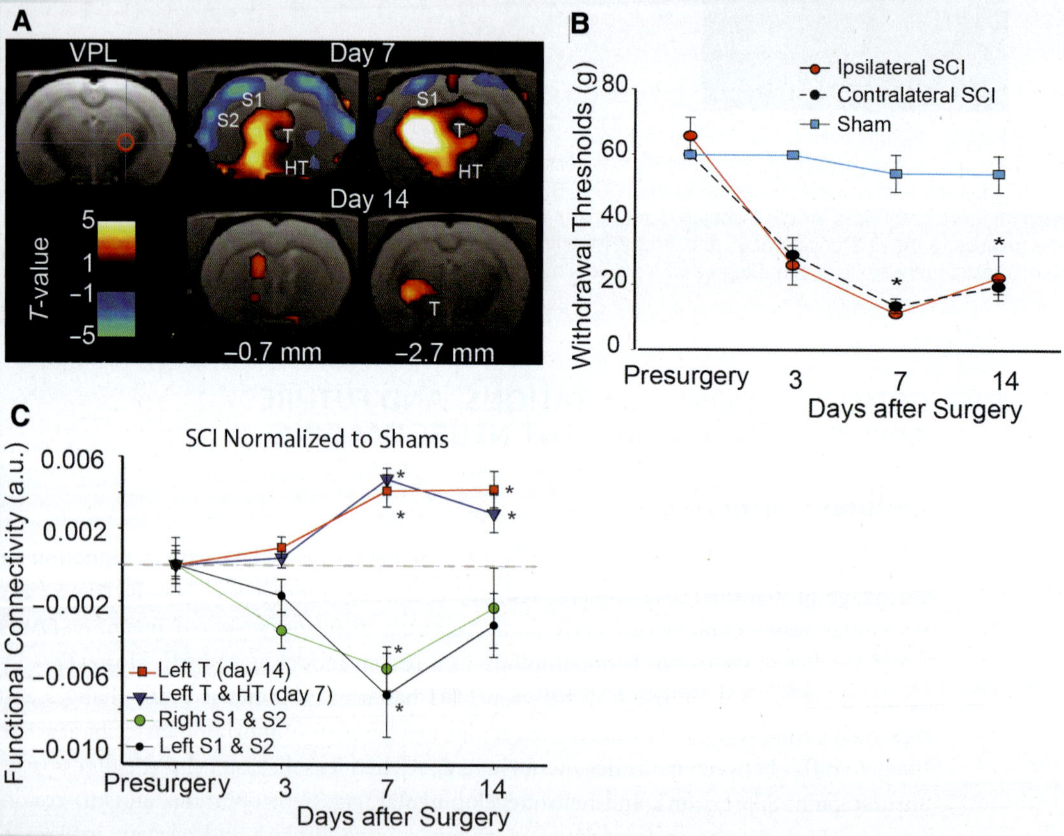

FIGURE 23-4 Ventroposterolateral thalamus (VPL) functional connectivity over time in an SCI model. **A:** Connectivity of the right VPL seed region (crosshair and *red circle*) and clusters that show increased (*red*) or decreased (*blue*) connectivity relative to sham animals at days 7 and 14 postinjury. The sections are referenced to Paxinos and Watson [60] atlas in terms of distance to bregma. **B:** Hindpaw (dorsal surface) mechanical withdrawal thresholds decrease over time, and hypersensitivity develops bilaterally after SCI. All values means ± 1 SEM; *statistically significant difference, $P < 0.001$. **C:** Plot of all clusters (shown in A) with increased or decreased functional connectivity at all time points in SCI relative to sham animals (*grey line*) and preinjury. *Significant cluster-corrected threshold at this time point compared with shams. a.u., arbitrary units; HT, hypothalamus; S1, primary somatosensory cortex; S2, secondary somatosensory cortex; T, thalamus. (Adapted from [66], with permission.)

Awake versus Anaesthetized

For practical reasons, rodent functional neuroimaging studies usually involve anaesthesia during scanning. However, several studies have examined fMRI brain activity in awake rats. Awake rat scanning requires either administering a partial paralytic agent or the use of restraint and training [21, 38]. This latter approach has been used in an fMRI experiment with thermal stimulation [6] and in a recent study employing magnetic resonance spectroscopy (MRS) [74]. Although the exact training procedures vary between studies, a common feature is to acclimate the animals incrementally to restraint in an attempt to reduce stress. In addition, the animals are routinely exposed to audio recordings of fMRI scan sequences as they would be heard in the scanner. This is important because increased stress in restrained animals can confound pain assessment and fMRI imaging results [5, 61, 64]. One group has shown that it takes repeated exposures (5–8 days of 90-minute training sessions) to the MR environment before stress-induced increases in corticosterone levels, autonomic activity, and movement-related artefacts are reduced during the MRI session [38], which supports the use of long training periods.

A major limitation of awake resting-state studies is the relatively high amount of movement, which is minimized in anaesthetized rats. A few studies have compared RSNs in awake and anaesthetized rats [45–47]. Although these studies tend to report on the advantages of awake procedures, it is clear upon examination of the literature that considerable overlap and stability exist between awake and anaesthetized rats at low levels of sedation. A recent study compared anaesthesia levels and showed that at isoflurane above 1.5% there is considerable loss of integrity of the BOLD fluctuations, with an overall increase in synchronicity [48], whereas at lower isoflurane levels much of the low-frequency BOLD fluctuations associated with various RSNs remained unaffected. We have worked with both awake and anaesthetized rats and generally feel comfortable examining RSNs in lightly anaesthetized animals. The tradeoff might be a loss of sensitivity, but the gains are fewer unusable datasets due to motion (and less motion overall), the lack of need to train animals for several days, the ability to apply strong noxious stimuli, and the circumvention of any interaction effect that might exist between training, stress, and the manipulation (e.g., nerve injury vs. sham) under investigation. There may be effects of repeated exposure to anaesthesia in longitudinal neuroimaging studies that have not yet been investigated.

In resting-state studies in human subjects, anaesthesia has some effect on brain connectivity. For example, Stamatakis et al. [69] examined the effects of propofol anaesthesia and found that, overall, the DMN—a network associated with the brain's baseline metabolic activity [62]—was intact in the three conditions of low, moderate, or no sedation. However, with light or moderate sedation, the DMN was connected with brain areas such as sensorimotor cortex and midbrain, which are not connected in the fully awake state. Others have found intact DMN connectivity under light anaesthetic [26] as well as other states marked by an absence of consciousness, such as sleep [10, 28]. These findings, combined with results from resting-state fMRI studies comparing DMN connectivity in awake versus anaesthetized rats, support the use of light sedation with certain anaesthetics for reducing movement-related artefacts in rodent neuroimaging.

Physiological and Nonphysiological Sources of Noise

Physiological (e.g., respiration and heart rate) and nonphysiological (i.e., scanner) noise can impart notable artefactual signals, decreasing signal-to-noise ratio (SNR), and potentially aliasing signals of interest. These concerns might be even greater in rodent imaging, where higher magnetic fields are typically used and much faster cardiac and respiratory rates are evident, even in deeply anaesthetized rodents. There are several available toolboxes for removing physiological artefact when simultaneous recordings of cardiac and respiratory rates are acquired.

Respiratory signals are highly correlated with resting-state fMRI signals [36]. However, sequential preprocessing of data—starting with motion correction—substantially decreases the effect of physiological noise contained within the fMRI signal [36]. Motion correction followed by regression of motion parameters removes much physiological noise (~35%), whereas sequential removal of respiration removes less (~5%) and cardiac less still (~1%) [36]. Thus, removal of motion and inclusion of motion regressors in the analysis are essential processing steps; even in the absence of concurrent physiological measures, most respiratory-related noise is removed with motion correction. Removal of cardiac and respiratory noise is less critical, but will lead to higher SNR and reproducibility. Also, global signal removal and bandpass filtering are insufficient for removal of physiological noise [36].

Other nonphysiological artefacts that frequently contaminate imaging data derive from instability in the scanner hardware system and/or MR environment, and include spike noise, gradient nonlinearities, static field inhomogeneities induced by ineffective shimming procedures, RF leakage, and low-frequency drift, all of which can severely degrade the fMRI signal. Most of these system-related artefacts can be minimized by the implementation of good quality control and assurance procedures, appropriate shielding of the scanner room from outside radiofrequencies, and daily calibration of scanner hardware with a phantom volume along with quality checks using specialized sequences to ensure the stability of the scanner hardware [78].

Statistical Considerations and Rules for Reporting Results

In general, we should apply the same rigor to statistical analysis in rodent neuroimaging papers as we do for those with human subjects. Several articles provide guidelines for human studies, such as the sample size required and rules for reporting results [22, 63]. Wherever possible, group results should be reported, as in human studies. As for sample size, one could argue that the better control of genetics and environment afforded by rodent studies would allow for smaller samples. The reduced anatomical variability across animals would also speak in favour of this. However, one could also argue that behavioural variability is greater in animals, and thus requires a larger sample. Moreover, the type of analysis to be performed and the effect size desired will determine the required sample size. For fMRI studies, it should be possible to use software applications such as fmripower.org to estimate the required sample size.

Results of neuroimaging data should be reported using coordinates for peak voxels, clusters, and regions of interest based on an anatomical atlas [33], such that replication and meta-analysis are possible. While there is currently no accepted standard rodent brain in the field such as the MNI152 for human imaging, several brain templates have recently been made available. One should consider that brain shape and size vary considerably by animal sex, weight, strain, and age.

Increasing SNR and Spatial Resolution

Spatial and temporal resolution in rodent fMRI studies can vary, with repetition times (TRs) as low as 100 ms and in-plane resolution less than 0.1 mm. Varying these factors will facilitate our ability to account for noise and better localize activations, and increase SNR. The advantage of high magnetic field (usually 4.7 to over 11.7 T in small animal scanners) fMRI is that SNR and spatial resolution are generally improved at the cost of greater distortions in the data. SNR and spatial resolution can also be improved by increasing the scan duration [17]. Because resting-state studies use time course data, the required duration of the functional scan is usually less than what is needed for an activation study, wherein several epochs must be averaged. Several other factors can influence spatial resolution and SNR, including the coil shape (e.g., saddle, surface, volume) and whether the coil is maintained at room temperature or cryogenic [4]. New technologies such as implanted surface coils will allow for image acquisition at even higher resolution and increase SNR [50].

A Challenge for Pain Research

Back to the question that we posed to open the chapter: what can we glean from rodent imaging that will inform the human condition? A recent article has suggested that parallel brain pathways could be identified in rats and humans [7]. This interpretation is appealing, but should be approached with skepticism. In that study, the analogous pathways were activated in rats and people through pain onset (aversion) and pain offset (relief). Do rats experience aversion and relief in the same way as people, especially people who know they are in an experiment, can stop at any time, and will not suffer injury? Yet, the procedures produced some overlapping activity in "analogous" brain regions in rats and people. While the experience in rats and humans is surely different, there is overlap in brain activity with identical paradigms. This opens the possibility of using invasive procedures to manipulate that activity in rats and examine the resultant behaviour. Supposing a desirable behaviour is achieved, one can move back to the human and test how noninvasive methods of manipulating either one of the behaviours or brain circuit of interest affect the other. In other words, the above example provides exactly the type of strength as that of rodent neuroimaging: a model from which to move back and forth to the human condition, a supplement to what we can identify in humans alone.

The future of rodent neuroimaging in the field of pain looks bright, with the use of innovative techniques such as MRS [74], integrating genetic and imaging data, and the use of optogenetics to directly stimulate brain areas while recording fMRI activity [35] or examine the effects of optogenetic manipulations on metabolic activity with PET imaging [70]. These and other innovations will allow the field to move forward, elucidating the intricate brain networks associated with various aspects of the pain experience. Careful assessments of behaviour and accounting for all possible variables and limitations will ensure fruitful progress.

REFERENCES

1. Afari N, Mostoufi S, Noonan C, Poeschla B, Succop A, Chopko L, Strachan E. C-reactive protein and pain sensitivity: findings from female twins. Ann Behav Med 2011;42:277–83.
2. Albensi BC, Knoblach SM, Chew BGM, O'Reilly MP, Faden AI, Pekar JJ. Diffusion and high resolution MRI of traumatic brain injury in rats: time course and correlation with histology. Exp Neurol 2000;162:61–72.
3. Baliki MN, Geha PY, Apkarian AV, Chialvo DR. Beyond feeling: chronic pain hurts the brain, disrupting the default-mode network dynamics. J Neurosci 2008;28:1398–403.
4. Baltes C, Radzwill N, Bosshard S, Marek D, Rudin M. Micro MRI of the mouse brain using a novel 400 MHz cryogenic quadrature RF probe. NMR Biomed 2009;22:834–42.
5. Bauer ME, Perks P, Lightman SL, Shanks N. Restraint stress is associated with changes in glucocorticoid immunoregulation. Physiol Behav 2001;73:525–32.

6. Becerra L, Chang PC, Bishop J, Borsook D. CNS activation maps in awake rats exposed to thermal stimuli to the dorsum of the hindpaw. NeuroImage 2011;54:1355–66.
7. Becerra L, Navratilova E, Porreca F, Borsook D. Analogous responses in the nucleus accumbens and cingulate cortex to pain onset (aversion) and offset (relief) in rats and humans. J Neurophysiol 2013;110:1221–6.
8. Becerra L, Pendse G, Chang PC, Bishop J, Borsook D. Robust reproducible resting state networks in the awake rodent brain. PLoS One 2011;6:e25701.
9. Biswal BB, Kannurpatti SS. Resting-state functional connectivity in animal models: modulations by exsanguination. Methods Mol Biol 2009;489:25–74.
10. Boly M, Tshibanda L, Vanhaudenhuyse A, Noirhomme Q, Schnakers C, Ledoux D, Boveroux P, Garweg C, Lambermont B, Phillips C, et al. Functional connectivity in the default network during resting state is preserved in a vegetative but not in a brain dead patient. Hum Brain Mapp 2009;30:2393–400.
11. Cauda F, D'Agata F, Sacco K, Duca S, Cocito D, Paolasso I, Isoardo G, Geminiani G. Altered resting state attentional networks in diabetic neuropathic pain. J Neurol Neurosurg Psychiatry 2010;81:806–11.
12. Cauda F, Sacco K, D'Agata F, Duca S, Cocito D, Geminiani G, Migliorati F, Isoardo G. Low-frequency BOLD fluctuations demonstrate altered thalamocortical connectivity in diabetic neuropathic pain. BMC Neurosci 2009;10:138.
13. Cauda F, Sacco K, Duca S, Cocito D, D'Agata F, Geminiani GC, Canavero S. Altered resting state in diabetic neuropathic pain. PLoS One 2009;4:e4542.
14. Chudasama Y. Animal models of prefrontal-executive function. Behav Neurosci 2011;125:327–43.
15. Davis KD, Moayedi M. Central mechanisms of pain revealed through functional and structural MRI. J Neuroimmune Pharmacol 2013;8(3):518–34.
16. Davoody L, Quiton RL, Lucas JM, Ji Y, Keller A, Masri R. Conditioned place preference reveals tonic pain in an animal model of central pain. J Pain 2011;12868–74.
17. Denic A, Macura S, Mishra P, Gamez J, Rodriguez M, Pirko I. MRI in rodent models of brain disorders. Neurotherapeutics 2011;8:3–18.
18. Draganski B, Gaser C, Busch V, Schuierer G, Bogdahn U, May A. Neuroplasticity: Changes in grey matter induced by training. Nature 2004;427:311–12.
19. Duerden EG, Albanese MC. Localization of pain-related brain activation: a meta-analysis of neuroimaging data. Hum Brain Mapp 2013;34:109–49.
20. Endo T, Spenger C, Hao J, Tominaga T, Wiesenfeld-Hallin Z, Olson L, Xu XJ. Functional MRI of the brain detects neuropathic pain in experimental spinal cord injury. Pain 2008;138:292–300.
21. Ferris CF, Febo M, Luo F, Schmidt K, Brevard M, Harder JA, Kulkarni P, Messenger T, King JA. Functional magnetic resonance imaging in conscious animals: a new tool in behavioural neuroscience research. J Neuroendocrinol 2006;18:307–18.
22. Friston KJ, Holmes AP, Worsley KJ. How many subjects constitute a study? NeuroImage 1999;10:1–5.
23. Galhardo V, Pais-Vieira M, Lima D. Prefrontal-based decision making impairment in rat models of chronic pain. J Pain 2007;4:S10.
24. Gear R, Becerra L, Upadhyay J, Bishop J, Wallin D, Pendse G, Levine J, Borsook D. Pain facilitation brain regions activated by nalbuphine are revealed by pharmacological fMRI. PLoS One 2013;8:e50169.
25. Governo RJM, Morris PG, Prior MJ, Marsden CA, Chapman V. Capsaicin-evoked brain activation and central sensitization in anaesthetised rats: a functional magnetic resonance imaging study. Pain 2006;126:35–45.
26. Greicius MD, Kiviniemi V, Tervonen O, Vainionpaa V, Alahuhta S, Reiss AL, Menon V. Persistent default-mode network connectivity during light sedation. Hum Brain Mapp 2008;29:839–47.
27. Herman P, Sanganahalli BG, Hyder F, Eke A. Fractal analysis of spontaneous fluctuations of the BOLD signal in rat brain. NeuroImage 2011;58:1060–9.
28. Horovitz SG, Fukunaga M, de Zwart JA, van GP, Fulton SC, Balkin TJ, Duyn JH. Low frequency BOLD fluctuations during resting wakefulness and light sleep: a simultaneous EEG-fMRI study. Hum Brain Mapp 2008;29:671–82.
29. Houston GC, Papadakis NG, Carpenter TA, Hall LD, Mukherjee B, James MF, Huang CL. Mapping of brain activation in response to pharmacological agents using fMRI in the rat. Magn Reson Imaging 2001;19:905–19.
30. Hutchison RM, Mirsattari SM, Jones CK, Gati JS, Leung LS. Functional networks in the anesthetized rat brain revealed by independent component analysis of resting-state FMRI. J Neurophysiol 2010;103:3398–406.
31. Ji G, Sun H, Fu Y, Li Z, Pais-Vieira M, Galhardo V, Neugebauer V. Cognitive impairment in pain through amygdala-driven prefrontal cortical deactivation. J Neurosci 2010;30:5451–64.
32. Jiang Y, Johnson GA. Microscopic diffusion tensor atlas of the mouse brain. NeuroImage 2011;56:1235–43.

33. Johnson GA, Calabrese E, Badea A, Paxinos G, Watson C. A multidimensional magnetic resonance histology atlas of the Wistar rat brain. NeuroImage 2012;62:1848–56.
34. Jonckers E, Van Audekerke J, De Visscher G, Van Der Linden A, Verhoye M. Functional connectivity fMRI of the rodent brain: comparison of functional connectivity networks in rat and mouse. PLoS One 2011;6:e18876.
35. Kahn I, Knoblich U, Desai M, Bernstein J, Graybiel AM, Boyden ES, Buckner RL, Moore CI. Optogenetic drive of neocortical pyramidal neurons generates fMRI signals that are correlated with spiking activity. Brain Res 2013;1511:33–45.
36. Kalthoff D, Seehafer JrU, Po C, Wiedermann D, Hoehn M. Functional connectivity in the rat at 11.7T: impact of physiological noise in resting state fMRI. Neuroimage 2011;54:2828–39.
37. Kim J, Eun LS, Sik MK, Jung HH, Lee JE, Kim SJ, Chang JW. Ventral posterolateral deep brain stimulation treatment for neuropathic pain shortens pain response after cold stimuli. J Neurosci Res 2013;91:997–1004.
38. King JA, Garelick TS, Brevard ME, Chen W, Messenger TL, Duong TQ, Ferris CF. Procedure for minimizing stress for fMRI studies in conscious rats. J Neurosci Methods 2005;148:154–60.
39. Kovacevic N, Henderson JT, Chan E, Lifshitz N, Bishop J, Evans AC, Henkelman RM, Chen XJ. A Three-dimensional MRI atlas of the mouse brain with estimates of the average and variability. Cereb Cortex 2005;15:639–45.
40. Lau JC, Lerch JP, Sled JG, Henkelman RM, Evans AC, Bedell BJ. Longitudinal neuroanatomical changes determined by deformation-based morphometry in a mouse model of Alzheimer's disease. NeuroImage 2008;42:19–27.
41. Lerch JP, Carroll JB, Dorr A, Spring S, Evans AC, Hayden MR, Sled JG, Henkelman RM. Cortical thickness measured from MRI in the YAC128 mouse model of Huntington's disease. NeuroImage 2008;41:243–251.
42. Lerch JP, Yiu AP, Martinez-Canabal A, Pekar T, Bohbot VD, Frankland PW, Henkelman RM, Josselyn SA, Sled JG. Maze training in mice induces MRI-detectable brain shape changes specific to the type of learning. NeuroImage 2011;54:2086–95.
43. Li N, Downey JE, Bar-Shir A, Gilad AA, Walczak P, Kim H, Joel SE, Pekar JJ, Thakor NV, Pelled G. Optogenetic-guided cortical plasticity after nerve injury. Proc Natl Acad Sci USA 2011;108:8838–43.
44. Liang Z, King J, Zhang N. Uncovering intrinsic connectional architecture of functional networks in awake rat brain. J Neurosci 2011;31:3776–83.
45. Liang Z, King J, Zhang N. Anticorrelated resting-state functional connectivity in awake rat brain. NeuroImage 2012;59:1190–9.
46. Liang Z, King J, Zhang N. Uncovering intrinsic connectional architecture of functional networks in awake rat brain. J Neurosci 2011;31:3776–83.
47. Liang Z, King J, Zhang N. Intrinsic organization of the anesthetized brain. J Neurosci 2012;32:10183–91.
48. Liu X, Zhu XH, Zhang Y, Chen W. The change of functional connectivity specificity in rats under various anesthesia levels and its neural origin. Brain Topogr 2013;26(3):363–77.
49. Majeed W, Magnuson M, Keilholz SD. Spatiotemporal dynamics of low frequency fluctuations in BOLD fMRI of the rat. J Magn Reson Imaging 2009;30:384–93.
50. Martin CJ, Kennerley AJ, Berwick J, Port M, Mayhew JE. Functional MRI in conscious rats using a chronically implanted surface coil. J Magn Reson Imaging 2013;38(3):739–44.
51. Masri R, Quiton RL, Lucas JM, Murray PD, Thompson SM, Keller A. Zona incerta: a role in central pain. J Neurophysiol 2009;102:181–91.
52. Metz AE, Yau HJ, Centeno MV, Apkarian AV, Martina M. Morphological and functional reorganization of rat medial prefrontal cortex in neuropathic pain. Proc Natl Acad Sci USA 2009;106:2423–8.
53. Millecamps M, Seminowicz DA, Laferriere AL, Stone LS, Bushnell MC. Histological brain changes associated with a rat model of long-term neuropathic pain. Paper presented at: International Association for the Study of Pain, 13th World Congress on Pain. Montreal; 2010.
54. Neugebauer V, Galhardo V, Maione S, Mackey SC. Forebrain pain mechanisms. Brain Res Rev 2009;60:226–42.
55. Pagano RL, Fonoff ET, Dale CS, Ballester G, Teixeira MJ, Britto LR. Motor cortex stimulation inhibits thalamic sensory neurons and enhances activity of PAG neurons: possible pathways for antinociception. Pain 2012;153:2359–69.
56. Pais-Vieira M, Lima D, Galhardo V. Sustained attention deficits in rats with chronic inflammatory pain. Neurosci Lett 2009;463:98–102.
57. Pais-Vieira M, Mendes-Pinto MM, Lima D, Galhardo V. Cognitive impairment of prefrontal-dependent decision-making in rats after the onset of chronic pain. Neuroscience 2009;161:671–9.
58. Pawela CP, Biswal BB, Cho YR, Kao DS, Li R, Jones SR, Schulte ML, Matloub HS, Hudetz AG, Hyde JS. Resting-state functional connectivity of the rat brain. Magn Reson Med 2008;59:1021–9.

59. Pawela CP, Biswal BB, Hudetz AG, Li R, Jones SR, Cho YR, Matloub HS, Hyde JS. Interhemispheric neuroplasticity following limb deafferentation detected by resting-state functional connectivity magnetic resonance imaging (fcMRI) and functional magnetic resonance imaging (fMRI). NeuroImage 2010;49: 2467–78.
60. Paxinos G, Watson R. The rat brain in stereotaxic coordinates. New York, NY: Elsevier Academic Press; 2005.
61. Porro CA, Carli G. Immobilization and restraint effects on pain reactions in animals. Pain 1988;32:289–307.
62. Raichle ME, Mintun MA. Brain work and brain imaging. Annu Rev Neurosci 2006;29:449–76.
63. Ridgway GR, Henley SMD, Rohrer JD, Scahill RI, Warren JD, Fox NC. Ten simple rules for reporting voxel-based morphometry studies. NeuroImage 2008;40:1429–35.
64. Rivat C, Laboureyras E, Laulin JP, Le RC, Richebe P, Simonnet G. Non-nociceptive environmental stress induces hyperalgesia, not analgesia, in pain and opioid-experienced rats. Neuropsychopharmacology 2007;32:2217–28.
65. Sawiak SJ, Wood NI, Williams GB, Morton AJ, Carpenter TA. Voxel-based morphometry in the R6/2 transgenic mouse reveals differences between genotypes not seen with manual 2D morphometry. Neurobiol Dis 2009;33:20–7.
66. Seminowicz DA, Jiang L, Ji Y, Xu S, Gullapalli RP, Masri R. Thalamocortical asynchrony in conditions of spinal cord injury pain in rats. J Neurosci 2012;32:15843–8.
67. Seminowicz DA, Laferriere AL, Millecamps M, Yu JSC, Coderre TJ, Bushnell MC. MRI structural brain changes associated with sensory and emotional function in a rat model of long-term neuropathic pain. NeuroImage 2009;47:1007–14.
68. Shehzad Z, Kelly AM, Reiss PT, Gee DG, Gotimer K, Uddin LQ, Lee SH, Margulies DS, Roy AK, Biswal BB, et al. The resting brain: unconstrained yet reliable. Cereb Cortex 2009;19:2209–9.
69. Stamatakis EA, Adapa RM, Absalom AR, Menon DK. Changes in resting neural connectivity during propofol sedation. PLoS ONE 2010;5:e14224.
70. Thanos PK, Robison L, Nestler EJ, Kim R, Michaelides M, Lobo MK, Volkow ND. Mapping brain metabolic connectivity in awake rats with μPET and optogenetic stimulation. J Neurosci 2013;33:6343–9.
71. Thompson SJ, Bushnell MC. Rodent functional and anatomical imaging of pain. Neurosci Lett 2012;520: 131–9.
72. Walton KD, Dubois M, Llinbs RR. Abnormal thalamocortical activity in patients with complex regional pain syndrome (CRPS) type I. Pain 2010;150:41–51.
73. Wang G, Thompson SM. Maladaptive homeostatic plasticity in a rodent model of central pain syndrome: thalamic hyperexcitability after spinothalamic tract lesions. J Neurosci 2008;28:11959–69.
74. Xu S, Ji Y, Chen X, Yang Y, Gullapalli RP, Masri R. In vivo high-resolution localized (1) H MR spectroscopy in the awake rat brain at 7 T. Magn Reson Med 2013;69:937–43.
75. Xu S, Zhuo J, Racz J, Shi D, Roys S, Fiskum G, Gullapalli R. Early microstructural and metabolic changes following controlled cortical impact injury in rat: a magnetic resonance imaging and spectroscopy study. J Neurotrauma 2011;28:2091–102.
76. Zhang N, Rane P, Huang W, Liang Z, Kennedy D, Frazier JA, King J. Mapping resting-state brain networks in conscious animals. J Neurosci Methods 2010;189:186–96.
77. Zhao F, Zhao T, Zhou L, Wu Q, Hu X. BOLD study of stimulation-induced neural activity and resting-state connectivity in medetomidine-sedated rat. NeuroImage 2008;39:248–60.
78. Zhuo J, Gullapalli RP. AAPM/RSNA physics tutorial for residents: MR artifacts, safety, and quality control. Radiographics 2006;26:275–97.
79. Zhuo J, Xu S, Proctor JL, Mullins RJ, Simon JZ, Fiskum G, Gullapalli RP. Diffusion kurtosis as an in vivo imaging marker for reactive astrogliosis in traumatic brain injury. NeuroImage 2012;59:467–77.

SECTION 6

The Brain Adapting with Chronic Pain

CHAPTER 24

Chronification of Back Pain: Causes and Consequences

A. Vania Apkarian and Marwan N. Baliki

Back pain affects a large sector of society and is the leading cause of disability in the United States. Also, it is one of the top seven leading causes of disability worldwide. When back pain becomes chronic, its cost to society is staggering. End organ–based studies of the condition have mostly been unproductive. Instead, human brain imaging studies are beginning to provide evidence for the essential role of the brain in its prediction, transition, and maintenance. These successes, by force, lead to a new exciting phase of pain research where circuitry and mechanisms identified in the human condition need to be back translated to animal model studies, which should in turn lead to a more precise molecular understanding of critical mechanisms and the potential for developing scientifically grounded effective therapies.

IMPACT OF BACK PAIN

Low back pain is a public health problem affecting between 70% and 85% of adults at some point in their lives [22]. The annual prevalence of chronic low back pain ranges from 15% to 45%, with point prevalence averaging 30% [1]. In the United States, chronic and acute back pain are the most common causes of activity limitation in people under 45, and the second most frequent reason for visits to physicians [25, 38]. Data from other Western countries are similar. The most recent analysis of the global burden of disease indicates that in the year 2010, low back pain was the number one condition for years lived in disability in the United States (n = 36,689), and the seventh leading cause of disability among all disease or injury conditions worldwide (across 187 countries) [35]. An article by Deyo [17] states:

> ". . . . Clearly, back pain is one of society's most significant non-lethal medical conditions. And yet the prevalence of back pain is perhaps matched in degree only by the lingering mystery accompanying it."

Current management of low back pain remains inadequate: Most individuals (>90%) with acute low back pain (0–7 days of back pain) recover full function in days or weeks with little or no lingering pain. Yet a small number of individuals with acute low back pain (~5% or less) go on to develop subacute back pain (SBP, 4–12 weeks of back pain), then chronic low back pain (CBP, >6 months of back pain) [22]. A high percentage of these patients fail treatment, continue to have significant degrees of pain, are significantly limited in their functional capacity, and become emotionally altered. A current longitudinal study has demonstrated that 50% of SBP patients continue to suffer from the same magnitude of back pain 1 year later [12]. Thus, this is the back pain population most vulnerable to pain chronicity, and unravelling mechanisms for transition to chronic pain within this group may have a large clinical impact.

Available treatments for back pain remain inadequate: Placebo-controlled trials conducted to date have found some support for the use of nonsteroidal anti-inflammatory drugs (NSAIDs) and antidepressants in treating back pain, but their results are usually not large enough to reach clinical effectiveness (>20% decrease in pain from placebo). A meta-analysis of NSAID studies found no evidence that these drugs were effective in treating low back pain once it has become chronic [46] (see also [16, 37]). A systematic review of antidepressants treatment for CBP also concluded that they produce only a moderate symptom reduction [44], and a review concluded: "Many drugs used for back pain are no more, or only slightly more, effective than placebos. . . no drug regimen can be legitimately recommended for back pain" [14]. The World Health Organization Advisory Panel likewise concluded that there is no single treatment superior to others for relieving CBP [18].

Existing biomarkers of back pain have low predictive power: (1) Anatomical and genetic risk factors: The probability that the cause of back pain can be identified by radiography is less than 1% [45]. Nevertheless, the histological composition of herniated disc material seems to correlate with clinical symptoms such as reported pain [49]. Another cause of pain and radicular symptoms seems to be due to pressure on the nerve from ligamentum flavum and facet joints [36]. Yet the low incidence of these biomarkers suggests they are unlikely to be important factors for explaining the condition.

Findings from two adult female twin studies indicate that 50–70% of the variation in disc degenerative processes is due to genetic factors [30, 41]. A similar Danish study also showed a genetic influence, albeit with more modest results [26]. Other experiments have identified a number of candidate genes that underlie disc degeneration and pain [31]. However, the extent to which these genetic factors are strong and reproducible enough to explain the condition remains to be determined.

(2) Psychosocial factors: As peripheral physical factors have failed to show a strong relationship with back pain, numerous psychosocial and demographic factors have been studied. Cumulatively, however, these factors provide weak predictions regarding chronic pain.

Depression is ranked as one of the strongest predictors of low back pain. This association is observed by multiple studies. One of the largest involved a national survey (n = 91,347) and a 2-year follow-up survey (n = 55,690), and indicates that depression and low back pain are interrelated (correlation of 0.4), with associational odds ratios increasing with the intensity of back pain and severity of depression [33]; see also [39]. The recent longitudinal brain imaging–based study indicates that 50% of SBP patients continue to experience persistent pain 1 year after the onset of symptoms, yet their depression values remain constant in this time period and do not differ from the subjects where the pain resolves [12]. Regarding psychosocial factors, the best predictors have been intensity and duration of pain, expectations of recovery and perception of health change, obesity, workplace risk factors [21, 42], and smoking [19]. Yet attempts to create models of CBP based upon psychosocial parameters have been unproductive [15, 28, 47, 50].

In summary, there is a long list of risk factors, but no dominant physical or psychosocial parameters that can substantially explain chronic pain. Given the large prevalence of back pain and its impact on society, it is not surprising that there is a large literature on the topic dominated by clinical observations and linked to the standard science of pain perception, that is, attempting to explain it by nociceptive activity in the periphery and also invoking gate theory and/or spinal cord sensitization [48].

CHRONIC BACK PAIN AS A FUNCTIONAL PAIN SYNDROME

About 15 years ago, I made the conscious decision that human brain imaging technology provides direct access to the human brain, and thus adapting such tools specifically to study clinical, chronic pain conditions has the potential to importantly advance our knowledge of underlying mechanisms. Implicit assumptions of this decision were as follows: (a) chronic and acute pain may have distinct underlying mechanisms, (b) studying the human brain in acute pain may in fact provide misleading information regarding chronic pain, (c) chronic pain is likely associated with brain reorganization, at least as a consequence of living with the condition, and (d) the brain may also possess predisposing characteristics, some due to genetics and others due to past experience, that predetermine the fate of subjects regarding transitioning to chronic pain. Our initial steps in this direction were done in chronic complex regional pain syndrome patients [6]. However, we quickly switched from this group to the study of back pain, mainly because it is the most prominent chronic pain condition (which should facilitate recruitment of needed participants) and because it seemed to be considered a mysterious state, where clinicians essentially put the blame on the patient by labelling them malingerers, seekers of disability compensation, or seekers of health industry in general, as drug or care dependents.

Our earliest human brain imaging reports showed that brain activity for different chronic pain conditions identifies quite distinct brain activity patterns [4, 7, 24], and even cognitive tests comparing across chronic pain conditions show specific properties [5]. As attested by the different chapters of this book, the pain research community is now engaged in unravelling the brain properties unique to each of the chronic pain conditions that in the past have been most often lumped into a single category. It is also remarkable to note that even we and many other groups have now shown a multiplicity of brain anatomical and functional differences between healthy subjects and chronic pain conditions. Even about 2 years ago, in a systematic review of the evidence regarding the contribution of peripheral processes in contrast to central parameters [40], we were equivocal and could not assert priority to either. This was mainly because the brain imaging studies were all cross-sectional in nature and thus they could not be used to identify causal relationships, and the end-organ viewpoint, although still highly popular with clinicians, lacks convincing evidence.

BRAIN ACTIVITY RELATED TO BACK PAIN

Our initial effort to unravel back pain–related brain activity was an attempt to provoke the back pain by using straight leg raising [4]. However, we quickly realized that the method guaranteed evoking head motion, tightly correlated with the task. Thus, head motion confound could not be corrected, and we abandoned the approach. In the process, we uncovered that simply rating spontaneous fluctuations of the back pain was sufficient to identify back pain–related brain activity. The approach had the advantage of its simplicity, with the additional bonus that we could claim to identify brain activity in proportion to the purely subjective perception of back pain, namely, the pain that subjects come to the clinic complaining about. The methodology could be generalized to assess a multiplicity of chronic pain conditions [7, 20, 23, 24], as well as distinguish between stimulus-related and perception-related brain activity for evoked thermal stimuli [10]. I had fully expected the approach would be adopted by other investigators, but to date although multiple laboratories have expressed interest in studying spontaneous pain, our laboratory remains the main source of such studies. One suspects small technical difficulties are the main roadblock, yet objections regarding the perfect control for such tasks have also been raised [34].

The primary observation of brain activity identified for spontaneous fluctuations of back pain was that it was represented primarily in the medial prefrontal cortex (mPFC), a brain region involved in self-monitoring and in emotional valuation, and not in somatosensory regions or regions most commonly seen for acute painful stimuli. We could observe this activity independently of the type of peripheral inciting event when we averaged across a small number group of 6–15 back pain patients, or when we averaged across a much larger group of 94 patients (Fig. 24-1). Surprisingly, when we averaged across 94 CBP patients, the only additional brain activity outside of mPFC was bilateral amygdala [27]. The latter study then establishes, beyond any serious doubt, the brain activity associated with subjective CBP.

Studying brain activity for chronic pain has been importantly advanced with the advent of the identification of resting-state activity, a methodology far simpler than examining activity for spontaneous pain, but the cost is the disadvantage that it is harder to link it to specific perceptual states. In the first study of the default-mode network (DMN) studied in CBP, we showed that it was diminished in extent, primarily because parts of mPFC fluctuated independently of the DMN [11]. Subsequently, we were able to show that resting-state mPFC activity has increased power in high-frequency brain activity and that these high-frequency fluctuations are in fact directly related to the spontaneous back pain [8]. This study, to our knowledge, remains the only illustration linking resting-state activity to perceptual properties. More recent studies provide additional evidence for the involvement of mPFC in CBP: Arterial spin label imaging (a technique capable of identifying metabolic rate of different brain regions) shows increased metabolic rate, most likely due to increased neuronal activity, in mPFC in such patients [29].

Yet, the pain research community continues to express skepticism about the notion that back pain activity is represented in mPFC, and not within the "pain matrix." This attitude is not very surprising because the field remains heavily dominated by Cartesian and Sherringtonian notions, with the cortex providing the real estate upon which sensory modalities are laid out. This specificity view of sensory information coding stipulates that pain has its dedicated representational real estate in the cortex, with the corollary that chronic pain simply sustains or enhances the activity within its own real estate [3]. Unique brain activity for distinct chronic pain conditions simply does not fit in the construct of specificity theory. We were recently able to directly address the issue by examining brain activity for back pain in subjects as they transition from an acute/subacute back pain state to chronicity over a 1-year span [27]. The study showed that the spontaneous pain of back pain is initially (within weeks after the onset of symptoms) represented in brain regions commonly observed to be activated for acute pain, and that in time this activity shifts away from these regions and engages the mPFC only in the subjects where the back pain was sustained for the year. Perhaps the largest surprise of this study was that the large-scale change in the location of back pain–related activity in the cortex, away from sensory and to emotional mPFC circuits, seems to occur in the absence of any significant change in the properties of the back pain or in mood parameters. The latter observation forces the conclusion that similar perceptions can result from distinct brain activity.

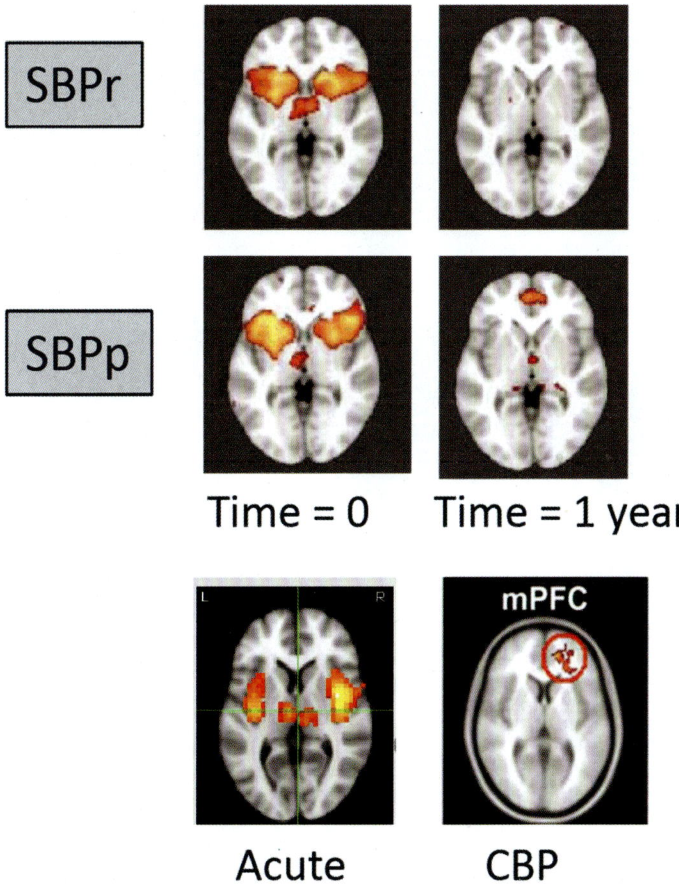

FIGURE 24-1 Brain activity in back pain shifts in time away from sensory regions of the brain and engages the medial prefrontal cortex (mPFC). The top two rows (adapted from Hashmi et al. [27]) show BOLD activity for rating spontaneous fluctuations of back pain in subacute back pain (SBP) subjects, subdivided into recovering (SBPr) and persisting (SBPp) based on a 20% decrease in intensity of back pain from entry into the study (time = 0) to 1 year later (time = 1 year). Brain activity collected at the time of entry into the study was identical for both groups and closely matched brain activity observed for acute pain. (Third row, acute, from *Neurosynth* [51]). One year later, in subjects recovering from back pain (SBPr), brain activity was essentially null, whereas in subjects transitioning to chronic pain (SBPp), BOLD activity shifted to mPFC, corresponding to brain activity observed in chronic back pain (CBP) patients. (Third row, CBP, adapted from Baliki et al. [9].)

ANATOMICAL REORGANIZATION OF CORTICAL GREY MATTER IN CHRONIC BACK PAIN

We and many other groups now show evidence that the cortical grey matter mantle is distinct in different chronic pain conditions. The cortical grey matter, when viewed as an anatomical network (Fig. 24-2), shows distinct patterns and distinct time constants of reorganization in different chronic pain conditions [13]. Some of this reorganization is reversed with successful therapy [43], and in CBP the reorganization seems to be mainly a decrease in regional grey density with persistence of pain. Underlying mechanisms remain unclear; however, when longitudinally tracking grey matter in acute/subacute back pain patients over 1 year, we observe its decrease to be limited to specific brain regions where functional connectivity (extent of information shared between the region and other brain areas) changes in proportion to the change in grey matter density and in relation to the intensity

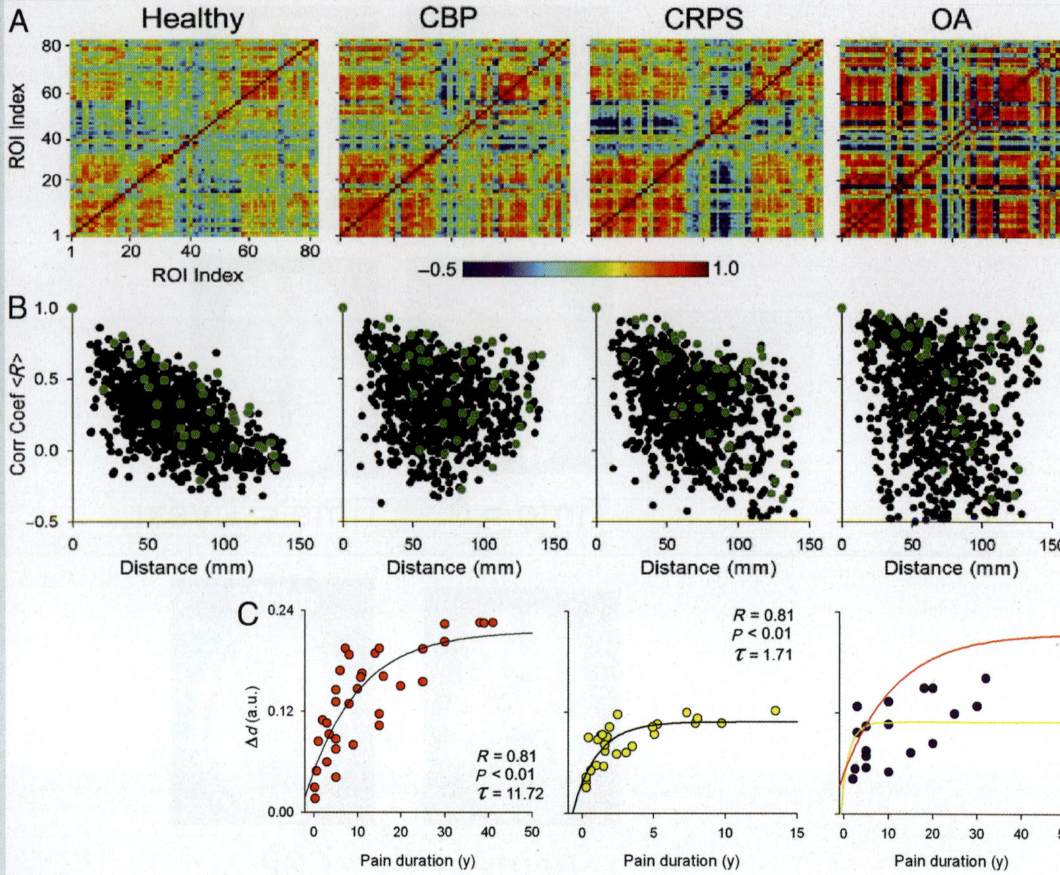

FIGURE 24-2 Brain neocortical grey matter density (GMD) properties, when envisioned as a network, exhibit chronic pain–type specific reorganization. **A:** Similarity matrices for GMD are shown for a group of healthy subjects (healthy), chronic back pain (CBP), complex regional pain syndrome (CRPS), and osteoarthritis (OA). Note the patterns are unique for each group. **B:** When the same data are presented as a function of distance between pairs of brain regions, we observe that the negative distance relationship seen in healthy subjects is uniquely disturbed in different types of chronic pain. **C:** When a global value was derived measuring the overall extent of reorganization of the neocortex in individual subjects, in comparison with healthy subjects, this parameter could be used to derive a time constant for brain reorganization in each group. Note each symbol is an individual subject. In CBP, GMD continues to reorganize for more than 10 years. (Figure adapted from [13].)

of the back pain only in subjects where the pain persists over 1 year but not in those where the back pain decreases [12]. Thus, we now consider the grey matter reorganization and the correlated functional connectivity changes as part and parcel of the back pain chronification. The latter provides a new definition of chronic pain, namely, reorganization of the cortex that sustains a persistent pain state.

CAUSAL PREDICTORS FOR TRANSITION TO CHRONIC BACK PAIN

Our longitudinal study of back pain transitioning from acute to a chronic condition has identified both functional and anatomical signatures that predict who will persist with back pain and who will recover from it [12]. The strength of functional connectivity between mPFC and nucleus accumbens (Fig. 24-3, top), determined from scans collected within

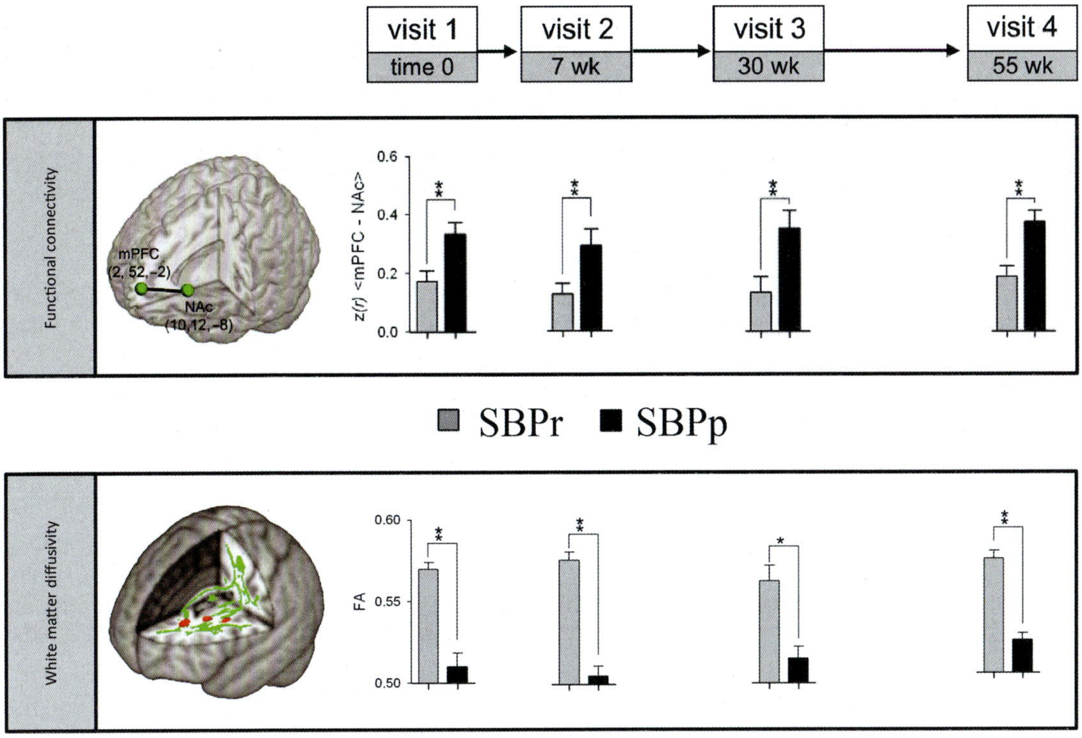

FIGURE 24-3 Brain functional properties and white matter myelination properties distinguish between back pain patients recovering (SBPr) from back pain or persisting (SBPp) with back pain. Thus, these unitary parameters causally determine transition to CBP. Top bar graphs: Functional connectivity strength (between medial prefrontal cortex [mPFC] and nucleus accumbens [NAc]) in SBPr and SBPp is shown for fMRI data collected at four times from entry into the study. Bottom bar graphs: White matter fractional anisotropy, a measure of myelination properties, identified to differ between SBPr and SBPp is shown for diffusion tensor imaging data collected at four times from entry into the study. (Data adapted from [12, 32].) $^*p < 0.05$, $^{**}p < 0.01$.

weeks from onset of back pain, predicts with better than 80% accuracy pain persistence 1 year later. We surmise that this functional connectivity is a critical link in the transition to chronic pain, as we have proposed that brain learning mechanisms (mediated through accumbens dopaminergic circuitry) control synaptic plasticity within large networks of the cerebral cortex, and thus actively participate in cortical reorganization and whether such a reorganization will or will not occur [2]. Similarly, white matter axonal track properties (Fig. 24-3, bottom) collected again at the time of entry into the study also predict with similar, or even better accuracy, pain persistence 1 year later [32]. These results, therefore, show that brain properties are causal predictors of the transition from acute to CBP. As such, this evidence is the first strong demonstration that changes the balance between end-organ properties versus brain properties regarding critical determinants of transition to CBP, and asserts that CBP is predicated on neurological predispositions.

IMPLICATIONS

In this chapter, we intentionally do not discuss the mechanisms underlying chronic pain, but, instead, concentrate on the role of the brain more generally in CBP and in the transition to CBP. Gross mechanistic implications are that brain predisposing factors are critical for pain chronification, which when coupled with an inciting event place such subjects at higher risk for the transition to chronic pain. This transition involves at least a cortical anatomical and functional change. Longer term living with chronic pain may underlie another set of mechanisms that reorganize the brain distinctly in different chronic pain conditions, reflecting specific properties of the condition and related suffering and coping mechanisms. These distinct mechanisms for the different phases of chronic pain in turn imply the possibility of different interventions for each of the phases of the transition to chronic pain.

CHALLENGES

A. Given that myriad of mechanisms seem to entail chronification of back pain, one wonders how many of these are common between different clinical pain conditions, and which are more specific to back pain.

B. In general, the outlined results show little evidence for the role of the end organ in back pain chronification. Is this specific to back pain, or does it generalize to other persistent pain conditions? An inciting event still seems necessary. Does this have to be a peripheral input, or can central disturbances also precipitate chronic pain? One suspects that higher intensity and/or longer duration of injury-induced pain increases the probability of chronification, yet most likely this also depends on specific brain predispositions as well; such interactions remain to be unravelled.

C. Reverse translational approaches are urgently necessary. Can we model components of the mechanisms observed in the human back pain in animal models, and use such models to then identify novel chemical and molecular targets?

REFERENCES

1. Andersson GBJ. The epidemiology of spinal disorders. In: Frymoyer JW, Ducker TB, Hadler NM, Kostuik JP, Weinstein JN, Whitecloud TS, editors. The adult spine: principles and practice, Vol. 2. Philadelphia, PA: Lippincott-Raven; 1997. pp. 93–141.
2. Apkarian AV. Pain perception in relation to emotional learning. Curr Opin Neurobiol 2008;18(4):464–8.
3. Apkarian AV. A brain signature for acute pain. Trends Cogn Sci 2013;17(7):309–10.
4. Apkarian AV, Krauss BR, Fredrickson BE, Szeverenyi NM. Imaging the pain of low back pain: functional magnetic resonance imaging in combination with monitoring subjective pain perception allows the study of clinical pain states. Neurosci Lett 2001;299(1–2):57–60.
5. Apkarian AV, Sosa Y, Krauss BR, Thomas PS, Fredrickson BE, Levy RE, Harden RN, Chialvo DR. Chronic pain patients are impaired on an emotional decision-making task Pain 2004;108:129–36.
6. Apkarian AV, Thomas PS, Krauss BR, Szeverenyi NM. Prefrontal cortical hyperactivity in patients with sympathetically mediated chronic pain. Neurosci Lett 2001;311(3):193–97.
7. Baliki M, Katz J, Chialvo DR, Apkarian AV. Single subject pharmacological-MRI (phMRI) study: modulation of brain activity of psoriatic arthritis pain by cyclooxygenase-2 inhibitor. Mol Pain 2005;1:32.
8. Baliki MN, Baria AT, Apkarian AV. The cortical rhythms of chronic back pain. J Neuroscience 2011;31(39):13981–90.
9. Baliki MN, Chialvo DR, Geha PY, Levy RM, Harden RN, Parrish TB, Apkarian AV. Chronic pain and the emotional brain: specific brain activity associated with spontaneous fluctuations of intensity of chronic back pain. J Neurosci 2006;26(47):12165–73.
10. Baliki MN, Geha PY, Apkarian AV. Parsing pain perception between nociceptive representation and magnitude estimation. J Neurophysiol 2009;101(2):875–87.
11. Baliki MN, Geha PY, Apkarian AV, Chialvo DR. Beyond feeling: chronic pain hurts the brain, disrupting the default-mode network dynamics. J Neurosci 2008;28(6):1398–403.
12. Baliki MN, Petre B, Torbey S, Herrmann KM, Huang L, Schnitzer TJ, Fields HL, Apkarian AV. Corticostriatal functional connectivity predicts transition to chronic back pain. Nat Neurosci 2012;15(8):1117–9.

13. Baliki MN, Schnitzer TJ, Bauer WR, Apkarian AV. Brain morphological signatures for chronic pain. PloS One 2011;6(10):e26010.
14. Bogduk N. Pharmacological alternatives for the alleviation of back pain1. Expert Opin Pharmacother 2004;5(10):2091–8.
15. Clays E, De Bacquer D, Leynen F, Kornitzer M, Kittel F, De Backer G. The impact of psychosocial factors on low back pain: longitudinal results from the Belstress study. Spine 2007;32(2):262–8.
16. Coats TL, Borenstein DG, Nangia NK, Brown MT. Effects of valdecoxib in the treatment of chronic low back pain: results of a randomized, placebo-controlled trial. Clin Ther 2004;26(8):1249–60.
17. Deyo RA. Low-back pain. Sci Am 1998;279(2):48–53.
18. Ehrlich GE. Low back pain. Bull World Health Organ 2003;81(9):671–6.
19. Feldman DE, Rossignol M, Shrier I, Abenhaim L. Smoking. A risk factor for development of low back pain in adolescents. Spine 1999;24(23):2492–6.
20. Foss JM, Apkarian AV, Chialvo DR. Dynamics of pain: fractal dimension of temporal variability of spontaneous pain differentiates between pain States. J Neurophysiol 2006;95(2):730–6.
21. Fransen M, Woodward M, Norton R, Coggan C, Dawe M, Sheridan N. Risk factors associated with the transition from acute to chronic occupational back pain. Spine 2002;27(1):92–8.
22. Frymoyer JW. Back pain and sciatica. N Engl J Med 1988;318(5):291–300.
23. Geha PY, Baliki MN, Chialvo DR, Harden RN, Paice JA, Apkarian AV. Brain activity for spontaneous pain of postherpetic neuralgia and its modulation by lidocaine patch therapy. Pain 2007;128(1–2):88–100.
24. Geha PY, Harden N, Paice J, Parrish T, Chialvo DR, Baliki M, Apkarian AV. Brain activity for modulation of spontaneous pain by topical lidocaine in post-herpetic neuropathy. J Pain 2005;6(5 Suppl):S51.
25. Hart LG, Deyo RA, Cherkin DC. Physician office visits for low back pain: frequency, clinical evaluation, and treatment patterns from a U.S. national survey. Spine 1995;20(1):11–9.
26. Hartvigsen J, Christensen K, Frederiksen H, Petersen HC. Genetic and environmental contributions to back pain in old age: a study of 2,108 danish twins aged 70 and older. Spine 2004;29(8):897–901.
27. Hashmi JA, Baliki MN, Huang L, Baria AT, Torbey S, Hermann KM, Schnitzer TJ, Apkarian AV. Shape shifting pain: chronification of back pain shifts brain representation from nociceptive to emotional circuits. Brain 2013;136(Pt 9):2751–68.
28. Keeley P, Creed F, Tomenson B, Todd C, Borglin G, Dickens C. Psychosocial predictors of health-related quality of life and health service utilisation in people with chronic low back pain. Pain 2008;135(1–2):142–50.
29. Loggia ML, Kim J, Gollub RL, Vangel MG, Kirsch I, Kong J, Wasan AD, Napadow V. Default mode network connectivity encodes clinical pain: an arterial spin labeling study. Pain 2013;154(1):24–33.
30. MacGregor AJ, Andrew T, Sambrook PN, Spector TD. Structural, psychological, and genetic influences on low back and neck pain: a study of adult female twins. Arthritis Rheum 2004;51(2):160–7.
31. Manek NJ, MacGregor AJ. Epidemiology of back disorders: prevalence, risk factors, and prognosis. Curr Opin Rheumatol 2005;17(2):134–40.
32. Mansour AR, Baliki MN, Huang L, Torbey S, Herrmann KM, Schnitzer TJ, Apkarian AV. Brain white matter structural properties predict transition to chronic pain. Pain 2013;154(10):2160–8.
33. Meyer T, Cooper J, Raspe H. Disabling low back pain and depressive symptoms in the community-dwelling elderly: a prospective study. Spine 2007;32(21):2380–6.
34. Moayedi M, Weissman-Fogel I. Is the insula the "how much" intensity coder? J Neurophysiol 2009;102(3): 1345-1347.
35. Murray CJ, Lopez AD. Measuring the global burden of disease. N Engl J Med 2013;369(5):448–57.
36. Okuda T, Baba I, Fujimoto Y, Tanaka N, Sumida T, Manabe H, Hayashi Y, Ochi M. The pathology of ligamentum flavum in degenerative lumbar disease. Spine 2004;29(15):1689–7.
37. Pallay RM, Seger W, Adler JL, Ettlinger RE, Quaidoo EA, Lipetz R, O'Brien K, Mucciola L, Skalky CS, Petruschke RA, et al. Etoricoxib reduced pain and disability and improved quality of life in patients with chronic low back pain: a 3 month, randomized, controlled trial1. Scand J Rheumatol 2004;33(4):257–66.
38. Praemer A, Furnes S, Rice DP. Musculoskeletal conditions in the United States, Vol. 1. Rosemont, IL: AAOS; 1992. pp. 1–99.
39. Reid MC, Williams CS, Gill TM. The relationship between psychological factors and disabling musculoskeletal pain in community-dwelling older persons. J Am Geriatr Soc 2003;51(8):1092–8.
40. Robinson JPA, A.V. Low back pain. In: Mayer EAB, Bushnell MC, editor. Functional pain syndromes: presentation and pathophysiology. Seattle, WA: International Association for the Study of Pain; 2009.
41. Sambrook PN, MacGregor AJ, Spector TD. Genetic influences on cervical and lumbar disc degeneration: a magnetic resonance imaging study in twins. Arthritis Rheum 1999;42(2):366–72.

42. Schultz IZ, Crook J, Meloche GR, Berkowitz J, Milner R, Zuberbier OA, Meloche W. Psychosocial factors predictive of occupational low back disability: towards development of a return-to-work model. Pain 2004;107(1–2):77–85.
43. Seminowicz DA, Wideman TH, Naso L, Hatami-Khoroushahi Z, Fallatah S, Ware MA, Jarzem P, Bushnell MC, Shir Y, Ouellet JA, et al. Effective treatment of chronic low back pain in humans reverses abnormal brain anatomy and function. J Neurosci 2011;31(20):7540–50.
44. Staiger TO, Gaster B, Sullivan MD, Deyo RA. Systematic review of antidepressants in the treatment of chronic low back pain. Spine 2003;28(22):2540–5.
45. van den Bosch MA, Hollingworth W, Kinmonth AL, Dixon AK. Evidence against the use of lumbar spine radiography for low back pain. Clin Radiol 2004;59(1):69–76.
46. van Tulder MW, Scholten RJ, Koes BW, Deyo RA. Nonsteroidal anti-inflammatory drugs for low back pain: a systematic review within the framework of the Cochrane Collaboration Back Review Group. Spine 2000;25(19):2501–13.
47. Vlaeyen JW, Linton SJ. Fear-avoidance and its consequences in chronic musculoskeletal pain: a state of the art. Pain 2000;85(3):317–32.
48. Waddell G. The back pain revolution. Edinburgh, Scotland: Churchill Livingstone; 1998.
49. Willburger RE, Ehiosun UK, Kuhnen C, Kramer J, Schmid G. Clinical symptoms in lumbar disc herniations and their correlation to the histological composition of the extruded disc material. Spine 2004;29(15):1655–61.
50. Woods MP, Asmundson GJ. Evaluating the efficacy of graded in vivo exposure for the treatment of fear in patients with chronic back pain: a randomized controlled clinical trial. Pain 2008;136(3):271–80.
51. Yarkoni T, Poldrack RA, Nichols TE, Van Essen DC, Wager TD. Large-scale automated synthesis of human functional neuroimaging data. Nat Methods 2011;8(8):665–70.

CHAPTER 25

Imaging Migraine

David Borsook, Lino Becerra, and Rami Burstein

MIGRAINE—A COMMON NEUROLOGICAL DISEASE

Migraine is the most common neurological disease. It is a disabling headache disorder characterized by intermittent attacks that may be associated with and without aura (ihs-classification.org). It is associated with a number of physiological and emotional processes, including pain, tiredness, nausea, vomiting, photophobia, or phonophobia. The global burden of migraine is reported to be 14.77% and is much higher compared with other chronic pain states such as chronic low back pain (9.17%) or osteoarthritis (3.6%) [34]. The World Health Organization (WHO) notes migraine to be among the top 20 causes of disability worldwide [13]. In many, it starts in childhood and affects people during the formative and most productive periods of their lives, between 25 and 55 [36, 37]. The condition affects some 45 million Americans [72].

The trigeminovascular system (TVS) is the major neural network involved in migraine. It comprises neurons located in the trigeminal ganglion that innervate the cerebral vasculature, including the dura mater. Afferent fibres that innervate these intracranial structures constitute the peripheral branches of trigeminal ganglion neurons whose cell somas are located in the ophthalmic division and central axons terminate in the spinal trigeminal nucleus. Pain transmission and vascular tone are modulated by several neurotransmitters, neuropeptides (e.g., calcitonin gene–related peptide [CGRP] and substance P [SP]) synthesized and secreted by trigeminal ganglion neurons.

THE MIGRAINE CONTINUUM

The disease we call migraine is an ongoing process that can begin in childhood and continue into old age. The continuum is also observed in the context of attack frequency—from 1 to 14 headache days per month in episodic migraine and more than 14 headache days a month in chronic migraine (ihs-classification.org).

MIGRAINE IMAGING METRICS

Imaging has changed our perception that migraine is an "event that comes and goes." Those affected by the disorder exhibit signs of brain function abnormalities before (peri-ictal), during (ictal), and after (postictal) attacks. The issue of "normal" is true in the context of no suffering, but the brains are different from healthy subjects and may thus be "at risk" for

BOX 25-1 Common Peri-ictal and Interictal Clinical Manifestations of Migraine

Preictal Changes/Prodrome

Sensory/Motor Changes
Visual aura
Sensory, motor, or verbal disturbances
Neck stiffness

Autonomic Changes
Appetitive changes
Dizziness
Yawning

Emotional Changes
Irritability or other mood changes

Other Changes
Confusion
Fatigue
Sleep disturbances
Difficulty concentrating

Ictal Changes/Attack

Sensory/Motor Changes
Head pain—lateralized or bilateral
Visual changes, including blurry and double vision
Hypersensitivity to sensory stimulation (photophobia, phonophobia, osmophobia, allodynia)
Neck pain and muscle tenderness

Autonomic Changes
Nausea and vomiting
Teary eyes, stuffy nose, and congestion
Yawning, frequent urination

Other Changes
Transient amnesia, expressive aphasia, motor clumsiness, depression

Postictal Changes/Postdrome

Other Changes
Tiredness

Interictal Changes
Anxiety, hypersensitivity to all sensory modalities

increased sensitivity to sound and light in their interictal period and perhaps more sensitive to attacks, particularly as these chronify. As noted in Fig. 25-1, multiple processes are involved in brain processing in migraine.

Ever since the exciting work published on the ictal migraine state using positron emission tomography by Weiller and colleagues [79], the field has been vigorously involved in

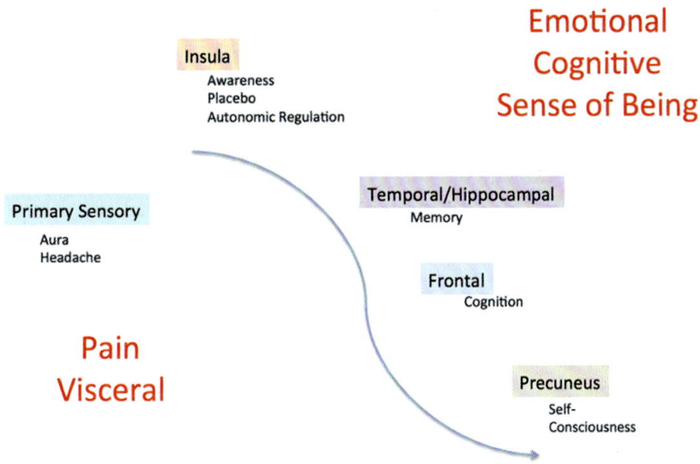

FIGURE 25-1 Migraine and the brain. The major manifestations of migraine may be sensory (e.g., pain, aura) and visceral symptoms (e.g., nausea and vomiting). Multiple processes, which are most salient in the peri-ictal period (Table 25-1), affect various neural circuits schematized in the cartoon. The constellation of processes alters neural processing that can be measured as perturbations in neural circuit grey matter volume and brain chemistry.

the use of imaging to try to better understand this neurological disorder. Below, we discuss what we consider some major research advances in the field of nuclear magnetic resonance (NMR) imaging during ictal or interictal episodic and chronic migraine in the past few years. Examples have been taken from our own work as well as from other groups; however, it is by no means comprehensive, but rather a view of some of those areas that NMR imaging has provided different and perhaps new insights into the field.

The Migraine Brain Connectivity

Resting-state networks (RSNs) and functional connectivity has been used to evaluate altered brain functional connectivity and, as such, has become a more common tool in studying chronic pain states including migraine [38, 39, 65, 80, 81]. Using these approaches, investigators have evaluated different components or networks in migraine patients, including those involved with pain modulation where a dysfunction of, or impairment of, the descending pain modulatory inputs from higher centres (prefrontal cortex, anterior cingulate, amygdala) to the periaqueductal grey (PAG) was noted [39]. This is consistent with other chronic pain conditions where dysfunctional descending systems, including the PAG, have been reported [25, 28]. Evaluation of RSNs in migraine patients without aura compared with healthy controls patients showed altered connectivity between networks (e.g., central executive network [CEN] and sensory salience network [SN]) and between both default-mode network (DMN) and CEN and the insula [80]. The data suggest that repeated migraine attacks alter the normal intrinsic brain network connectivity and provide potential measures for assessing reversal of these networks with treatment. The changes in these networks are associated with structural changes (see below) in many brain regions. A number of authors have noted specific correlation of structure and function in different brain regions that may contribute to the aberrant connectivity [29, 38, 42]. As with the rest of the field, the actual harnessing and modulation of these networks in the migraine brain is not fully understood and awaits a better delineation of those components that are most salient [69]. Further work in the ensuing years will undoubtedly add further insights into the utility of such networks as markers of disease state and treatment effects.

Migraine and the Basal Ganglia

The basal ganglia have been shown to play a more important role in chronic pain than previously thought [9]. A number of reports have shown alterations in basal ganglia structure and function in migraineurs [43] and also other changes such as increased iron deposition in the globus pallidus that may contribute to these changes [73]. Two recent publications have noted both functional and morphological alterations in the basal ganglia. One from our group noted differences between low-frequency (LF) and high-frequency (HF) migraineurs, where responses to pain in HF compared with LF patients were significantly lower in the caudate, putamen, and pallidum (Fig. 25-2). In addition, decreased grey matter volume was observed in the caudate nucleus [43]. In another study, resting-state functional connectivity in migraine patients without aura was compared with healthy controls. The work also found decreased volume in the caudate (left) as well as the right nucleus accumbens (NAc) [81]. Importantly, alterations in functional connectivity were correlated with the anatomical changes in these regions: increased migraine frequency was correlated with increased functional connectivity between both right and left caudate nuclei and the left insula. Disease duration correlated with increased functional connectivity between the right NAc and bilateral anterior cingulate cortex [81]. Taken together with alterations in functional activity, the data contribute to our notion that these brain regions play a role in migraine. These regions are also involved in the integration of information between cortical

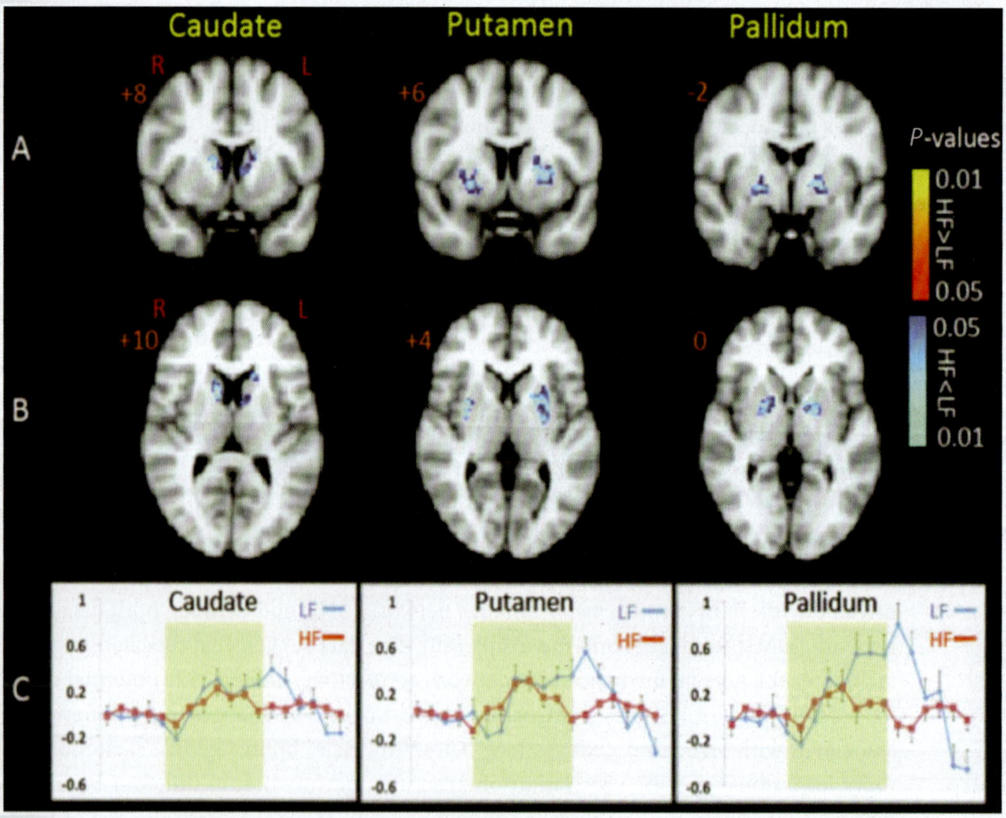

FIGURE 25-2 Functional activation in basal ganglia in response to noxious heat in migraineurs. Contrast analysis of the HF versus LF migraine group in response to the "pain threshold +1°C" stimuli revealed significant ($P < 0.05$, corrected) differences in the basal ganglia nuclei in coronal **(A)** and axial **(B)** views. In **(C)**, single trial averages for the response to painful heat stimulation in caudate, putamen, and pallidum are presented. Yellow represents the stimulus application period. (From Maleki et al. [43], with permission.)

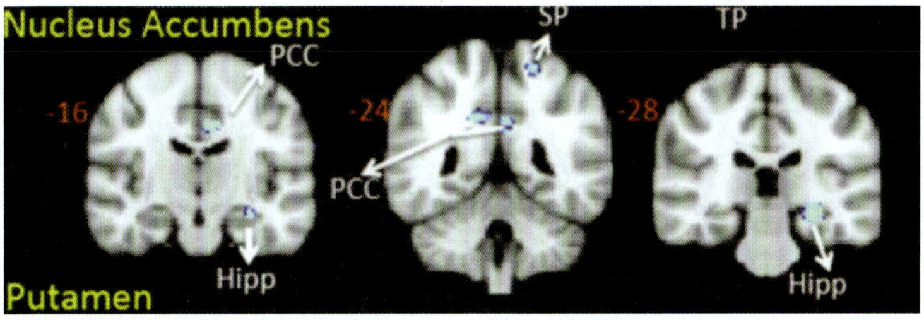

FIGURE 25-3 Functional connectivity contrast maps of the nucleus accumbens (NAc). Functional connectivity contrast maps of the NAc nuclei during intermittent heat stimuli (pain threshold +1°C on hand) in HF versus LF migraine patients. PCC, posterior cingulate cortex; SP, superior parietal; Hipp, hippocampus. (From Maleki et al. [43], with permission.)

and thalamic regions involved in sensory (pain), emotional, and cognitive processing and may become dysfunctional in migraine patients even during their interictal period (Fig. 25-3).

Migraine, Stress, and the Hippocampus

The hippocampus is classically known to be involved in memory and learned behaviour [22, 76] and seizure activity [68]. It is also intimately affected by stress and stress hormones (glucocorticoids) [48, 49, 62] that, as a consequence of increased levels, may alter the hippocampus functionally and anatomically [63]. Electrophysiological and imaging studies support a role for the hippocampus in pain processing [1, 31, 45, 50, 58, 59]. Studies in migraineurs have shown bilateral morphometric decreased volume in the hippocampus of HF versus LF patients, greater activation in HF than in LF patients, and reduction in functional connectivity of the hippocampus with brain regions involved in pain processing (temporal lobe, nucleus accumbens, and insula) [42]. Functional studies indicate an increased sensitivity to stimulation in the hippocampus for HF versus LF migraineurs, whereas connectivity studies would indicate diminished functional outputs. These may have significant consequences on other brain systems, for example, hippocampal–accumbens systems [53].

Dynamic Grey Matter Changes

Voxel-based morphology has been used to measure changes in cortical and subcortical brain regions in migraine patients across a number of studies (Table 25-1). Brain changes in migraine are assumed to be responses to the acute pain processing, repeated attacks, and also other changes produced by the migraine state.

Table 25-1 describes several brain regions showing alteration in grey matter volume. A number of interesting features have been noted. First, there are significant changes in a diffuse number of brain regions. Second, medication-overuse headache in migraineurs seems to have an objective basis, at least in terms of alteration of grey matter volume [60]; third, there are gender differences in grey matter volume (see below); fourth, grey matter volume in some regions (e.g., anterior cingulate cortex) correlates with disease duration and lifetime headache and frequency [29, 32, 75] in migraine patients. In addition, grey matter changes with a specific area may show dynamic changes when evaluated in terms of migraine frequency with increased grey matter volume (e.g., in the caudate) in low frequency migraineurs (compared with controls) and decreased grey matter volume back to control levels compared with LF migraineurs [43]. Similarly in the primary somatosensory

TABLE 25-1 **Alterations in Grey Matter Volume in Cortical and Subcortical Brain Regions**

Region	Changes	Condition	Reference
Cortical Regions			
S1	+	M vs. C	[19]
	+	LF vs. HF	[41]
Anterior cingulate cortex	−	LF vs. HF	[41]
Middle cingulate cortex	−	LF vs. HF	[41]
Posterior cingulate cortex	−	LF vs. HF	[41]
	−	MOH	[60]
	−	M vs. C	[32]
	−	CM vs. EM	[75]
Orbitofrontal cortex	−	M vs. C	[32]
	−		[29]
MPF	−		[29]
Medial frontal gyrus	−	CM vs. EM	[75]
Inferior frontal gyrus	−	CM vs. EM	[75]
	+	F vs. M	[46]
	−	M vs. C	[32]
	−	CM vs. EM	[75]
Frontal lobe	−	M vs. C	[66]
Precuneus	+	F vs. M	[46]
	−	MOH	[60]
Occipital cortex	−		[29]
Hippocampus	+	LF vs. HF	[42]
Subcortical Regions			
Thalamus	+	MOH	[60]
Caudate	+	LF < HF	[43]
Nucleus accumbens	+	LF < HF	[43]
Ventral striatum	+	MOH	[60]
Periaqueductal grey	+	MOH	[60]
Amygdala	−	CM vs. EM	[75]

Abbreviations: C, healthy controls; CM, chronic migraine; EM, episodic migraine; F, female; LF, low frequency (<4); HF, high frequency (>8); M, male; MOH, medication-overuse headache; MPF, medial prefrontal.

cortex, there is an increase in cortical grey matter thickness in migraineurs versus controls [19, 41]. Such dynamic changes offer several models to evaluate the progression of migraine over time/frequency/age, etc.

Migraine and the Insula—A Potential Gateway to Conscious Perception of Migraine Processes

The insula is in a prominent position to be part of the cortical expression and integration of many of the symptoms that occur during migraine—from pain to autonomic dysfunction to exaggerated perceptual responses to light (photophobia), sound (phonophobia), smell (osmophobia), and motion (vestibular). One explanation could be the abundance of the von Economo neurons (VEN) in the insula and the putative role they play in facilitating functional connectivity between the insula (as a hub) and the rest of the brain [15] for integration of salience [51]; interoception [17]; multisensory processing including pain, gustatory, olfactory, and auditory processes; as well as autonomic functions. Imaging studies have reported functional and structural changes in the insula in migraine patients [26, 46]. The anterior insula is involved in interoception [82], a basis for self-awareness, and may be involved in impending stimulus significance [7]. The posterior insula is involved in sensory perception [24]. Repetitive stimuli-produced "experience and familiarity" may explain why patients with HF migraine exhibit a blunted response to interoceptive processing of pain, which, from a neurological perspective, may be a consequence of an adaptation process. The awareness of perturbations thus occurs in the preictal migraine and perhaps the interictal migraine state. This view is supported by the connectivity analysis of the insula reported in our results, where HF patients show a stronger connectivity with sensory processing regions, including the postcentral gyrus compared with LF patients. In addition, behavioural changes in migraine patients include disturbances of body image and physical sensations, including alteration of time sense, which are indicative of alteration of self-perception/interoception.

Migraine and Vegetative Changes

As noted in the section above, many components of the clinical phenotype include autonomic and "vegetative" processing. In a recent neuroimaging report, resting-state measures of patients with migraine (both with and without aura) were compared with healthy controls and other pain syndromes, including pain affecting the head/face [26]. Only those with migraine had increased connectivity between the amygdala and visceral insula (a putative limbic/viscerosensory network) [40]. Interestingly, little is known about brain processing in the preheadache phase of migraineurs where many vegetative processes may be active including altered sleep, altered mood, and gastrointestinal changes [30]. Indeed, some have described migraine as a primary sympathetic disorder [57].

Migraine and Gender

Women suffer disproportionately from migraine. Migraine is two times as common in women versus men [12]. We recently reported significant changes in grey matter volume in the posterior insula and precuneus (thicker) in women migraineurs, and decreased volume of the parahippocampus in men versus healthy subjects (in women it remained stable vs. healthy) as well as altered functional responses and connectivity (female migraineurs showed significantly stronger negative functional connectivity between the insular region of interest and brain areas such as S1, posterior cingulate, precuneus, and temporal pole) across gender in response to a noxious heat stimulus [46] (Fig. 25-4).

Of interest, psychophysical measures showed increased pain unpleasantness in women versus men, and the functional data suggested that emotional circuitry compared with sensory processing appears involved to a greater degree in female than male migraineurs. Clearly, the issue of gender and understanding changes in the female versus the male brain as we age (going through puberty and in women, menarche) should provide very useful insights on the brain's susceptibility to migraine.

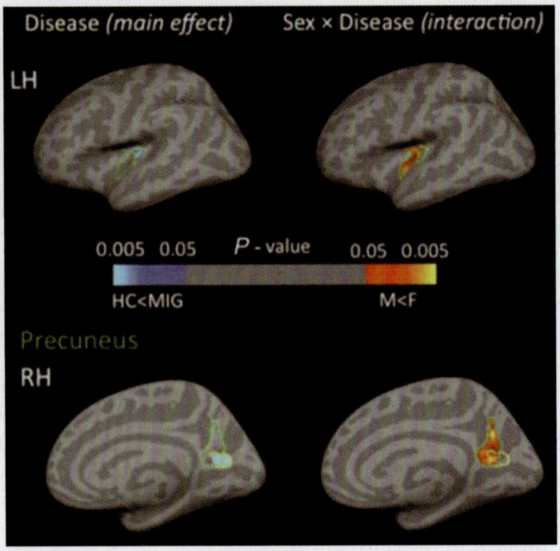

FIGURE 25-4 Gender differences in precuneus and insula. Significant clusters from vertex-wise cortical thickness comparisons conducted on all of the subjects (migraine male and female, and healthy control male and female) to determine the main effect (disease) effect and interaction effect (sex × disease). The disease effect (*blue–light blue* colour map) and sex × disease interaction (*red–yellow* colour map) are shown. (From Maleki et al. [46], with permission.)

Migraine and the Hypothalamus

Obviously, regions such as the hypothalamus are clear targets for imaging studies: the focus on the hypothalamus is rationalized by the role it plays in regulating circadian cyclicity, appetite, sleep, energy, mood, yawning, urination, body temperature, tiredness, altered mood, and other symptoms associated with the different phases of a migraine attack. In addition, the hypothalamus is involved in the stress response. Imaging studies have shown clear hypothalamic changes in patients with cluster headache [21]. Hypothalamic volume is increased in hypnic headache, and activation is present in cluster headache [47], but less defined in classical migraine.

Migraine and Brain Excitability

The preponderance of evidence shows a hyperexcitable brain in migraineurs during both ictal and interictal periods [67]. These changes are evident in primary sensory systems, including visual, auditory, and pain processing. It is unclear whether these are genetically derived or driven in part by repeated headache, or cortical spreading depression (that may not be limited to the cortex [23]), migraine frequency, and chronification of the disease. Psychophysical and functional neuroimaging studies showed increased sensitivity to smell [20], noise [77], visual stimuli [33], or diminished modulatory tone [52]. Below, we discuss some examples of how imaging has contributed to our insights of brain hyperexcitability.

Photophobia. Bright light that produces exacerbation of pain is perhaps the best example of the hyperexcitable state. Photophobia in blind migraine patients who had no visual perception, and blind migraine patients capable of detecting light led to the discovery of the retino-thalamo-cortical pathway [54]. This pathway defined in rats transmits nonvisual forming light signals from the retina to posterior thalamic regions and putatively to the pulvinar in humans [44]. It is this region of the thalamus that is involved in extracephalic allodynia [10]. An optic tract pathway could also be traced in humans to the pulvinar, utilizing diffusion tensor tractography [45] (Fig. 25-4).

Allodynia: One of the sensory features in migraine is the process of allodynia in patients that may affect the face or whole body [11]. The process of allodynia is thought to involve progressive changes along the trigeminovascular pathway (trigeminal nucleus in facial allodynia; and thalamus in generalized allodynia). These clinical observations have led to animal and human imaging studies. The pulvinar is the posterior nuclear complex in the thalamus most frequently associated with processing of visual information [74], but is considered to be important in two aspects of transmission of information from layer 5 of one cortical area to another cortical area and also in integrating multisensory information [70]. Activation in the pulvinar during migraine corresponds with extended allodynia, presumably as a result of converging afferent nociceptive neurons onto cells that drive secondary responses (i.e., allodynia) [10]. In addition, nonvisual forming retinal projections to the pulvinar may contribute to light-induced hypersensitivity in migraine patients [56]. Taken together, the concept is that during migraine, nociceptive information travels directly rather than indirectly from one cortical area to another [55]. Fig. 25-5 shows human brain activity relating to posterior thalamus hyperexcitability in migraine [10].

Trigeminal Nuclei and Brainstem

The TVS is clearly central to migraine [14]. Within the system, attention has been focused on trigeminal nuclei to try to dissect their role in the peri-ictal migraine state [6]. The most recent evaluation of trigeminal nuclei in migraine has come from recent imaging studies. In one, the authors reported that a "cycling of activity of the spinal trigeminal nuclei in response to nociceptive stimulation showed a cycling behaviour over the migraine interval" [71]. The data provide two important insights; the first is that the measures of brainstem (trigeminal) nuclei as previously found in healthy subjects [18] can be shown in migraine patients, and, given that this may be an "entry point" following peripheral activation or altered central modulation, this site may provide further insights into the mechanism that regulates attack onset.

The second is that brainstem activations have been the focus of migraine research since the initial positron emission tomography study of spontaneous migraine by Weiller and colleagues [79]. Recent studies have reported activation in the pons following a noxious heat stimulus during the interictal state, correlated with headache disability [61]. The technical challenges of brainstem measures including the PAG [35] are being resolved with new standards and new imaging approaches. The issue of brainstem including the pons contribution to headache onset is still a debate and has recently been reviewed [5].

CONCLUSION

Imaging may contribute to some fundamental changes in the way we currently think about migraine as a disease and in clinical practice. A few examples are noted below:

1. The field has begun to look at the use of fMRI in the development of biomarkers for pain and analgesia [2–4]. Some specific suggestions have included cortical hyperexcitability [27], basal ganglia changes [43], or measures in more "obvious" structures such as the hypothalamus [61]. By having clinical markers, the evaluation of peripherally or centrally acting drugs may be more critically evaluated.

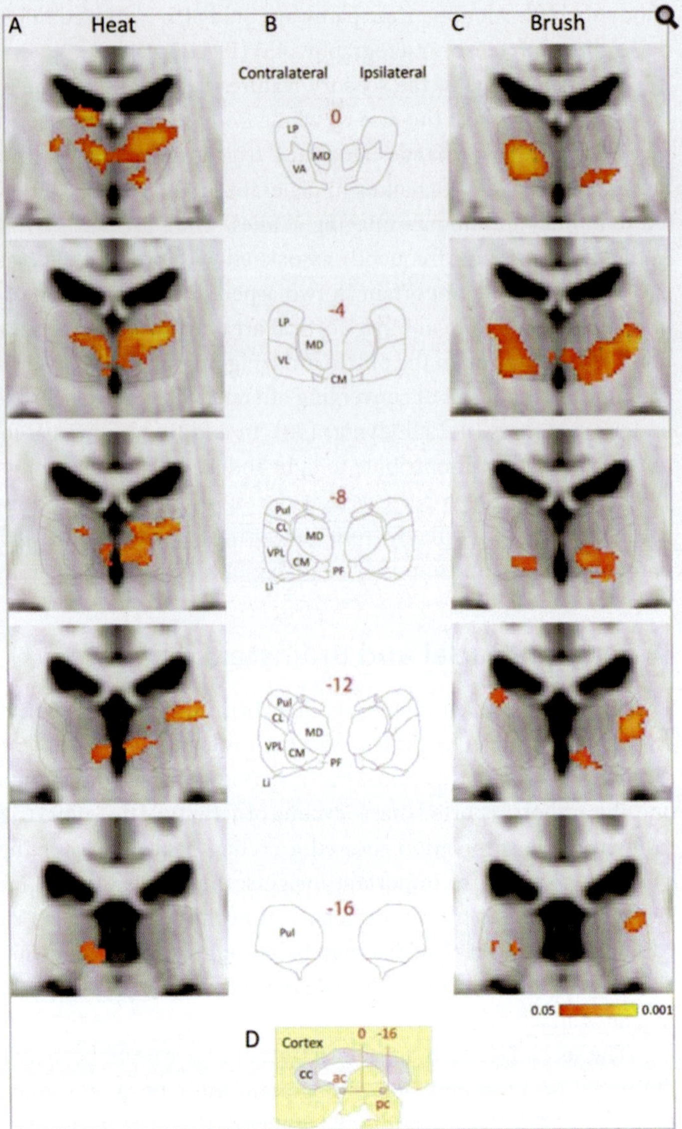

FIGURE 25-5 **Thalamic central sensitization in migraine.** Contrast analysis of blood oxygenation level–dependent (BOLD) signals registered in fMRI scans of the human posterior thalamus following innocuous and noxious skin stimuli during migraine attacks that were associated with extracephalic allodynia. **A, C:** Pooled statistical maps ($n = 8$) of responses to stimulation of the back of the hand using heat **(A)** and brush **(C)**. Activation mapping probabilities are coded as indicated by the colour bar at the bottom of **(C)**. **B:** Drawings of the corresponding coronal planes (numbers in *red*) traced from Schaltenbrand and Wahren's atlas of the human brain. D**:** A sagittal perspective of the area of interest. Anterior–posterior coordinates (*red numbers* in **B, D**) indicate distance in mm from the midpoint (*arrow* in **D**) between the anterior and posterior commissures. BOLD signals were pooled according to their ipsilateral/contralateral position in relation to the side of the headache (this normalized orientation is indicated at the top of **B**). BOLD signals were fitted onto Montreal Neurological Institute (MNI) standard brain images, using FSL Linear Registration Tool (FLIRT). Schematic atlas drawings were size-fitted onto the corresponding MNI images to facilitate anatomical localization of BOLD signals. *Abbreviations*: ac, anterior commissure; cc, corpus callosum; CL, centrolateral thalamic nucleus; CM, centromedian thalamic nucleus; LI, limitans nucleus; LP, lateral posterior thalamic group; MD, mediodorsal thalamic group; pc, posterior commissure; PF, parafascicular thalamic nucleus; Pul, pulvinar; VA, ventral anterior thalamic nucleus; VL, ventral lateral posterior thalamic group; VPL, ventral posterior lateral thalamic nucleus. (From Burstein et al. [10] with permission.)

2. Imaging should be able to help define a more rational approach to migraine definition—such as what differentiates episodic migraine from chronic daily headache since this is a clinical definition at this time. Methods that include machine vector learning can be deployed for this approach [78].
3. A renewed view of the neurobiology of migraine as evaluated by neuroimaging should contribute to further mechanistic understanding of the disease [8, 16].
4. Imaging should be able to contribute to clinical evaluation in several ways including diagnosis, stage of disease, and prediction for chronification.

ACKNOWLEDGEMENT

This work was supported by grants from NINDS R01 NS073997, R01 NS075018, and NCCAM R21 AT007530 to DB; and grants R01 NS069847, R01 NS051484, and R37 NS079778 to RB.

REFERENCES

1. Becerra L, Breiter HC, Wise R, Gonzalez RG, Borsook D. Reward circuitry activation by noxious thermal stimuli. Neuron 2001;32(5):927–46.
2. Borsook D, Becerra L, Fava M. Use of functional imaging across clinical phases in CNS drug development. Transl Psychiatry 2013;3:e282.
3. Borsook D, Becerra L, Hargreaves R. Biomarkers for chronic pain and analgesia, part 1: the need, reality, challenges, and solutions. Discov Med 2011;11(58):197–207.
4. Borsook D, Becerra L, Hargreaves R, Biomarkers for chronic pain and analgesia, part 2: how, where, and what to look for using functional imaging. Discov Med 2011;11(58):209–19.
5. Borsook D, Burstein R. The enigma of the dorsolateral pons as a migraine generator. Cephalalgia 2012. 32(11): 803–12.
6. Borsook D, Burstein R, Moulton E, Becerra L. Functional imaging of the trigeminal system: applications to migraine pathophysiology. Headache 2006;46(Suppl 1):S32–8.
7. Borsook D, Edwards R, Elman I, Becerra L, Levine J. Pain and analgesia: the value of salience circuits. Prog Neurobiol 2013;104:93–105.
8. Borsook D, Hargreaves R. Brain imaging in migraine research. Headache 2010;50(9):1523–7.
9. Borsook D, Upadhyay J, Chudler EH, Becerra L. A key role of the basal ganglia in pain and analgesia—insights gained through human functional imaging. Mol Pain 2010;6:27.
10. Burstein R, Jakubowski M, Garcia-Nicas E, Kainz V, Bajwa Z, Hargreaves R, Becerra L, Borsook D. Thalamic sensitization transforms localized pain into widespread allodynia. Ann Neurol 2010;68(1):81–91.
11. Burstein R, Yarnitsky D, Goor-Aryeh I, Ransil BJ, Bajwa ZH. An association between migraine and cutaneous allodynia. Ann Neurol 2000;47(5):614–24.
12. Buse DC, Loder EW, Gorman JA, Stewart WF, Reed ML, Fanning KM, Serrano D, Lipton RB. Sex differences in the prevalence, symptoms, and associated features of migraine, probable migraine and other severe headache: results of the American Migraine Prevalence and Prevention (AMPP) Study. Headache 2013;53(8):1278–99.
13. Buse DC, Rupnow MF, Lipton RB. Assessing and managing all aspects of migraine: migraine attacks, migraine-related functional impairment, common comorbidities, and quality of life. Mayo Clin Proc 2009;84(5):422–35.
14. Buzzi MG, Moskowitz MA. The trigemino-vascular system and migraine. Pathol Biol (Paris), 1992;40(4): 313–7.
15. Cauda F, Torta DM, Sacco K, D'Agata F, Geda E, Duca S, Geminiani G, Vercelli A. Functional anatomy of cortical areas characterized by Von Economo neurons. Brain Struct Funct 2013;218(1):1–20.
16. Charles A. Migraine: a brain state. Curr Opin Neurol 2013;26(3):235–9.
17. Craig AD. How do you feel—now? The anterior insula and human awareness. Nat Rev Neurosci 2009;10(1): 59–70.
18. DaSilva AF, Becerra L, Makris N, Strassman AM, Gonzalez RG, Geatrakis N, Borsook D. Somatotopic activation in the human trigeminal pain pathway. J Neurosci 2002;22(18):8183–92.

19. DaSilva AF, Granziera C, Snyder J, Hadjikhani N. Thickening in the somatosensory cortex of patients with migraine. Neurology 2007;69(21):1990–5.
20. Demarquay G, Royet JP, Mick G, Ryvlin P. Olfactory hypersensitivity in migraineurs: a $H_2^{15}O$-PET study. Cephalalgia 2008;28(10):1069–80.
21. Dunckley P, Wise RG, Fairhurst M, Hobden P, Aziz Q, Chang L, Tracey I. A comparison of visceral and somatic pain processing in the human brainstem using functional magnetic resonance imaging. J Neurosci 2005;25(32):7333–41.
22. Eichenbaum H, Dudchenko P, Wood E, Shapiro M, Tanila H. The hippocampus, memory, and place cells: is it spatial memory or a memory space? Neuron 1999;23(2):209–26.
23. Eikermann-Haerter K, Negro A, Ayata C. Spreading depression and the clinical correlates of migraine. Rev Neurosci 2013;24(4):353–63.
24. Garcia-Larrea L. The posterior insular-opercular region and the search of a primary cortex for pain. Neurophysiol Clin 2012;42(5):299–313.
25. Giesecke T, Gracely RH, Clauw DJ, Nachemson A, Duck MH, Sabatowski R, Gerbershagen HJ, Williams DA, Petzke F. Central pain processing in chronic low back pain. Evidence for reduced pain inhibition. Schmerz 2006;20(5):411–4, 416–7.
26. Hadjikhani N, Ward N, Boshyan J, Napadow V, Maeda Y, Truini A, Caramia F, Tinelli E, Mainero C. The missing link: enhanced functional connectivity between amygdala and visceroceptive cortex in migraine. Cephalalgia 2013;33(15):1264–8.
27. Huang J, Cao Y. Functional MRI as a biomarker for evaluation and prediction of effectiveness of migraine prophylaxis. Biomark Med 2012;6(4):517–27.
28. Jensen KB, Loitoile R, Kosek E, Petzke F, Carville S, Fransson P, Marcus H, Williams SC, Choy E, Mainguy Y. Patients with fibromyalgia display less functional connectivity in the brain's pain inhibitory network. Mol Pain 2012;8:32.
29. Jin C, Yuan K, Zhao L, Yu D, von Deneen KM, Zhang M, Qin W, Sun W, Tian J. Structural and functional abnormalities in migraine patients without aura. NMR Biomed 2013;26(1):58–64.
30. Kelman L. The premonitory symptoms (prodrome): a tertiary care study of 893 migraineurs. Headache 2004;44(9):865–72.
31. Khanna S, Sinclair JG. Noxious stimuli produce prolonged changes in the CA1 region of the rat hippocampus. Pain 1989;39(3):337–43.
32. Kim JH, Suh SI, Seol HY, Oh K, Seo WK, Yu SW, Park KW, Koh SB. Regional grey matter changes in patients with migraine: a voxel-based morphometry study. Cephalalgia 2008;28(6):598–604.
33. Lang E, Kaltenhauser M, Neundorfer B, Seidler S. Hyperexcitability of the primary somatosensory cortex in migraine—a magnetoencephalographic study. Brain 2004;127(Pt 11):2459–69.
34. Lim SS, Vos T, Flaxman AD, Danaei G, Shibuya K, Adair-Rohani H, Amann M, Anderson HR, Andrews KG, Aryee M. A comparative risk assessment of burden of disease and injury attributable to 67 risk factors and risk factor clusters in 21 regions, 1990–2010: a systematic analysis for the Global Burden of Disease Study 2010. Lancet 2012;380(9859):2224–60.
35. Linnman C, Moulton EA, Barmettler G, Becerra L, Borsook D. Neuroimaging of the periaqueductal gray: state of the field. NeuroImage 2012;60(1)505–22.
36. Lipton RB, Stewart WF, Diamond S, Diamond ML, Reed M. Prevalence and burden of migraine in the United States: data from the American Migraine Study II. Headache 2001;41(7):646–57.
37. Lipton RB, Stewart WF, Reed M, Diamond S. Migraine's impact today: burden of illness, patterns of care. Postgrad Med 2001;109(1):38–40, 43–5.
38. Liu J, Zhao L, Li G, Xiong S, Nan J, Li J, Yuan K, von Deneen KM, Liang F, Qin W, et al. Hierarchical alteration of brain structural and functional networks in female migraine sufferers. PLoS One 2012;7(12):e51250.
39. Mainero C, Boshyan J, Hadjikhani N. Altered functional magnetic resonance imaging resting-state connectivity in periaqueductal gray networks in migraine. Ann Neurol 2011;70(5):838–45.
40. Maizels M, Aurora S, Heinricher M. Beyond neurovascular: migraine as a dysfunctional neurolimbic pain network. Headache 2012;52(10):1553–65.
41. Maleki N, Becerra L, Brawn J, Bigal M, Burstein R, Borsook D, Concurrent functional and structural cortical alterations in migraine. Cephalalgia 2012;32(8):607–20.
42. Maleki N, Becerra L, Brawn J, McEwen B, Burstein R, Borsook D. Common hippocampal structural and functional changes in migraine. Brain Struct Funct, 2013;218(4):903–12.
43. Maleki N, Becerra L, Nutile L, Pendse G, Brawn J, Bigal M, Burstein R, Borsook D. Migraine attacks the basal ganglia. Mol Pain 2011;7:71.

44. Maleki N, Becerra L, Upadhyay J, Burstein R, Borsook D. Direct optic nerve pulvinar connections defined by diffusion MR tractography in humans: implications for photophobia. Hum Brain Mapp 2012;33(1):75–88.
45. Maleki N, Brawn J, Barmettler G, Borsook D, Becerra L. Pain response measured with arterial spin labeling. NMR Biomed 2013;26(6):664–73.
46. Maleki N, Linnman C, Brawn J, Burstein R, Becerra L, Borsook D. Her versus his migraine: multiple sex differences in brain function and structure. Brain 2012;135(Pt 8):2546–59.
47. May A, Bahra A, Buchel C, Frackowiak RS, Goadsby PJ. Hypothalamic activation in cluster headache attacks. Lancet 1998;352(9124):275–8.
48. McEwen BS. Plasticity of the hippocampus: adaptation to chronic stress and allostatic load. Ann N Y Acad Sci, 2001;933:265–77.
49. McEwen BS. Stress, sex, and neural adaptation to a changing environment: mechanisms of neuronal remodeling. Ann N Y Acad Sci 2010;1204(Suppl):E38–59.
50. McKenna JE, Melzack R. Analgesia produced by lidocaine microinjection into the dentate gyrus. Pain 1992;49(1):105–12.
51. Menon V, Uddin LQ. Saliency, switching, attention and control: a network model of insula function. Brain Struct Funct 2010;214(5–6):655–67.
52. Moulton EA, Becerra L, Maleki N, Pendse G, Tully S, Hargreaves R, Burstein R, Borsook D. Painful heat reveals hyperexcitability of the temporal pole in interictal and ictal migraine states. Cereb Cortex 2011;21(2):435–48.
53. Nason MW Jr, Adhikari A, Bozinoski M, Gordon JA, Role LW. Disrupted activity in the hippocampal-accumbens circuit of type III neuregulin 1 mutant mice. Neuropsychopharmacology 2011;36(2):488–96.
54. Noseda R, Burstein R. Advances in understanding the mechanisms of migraine-type photophobia. Curr Opin Neurol 2011;24(3):197–202.
55. Noseda R, Jakubowski M, Kainz V, Borsook D, Burstein R. Cortical projections of functionally identified thalamic trigeminovascular neurons: implications for migraine headache and its associated symptoms. J Neurosci 2011;31(40):14204–17.
56. Noseda R, Kainz V, Jakubowski M, Gooley JJ, Saper CB, Digre K, Burstein R. A neural mechanism for exacerbation of headache by light. Nat Neurosci 2010;13(2):239–45.
57. Peroutka SJ. Migraine: a chronic sympathetic nervous system disorder. Headache 2004;44(1):53–64.
58. Ploghaus A, Becerra L, Borras C, Borsook D. Neural circuitry underlying pain modulation: expectation, hypnosis, placebo. Trends Cogn Sci 2003;7(5):197–200.
59. Prado WA, Roberts MH. An assessment of the antinociceptive and aversive effects of stimulating identified sites in the rat brain. Brain Res 1985;340(2):219–28.
60. Riederer F, Marti M, Luechinger R, Lanzenberger R, von Meyenburg J, Gantenbein AR, Pirrotta R, Gaul C, Kollias S, Sandor PS. Grey matter changes associated with medication-overuse headache: correlations with disease related disability and anxiety. World J Biol Psychiatry 2012;13(7):517–25.
61. Robert C, Bourgeais L, Arreto CD, Condes-Lara M, Noseda R, Jay T, Villanueva L. Paraventricular hypothalamic regulation of trigeminovascular mechanisms involved in headaches. J Neurosci 2013;33(20):8827–40.
62. Rodrigues SM, LeDoux JE, Sapolsky RM. The influence of stress hormones on fear circuitry. Annu Rev Neurosci 2009;32:289–313.
63. Rothman SM, Mattson MP. Adverse stress, hippocampal networks, and Alzheimer's disease. Neuromolecular Med 2010;12(1):56–70.
64. Russo A, Tessitore A, Esposito F, Marcuccio L, Giordano A, Conforti R, Truini A, Paccone A, d'Onofrio F, Tedeschi G. Pain processing in patients with migraine: an event-related fMRI study during trigeminal nociceptive stimulation. J Neurol 2012;259(9):1903–12.
65. Russo A, Tessitore A, Giordano A, Corbo D, Marcuccio L, De Stefano M, Salemi F, Conforti R, Esposito F, Tedeschi G. Executive resting-state network connectivity in migraine without aura. Cephalalgia 2012;32(14):1041–8.
66. Schmitz N, Arkink EB, Mulder M, Rubia K, Admiraal-Behloul F, Schoonman GG, Kruit MC, Ferrari MD, van Buchem MA. Frontal lobe structure and executive function in migraine patients. Neurosci Lett 2008;440(2):92–6.
67. Schoenen J. Neurophysiological features of the migrainous brain. Neurol Sci 2006;27(Suppl 2):S77–81.
68. Schwartzkroin PA. Role of the hippocampus in epilepsy. Hippocampus 1994;4(3):239–42.
69. Sepulcre J, Sabuncu MR, Johnson KA. Network assemblies in the functional brain. Curr Opin Neurol 2012;25(4):384–91.
70. Sherman SM. The thalamus is more than just a relay. Curr Opin Neurobiol 2007;17(4):417–22.

71. Stankewitz A, Aderjan D, Eippert F, May A. Trigeminal nociceptive transmission in migraineurs predicts migraine attacks. J Neurosci 2011;31(6):1937–43.
72. Stewart WF, Shechter A, Rasmussen BK. Migraine prevalence: a review of population-based studies. Neurology 1994;44(6 Suppl 4):S17–23.
73. Tepper SJ, Lowe MJ, Beall E, Phillips MD, Liu K, Stillman MJ, Horvat M, Jones SE. Iron deposition in pain-regulatory nuclei in episodic migraine and chronic daily headache by MRI. Headache, 2012;52(2):236–43.
74. Toosy AT, Ciccarelli O, Parker GJ, Wheeler-Kingshott CA, Miller DH, Thompson AJ. Characterizing function-structure relationships in the human visual system with functional MRI and diffusion tensor imaging. Neuroimage 2004;21(4):1452–63.
75. Valfre W, Rainero I, Bergui M, Pinessi L. Voxel-based morphometry reveals gray matter abnormalities in migraine. Headache 2008;48(1):109–17.
76. van der Flier WM, Scheltens P. Alzheimer disease: hippocampal volume loss and Alzheimer disease progression. Nat Rev Neurol 2009;5(7):361–2.
77. Vingen JV, Pareja JA, Storen O, White LR, Stovner LJ. Phonophobia in migraine. Cephalalgia 1998;18(5): 243–9.
78. Wager TD, Atlas LY, Lindquist MA, Roy M, Woo CW, Kross E. An fMRI-based neurologic signature of physical pain. N Engl J Med 2013;368(15):1388–97.
79. Weiller C, May A, Limmroth V, Juptner M, Kaube H, Schayck RV, Coenen HH, Diener HC. Brain stem activation in spontaneous human migraine attacks. Nat Med 1995;1(7):658–60.
80. Xue T, Yuan K, Zhao L, Yu D, Zhao L, Dong T, Cheng P, von Deneen KM, Qin W, Tian J. Intrinsic brain network abnormalities in migraines without aura revealed in resting-state fMRI. PLoS One, 2012;7(12):e52927.
81. Yuan K, Zhao L, Cheng P, Yu D, Zhao L, Dong T, Xing L, Bi Y, Yang X, von Deneen KM, et al. Altered structure and resting-state functional connectivity of the basal ganglia in migraine patients without aura. J Pain 2013;14(8):836–44.
82. Zaki J, Davis JI, Ochsner KN. Overlapping activity in anterior insula during interoception and emotional experience. NeuroImage 2012;62(1):493–9.

CHAPTER 26

Chronic Visceral Pain

Emeran A. Mayer, Arpana Gupta, Yasser Al Omran, and Qasim Aziz

Chronic visceral pain syndromes, in particular those related to the gastrointestinal (GI) and the urinary tract, are important clinical problems with largely unmet medical needs [12]. Some of the most prevalent of these disorders are irritable bowel syndrome (IBS), functional dyspepsia (FD), and functional esophageal disorders, which all fall under the general category of functional gastrointestinal disorders (FGIDs). In the absence of generally agreed upon biomarkers, these disorders remain defined by symptom criteria and the absence of organic disease [12]. On the basis of the common overlap with other chronic disorders of visceral or somatic pain, mood and affect, and the shared responsiveness of these disorders to centrally targeted treatments, there is a growing consensus that alterations of the central nervous system (CNS) play an important role in their pathophysiology and symptom generation [42].

In order to understand and treat the complex human pain experience, it is crucial to understand that there is no linear relationship between the information that is encoded by primary afferents in the GI tract and the complex subjective experience of pain. Multiple factors including cognitive, emotional, and reward processes, as well as memories of past experiences, and prediction of future experiences are integrated with sensory information in specific brain circuits (including the saliency and emotional arousal circuits), and this integrated information will ultimately determine a patient's experience. The only currently available technique to dissect the various components of this subjective human experience into biological substrates is multimodal brain imaging. Functional brain imaging allows for the quantification of the viscerosensory input reaching the brain, and of an understanding of how nonsensory factors contribute to the overall phenotype. Together with structural and diffusion tensor imaging (DTI), multimodal brain imaging makes it possible to identify human brain circuits that correlate with various phenotypic and behavioural manifestations of FGIDs, such as psychological states, traits, symptoms, and dysregulations of the hypothalamic pituitary adrenal axis and the autonomic nervous system (ANS) [14].

In this chapter, we provide a brief review of structural and functional brain imaging studies published during the past 5 years, which have been performed in healthy subjects and in those reporting chronic visceral pain. On the basis of the published literature and the rapid progress made in the understanding of the CNS in the pathophysiology of different chronic pain states, we will suggest possible future directions for this exciting field of neuroscience.

OVERVIEW OF fMRI STUDIES PUBLISHED BETWEEN 1997 AND 2008

A growing number of reports on brain imaging results obtained in patients with chronic abdominal pain have been published during the last decade [43, 51], and have led to some insights into the understanding of central aspects of visceral pain modulation in humans. A previous review, on studies published between 1997 and 2008, found that even though there were wide variations in terms of methods of stimulation, study procedures, study populations, and number of subjects and image analysis, the most consistently activated brain regions in all reports were the insular cortex (INS) and anterior cingulate cortex (ACC), followed in order of reported frequency by the primary sensory cortex (S1), prefrontal cortex (PFC), posterior parietal cortex (PPC), and thalamus (THAL) [43]. Results from two recent meta-analyses of fMRI studies in IBS patients and healthy control subjects (HCs) using controlled rectal balloon distension as a stimulus have reported consistent activation of INS, ACC, and THAL in both populations [49, 52]. However, IBS patients differed from HCs by showing activation in regions associated with emotional arousal (including the pregenual anterior cingulate cortex [pgACC] and the amygdala [AMG]) and activation of a midbrain cluster, possibly related to endogenous pain inhibition systems. In contrast, HCs showed more activation of the medial and lateral PFC, possibly related to greater engagement of cortico-pontine-spinal pain inhibition systems. Despite wide variations in experimental protocols and analyses used, these findings demonstrated alterations in emotional arousal, cognitive control, and endogenous pain modulation systems [14, 20, 28] involving THAL, INS, and ACC subregions. This consistent pattern led to the erroneous concept of a "pain matrix," with greater engagement in patient populations. However, it soon became obvious that the great majority of brain imaging studies in HCs and various disease states showed activation of the same brain regions, suggesting that these brain regions are part of a saliency network that is engaged in response to any salient stimulus, not limited to pain.

RESULTS PUBLISHED BETWEEN 2009 AND 2014

Evoked Brain Responses

Modulation by Emotional Factors

Although the close relationship between emotion and visceral pain is well known to clinicians seeing patients with FGIDs, and such a relationship is strongly supported by extensive epidemiological data [50], neuroimaging studies have demonstrated an interaction between experimental visceral stimulus (e.g., painful or nonpainful esophageal stimulation), emotional state (e.g., neuroticism), subjective perception, and brain activation. For example, nonpainful balloon distension of the esophagus during a negative emotional state was perceived more intensely than that in a neutral emotional state, and this enhanced perception was associated with increased activation of the dorsal ACC and the anterior INS, key regions of a saliency network [46]. More recently, exposure to both nonpainful and painful esophageal distension in negative emotional states confirmed the original results [11]. Another study found that during pain expectation, there was a positive correlation between neuroticism and brain activity in regions of the saliency network and the parahippocampal gyrus. In contrast, when the noxious stimulus was delivered, neuroticism showed a negative correlation with these regions. One interpretation of these findings is that individuals with high trait anxiety/neuroticism attribute greater saliency and exhibit increased emotional arousal during pain expectation, but inhibit these brain networks during the experience of pain [10]. In a later study, these results were expanded with the demonstration that personality traits might affect visceral sensation [18]. In this study, subjects underwent real-time ANS testing and had serum cortisol measured at baseline and following painful somatic and visceral stimulation, and fMRI was used to determine brain processing of the visceral pain. Two distinct patient clusters were identified. The first can be described as being more neurotic, having greater baseline sympathetic tone and higher cortisol release. These subjects had increased parasympathetic response to pain, had lower pain thresholds, and habituated less to pain. The other cluster had the opposite profile both at baseline and during pain [18].

Brain imaging studies in IBS patients have confirmed the close relationship between increased affect, enhanced visceral stimulus perception, and altered brain responses, where increased intensity ratings of rectal distension-induced pain and discomfort were correlated with symptoms of anxiety and depression. Anxiety symptoms were significantly correlated with stimulus-induced activation of midcingulate cortex (MCC) and pgACC, whereas depression symptoms were correlated with the cerebellum and PFC regions. However, group differences between patients and HCs (in PFC and anterior INS) were no longer seen after correcting for anxiety and depression scores [15, 16].

These results confirm the close interactions between trait anxiety/neuroticisms and symptoms of anxiety and depression with behavioural and brain responses to a visceral stimulus and implicate alterations in emotional processing and modulation as an important factor in the pathophysiology of chronic visceral pain conditions affecting the upper and lower GI tract. These findings are also consistent with the increased engagement of an emotional arousal circuit in IBS patients, especially during pain expectation [37, 38].

Modulation by Cognitive Factors and Expectations

Alterations in cognitive mechanisms, such as attention, salience attribution, and prediction, play an important role in chronic pain, including FGIDs [28]. Selective attention to threat, hypervigilance, increased salience attribution to somatic sensation, and the failure to correct prediction error ("catastrophizing") have all been demonstrated in chronic pain populations including those with IBS patients, and some of these measures have been shown to correlate with symptom severity [28, 32].

Pain Expectation

In a study with IBS patients divided into normosensitive and hypersensitive subgroups, Lowen et al. found that even though the two IBS groups did not differ in reported symptom severity or psychological symptoms, the hypersensitive group had greater activation in the INS, and reduced deactivation in the pgACC. Brain responses during expectation were similar to those during actual distension, with both IBS groups showing greater responses than the HC group [39]. Schmid et al. [47] studied HCs during controlled aversive rectal distension while subjects received an intravenous application of an inert substance combined with either instructions about pain relief (placebo) or negative instructions of pain increase (nocebo effect) compared with neutral instructions. Expected and perceived pain intensity were significantly increased in the nocebo group, and significantly decreased in the placebo group. The placebo response was associated with reduced activation of the somatosensory cortex during expectation, and of the INS, somatosensory cortex, and amygdala during the aversive distension compared with neutral expectations. Negative expectations were associated with increased INS activation during the aversive stimulus. When brain responses were compared between groups, negative expectation was associated with an increased response in the somatosensory cortex. Using a similar design, Lee et al. [40] studied brain responses in IBS patients and HCs during aversive rectal distension and its expectation while receiving an inert intravenous infusion and while receiving suggestions about the therapeutic effect of the infusion. Patients and HCs showed similar subjective placebo analgesia. The placebo during distension was associated with greater activation of INS, MCC, and ventrolateral PFC in IBS subjects than in the control group.

These studies support the concept that expected severity of an announced stimulus, based either on a cue preceding the stimulus or on verbal instructions about the effectiveness of an intervention (placebo), can result in differences in the subjective experience of visceral pain. These expectations are associated with the engagement of brain regions of prefrontal, affective, and sensory brain regions. Interestingly, negative expectations (induced by either a cue or negative instructions) were associated with greater activation of somato- and viscerosensory brain regions, providing for a possible neurobiological mechanism by which pain catastrophizing (prediction of a high likelihood of worst symptom outcomes) is influencing symptom severity. The mechanism by which expectations increase the activity in sensory brain regions is unclear, but may be mediated by greater engagement of descending facilitatory pathways increasing dorsal horn excitability and activity in ascending viscerosensory pathways.

Prediction Error

Several factors may underlie the persistence of prediction errors about the severity of future pain in chronic pain conditions, including alterations in the ability to extinguish aversive memories, and the cognitive inability to correct erroneous pain predictions. In asymptomatic subjects, erroneous expectations about pain are corrected once the individual realizes that the expected outcome is not as severe as predicted and this ability is based on cognitive flexibility and set shifting in response to error feedback. To test the hypothesis that the persistence of prediction error regarding abdominal pain and discomfort in IBS patients is related to a compromised ability to employ these cognitive strategies, Aizawa et al. [2] studied brain responses in IBS patients and HCs during the Wisconsin Card Sorting Test [45]. IBS subjects had more perseverative errors and set-maintenance difficulties than HCs. This was accompanied by decreased activity of the right dorsolateral PFC and right hippocampus, and increased activity in the left posterior INS at error feedback during set shifting. Dynamic causal modelling showed reduced prefrontal to presupplementary motor area connectivity in IBS patients. These findings are consistent with previously demonstrated alterations in PFC and INS activation and connectivity during aversive visceral stimulation and support the concept that prediction error and the inability to correct such errors plays an important part in chronic visceral pain and IBS pathophysiology.

Another mechanism that may be involved in the persistence of prediction error about pain involves the enhanced learning of a conditioned response (acquisition) and the inability to correct the error if the expected negative outcome does not happen (extinction learning). Kattoor et al. [26] found that fear conditioning resulted in learned unpleasantness of a previously neutral visual stimulus, and this was associated with anticipatory activation of the ACC, somatosensory cortex, cuneus, and amygdala. During extinction learning, anticipatory engagement of the dorsolateral PFC was observed, while in the reinstatement phase, a trend for parahippocampal activation was observed. In a separate report, the involvement of the cerebellum in aversive extinction learning was demonstrated [27]. These results demonstrate that in HCs, conditioned responses quickly disappear, and learning of new predictive cue properties is paralleled by prefrontal activation. Labus et al. [35] found that the corticotropin-releasing factor type 1 receptor (CRF-R1) antagonist GW876008, compared with placebo, significantly reduced activity in the THAL in both IBS and HC women during acquisition, while it produced greater suppression of brain activity in the patient group in a wide range of regions, including the medial PFC, anterior INS, hippocampus, and pons, supporting an alteration primarily in the extinction process.

Modulation by Heterotopic Stimulation

Several psychophysical and brain imaging studies support the concept that IBS patients have an altered engagement of endogenous pain modulation systems during heterotypic stimulation, for example, while receiving an aversive stimulus at a site distant from the chronic visceral pain [8]. These findings point towards an important role of alterations in spinal and/or supraspinal endogenous pain modulation mechanisms, and involved brain networks in the pathophysiology of chronic visceral pain. It is conceivable that chronically engaged descending pain facilitatory pathways result in chronically enhanced ascending input to primary sensory brain regions (posterior INS, primary somatosensory cortex), which in turn results in neuroplastic grey and white matter changes, as well as alterations in intrinsic oscillations in these sensory pathways and brain regions as observed in several studies [24].

Imaging Genetics

Two studies evaluated the role of gene polymorphisms related to the serotonin (5-HT) signalling system on brain responses to emotional and nonemotional tasks. Using an emotion recognition task, Kilpatrick et al. [29] showed that regardless of IBS diagnosis, the C/C genotype of the c.−42C>T polymorphism in serotonin receptor gene *HTR3A* compared with T carrier status was associated with greater anxiety and amygdala responsiveness during emotional and nonemotional tasks. Fukudo et al. [21] found that individuals with the s/s genotype of the 5-HTTLPR polymorphism showed greater distension-induced increases in regional cerebral blood flow (rCBF) in emotional regulation regions, including the ACC, parahippocampal gyrus, and orbitofrontal cortex compared with those with the l allele. The results of these studies are consistent with the well-known role of the serotonin signalling system in brain–gut interactions and in the modulation of affective behaviour [20].

Pharmacological and Nonpharmacological Modulation of Brain Activity

Several studies have evaluated functional brain responses to pharmacological and nonpharmacological interventions in IBS subjects and HCs.

Pharmacological Modulation

On the basis of the preclinical studies in rodent models of IBS and other stress-sensitive disorders, several central signalling mechanisms have been implicated in the pathophysiology of IBS, including those involving serotonin (5-HT), norepinephrine, and CRF [20, 44]. Several fMRI studies have used pharmacological manipulation of these systems to probe involved brain mechanisms. Labus et al. [36] found that acute tryptophan depletion (ATD) resulted in an increased response of an extensive brain network to rectal distension, including nodes of the emotional arousal and homeostatic afferent network. The effect was greater during high inflation pressures, suggesting greater engagement of the central 5-HT system with more aversive visceral stimuli. ATD was also associated with a loss of negative feedback inhibition of the amygdala. When viewed together with earlier 5-HT-related brain imaging studies [6] and those reviewed in this chapter [21, 29], there is strong evidence supporting the role of the central 5-HT signalling system in the inhibition of the emotional arousal system in IBS, and this inhibition is likely to play a central role in the therapeutic benefits of 5-HT-modulating drugs in IBS symptoms [9]. Another monoaminergic system that has been implicated in the pathophysiology of chronic visceral pain is the noradrenergic system. Berman et al. [5] found that IBS patients showed higher plasma norepinephrine levels and reduced yohimbine-mediated reduction of activity in a central arousal circuit, consistent with fewer functional presynaptic α_2-adrenergic receptors. Yohimbine-mediated reduction of brainstem and amygdala activity was inversely correlated with early life trauma, an event that has been linked to increased responsiveness of central stress circuits. These findings demonstrate increased noradrenergic activity in IBS subjects, which may be related to a downregulation of presynaptic inhibitory α_2-adrenergic receptors in the brain.

Nonpharmacological Modulation

Several studies reported on the effects of interventions (hypnosis and acupuncture) with possible therapeutic values for IBS patients. The effectiveness of gut-directed hypnotherapy has been demonstrated in well-controlled trials [53]. To identify the brain correlates of this intervention, Lowen et al. [41] found that clinically successful treatment (combined responders from hypnotherapy and the educational intervention) was associated with significant attenuation during distension in the dorsal and ventral anterior INS. Hypnotherapy responders showed a reduction in posterior INS activation during distension, and significant reductions in brain activation during the expectation condition. Following treatment, the IBS brain response to distension was similar to that observed in the HCs.

Nonevoked Brain Alterations

Resting-State Imaging

Rather than evaluate task-dependent brain activity or brain regions activated poststimulation, resting-state (RS) fMRI evaluates brain activity independent of visceral stimulation. A small number of studies have employed RS analysis to study HCs and those with IBS and FD. Using task-free RS-fMRI and an analysis technique aimed at measuring power spectrum intensity of spontaneous brain oscillations, Hong et al. [22] found that both female HCs and female IBS subjects had a frequency power distribution skewed towards high frequency to a greater extent in the amygdala and hippocampus compared with male subjects. In addition, female IBS subjects had a frequency power distribution skewed towards high frequency in the INS and towards low frequency in the sensorimotor cortex to a greater extent than in male subjects. In the upper GI tract, this approach has been used recently to study the functional connectivity of a distributed network of brain regions involved in swallowing, referred to as the brain-swallowing network (BSN). Using RS-fMRI, it was found that esophageal acid stimulation in healthy volunteers augmented the overall functional connectivity of the right anterior INS [3]. As the INS is believed to act as the central cortical processing area of visceral afferents, these findings suggest that the BSN is responsive to unperceived esophageal chemical stimulation [3]. Therefore, it may be possible that this modulation of the BSN may explain esophageal hypersensitivity that can occur in response to acid exposure and may lead to chest pain.

Structural Imaging

Recently, there has been a move towards the use of other MRI techniques, such as DTI, and measurement of cortical, grey matter (GM) densities to obtain structural information on the neural structures and networks between the centres involved in pain processing.

Grey Matter Alterations

Seminowicz et al. [48] used voxel-based morphometry and cortical thickness analysis to identify disease-related differences in GM between IBS and HCs and found regional GM density reductions in PFC, PPC, ventral striatum, and THAL, while regional increases were observed in pgACC and posterior INS/secondary sensory cortex. Jiang et al. [24] reported results from a cortical thickness analysis in IBS and HCs showing that although the two groups did not differ from each other, female patients showed both regional increases (somatosensory and primary motor cortices) and decreases (bilateral INS and pgACC) compared with female HCs. In a larger follow-up study, group differences in grey matter volume (GMV) were identified in many brain regions, including IBS-related GMV reductions in frontal, prefrontal, and anterior cingulate regions; basal ganglia; affective regions (amygdala and hippocampus); and INS [33]. Similar to the CT findings by Jiang et al. [24], GMV increases were seen in the left postcentral gyrus [33]. Using graph theoretical analysis of the structural data, Labus et al. [33] showed that the regional alterations were associated with altered global and regional properties of large-scale brain volumetric networks.

White Matter Abnormalities

Ellingson et al. [13] studied 126 subjects (33 IBS subjects) using DTI and probabilistic tractography. They found microstructural white matter abnormalities in the IBS group in the THAL, basal ganglia, and sensorimotor integration areas. In addition, they reported altered connectivity between the THAL and PFC, and between thalamic subnuclei and the ACC. The observed changes showed no significant correlations with subjective symptoms. When viewed together, these findings support the hypothesis of long-term microstructural changes in brain regions associated with integration of sensory information and corticothalamic modulation. Zhou et al. [54] used DTI to study white matter abnormalities in 36 HCs and 36 patients with postprandial distress syndrome, a subcategory of FD. They reported widespread changes in white matter integrity, even though most group differences disappeared when correcting for depression and anxiety. No significant correlations between white matter changes and subjective symptom measures were observed.

Structural imaging approaches have also been used to identify abnormal central pain processing in patients with chronic inflammatory conditions of the viscera (chronic pancreatitis, inflammatory bowel disorders), for example, disorders that differ from functional GI disorders by the presence of a documented peripheral pathology. Using DTI, it was found that chronic pancreatitis patients had microstructural changes in the somatosensory (S2), prefrontal, frontal, and midcingulate cortical regions and that some of these abnormalities correlated with patients' clinical pain scores [19]. Agostini et al. [1] reported results in patients with Crohn disease in remission and HCs, and found GMV reductions in frontal cingulate cortex and MCC, and a negative correlation between GMV of several brain regions and disease duration. In a recent study, Hong et al. [23] studied cortical thickness in ulcerative colitis (UC) subjects, IBS subjects, and HCs. UC subjects showed greater cortical thickness in ACC and in primary somatosensory cortex compared with both IBS subjects and HCs. Compared with HCs, UC subjects showed lower cortical thickness in orbitofrontal cortex and in primary interoceptive regions (mid- and posterior INS), whereas IBS subjects showed lower cortical thickness in the anterior INS, an association area receiving cognitive, affective, and interoceptive input. Strong correlations between thickness in the orbitofrontal cortex and postcentral gyrus and with symptom duration were observed only in UC subjects.

When viewed together, some general conclusions can be drawn from the published reports on structural brain alterations, even though many details remain unclear. While most studies report both increases and decreases in GM, and evidence for microstructural remodelling of the brain in subjects with functional and organic GI disorders, many of the differences are no longer present after controlling for symptoms of anxiety and depression, and strong correlations of these structural changes with subjective symptoms are present only in subjects with chronic inflammatory pain. In general, structural abnormalities (both in terms of grey and white matter) have been observed in regions involved in sensory processing, integration, and modulation (THAL, basal ganglia, somatosensory cortex), in prefrontal modulatory regions and in regions of the saliency network (ACC, INS). Furthermore, regional GM differences correlate with perceptual sensitivity to visceral and to somatic experimental stimuli in HCs [17], suggesting that such changes are not related to nociceptive input to the brain, but may be genetically or epigenetically determined differences in regional brain structure, which may predispose to chronic pain disorders. By studying differences in structural brain alterations between functional (IBS, FD) and chronic inflammatory conditions (chronic pancreatitis, inflammatory bowel disease), it may be possible in the future to differentiate between brain changes secondary to increased nociceptive input to the brain and those secondary to other factors.

Sex-Related Differences

Although subjective responses to experimental visceral distension are similar in healthy men and women, female IBS patients are more sensitive to such stimuli, and show greater sensitization by repeated delivery of such stimuli than both male patients and male and female controls [38]. On the basis of a small number of earlier functional brain imaging studies using rectal balloon distension and expectation of such distension, it appeared that male and female IBS subjects showed largely similar activation of brain regions to both stimuli, even though some sex-related differences were observed in the engagement of emotional arousal regions (greater in women) and greater engagement in prefrontal regions (greater in men) [7]. These differences were most pronounced during expectation (rather than actual delivery) of rectal discomfort [31]. Using prepulse inhibition (PPI) of the acoustic startle response (a measure of sensorimotor gating), Kilpatrick et al. [30] showed that male IBS patients had significantly reduced PPI compared with healthy males. In contrast, female patients had significantly enhanced PPI responses, suggesting hypervigilance. When viewed together with previous reports on sex-related differences in visceral perception and brain responses, the authors speculated that compromised filtering of visceral signals in male patients may be due to compromised top-down cortical control mechanisms, whereas increased attention to threat due to increased emotional arousal circuits may be characteristic of female IBS patients. Sex-related differences in brain responses were also demonstrated in a recent study of male and female HCs, using esophageal distension and its expectation as stimuli. In this study, women showed significantly greater regional activations in cuneus, precuneus and supplementary motor area, and stronger deactivation in amygdala and parahippocampal gyrus during expectation, whereas men demonstrated greater activation of the cerebellum [25]. The greater inhibition by the female subjects of affective brain regions during pain expectation may be considered to be a cognitive coping strategy for imminent painful stimulation. Benson et al. [4] studied brain responses in 30 healthy subjects (15 women) during aversive visceral learning, extinction, and reactivation of fear memory (e.g., reinstatement). They found enhanced brain responses during reinstatement in key brain regions relevant for memory processes (hippocampus, cerebellum, THAL), suggesting enhanced reactivation of fear memory traces in women. Using an emotion recognition paradigm (viewing of emotionally valenced faces depicting fear and anger) in an fMRI study of 47 IBS patients and 67 HCs, Labus et al. [34] showed that male subjects regardless of disease showed overall greater brain responses to this particular visual stimulus than female subjects. Using an effective connectivity analysis, male IBS subjects were shown to demonstrate greater engagement of cortical and affect-related brain circuits compared with male control subjects and female patients.

In summary, a limited number of brain imaging studies performed during the past 5 years confirm sex-related differences in spontaneous and evoked brain activity, as well as in brain grey and white matter in large samples of IBS and HCs. Some of the results of these studies are consistent with earlier reports of greater engagement of emotional brain circuits in female subjects, and greater engagement of prefrontal circuits in male subjects. However, when using stimuli that elicit greater behavioural responses in male subjects (emotions of fear and anger), males showed greater responses and male IBS subjects showed increased connectivity of cortical and emotional arousal circuits. In addition to these differences seen in evoked brain responses, structural and RS analyses indicate sex-related differences in brain systems involved in sensory integration and motor responses.

CRITICAL ASSESSMENT, RECOMMENDATIONS, AND FUTURE DIRECTIONS

This brief review of the literature on brain imaging studies in chronic GI pain during the past 5 years clearly demonstrates the tremendous progress in study design, methodology, and analysis techniques that this field has experienced. Even though different paradigms have been used by different investigators, a significant consensus is evolving in some areas (including the role of cognitive and emotional modulation of pain perception, and the underlying brain regions and circuits). Differences in reported results remain in other areas, including differences between control subjects and IBS subjects in functional and structural brain imaging results and sex-related differences in brain activation. However, given the rapid advances that are being made in other areas of chronic pain research, emotion regulation, and imaging genetics, the application of existing and emerging neuroimaging techniques to the study of brain–gut interactions in health and disease may lead to breakthroughs in the understanding of pathophysiology of chronic visceral pain conditions, in the identification of similarities and differences with other chronic pain conditions, and in the prediction of treatment responses in the near future. However, some of the limitations (described subsequently) inherent in current studies will need to be overcome to make significant progress.

Many of the studies described in this review have involved detecting and determining the extent of regional brain activation across levels of an independent variable such as stimulus intensity or group. This is essentially a univariate analysis in that each brain volume or *a priori* chosen region is examined separately and the statistical threshold is adjusted for many individual comparisons made. While important for generating hypotheses about what parts of the brain might be involved in visceral sensation and the response to these sensations, this descriptive approach to imaging clearly does not capture the critical interrelationships among structures that form the foundation of brain function. The brain operates as functional networks, and activations in specific brain areas may have very different interpretations based on the coactivation of other regions that are connected via a network of inputs and projections. Much more sophisticated connectivity analyses that include a much larger set of highly specific brain regions (including large-scale network analyses and machine learning approaches) are now becoming possible and they go hand in hand with other advances in brain imaging, including increased spatial and temporal scanner resolution, use of radioligand tracers specific to molecules of interest, and the application of genetic analyses related to the development of specific brain circuitry. When combined with large data sets of well-phenotyped subjects (standardized brain imaging and behavioural and biological metadata), these new analytical tools should yield important breakthroughs in our understanding of central processes related to the pathophysiology of visceral pain disorders.

It is clear from the discussion above that in order to perform meaningful functional brain imaging studies, investigators must be mindful of the numerous factors that are likely to influence results. For example, it is important to pay particular attention to subject selection. Comparison of two groups, for instance, where age, sex, previous imaging experience, or experience of stimulation techniques used in the study, or where psychological state and trait measures including personality and psychiatric comorbidity are not controlled for will mean that differences in brain areas activated may well reflect the differences in the variables described rather than a reflection of the disease state or condition being studied. Many of the studies published during the past 5 years continue to pool male and female subjects and do not take into account important sex-related differences in brain and behavioural approaches. Particular care must be taken when studying patients especially those with FGIDs, which are inherently heterogenous. Every effort must be made to ensure that patients are as psychophysiologically homogenous as possible. An important exception to this rule of studying homogenous populations is, of course, when the variability in certain psychophysiological parameters between subjects is itself under study. These measures can then be used as covariates of the imaging findings. One might predict, for example, that opposite findings in a given area of the ACC may be observed as a function of whether the individuals being studied score high or low in anxiety state.

It is desirable that each new laboratory should undertake studies to develop normal values and reproducibility in healthy volunteers for the stimulation modality and parameters, sex and age before embarking upon patient studies. This will allow investigators to gain experience and establish normal values for their laboratory for variables that are important for their studies. It must be remembered that all studies must be powered to detect differences in the variables under study, for example, sex of the subject. In some cases, it may be more appropriate to study one parameter alone (e.g., female subjects only) if the study cannot be powered well enough to comment on multiple parameters.

Adequate behavioural measures must be used during studies involving experimental stimulation of the GI tract. For instance, when studying pain, it is desirable to control not only for intensity but also for unpleasantness when comparing two study populations. This could be achieved by titrating groups to a chosen level of either intensity or unpleasantness on a well-characterized visual analogue scale. Visual analogue scales and verbal descriptors of sensory experience and psychological state such as anxiety should be used in a controlled manner throughout the study so that acquisition of these variables does not interfere with data analysis and does not confound the results. Independent physiological measures of stress responsiveness during the study of visceral sensation such as ANS measures and cortisol levels may also be helpful in subsequent data interpretation. Correlation of the psychophysiological state with the imaging results can provide important information, which would be missed if the above measures are ignored.

The experimental environment within the brain imaging suite and the mental state of the subject must be adequately controlled. For instance, different brain areas will be activated if subjects attend to bodily sensations versus emotional feelings. This is particularly important during rest or baseline conditions when volunteers quite often have no control task to perform. The extent to which psychological factors are controlled and the extent to which behavioural measures are obtained during imaging to verify that the instructions were followed (e.g., measuring reactions times during an attention task) are essential for the conduct of good-quality studies. In some of the previously published studies, no specific instructions had been given, and this may well be the reason why there are sometimes "contradictory" findings across studies.

With the availability of imaging techniques, which can be standardized across sites (such as RS-functional imaging, MR spectroscopy, structural imaging, and DTI), it is now possible to collect large data sets (standardized brain imaging and metadata) from multiple sites in the form of brain imaging repositories. Such an approach has been successfully pioneered by the NIDDK-funded MAPP (Multidisciplinary Approaches to Pelvic Pain), and efforts are under way to create much larger repositories based on international collaborations (painrepository.org). Such repositories, when combined with standardized biological metadata (genomics, transcriptomics, microbiome), will provide unprecedented research opportunities into the pathophysiology of chronic visceral pain.

REFERENCES

1. Agostini A, Benuzzi F, Filippini N, Bertani A, Scarcelli A, Farinelli V, Marchetta C, Calabrese C, Rizzello F, Gionchetti P, et al. New insights into the brain involvement in patients with Crohn's disease: a voxel-based morphometry study. Neurogastroenterol Motil 2013;25(2):147–e82.
2. Aizawa E, Sato Y, Kochiyama T, Saito N, Izumiyama M, Morishita J, Kanazawa M, Shima K, Mushiake H, Hongo M, et al. Altered cognitive function of prefrontal cortex during error feedback in patients with irritable bowel syndrome, based on fMRI and dynamic causal modeling. Gastroenterology 2012;143(5):1188–98.
3. Babaei A, Siwiec RM, Kern M, Douglas Ward B, Li SJ, Shaker R. Intrinsic functional connectivity of the brain swallowing network during subliminal esophageal acid stimulation. Neurogastroenterol Motil 2013;25(12):992–e779.
4. Benson S, Kattoor J, Kullmann JS, Hofmann S, Engler H, Forsting M, Gizewski ER, Elsenbruch S. Towards understanding sex differences in visceral pain: enhanced reactivation of classically-conditioned fear in healthy women. Neurobiol Learn Mem 2014;109C:113–21.
5. Berman S, Suyenobu B, Naliboff BD, Bueller J, Stains J, Wong H, Mandelkern M, Fitzgerald L, Ohning G, Gupta A, et al. Evidence for alterations in central noradrenergic signaling in irritable bowel syndrome. NeuroImage 2012;63(4):1854–63.
6. Berman SM, Chang L, Suyenobu B, Derbyshire SW, Stains J, Fitzgerald L, Mandelkern M, Hamm L, Vogt B, Naliboff BD, et al. Condition-specific deactivation of brain regions by 5-HT(3) receptor antagonist alosetron. Gastroenterology 2002;123(4):969–77.

7. Berman SM, Naliboff BD, Suyenobu B, Labus JS, Stains J, Bueller JA, Ruby K, Mayer EA. Sex differences in regional brain response to aversive pelvic visceral stimuli. Am J Physiol Regul Integr Comp Physiol 2006;291(2):R268–76.
8. Bouhassira D, Moisset X, Jouet P, Duboc H, Coffin B, Sabate JM. Changes in the modulation of spinal pain processing are related to severity in irritable bowel syndrome. Neurogastroenterol Motil 2013;25(7):623–e468.
9. Camilleri M, Chang L. Challenges to the therapeutic pipeline for irritable bowel syndrome: end points and regulatory hurdles. Gastroenterology 2008;135(6):1877–91.
10. Coen SJ, Kano M, Farmer AD, Kumari V, Giampietro V, Brammer M, Williams SCR, Aziz Q. Neuroticism influences brain activity during the experience of visceral pain. Gastroenterology 2011;141(3):909–U639.
11. Coen SJ, Yaguez L, Aziz Q, Mitterschiffthaler MT, Brammer M, Williams SC, Gregory LJ. Negative mood affects brain processing of visceral sensation. Gastroenterology 2009;137(1):253–61, 261.e251–2.
12. Drossman DA, Dumitrascu DL. Rome III: new standard for functional gastrointestinal disorders. J Gastrointestin Liver Dis 2006;15(3):237–41.
13. Ellingson BM, Mayer E, Harris RJ, Ashe-McNally C, Naliboff BD, Labus JS, Tillisch K. Diffusion tensor imaging detects microstructural reorganization in the brain associated with chronic irritable bowel syndrome. Pain 2013;154(9):1528–41.
14. Elsenbruch S. Abdominal pain in irritable bowel syndrome: a review of putative psychological, neural and neuro-immune mechanisms. Brain Behav Immu 2011;25(3):386–94.
15. Elsenbruch S, Rosenberger C, Bingel U, Forsting M, Schedlowski M, Gizewski ER. Patients with irritable bowel syndrome have altered emotional modulation of neural responses to visceral stimuli. Gastroenterology 2010;139(4):1310–19.
16. Elsenbruch S, Rosenberger C, Enck P, Forsting M, Schedlowski M, Gizewski ER. Affective disturbances modulate the neural processing of visceral pain stimuli in irritable bowel syndrome: an fMRI study. Gut 2010;59(4):489–95.
17. Elsenbruch S, Schmid J, Kullmann JS, Kattoor J, Theysohn N, Forsting M, Kotsis V. Visceral sensitivity correlates with decreased regional gray matter volume in healthy volunteers: a voxel-based morphometry study. Pain 2014;155(2):244–9.
18. Farmer AD, Coen SJ, Kano M, Paine PA, Shwahdi M, Jafari J, Kishor J, Worthen SF, Rossiter HE, Kumari V, et al. Psychophysiological responses to pain identify reproducible human clusters. Pain 2013;154(11):2266–76.
19. Frokjaer JB, Olesen SS, Gram M, Yavarian Y, Bouwense SAW, Wilder-Smith OH, Drewes AM. Altered brain microstructure assessed by diffusion tensor imaging in patients with chronic pancreatitis. Gut 2011;60(11):1554–62.
20. Fukudo S. Stress and visceral pain: focusing on irritable bowel syndrome. Pain 2013;154(Suppl 1):S63–70.
21. Fukudo S, Kanazawa M, Mizuno T, Hamaguchi T, Kano M, Watanabe S, Sagami Y, Shoji T, Endo Y, Hongo M, et al. Impact of serotonin transporter gene polymorphism on brain activation by colorectal distention. NeuroImage 2009;47(3):946–51.
22. Hong JY, Kilpatrick LA, Labus J, Gupta A, Jiang ZG, Ashe-McNalley C, Stains J, Heendeniya N, Ebrat B, Smith S, et al. Patients with chronic visceral pain show sex-related alterations in intrinsic oscillations of the resting brain. J Neurosci 2013;33(29):11994–2002.
23. Hong JY, Labus JS, Jiang Z, Ashe-McNalley C, Dinov I, Gupta A, Shi Y, Stains J, Heendeniya N, Smith SR, et al. Regional neuroplastic brain changes in patients with chronic inflammatory and non-inflammatory visceral pain. PloS One 2014;9(1):e84564.
24. Jiang Z, Dinov ID, Labus J, Shi Y, Zamanyan A, Gupta A, Ashe-McNalley C, Hong JY, Tillisch K, Toga AW, et al. Sex-related differences of cortical thickness in patients with chronic abdominal pain. PloS One 2013;8(9):e73932.
25. Kano M, Farmer AD, Aziz Q, Giampietro VP, Brammer MJ, Williams SC, Fukudo S, Coen SJ. Sex differences in brain response to anticipated and experienced visceral pain in healthy subjects. Am J Physiol Gastrointest Liver Physiol 2013;304(8):G687–99.
26. Kattoor J, Gizewski ER, Kotsis V, Benson S, Gramsch C, Theysohn N, Maderwald S, Forsting M, Schedlowski M, Elsenbruch S. Fear conditioning in an abdominal pain model: neural responses during associative learning and extinction in healthy subjects. PloS One 2013;8(2):e51149.
27. Kattoor J, Thurling M, Gizewski ER, Forsting M, Timmann D, Elsenbruch S. Cerebellar contributions to different phases of visceral aversive extinction learning. Cerebellum 2014;13(1):1–8.
28. Kennedy PJ, Clarke G, Quigley EMM, Groeger JA, Dinan TG, Cryan JF. Gut memories: towards a cognitive neurobiology of irritable bowel syndrome. Neurosci Biobehav Rev 2012;36(1):310–40.

29. Kilpatrick LA, Labus JS, Coveleskie K, Hammer C, Rappold G, Tillisch K, Bueller JA, Suyenobu B, Jarcho JM, McRoberts JA, et al. The *HTR3A* polymorphism c. −42C>T is 25 associated with amygdala responsiveness in patients with irritable bowel syndrome. Gastroenterology 2011; 140(7): 1943–51.
30. Kilpatrick LA, Ornitz E, Ibrahimovic H, Treanor M, Craske M, Nazarian M, Labus JS, Mayer EA, Naliboff BD. Sex-related differences in prepulse inhibition of startle in irritable bowel syndrome (IBS). Biol Psychol 2010;84(2):272–8.
31. Labus J, Mayer EA, Berman S, Suyenobu B, Chang L, Naliboff BD. Sex-specific differences in a brain network functioning during anticipation of rectal discomfort in irritable bowel syndrome patients (IBS). Gastroenterology 2006;130(4):A93.
32. Labus JS, Bolus R, Chang L, Wiklund I, Naesdal J, Mayer EA, Naliboff BD. The Visceral Sensitivity Index: development and validation of a gastrointestinal symptom-specific anxiety scale. Aliment Pharmacol Ther 2004;20(1):89–97.
33. Labus JS, Dinov ID, Jiang Z, Ashe-McNalley C, Zamanyan A, Shi Y, Hong JY, Gupta A, Ebrat B, Tillisch K, et al. Irritable bowel syndrome in female patients is associated with alterations in structural brain networks. Pain 2014;155(1):137–49.
34. Labus JS, Gupta A, Coveleskie K, Tillisch K, Kilpatrick L, Jarcho J, Feier N, Bueller J, Stains J, Smith S, et al. Sex differences in emotion-related cognitive processes in irritable bowel syndrome and healthy control subjects. Pain 2013;154(10):2088–99.
35. Labus JS, Hubbard CS, Fanselow MS, Chen MP, Ebrat B, Bueller JA, Tillisch K, Stains J, Dukes GE, Kelleher D, et al. The corticotropin releasing factor 1 receptor (CRF-R1) antagonist Gw876008 differentially modulates brain response during acquisition and extinction of conditioned fear in irritable bowel syndrome (IBS) patients and healthy control subjects (HCS). Gastroenterology 2012;142(5):S71–2.
36. Labus JS, Mayer EA, Jarcho J, Kilpatrick LA, Kilkens TO, Evers EA, Backes WH, Brummer RJ, van Nieuwenhoven MA. Acute tryptophan depletion alters the effective connectivity of emotional arousal circuitry during visceral stimuli in healthy women. Gut 2011;60(9): 1196–203.
37. Labus JS, Naliboff BD, Berman SM, Suyenobu B, Vianna EP, Tillisch K, Mayer EA. Brain networks underlying perceptual habituation to repeated aversive visceral stimuli in patients with irritable bowel syndrome. NeuroImage 2009;47(3):952–60.
38. Labus JS, Naliboff BN, Fallon J, Berman SM, Suyenobu B, Bueller JA, Mandelkern M, Mayer EA. Sex differences in brain activity during aversive visceral stimulation and its expectation in patients with chronic abdominal pain: a network analysis. NeuroImage 2008;41(3):1032–43.
39. Larsson MB, Tillisch K, Craig AD, Engstrom M, Labus J, Naliboff B, Lundberg P, Strom M, Mayer EA, Walter SA. Brain responses to visceral stimuli reflect visceral sensitivity thresholds in patients with irritable bowel syndrome. Gastroenterology 2012;142(3):463–U111.
40. Lee HF, Hsieh JC, Lu CL, Yeh TC, Tu CH, Cheng CM, Niddam DM, Lin FY, Chang FY. Enhanced affect/cognition-related brain responses during visceral placebo analgesia in irritable bowel syndrome patients. Pain 2012;153(6): 1301–10.
41. Lowen MB, Mayer EA, Sjoberg M, Tillisch K, Naliboff B, Labus J, Lundberg P, Strom M, Engstrom M, Walter SA. Effect of hypnotherapy and educational intervention on brain response to visceral stimulus in the irritable bowel syndrome. Aliment Pharmacol Ther 2013;37(12): 1184–97.
42. Mayer EA, Bushnell, CM. Functional pain syndromes: presentation and pathophysiology, Vol. 1. Seattle, WA: International Association for the Study of Pain; 2009.
43. Mayer EA, Aziz Q, Coen S, Kern M, Labus JS, Lane R, Kuo B, Naliboff B, Tracey I. Brain imaging approaches to the study of functional GI disorders: a Rome working team report. Neurogastroenterol Motil 2009;21(6): 579–96.
44. Mayer EA, Collins SM. Evolving pathophysiological models of functional GI disorders: implications for new drug development. New York, NY: Health Education Alliance; 2000.
45. Nelson HE. A modified card sorting test sensitive to frontal lobe defects. Cortex 1976;12(4):313–24.
46. Phillips ML, Gregory LJ, Cullen S, Coen S, Ng V, Andrew C, Giampietro V, Bullmore E, Zelaya F, Amaro E, et al. The effect of negative emotional context on neural and behavioural responses to oesophageal stimulation. Brain 2003;126(Pt 3):669–84.
47. Schmid J, Theysohn N, Gass F, Benson S, Gramsch C, Forsting M, Gizewski ER, Elsenbruch S. Neural mechanisms mediating positive and negative treatment expectations in visceral pain: a functional magnetic resonance imaging study on placebo and nocebo effects in healthy volunteers. Pain 2013;154(11):2372–80.
48. Seminowicz DA, Labus JS, Bueller JA, Tillisch K, Naliboff BD, Bushnell MC, Mayer EA. Regional gray matter density changes in brains of patients with irritable bowel syndrome. Gastroenterology 2010;139(1):48–U82.

49. Sheehan J, Gaman A, Vangel M, Kuo B. Pooled analysis of brain activity in irritable bowel syndrome and controls during rectal balloon distension. Neurogastroenterol Moti 2011;23(4):336–46, e158.
50. Talley NJ. Functional gastrointestinal disorders as a public health problem. Neurogastroenterol Motil 2008;20(Suppl 1):121–9.
51. Tillisch K, Labus JS. Advances in imaging the brain-gut axis: functional gastrointestinal disorders. Gastroenterology 2011;140(2):407–U499.
52. Tillisch K, Mayer EA, Labus JS. Quantitative meta-analysis identifies brain regions activated during rectal distension in irritable bowel syndrome. Gastroenterology 2011;140(1):91–100.
53. Whorwell PJ. IBS: hypnotherapy—a wasted resource? Nat Rev Gastroenterol Hepatol 2012;9(1):12–3.
54. Zhou G, Qin W, Zeng F, Liu P, Yang X, von Deneen KM, Gong Q, Liang F, Tian J. White-matter microstructural changes in functional dyspepsia: a diffusion tensor imaging study. Am J Gastroenterol 2013;108(2):260–9.

CHAPTER 27

Brain Imaging and Chronic Visceral Pain

Yasser Al Omran and Qasim Aziz

When dysfunctional, the gastrointestinal (GI) tract may cause chronic visceral pain. Brain imaging research on the gut–brain interaction has significantly enhanced our understanding of the mechanisms involved in perceiving and processing visceral pain, in both health and disease, especially in functional gastrointestinal disorders (FGIDs). However, these studies present some inconsistencies with respect to one another. This may be partly due to the insufficient integration of cognitive and psychological processes, which contribute to the intrinsic heterogeneity of chronic visceral pain, in visceral pain brain imaging research. By dealing with the current limitations of brain imaging studies in visceral pain studies, we should see greater advancements in the field, and this may even provide the crucial first step towards developing patient-tailored treatments for chronic pain, with better efficacy than ever before.

The GI tract is involved in the ingestion, digestion and absorption of food, and the subsequent defecation of waste. This organ system also possesses an elaborate arrangement of nerves and adjuvant cells that have the potential to provide conscious awareness of injury and can generate painful responses. This may be advantageous in certain circumstances, as it allows the subject to react appropriately to noxious stimuli, and may thus be protective. However, when dysfunctional, especially on a chronic basis, the same system can lead to substantial morbidity.

Brain imaging research on the gut–brain interaction, involving relatively new techniques such as functional magnetic resonance imaging (fMRI) and positron emission tomography (PET), has significantly enhanced our understanding of the neuronal mechanisms behind the perception of visceral sensations in both health and disease. This research has focused predominantly on visceral pain, especially in FGID, a constellation of disorders characterized by chronic discomfort and pain in various locations of the GI tract that occur without discernible physical, biological, or anatomical abnormalities that would explain their symptoms [1]. However, results from this research have at times been heterogeneous. This may be due to methodological differences in stimulation method (stimulating at a fixed intensity or at titrated intensity depending on perception thresholds), image modality (fMRI vs. PET), or image processing and analysis [2]. Additionally, these inconsistencies may be a result of the heterogeneity of FGID, as their definition is based on symptoms as opposed to a specific pathophysiology [1]. However, comorbidity with other psychiatric disorders and "functional pain syndromes" (FPS), such as fibromyalgia (a condition with chronic widespread somatic pain), is common, suggesting that these disorders may share psychobiological processes in their cause [3].

Despite the developing notion of the importance of psychobiological processes in visceral pain, the methodology, design, and results from most brain imaging studies have not been incorporated with behavioural and epidemiological evidence on the psychological

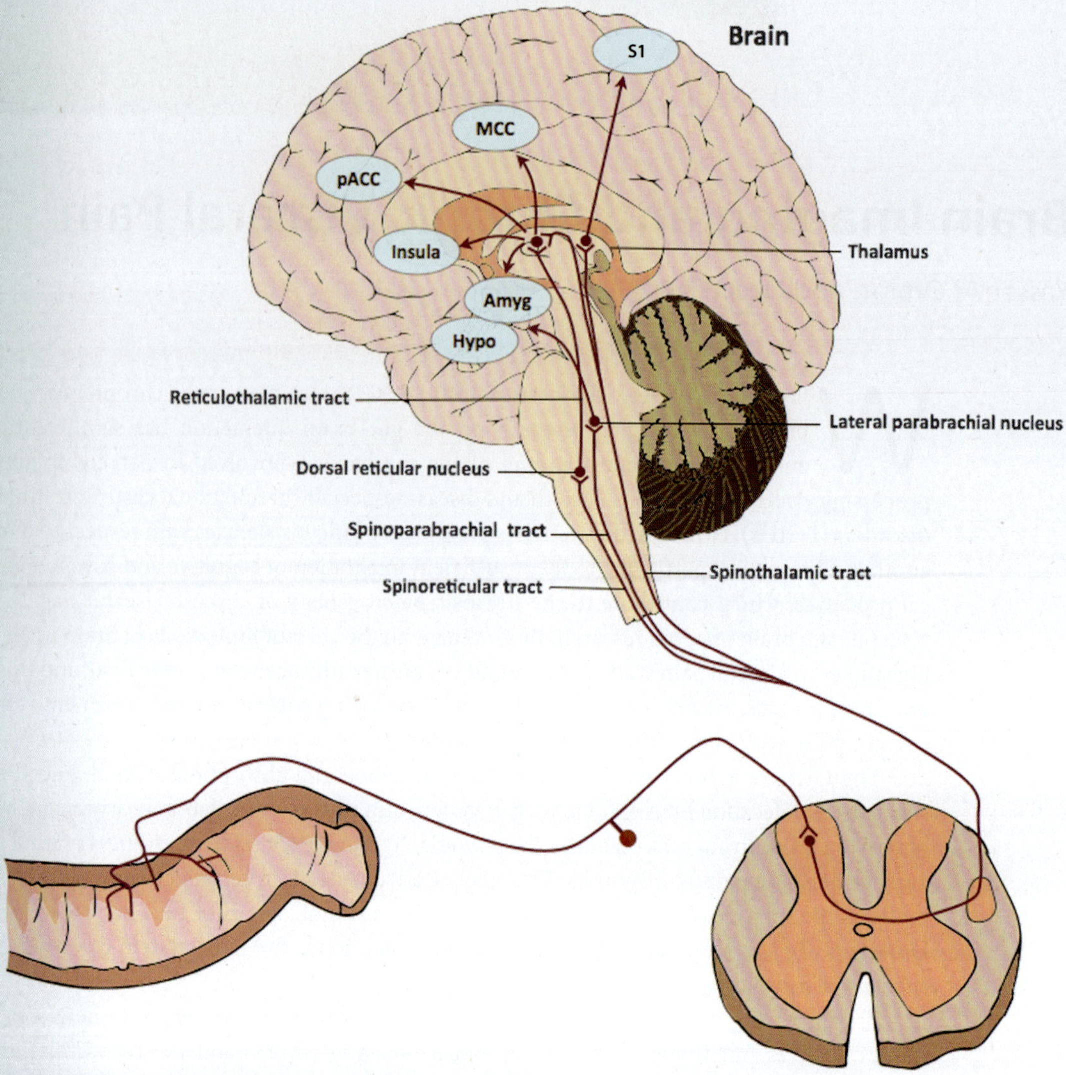

FIGURE 27-1 Ascending visceral pain pathways. After nociceptive activity has been transduced into electrical signals, and then transmitted from viscera to the spinal cord, it ascends to supraspinal structures by means of three pathways: the spinothalamic, the spinoparabrachial, and the spinoreticular pathways. The spinothalamic tract terminates in the medial and posterior thalamus. From here, the thalamocortical tract then projects to the primary and secondary somatosensory cortices (S1, S2), and is involved in pain localization and discrimination. The spinoparabrachial tract projects to the lateral parabrachial nucleus in the pons. From here, it projects to areas such as the hypothalamus and amygdala for the emotional processing of pain. The spinoreticular tract terminates in the dorsal reticular nucleus in the medulla. The reticulothalamic tract then transmits pain signals to the medial and intralaminar nuclei in the thalamus, before thalamocortical fibres project these signals to regions in the PFC, such as the insula, amygdala, and anterior cingulate cortex (ACC), which can be subdivided into the perigenual ACC (pACC) and mid-cingulate cortex (MCC). These areas are involved in motivational, reflexive, and affective aspects of pain. Other ascending pain-signalling pathways exist, but have not been shown. *Abbreviations*: Amyg, amygdala; Hypo, hypothalamus. (Adapted from Sharma et al. [49].)

processes of pain, nor with other branches of neuroscience such as cognitive and psychiatric neuroscience, which have utilized brain imaging. In contrast, somatic pain research has made substantial headway in this regard by trying to take into consideration and integrate cognitive (e.g., expectation and anticipation), emotional (e.g., sadness), and psychological aspects into experimental design, and to see how they may affect pain processing. Therefore, similar integration of other brain imaging neuroscience modalities into visceral pain

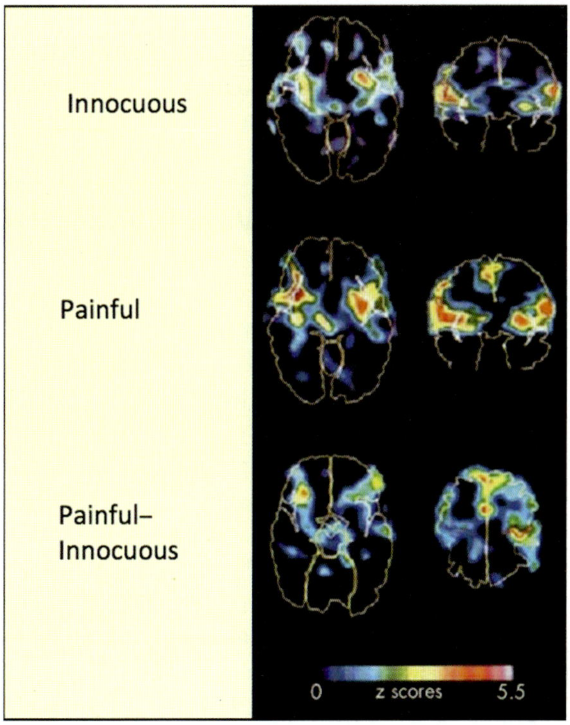

FIGURE 27-2 **Positron emission tomography (PET) scans displaying some aspects of the pain neuromatrix.** Group mean PET scans illustrating *z*-score maps for innocuous **(top panel)**, noxious **(middle panel)**, and both painful and innocuous **(bottom panel)** sensation contrasts. Innocuous stimulation elicited bilateral activity in the primary somatosensory, insular, and motor cortices **(top panel)**. Painful stimulation produced more intense activity in the same areas, and additional activity in the right anterior insular cortex and the anterior cingulate gyrus **(middle panel)**. Multiple areas of decreased activity were also observed; prominent among these was the right prefrontal cortex, which was inhibited during both innocuous and painful stimulation **(middle panel)**. (Adapted from Aziz et al. [7].)

studies may be equally fruitful and should be adopted. The purpose of this chapter is to summarize how brain imaging techniques have shaped our understanding of chronic visceral pain, especially in FGID, and address potential limitations and ways of enhancing brain imaging research in chronic visceral pain.

THE PAIN NEUROMATRIX

Pain has been described as a "homeostatic emotion" that is different from other senses in that it is multidimensional and complex [4]. This complexity is highlighted in early PET studies of somatic pain [5, 6], which showed activation of an elaborate network of cortical and subcortical structures following noxious, thermal stimulation of the skin, and which have helped establish some of the ascending pain pathways (Fig. 27-1). But is the "visceral pain neuromatrix" the same? One of the earliest studies that aimed to describe the visceral pain neuromatrix activated following GI stimulation used PET to study cortical activation to esophageal stimulation at noxious and innocuous (physiological) intensities [7]. They reported that the supraspinal structures involved in processing GI pain paralleled those previously reported from somatic studies (Fig. 27-2). In short, innocuous esophageal stimulation caused bilateral activity in the primary and secondary somatosensory cortices (S1 and S2) and insula. Noxious, painful esophageal stimulation not only generated greater activity in these regions but also activated the anterior cingulate cortex (ACC) [7]. Other studies have subsequently confirmed that these four supraspinal structures are activated during both somatic and visceral pain paradigms [8–11].

BRAIN IMAGING TO PROVIDE INSIGHT INTO FGID

A concept that has arisen, particularly, as a result of brain imaging, is that the perception of pain has a huge impact on the experience of pain. In FGID, psychological disorders such as dysthymia, depression, and heightened anxiety have been reported [12]. This prompted the investigation of the effects of different psychological states on the intensity and distribution of cortical activation. A negative emotional state may be studied as an example using fMRI; it was demonstrated that esophageal (nonpainful balloon) distension during a negative emotional state (elicited by presenting the subject with fearful facial expressions) was associated with increased cortical activation of the dorsal ACC and the anterior insula [13]. Esophageal sensation was perceived more intensely and generated greater anxiety compared with distension in a neutral emotion state (elicited by presenting the subject with neutral facial expressions) [13]. Additionally, exposure to both nonpainful and painful esophageal distension using emotionally valent music to induce negative emotional states also showed increased activity in the right ACC and anterior insula [14]. These findings highlight that psychobiological changes have a profound effect on patterns of cortical activity. Consistent with this, as many FGID patients have been reported to feel depressed and anxious, and associate GI sensations with negative feelings [15], these findings have suggested a means by which psychobiology can influence our perception of pain in both health and FGID and validate the importance of controlling for these factors in brain imaging studies.

Moreover, studies have shown that the intensity of pain may be attenuated when the subject is distracted or focusing on other tasks, and heightened when focusing upon the stimulus that causes the pain [16]. Therefore, how much attention we pay may influence the intensity of sensations. In FGID, patients may be more attentive to their visceral sensations, and this may in part be responsible for their persistent symptoms [17].

Additionally, as most GI sensations are not consciously perceived in health like other modalities such as touch, this may be due to decreased selective attention compared with the other modalities. This was validated in a study in which subjects were exposed to either visual or nonpainful esophageal distension simultaneously, but had their attention either divided between the two sensory modalities or selectively focused on one sensory modality at a time. Using fMRI, selective attention to esophageal stimuli was shown to activate visceral sensory (S1 and S2) as well as cognitive and emotional regions (ACC and insula), whereas selective attention to visual stimuli mainly activated the visual cortex [18]. Notably, while selectively focusing on visual stimuli, cortical activity associated with esophageal distension was significantly attenuated [18]. The same group further supported these results with later studies [19]. They showed that the decrease in pain rating when distracted from a painful esophageal distension was associated with attenuation in neural activity in the right mid-ACC and the right dorsolateral and ventrolateral prefrontal cortex (PFC) (Fig. 27-3). Moreover, the same group recently showed that personality traits may affect visceral sensations as subjects that were neurotic and more anxious demonstrated lower pain thresholds, perhaps because of increased attention to sensations, compared with subjects with opposite profiles [20]. They also showed that these neurotic and anxious subjects had a predominant

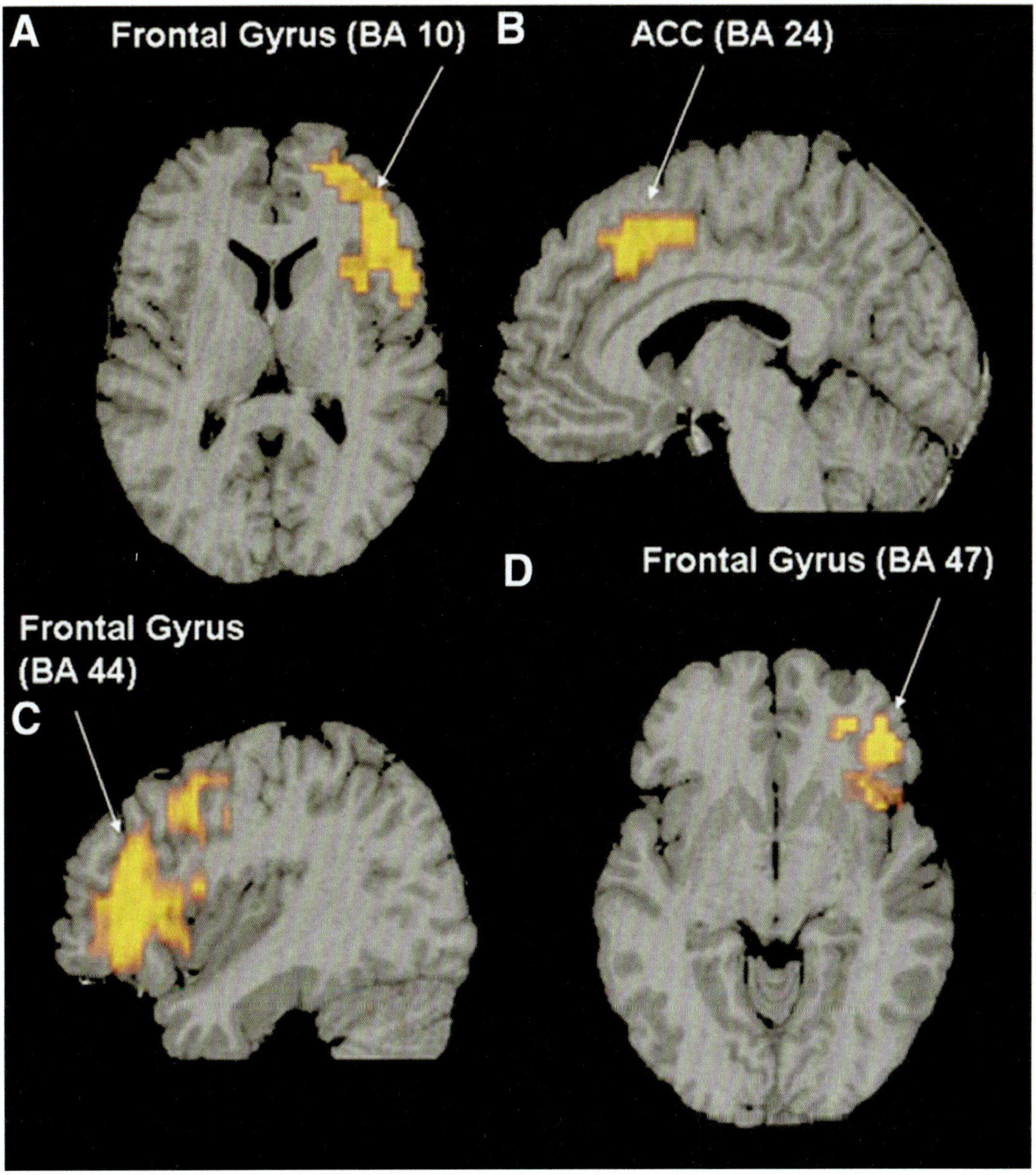

FIGURE 27-3 Functional magnetic resonance imaging and selective attention. The represented brain regions that show significantly increased activity during painful esophageal stimulation alone, compared with pain during distraction. **A:** *BA10* of the right frontal gyrus, **B:** the right ACC (*BA24*), **C:** *BA44* of the right frontal gyrus, and **D:** right frontal gyrus (*BA47*). (Adapted from Coen et al. [19].)

parasympathetic response to pain, suggesting that physiological factors can also influence the processing of visceral pain [20]. Taken together, these findings suggest that selective attention of visceral sensations increases neural resources necessary to process this information, which may exaggerate visceral sensations and subsequently lead to increased emotional responsiveness. It is possible that these processes can occur in FGID, and may explain why FGID patients have amplified sensory awareness as has been seen in numerous FGID studies [17]. This is further supported by the success of hypnosis, both in somatic pain and in irritable bowel syndrome (IBS, the most common disorder of FGID) [21].

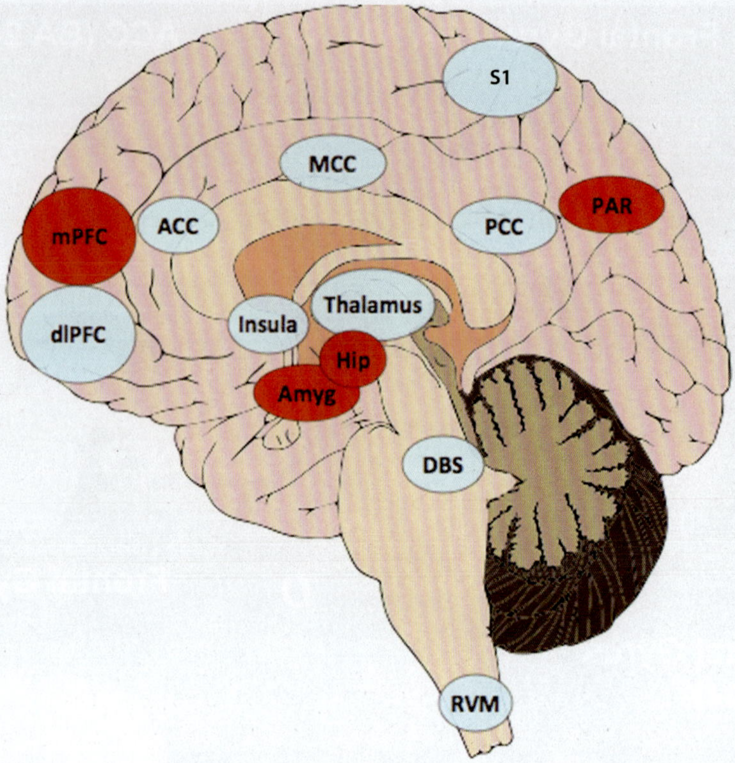

FIGURE 27-4 Supraspinal structures activated after heterotopic stimulation. Heterotopic stimulation refers to the modulation of a primary pain stimulus by another, distant, stimulus (i.e., esophageal distension and thermal foot stimulation), which usually causes a decrease in pain sensitivity. The regions depicted above are the ones most consistently activated after heterotopic stimulation in healthy subjects (*blue*) and in patients with IBS (*red*). *Abbreviations*: ACC, anterior cingulate cortex; Amyg, amygdala; DBS, dorsal brainstem; Hip, hippocampus; PAR, parietal cortex; PCC, posterior cingulate cortex; dlPFC, dorsolateral prefrontal cortex; mPFC, medial prefrontal cortex; RVM, rostroventral medulla; S1, primary somatosensory cortex; THAL, thalamus. (Adapted from Wilder-Smith [50].)

In both somatic pain syndromes and IBS, hypnosis has been shown to lead to the activation of the PFC, an area attributed to increased sensory perception in chronic pain patients, and so may thus modulate responses and distance subjects from the emotional effect of pain and result in pain reduction [22]. However, activation of particular brain regions may be dependent on the type of hypnosis, as autogenic training (a clinically used, self-hypnosis technique) has been shown to activate the left insular and supplementary cortices only, and not the PFC [23]. Nevertheless, as pain reduction was achieved regardless of regional brain activity, the efficacy of hypnosis in reducing pain has supported the role of selective attention in FGID.

Although the aforementioned studies provide convincing evidence for the effect of psychological factors on visceral pain, they were conducted mainly in healthy subjects. To provide further insight, brain imaging studies of visceral pain in FGID patients have also been explored. The first comparison of GI-associated cortical activity between healthy subjects and FGID patients used PET and implied that activation of the ACC was attenuated in IBS, but activation of the PFC was heightened [24]. The reduced activity in the ACC was originally thought to be because of aberrant modulatory effects of the endogenous opioid system, whereas enhanced activity in the PFC was thought to be because of increased awareness of GI stimulation. Another group supported the notion of endogenous pain modulation [25]. By using heterotopic stimulation (two distant but simultaneously occurring painful stimulations), they showed that noxious stimulation of the foot significantly reduces rectal pain during balloon distension in healthy controls and increases pain in patients with IBS. Specifically, healthy controls demonstrate a bilateral activation of supraspinal structures, including the ACC and the ventral and dorsal PFC [26]. Activity in these areas was reduced in constipation-predominant IBS (IBS-C) patients and absent in diarrhoea-predominant IBS (IBS-D) patients. Healthy controls showed decreased activity in areas of the pain neuromatrix, including the thalamus and insula, whereas in IBS-C and IBS-D patients, these regions showed no change and increased activity, respectively, while the amygdala and orbitofrontal cortex, which are pain modulatory regions, showed increased activity [27]. Other IBS studies using heterotopic stimulation have validated the altered activity in these regions and have demonstrated the activation of other regions (Fig. 27-4) [27, 28].

fMRI studies of chronic visceral pain show considerable variation in the brain areas that are activated. For example, IBS patients exhibit variable activity in ACC compared with healthy subjects [29]. Some studies using fMRI in colorectal pain demonstrated greater neural activity in several brain regions, including those relating to sensory as well as cognitive and emotional regions in IBS patients compared with age- or sex-matched controls [30]. Furthermore, they show that visceral hypersensitivity in IBS patients is followed by further increases in neural activity within the same brain structures. This implies that the increased visceral pain may be due to increased afferent processing, perhaps because of increased sensitization by previous infectious or inflammatory events, as opposed to selectively increased activity in supraspinal structures [30]. Further research has reported both decreased and increased cortical activation in patients with IBS and has either supported or opposed the two main hypotheses (sensitization of afferent pathways or amplification of GI signals due to selective attention) as potential mechanisms of increased hypersensitivity in FGID patients (for in-depth meta-analysis, see [31]). This sets up a problem because both mechanisms are possible, and have sufficient evidence from brain imaging studies to support them [32].

LIMITATIONS

As both sensitization of afferents and selective attention have been supported by brain imaging as possible underlying mechanisms to increase visceral pain in FGID, it is conceivable to think that faults in methodology may explain the results of brain imaging studies rather than the results being mechanistically important. For instance, for the selective attention hypothesis of visceral pain, the mid-ACC has been shown to be important in the processing of pain, and is assumed to have enhanced activation of this region [18, 19]. It is nevertheless possible that a subject used in these studies may be claustrophobic and anxious lying inside a noisy magnetic resonance scanner, and perhaps made more anxious by a balloon about to be painfully inserted into their rectum and inflated. As a result, the mid-ACC of that patient may be more active throughout the length of the study. This fear and anxiety may exaggerate visceral pain in a process known as pain catastrophizing [33] and may thus act to produce erroneous results in subtraction analysis. Because these methodological issues are universal among all brain imaging studies, this implies that we are no closer to coming to the clinical reality behind why chronic visceral pain occurs in FGID and other visceral disorders.

Consequently, it seems that the limitations of current brain imaging studies as a whole need to be addressed. First, individual brain imaging studies employ relatively small sample sizes, making it difficult to control the multiple covariates (such as the psychological covariate). Although meta-analytical methods for brain imaging have helped to limit these covariates [31], brain imaging research studies of GI hypersensitivity are still limited by methodological restraints and by the heterogeneity and quality of individual studies. A possible solution to this may be to develop multicentre partnerships with standardized protocols to enable comparable results and the pooling of these results between centres. This tactic will allow for clearer conclusions and will allow potential confounders to be controlled more appropriately.

Additionally, the nature of inferences in brain imaging studies of visceral sensations is often weakly supported by functional brain imaging studies. For example, the identification of different anatomical brain regions during different cognitive processes (e.g., the experience of pain vs. no pain) is inferred as being involved in those processes. However, such an approach is essentially correlational in nature, making it difficult to determine whether the brain regions activated during the different mental/perceptual processes are required for the occurrence of those processes [33]. Nevertheless, inferences about the involvement of specific anatomical areas are made and so may naturally be unsubstantiated. Moreover, such inferences have unfortunately been often used as a direct means to analyze brain imaging results, instead of guiding succeeding brain imaging and behavioural studies, which may be its best function [34, 35].

These inferences may be better substantiated if the experimental paradigm includes functional and anatomical analyses. Functional connectivity gives information on the effect one brain region has on another. However, previous functional connectivity studies have been founded on *a priori* knowledge, based mainly on use of neuronal tracers in animal studies to determine pathways [36]. This suggests that these neuronal circuits or networks have not been firmly characterized in human studies and are therefore subject to bias. However, this limitation may be overcome by using novel structural connectivity imaging such as diffusion tensor imaging (DTI). DTI uses the diffusivity of water as a probe to infer the anatomy and integrity of different white matter tracts. This has already helped researchers to define anatomical borders between cortical and subcortical regions [36, 37], and has already been incorporated into somatic pain studies. For example, a recent DTI-based study reported that increased pain intensity in patients with fibromyalgia was correlated with microstructural changes in the thalamus, the thalamocortical tracts, and both insular regions [38]. Although DTI is beginning to be used in visceral pain studies [39], such an approach should allow researchers to better delineate networks in functional connectivity analysis, allowing them to better interpret the brain domains activated by such networks.

Finally, a preponderance of brain imaging, pain research studies use healthy volunteers who are subjected to superficial acute pain. Therefore, these results may not be clinically translatable, as this pain differs from the deep (e.g., neuropathic, muscular) pain seen in clinical practice and sometimes experienced by healthy volunteers. A shift to using more patients with chronic pain may be a possible solution.

LESSONS FROM SOMATIC PAIN STUDIES (DEPRESSION AS AN EXAMPLE)

Like the use of DTI in pain studies, there are other approaches undertaken in somatic pain research that could be adopted in visceral pain research to further enhance our understanding. Although such approaches are beyond the scope of this chapter (for reviews, see [40, 41]), research on depression and pain processing will be briefly reviewed as an example.

fMRI was utilized to examine the neurophysiological interface between depression and disease-related pain in rheumatoid arthritis. It suggested that depression correlated significantly with joint pain and with medial PFC (mPFC) activity when joint pain was provoked [42]. This indicates that the mPFC may have an important role in facilitating the interactions between depression and the clinical severity of pain in rheumatoid arthritis, perhaps by activation of pain modulatory brain regions such as the hippocampus, amygdala, and dorsolateral PFC [43]. Similar interactions have been seen in heat pain and depression. Major depressive disorder patients showed greater engagement of brain regions involved in anticipation of pain such as the amygdala and areas involved in pain processing such as the anterior insula and the anterior mid-cingulate cortex (aMCC). Following exposure to pain, patients with major depressive disorder showed abnormal activity in pain modulatory regions such as the perigenual ACC (pACC) and the dorsolateral PFC [43].

Taken together, these results signify the importance of comorbid depressive symptoms in influencing pain perception, specifically by interfering with the mechanisms behind pain processing and pain modulation, and also suggest the need to register and control psychiatric comorbidities in visceral pain brain imaging studies, especially when comparing FGID patients with healthy controls, as the former have commonly reported having comorbidity with other psychiatric disorders [3]. Fortunately, this approach may be adopted more in pain research as the use of psychotropic drugs in FGID patients has shown to be effective in reducing pain levels, further validating the link between depression and visceral pain [44, 45].

FUTURE DIRECTIONS AND CONCLUSIONS

In conclusion, although brain imaging has revealed a great deal behind the mechanisms of visceral pain, there are problems with the field (as previously highlighted). Alternatively, the integration of research from affective, cognitive, and psychiatric neuroscience as well as research from behavioural and epidemiological evidence relating to the involvement of psychological processes has offered great insight in the field of somatic pain; this is particularly true with regard to the psychobiological mechanisms that seem to determine the subjective experience of pain. This integrative approach should be adopted by future visceral pain studies utilizing brain imaging resources; although this chapter has highlighted a few ways in which this has improved, it has been limited thus far. This integration has to be applied at all stages: data design, collection, and analysis. Moreover, researchers need to be aware of the limitations of brain imaging studies (some of which have been highlighted in this chapter), and researchers need to try avoiding them in order to obtain results that best relate and reflect clinical situations.

Moreover, although not really mentioned in this chapter, peripheral mechanisms at the level of the gut need to be acknowledged and integrated into brain visceral pain as the gut forms a bidirectional interface with the brain via hormonal, immune, and neural routes [46], and can form clearer associations between peripheral and central mechanisms to complete the integrated picture of the pathophysiology and clinical reality of visceral pain. These three routes can be studied through a variety of means and are starting to be used in unison with functional brain imaging [20, 47, 48].

Overall, by adopting an integrative approach, we should soon be able to identify psychophysiological vulnerable factors and subgroups (as opposed to symptom-based ones), not only in FGID but in any chronic visceral disorders. These approaches may provide the crucial first step towards developing patient-tailored treatments, with better efficacy than ever before, in lowering chronic visceral pain levels.

REFERENCES

1. Tillisch K, Labus JS. Advances in imaging the brain-gut axis: functional gastrointestinal disorders. Gastroenterology 2011;140(2):407–11.e1.
2. Mayer EA, Aziz Q, Coen S, Kern M, Labus JS, Lane R, Kuo B, Naliboff B, Tracey I. Brain imaging approaches to the study of functional GI disorders: a Rome working team report. Neurogastroenterol Motil 2009;21(6): 579–96.
3. Van Oudenhove L, Aziz Q. Recent insights on central processing and psychological processes in functional gastrointestinal disorders. Dig Liver Dis 2009;41(11):781–7.
4. Craig AD. A new view of pain as a homeostatic emotion. Trends Neurosci 2003;26(6):303–7.
5. Jones AK, Brown WD, Friston KJ, Qi LY, Frackowiak RS. Cortical and subcortical localization of response to pain in man using positron emission tomography. Proc Biol Sci 1991;244(1309):39–44.
6. Talbot JD, Marrett S, Evans AC, Meyer E, Bushnell MC, Duncan GH. Multiple representations of pain in human cerebral cortex. Science 1991;251(4999):1355–8.
7. Aziz Q, Andersson JL, Valind S, Sundin A, Hamdy S, Jones AK, Foster ER, Långström B, Thompson DG. Identification of human brain loci processing esophageal sensation using positron emission tomography. Gastroenterology 1997;113(1):50–9.
8. Aziz Q, Thompson DG, Ng VW, Hamdy S, Sarkar S, Brammer MJ, Bullmore ET, Hobson A, Tracey I, Gregory L, et al. Cortical processing of human somatic and visceral sensation. J Neurosci 2000;20(7):2657–63.
9. Peyron R, Laurent B, Garcia-Larrea L. Functional imaging of brain responses to pain: a review and meta-analysis (2000). Neurophysiol Clin 2000;30(5):263–88.
10. Hobday DI, Aziz Q, Thacker N, Hollander I, Jackson A, Thompson DG. A study of the cortical processing of ano-rectal sensation using functional MRI. Brain 2001;124(Pt 2):361–8.
11. Lotze M, Wietek B, Birbaumer N, Ehrhardt J, Grodd W, Enck P. Cerebral activation during anal and rectal stimulation. NeuroImage 2001;14(5):1027–34.
12. Talley NJ. Functional gastrointestinal disorders as a public health problem. Neurogastroenterol Motil 2008;20(Suppl 1):121–9.
13. Phillips ML, Gregory LJ, Cullen S, Coen S, Ng V, Andrew C, Giampietro V, Bullmore E, Zelaya F, Amaro E, et al. The effect of negative emotional context on neural and behavioural responses to oesophageal stimulation. Brain 2003;126(Pt 3):669–84.
14. Coen SJ, Yaguez L, Aziz Q, Mitterschiffthaler MT, Brammer M, Williams SC, Gregory LJ. Negative mood affects brain processing of visceral sensation. Gastroenterology 2009;137(1):253–61, 61.e1–2.
15. Kim SE, Chang L. Overlap between functional GI disorders and other functional syndromes: what are the underlying mechanisms? Neurogastroenterol Motil 2012;24(10):895–913.
16. Johnston NE, Atlas LY, Wager TD. Opposing effects of expectancy and somatic focus on pain. PLoS One 2012;7(6):e38854.
17. Whitehead WE, Palsson OS. Is rectal pain sensitivity a biological marker for irritable bowel syndrome: psychological influences on pain perception. Gastroenterology 1998;115(5):1263–71.
18. Gregory LJ, Yaguez L, Williams SC, Altmann C, Coen SJ, Ng V, Brammer MJ, Thompson DG, Aziz Q. Cognitive modulation of the cerebral processing of human oesophageal sensation using functional magnetic resonance imaging. Gut 2003;52(12):1671–7.
19. Coen SJ, Aziz Q, Yaguez L, Brammer M, Williams SC, Gregory LJ. Effects of attention on visceral stimulus intensity encoding in the male human brain. Gastroenterology 2008;135(6):2065–74, 74.e1
20. Farmer AD, Coen SJ, Kano M, Paine PA, Shwahdi M, Jafari J, et al. Psychophysiological responses to pain identify reproducible human clusters. Pain 2013;154(11):2266–76.
21. Raij TT, Numminen J, Narvanen S, Hiltunen J, Hari R. Strength of prefrontal activation predicts intensity of suggestion-induced pain. Hum Brain Mapp 2009;30(9):2890–7.
22. Wilson S, Maddison T, Roberts L, Greenfield S, Singh S. Systematic review: the effectiveness of hypnotherapy in the management of irritable bowel syndrome. Aliment Pharmacol Ther 2006;24(5):769–80.
23. Naglatzki RP, Schlamann M, Gasser T, Ladd ME, Sure U, Forsting M, et al. Cerebral somatic pain modulation during autogenic training in fMRI. Eur J Pain. 2012;16(9):1293-301.
24. Silverman DH, Munakata JA, Ennes H, Mandelkern MA, Hoh CK, Mayer EA. Regional cerebral activity in normal and pathological perception of visceral pain. Gastroenterology 1997;112(1):64–72.
25. Wilder-Smith CH, Robert-Yap J. Abnormal endogenous pain modulation and somatic and visceral hypersensitivity in female patients with irritable bowel syndrome. World J Gastroenterol 2007;13(27): 3699–704.

26. Wilder-Smith CH, Schindler D, Lovblad K, Redmond SM, Nirkko A. Brain functional magnetic resonance imaging of rectal pain and activation of endogenous inhibitory mechanisms in irritable bowel syndrome patient subgroups and healthy controls. Gut 2004;53(11):1595–601.
27. Song GH, Venkatraman V, Ho KY, Chee MW, Yeoh KG, Wilder-Smith CH. Cortical effects of anticipation and endogenous modulation of visceral pain assessed by functional brain MRI in irritable bowel syndrome patients and healthy controls. Pain 2006;126(1–3):79–90.
28. Bishop SJ. Trait anxiety and impoverished prefrontal control of attention. Nat Neurosci 2009;12(1):92–8.
29. Mertz H, Morgan V, Tanner G, Pickens D, Price R, Shyr Y, Kessler R. Regional cerebral activation in irritable bowel syndrome and control subjects with painful and nonpainful rectal distention. Gastroenterology 2000;118(5):842–8.
30. Verne GN, Himes NC, Robinson ME, Gopinath KS, Briggs RW, Crosson B, Price DD. Central representation of visceral and cutaneous hypersensitivity in the irritable bowel syndrome. Pain 2003;103(1–2):99–110.
31. Tillisch K, Mayer EA, Labus JS. Quantitative meta-analysis identifies brain regions activated during rectal distension in irritable bowel syndrome. Gastroenterology 2011;140(1):91–100.
32. Hobson AR, Aziz Q. Brain imaging and functional gastrointestinal disorders: has it helped our understanding? Gut 2004;53(8):1198–206.
33. Garland EL, Gaylord SA, Palsson O, Faurot K, Douglas Mann J, Whitehead WE. Therapeutic mechanisms of a mindfulness-based treatment for IBS: effects on visceral sensitivity, catastrophizing, and affective processing of pain sensations. J Behav Med 2012;35(6):591–602.
34. Poldrack RA. Can cognitive processes be inferred from neuroimaging data? Trends Cogn Sci 2006;10(2): 59–63.
35. Poldrack RA. The role of fMRI in cognitive neuroscience: where do we stand? Curr Opin Neurobiol 2008;18(2):223–7.
36. Johansen-Berg H, Rushworth MF. Using diffusion imaging to study human connectional anatomy. Annu Rev Neurosci 2009;32:75–94.
37. Zuo N, Cheng J, Jiang T. Diffusion magnetic resonance imaging for Brainnetome: a critical review. Neurosci Bull 2012;28(4):375–88.
38. Lutz J, Jager L, de Quervain D, Krauseneck T, Padberg F, Wichnalek M, Beyer A, Stahl R, Zirngibl B, Morhard D, et al. White and gray matter abnormalities in the brain of patients with fibromyalgia: a diffusion-tensor and volumetric imaging study. Arthritis Rheum 2008;58(12):3960–9.
39. Ellingson BM, Mayer E, Harris RJ, Ashe-McNally C, Naliboff BD, Labus JS, et al. Diffusion tensor imaging detects microstructural reorganization in the brain associated with chronic irritable bowel syndrome. Pain 2013;154(9):1528–41.
40. Tracey I. Can neuroimaging studies identify pain endophenotypes in humans? Nat Rev Neurol 2011;7(3): 173–81.
41. Van Oudenhove L. Understanding gut-brain interactions in gastrointestinal pain by neuroimaging: lessons from somatic pain studies. Neurogastroenterol Motil 2011;23(4):292–302.
42. Schweinhardt P, Kalk N, Wartolowska K, Chessell I, Wordsworth P, Tracey I. Investigation into the neural correlates of emotional augmentation of clinical pain. NeuroImage 2008;40(2):759–66.
43. Strigo IA, Simmons AN, Matthews SC, Craig AD, Paulus MP. Association of major depressive disorder with altered functional brain response during anticipation and processing of heat pain. Arch Gen Psychiatry 2008;65(11):1275–84.
44. Dekel R, Drossman DA, Sperber AD. The use of psychotropic drugs in irritable bowel syndrome. Expert Opin Investig Drugs 2013;22(3):329–39.
45. Vogt BA. Inflammatory bowel disease: perspectives from cingulate cortex in the first brain. Neurogastroenterol Motil 2013;25(2):93–8.
46. Mayer EA. Gut feelings: the emerging biology of gut-brain communication. Nat Rev Neurosci 2011;12(8): 453–66.
47. Kindt S, Van Oudenhove L, Broekaert D, Kasran A, Ceuppens JL, Bossuyt X, Fischler B, Tack J. Immune dysfunction in patients with functional gastrointestinal disorders. Neurogastroenterol Motil 2009;21(4): 389–98.
48. Sharma A, Paine P, Rhodes S, Warburton F, Chua YC, Aziz Q. The autonomic response to human esophageal acidification and the development of hyperalgesia. Neurogastroenterol Motil 2012;24(7):e285–93.
49. Sharma A, Lelic D, Brock C, Paine P, Aziz Q. New technologies to investigate the brain-gut axis. World J Gastroenterol 2009;15(2):182–91.
50. Wilder-Smith CH. The balancing act: endogenous modulation of pain in functional gastrointestinal disorders. Gut 2011;60(11):1589–99.

CHAPTER 28

In Search of Pelvic Pain

Melissa A. Farmer

The pelvis cradles the reproductive machinery necessary for our species to evolve. As such, pelvic pain represents a critical threat to the survival of the individual and future offspring. Acute pelvic pain signals the presence of bacterial, fungal, or viral infection, or frank tissue damage. Accordingly, traditional assessment and treatment of pelvic pain target the end organs as the primary source(s) of pathology. However, when pelvic pain outlasts the normal healing period, a patient's diagnosis will often depend on the treating physician rather than the unique configuration of symptoms. Gynaecologists investigate potential anatomical, hormonal, and pathophysiological causes; physical therapists assess the tension, controllability, and strength of pelvic floor muscles; urologists biopsy tissue and test the functional capacity of involved organs; neurologists explore potential nerve entrapment or injury; sex therapists focus on anxiety and distraction to enhance sexual function; and psychiatrists seek psychosomatic causes with limited consideration of physical pathology. Like the Indian parable of the blind men and the elephant, each type of clinician emphasizes a narrow aspect of chronic pelvic pain (CPP) to guide diagnosis.

This specialization approach has given rise to three clinical obstacles that influence our understanding of CPP: (a) etiological theories outside a clinician's specialty may not be considered; (b) clinicians rarely communicate across theoretical camps, leading CPP research to evolve as cross-disciplinary islands of unintegrated knowledge; and (c) such specialized approaches have seldom identified physical findings that explain the common symptom of pelvic pain. Indeed, CPP conditions are referred to as a family of clinical "wastebasket" diagnoses because, as diagnoses of exclusion, they are mutually defined by the lack of identifiable pathology. This atheoretical diagnostic approach fails to acknowledge the heterogeneity within each condition that likely points to multiple underlying pain subgroups.

In the context of the pain research field, this fragmented approach to studying pelvic pain is a symptom of long-standing ideological biases within the medical profession. An obsession with end-organ pain mechanisms restricts inquiry to local phenomena (i.e., pelvic pathology, local inflammation, pelvic floor muscles). Similarly, a poor understanding of spinally mediated referred pain and viscerovisceral hyperalgesia reinforces a focus on misleading clinical symptoms characteristic of visceral pain. The common missing element is supraspinal involvement in processing chronic nociceptive input. Perhaps the last place one seeks to find the pelvis is in the brain.

The traditional view of peripheral and central nervous system (CNS) pain mechanisms as independent contributors to CPP reflects an artificial distinction that, surprisingly, continues to fuel controversy within the field [28, 58]. Peripheral and central input may compete, certainly, yet it is more likely that the respective roles of peripheral and central processes shift with pain chronification as the organism adapts to a new baseline state of chronic pain [9, 27]. As a "sentient neural hub," the brain mediates pain perception by iteratively integrating environmental, nociceptive, and psychological inputs [38]. These inputs culminate in an ongoing neural representation of pain that serves many purposes, including the recruitment of protective behavioural responses such as escape, avoidance, or guarding [14]. The brain is uniquely suited to facilitate these adaptations through experience-dependent neuroplasticity.

LEARNING TO LIVE WITH PELVIC PAIN

Chronic pain has recently been conceptualized as a learned state of suffering [6]. CPP can therefore be characterized as an experience-dependent learned association between pelvic pain perception and functional disability. Functional disability secondary to CPP may take many forms, including hypervigilance to bodily sensations (digestive, urological, and sexual function), restricted movement, limited social interaction, and disrupted sleep, as well as negative emotional states that may diminish motivation to seek reward. By facilitating modified behaviour and motivation, chronic pain essentially redefines how an organism interacts with the environment. The brain adapts to this changing environment through learning, which requires long-term potentiation (LTP), an activity- and postsynaptic NMDA-dependent enhancement of neural synchrony that underlies memory formation (i.e., *consolidation*) and memory revision (i.e., *reconsolidation*), which drives synaptic plasticity throughout the CNS [15], and potentially in the spinal cord [18]. Chronic pain must then be subject to the rules of memory formation and maintenance.

Arousal mechanisms inherent to pelvic pain ensure that a pain memory is strongly encoded from its inception. Pelvic visceral pain—or any visceral pain, for that matter—is inherently emotional because it is accompanied by increased autonomic arousal and strong negative emotional responses. McGaugh and others [35, 37] have hypothesized that memory consolidation relies on arousal mechanisms to modulate memory strength, such that memories encoded during stressful situations will be well remembered for future adaptive purposes. The basolateral amygdala plays a pivotal role in emotional (fear) memory formation because it is optimally responsive to norepinephrine produced during the stress response [39]. When paired with nociceptive input funnelled through the central nuclei of the amygdala, the negatively valenced sensory information can modulate (and amplify) pain behaviour. Conversely, the pharmacological inhibition of amygdala activity inhibits spinally mediated pain behaviour, suggesting that spinally mediated central sensitization may be dependent on supraspinal mechanisms [16, 42]. Furthermore, the reactivation of established emotional memory pathways with each subsequent episode of intense pain may facilitate reconsolidation (and further strengthening) of the salient pain memory [21] (but see [1]). CPP patients are then left with repetitive exposure to stress-enhanced pelvic pain.

Repeated emotional experiences with pelvic pain may alter the perception of other emotionally salient situations. Pelvic pain disrupts some of the most intrinsically rewarding physiological processes: sexual arousal, orgasm, urination, and defecation. The literature is rife with examples of how pelvic pain can frequently interfere with these rewarding processes. A subset of men with chronic prostatitis (CP) or chronic pelvic pain syndrome (CPPS) experience excruciating pain with ejaculation during masturbation and/or intercourse, thereby dampening sexual motivation for future sexual encounters [5, 52]. Similarly, women with vulvodynia report exquisite pain with light vulvar touch, and also diminished sexual pleasure and sexual motivation [56]. The latter results are consistent with an animal model showing suppressed pacing mating behaviour—and therefore reduced sexual

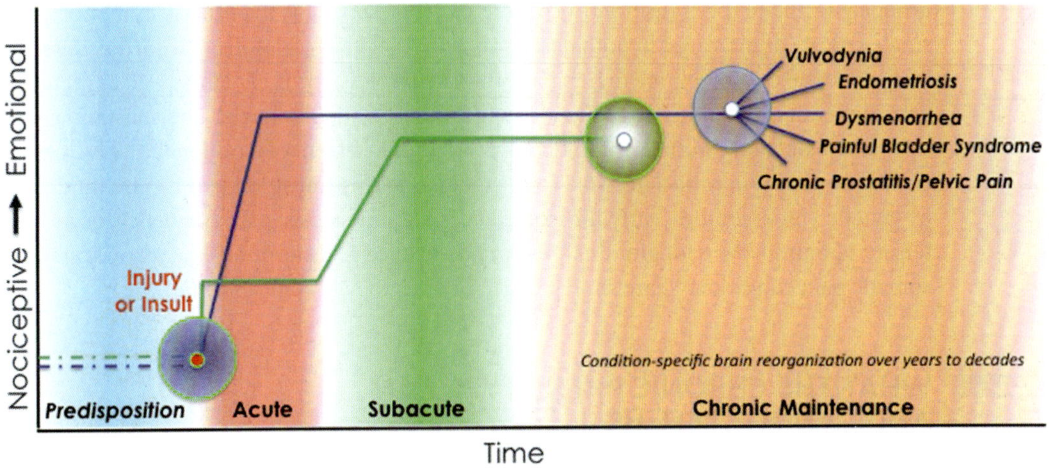

FIGURE 28-1 Hypothesized divergence of pain chronification for pelvic visceral versus somatic pain. Pain chronification is depicted across time (*y* axis) and by dominant cortical systems involved in pain processing (*x* axis), ranging from regions mediating nociceptive processing (including primary and secondary somatosensory cortices, insula, anterior cingulate cortex, prefrontal cortex, and thalamus) to regions mediating emotion processing (limbic and mesocortical regions). In addition to the impact of predisposing factors (*blue shading*) prior to injury onset, it is hypothesized that the type of pain properties can also determine the trajectory of pain chronification. Acute pelvic visceral pain (*red shading*), defined by strong negative emotion and autonomic arousal, creates optimal conditions for arousal-enhanced fear learning of pelvic pain. In contrast, existing evidence suggests that emotional learning during the subacute phase (*green shading*) drives chronification of chronic low back pain—a prevalent form of somatic pain. Further changes in brain function and structure that characterize unique pelvic pain diagnoses emerge during the chronic pain phase (*orange shading*), forging condition-specific trajectories.

encounters—in female mice with inflammatory genital pain [24]. In addition to sexual disturbances, previously rewarding processes such as urination and defecation are disrupted with pelvic pain. Individuals with bladder pain syndrome may report ongoing or intermittent lack of relief or pain with urination, pain with bladder filling, and heightened urinary urgency that persists [55]. Similarly, some men with CPP report a "golf ball in the anus" sensation that worsens with defecation and may trigger additional pelvic pain. These clinical reports suggest that, when previously pleasurable events become painful, the emotional valence of reward may shift, as well. Such a phenomenon has been observed in chronic back pain patients who show abnormal nucleus accumbens activity associated with pain relief [11]. It is feasible that a maladaptive limbic circuit maintaining CPP may also influence processing of hedonic information.

Considering the emotionally salient origins of pelvic pain, it is reasonable to assume that factors driving the transition to CPP chronicity may differ from somatic pain conditions, for which pain is localized to the skin, muscles, and/or bone (Fig. 28-1). In the first longitudinal neuroimaging study examining brain changes that parallel the transition to a common somatic pain condition, chronic back pain, functional representation of pain shifted from sensory nociceptive brain regions to limbic regions as pain persisted [9, 27]. These observations support the hypothesis that back pain is increasingly processed through more emotion-related regions as it becomes chronic. In contrast, pelvic visceral pain begins with strong nociceptive and emotional involvement, suggesting that limbic circuitry would likely be recruited soon after pelvic pain onset. It has been established that a predisposition to emotional learning can manifest in altered features of brain function and structure [13]. One possibility is that larger volumes of subcortical regions prior to visceral pain onset may uniquely facilitate the transition to chronic visceral pain. This hypothesis is supported by single reports of increased hypothalamic, anterior cingulate, orbitofrontal cortex, dorsolateral prefrontal cortex volume in irritable bowel syndrome (IBS) [17, 48], as well as increased grey matter density limited to bilateral hippocampus, lenticular nuclei, and substantia nigra in a sample of young women with vulvodynia [46]. The extent of emotional involvement in pelvic pain onset may be a decisive factor mediating this transition and can be influenced by genetic vulnerabilities, early life experiences, chronic stress, pain frequency, and/or intensity of pain. Future longitudinal research is needed to determine whether visceral and somatic pain conditions share similar trajectories as they become chronic.

WHAT THE CHRONIC PHENOTYPE CAN AND CANNOT TELL US

The neuroimaging of pelvic pain is a young field. Unfortunately, the field has inherited ideological biases that will continue to limit the advancement of pain neuroimaging if left unchallenged. For instance, it is commonly assumed in pain neuroimaging that the chronic brain phenotype can reflect the etiological mechanisms that initiated the pain. This assumption has evolved across many clinical and scientific environments that were limited by many unknowns: (a) the inciting factors triggering pelvic pain are frequently unknown; (b) the extent of peripheral injury rarely correlates with the features of chronic pain; (c) the few clinically relevant animal models of pelvic pain have yet to experimentally validate popular etiological theories (with the exception of [23]); and (d) a general disinterest in supraspinal mechanisms of pain chronification has focused inquiry to primary afferents and their spinal terminations. It is therefore critical to recognize that distinct mechanisms underlie the initiation and maintenance of chronic pain. This distinction has clear significance for assessment and treatment approaches for CPP, as clinicians often obsess about how the pain began rather than how the body has adapted to maintain persistent pelvic pain.

Most pain neuroimaging literature is based on the chronic phenotype. Unique configurations of grey matter changes distinguish between chronic pain diagnoses, including chronic IBS, CP/CPPS, vulvodynia, interstitial cystitis/painful bladder syndrome, low back pain, osteoarthritis, phantom limb, chronic regional pain syndrome, temporomandibular pain, and others [4, 19, 29]. These robust differences across pain populations suggest that neuronal changes driving unique patterns of grey matter reorganization are condition-specific. However, the lack of consistent grey matter changes between—and sometimes within—conditions has frustrated efforts to delineate the meaning of these structural changes. Unreplicated studies of women with chronic vulvar pain [46], interstitial cystitis/painful bladder syndrome [29], and dysmenorrhea [59, 60] have noted regional increases in subcortical grey matter, yet the finding of increased GM is far less common in other pelvic pain neuroimaging studies in men and women [8, 23, 40]. In men with CPP, Farmer and colleagues [23] found that anterior insula activity and grey matter density were associated with the magnitude of pelvic pain. In a separate male CPP cohort, significant reductions in anterior cingulate cortex volume also correlated with pelvic pain severity [40].

We know that it takes time to translate brain activity, which fuels the synaptic strengthening of pain memory traces, into anatomical changes that can sustain these memories. The formation of lasting memories requires late-phase LTP in the hippocampus to induce the protein synthesis necessary to initiate lasting structural changes (i.e., of terminal boutons, dendrite morphology, etc.). The rate of hippocampal protein synthesis regulates the time course of these early anatomical changes, and the hippocampus requires approximately 2 weeks to establish long-term cortical networks needed to encode and sustain a pain memory trace. During the early stages of pain chronification, the hippocampus remains continuously engaged via upregulated hippocampal–medial prefrontal connectivity that directly covaries with pain intensity [41], and this ongoing activity may account for incremental voxel-wise changes in neocortical grey matter observed in chronic pain patients over the course of weeks, months, and years [9, 12]. The time frame of this latter process, which is consistent with the timescale of systems memory consolidation [22, 53], strongly suggests that observed alterations in regional grey matter reflect mechanisms underlying the chronic maintenance of pain memories, rather than the inciting processes that initially triggered LTP.

Interestingly, the hippocampus may play a prolonged role in the development of chronic pain. Under normal circumstances, a memory shifts from a hippocampus-dependent to -independent state in which the memory becomes a striatum-maintained habit modulated by the amygdala, which provides an emotional volume control for the memory [3, 30, 36, 50, 57]. Only when novel or high-arousal experiences are paired with a consolidated memory does the hippocampus competitively re-engage the memory [34]. Hypothetically, ongoing hippocampal involvement implies that the pain memory trace is continually reactivated and thus rendered vulnerable to change. Recent longitudinal data support this hypothesis and suggest that ongoing, severe pain is a sufficiently novel stimulus to maintain hippocampal involvement [41], and by extension, the amygdala–striatal modulatory loop that competes with the hippocampus for information [34]. Importantly, reactivated pain memories are susceptible to synaptic strengthening as well as the disruption of the memory trace through the process of memory reconsolidation. Compounds that mediate context-specific memory disruption and/or pain-specific emotional dampening may be promising therapies for central modulation of pelvic pain.

Consistent with evidence that regional grey matter changes in pain patients take months to years to develop, the extent of grey matter changes consistently correlates with the duration of pain. Pain duration correlates with grey matter density of the anterior insula in men with CPP [23], and similar findings have been found in other chronic pain populations [10, 17, 45, 48]. Global grey matter reorganization may continue to shift across the course of years, suggesting that the magnitude of structural changes will evolve as pain persists [12]. Conversely, the reversal of pain-related alterations in grey matter is observed with successful treatment, such that the reduction of clinical pain is accompanied by a partial reversal of regional grey matter changes [44, 49]. For these reasons, grey matter properties may best be viewed as indicators of ongoing clinical severity related to pain maintenance. As such, grey matter properties may be used to track the progression of pain chronification, as well as confirm successful treatment.

The close temporal relationship between pain maintenance and neocortical grey matter properties suggests that these structural changes reflect ongoing neuroplastic processes as pain ebbs and flows. This pattern has been observed across numerous chronic pain conditions [7, 12, 33, 51]. Even rapid fluctuations in grey matter properties closely correlate with symptom severity in women with cyclic menstrual pain [60]. Neural correlates of short-term pain fluctuations in CPP are of special clinical interest, given our poor understanding of pain "flares," a term used to describe exacerbations of pain that may last minutes, days, or weeks [54, 55]. Rapid brain structural changes over the timescale of weeks are suggestive of greater cortical reorganization with increased pain frequency and severity.

TRANSLATING THEORY INTO DATA

The pelvic pain field, as a specialty that frequently deals with diagnoses of exclusion, lacks a strong theoretical framework for assessment, diagnosis, and treatment. By conceptualizing CPP as a collection of heterogeneous chronic disease states rooted in emotional learning, unanswered questions about pelvic pain etiology and disease maintenance become accessible and testable. Furthermore, multimodal neuroimaging can be combined to identify the mechanistic interactions between brain function and structure in CPP.

Functional scanning of CPP has yet to be tailored to the stage of chronicity. Given the hypothesis that emotional learning plays a prominent role in the initiation and maintenance of CPP, it follows that brain functional representations of pelvic pain should preferentially reflect limbic involvement. However, emotional involvement may be more pronounced during the initial transition phase to CPP as novel pain information is consolidated and new memories are strengthened. In contrast, most CPP fMRI studies—as well as in the pain field in general—evaluate the chronic phenotype and may not capture the "critical window" of the greatest limbic involvement. To date, functional imaging of CPP has typically yielded nociceptive activity maps consistent with acute pain. For example, painful heat applied to the lower abdomen and arm evokes similar activation patterns in women with and without dysmenorrhea, including the secondary somatosensory cortex, premotor cortex, insula, anterior cingulate cortex, posterior cingulate cortex, orbitofrontal cortex, and subcortical regions (e.g., putamen, thalamus, caudate, and brainstem) [61]. Such approaches have drawn criticism because they have not captured brain activity related to the clinical experience of spontaneous visceral pelvic pain. Even studies that manage to evoke clinically relevant pain, such as provoked vulvar pain in women with vulvodynia, have yielded spatially identical activity maps in vulvodynia and pain-free women [26, 43]. One strategy hypothesized to better capture CPP-related brain activity is to have patients continuously report spontaneous pelvic pain intensity throughout a scan. Continuous ratings of pelvic pain intensity in men with CPP elicited activity that was consistent with acute nociceptive encoding (e.g., insula, dorsolateral prefrontal cortex, posterior parietal cortex, primary somatosensory cortex, primary motor cortex, and precuneus regions) yet lacked involvement of key nociceptive encoding regions (e.g., anterior cingulate cortex, secondary somatosensory cortex, medial prefrontal cortex, thalamus). This activation profile is consistent with other clinical pain conditions that show less frequent involvement of these classic "pain" regions [7].

Collectively, these findings strongly suggest that functional imaging in CPP populations has yet to produce new information about pelvic pain, with the exception of legitimizing pelvic pain as an objectively measurable clinical state. Methodological and/or analytic limitations can certainly account for a lack of CPP-specific functional activations, whereas other explanations should be considered in future research. (a) A greater magnitude of functional resources recruited for acute pain processing, which is essentially a task-related activity, may overpower our ability to detect lesser underlying CPP-related activity. (b) Pain perception may occur at a network rather than a brain regional level, therefore requiring an analysis of task and task-free (resting-state) activity to identify CPP-specific network dynamics (as seen in [31]). Network connectivity is critical in differentiating transient states of mind, including intrinsic and task-related states [25], as well as developmental processes and the presence of chronic disease [2, 47]. (c) Finally, abnormal brain activity may be more prominent during the initial transition from acute to chronic CPP, as suggested by early changes in nucleus accumbens and prefrontal cortical functional connectivity in predicting pain chronicity in subacute back pain patients [9]. In the latter case, functional imaging of the chronic phenotype may simply be insufficient to detect the critical brain activity underlying CPP. Future work that samples CPP groups at different stages of chronicity, as well as longitudinal neuroimaging studies, are required to detect the "critical window" when CPP-specific brain activity is a dominant feature.

The impact of prior brain activity can be estimated, albeit indirectly, by examining abnormalities in neuronal and axonal structure in the chronic CPP phenotype. The Hebbian axiom "Neurons that fire together wire together" reminds us that observable changes in brain structure result from novel communication patterns that are forged over time. Therefore, voxel-wise grey matter changes, which take weeks to months to develop, likely reflect long-term patterns of activity that have maintained the chronic phenotype of CPP. Perhaps the greatest danger in moving forward is to underestimate the heterogeneity in CPP populations, as this oversight would enhance noise in data and make it more difficult to detect real structural changes that result from specific disease processes leading to CPP.

Moving forward, the priority for pelvic pain neuroimaging is a thorough assessment of brain functional and structural abnormalities that differentiate CPP diagnoses, as well as subtypes within each diagnosis. A longitudinal characterization of brain structure is required to dissociate mechanisms underlying chronic pain initiation versus maintenance. Data-driven approaches should be used to distinguish features of subacute/early chronification from the chronic phenotype (as opposed to the clinical convention of arbitrarily defining chronic pain as a 3- or 6-month process). These priorities are cornerstones of the first multicentre longitudinal neuroimaging study of CPP populations, the Multidisciplinary Approach to the Study of Chronic Pelvic Pain (MAPP) Research Network, conceived by the National Institute of Diabetes and Digestive and Kidney Diseases (NIDDK) with collaborations between Northwestern University, University of California at Los Angeles, Stanford University, University of Michigan, University of Alabama, and University of Washington, and Washington University in St. Louis, with the University of Colorado at Denver leading tissue analysis and the University of Pennsylvania coordinating data [20, 32]. Pairing detailed MAPP epidemiological data with multimodal neuroimaging data, including resting-state functional, T1-weighted anatomical, and diffusion tensor imaging scans, will drive the identification of behavioural proxies that can be rapidly assessed by clinicians who treat CPP. Such proxies are critical to guiding early interventions in those who are vulnerable to developing CPP, as well as guiding therapeutic use of centrally acting agents and/or psychotherapy in patients who are most likely to respond to these treatment modalities.

ACKNOWLEDGEMENT

This work was supported by the National Vulvodynia Association and the National Institutes of Health (NIH) National Institute for Diabetes and Digestive and Kidney Diseases (NIDDK) U01 DK082342, in collaboration with the Multidisciplinary Approach to the Study of Chronic Pelvic Pain (MAPP) Research Network.

CONFLICT OF INTEREST

The author has no conflicts of interest.

REFERENCES

1. Akirav I, Maroun M. Stress modulation of reconsolidation. Psychopharmacology 2013;226(4):747–61.
2. Alexander-Bloch A, Raznahan A, Bullmore E, Giedd J. The convergence of maturational change and structural covariance in human cortical networks. J Neurosci 2013;33(7):2889–99.
3. Alvarez P, Squire LR. Memory consolidation and the medial temporal lobe: a simple network model. Proc Natl Acad Sci USA 1994;91(15):7041–5.
4. Alzahrani K, Gandhi R, Debeer J, Petruccelli D, Mahomed NN. Prevalence of clinically significant improvement following total knee replacement. J Rheumatol 2011;38(4):753–9.
5. Anderson RU, Wise D, Sawyer T, Chan CA. Sexual dysfunction in men with chronic prostatitis/chronic pelvic pain syndrome: improvement after trigger point release and paradoxical relaxation training. J Urol 2006; 176(4 Pt 1):1534–8; discussion 1538–9.
6. Apkarian AV, Baliki MN, Geha PY. Towards a theory of chronic pain. Prog Neurobiol 2009;87(2):81–97.
7. Apkarian AV, Hashmi JA, Baliki MN. Pain and the brain: specificity and plasticity of the brain in clinical chronic pain. Pain 2011;152(3):s49–64.
8. As-Sanie S, Harris RE, Napadow V, Kim J, Neshewat G, Kairys A, Williams D, Clauw DJ, Schmidt-Wilcke T. Changes in regional gray matter volume in women with chronic pelvic pain: a voxel-based morphometry study. Pain 2012;153(5):1006–14.
9. Baliki M, Petre B, Torbey S, Herrmann KM, Huang LS, Schnitzer TJ, Fields HL, Apkarian AV. Corticostriatal functional connectivity predicts transition to chronic back pain. Nat Neurosci 2012;15(8):1117–9,
10. Baliki MN, Chialvo DR, Geha PY, Levy RM, Harden RN, Parrish TB, Apkarian AV. Chronic pain and the emotional brain: specific brain activity associated with spontaneous fluctuations of intensity of chronic back pain. J Neurosci 2006;26(47):12165–73.
11. Baliki MN, Geha PY, Fields HL, Apkarian AV. Predicting value of pain and analgesia: nucleus accumbens response to noxious stimuli changes in the presence of chronic pain. Neuron 2010;66(1):149–60.
12. Baliki MN, Schnitzer TJ, Bauer WR, Apkarian AV. Brain morphological signatures for chronic pain. PloS One 2011;6(10):e26010.
13. Baria AT, Baliki MN, Parrish T, Apkarian AV. Anatomical and functional assemblies of brain BOLD oscillations. J Neurosci 2011;31(21):7910–19.
14. Baumgartner U, Iannetti GD, Zambreanu L, Stoeter P, Treede RD, Tracey I. Multiple somatotopic representations of heat and mechanical pain in the operculo-insular cortex: a high-resolution fMRI study. J Neurophysiol 2010;104(5):2863–72.
15. Besnard A, Caboche J, Laroche S. Reconsolidation of memory: a decade of debate. Prog Neurobiol 2012;99(1):61–80.
16. Bird GC, Lash LL, Han JS, Zou X, Willis WD, Neugebauer V. Protein kinase A-dependent enhanced NMDA receptor function in pain-related synaptic plasticity in rat amygdala neurones. J Physiol 2005;564(Pt 3):907–21.
17. Blankstein U, Chen J, Diamant NE, Davis KD. Altered brain structure in irritable bowel syndrome: potential contributions of pre-existing and disease-driven factors. Gastroenterology 2010;138(5):1783–9.
18. Bonin RP, De Koninck Y. A spinal analog of memory reconsolidation enables reversal of hyperalgesia. Nat Neurosci 2014;17(8):1043–5.
19. Chappell AS, Desaiah D, Liu-Seifert H, Zhang S, Skljarevski V, Belenkov Y, Brown JP. A double-blind, randomized, placebo-controlled study of the efficacy and safety of duloxetine for the treatment of chronic pain due to osteoarthritis of the knee. Pain Pract 2010;11(1):33–41.
20. Clemens JQ, Mullins C, Kusek JW, Kirkali Z, Mayer EA, Rodriguez LV, Klumpp DJ, Schaeffer AJ, Kreder KJ, Buchwald D, et al. The MAPP research network: a novel study of urologic chronic pelvic pain syndromes. BMC Urol 2014;14:57.
21. Diamond DM, Campbell AM, Park CR, Halonen J, Zoladz PR. The temporal dynamics model of emotional memory processing: a synthesis on the neurobiological basis of stress-induced amnesia, flashbulb and traumatic memories, and the Yerkes-Dodson law. Neural Plast 2007;2007:60803.
22. Dudai Y. The neurobiology of consolidations, or, how stable is the engram? Ann rev Psychol 2004;55:51–86.
23. Farmer MA, Chanda ML, Parks EL, Baliki MN, Apkarian AV, Schaeffer AJ. Brain functional and anatomical changes in chronic prostatitis/chronic pelvic pain syndrome. J Urol 2011;186(1):117–24.
24. Farmer MA, Leja A, Foxen-Craft E, Chan L, MacIntyre LC, Niaki T, Chen M, Mapplebeck JC, Tabry V, Topham L, et al. Pain reduces sexual motivation in female but not male mice. J Neurosci 2014;34(17):5747–53.
25. Gusnard DA, Raichle ME, Raichle ME. Searching for a baseline: functional imaging and the resting human brain. Nat Rev Neurosci 2001;2(10):685–94.

26. Hampson JP, Reed BD, Clauw DJ, Bhavsar R, Gracely RH, Haefner HK, Harris RE. Augmented central pain processing in vulvodynia. J Pain 2013;14(6):579–89.
27. Hashmi JA, Baliki MN, Huang L, Baria AT, Torbey S, Hermann KM, Schnitzer TJ, Apkarian AV. Shape shifting pain: chronification of back pain shifts brain representation from nociceptive to emotional circuits. Brain 2013;136(Pt 9):2751–68.
28. Julius D, Basbaum AI. Molecular mechanisms of nociception. Nature 2001;413(6852):203–10.
29. Kairys AE, Schmidt-Wilcke T, Puiu T, Ichesco E, Labus JS, Martucci K, Farmer MA, Ness TJ, Deutsch G, Mayer EA, et al. Increased brain gray matter in the primary somatosensory cortex is associated with increased pain and mood disturbance in interstitial cystitis/painful bladder syndrome patients. J Urol 2015;193(1):131–7.
30. Kensinger EA, Corkin S. Two routes to emotional memory: distinct neural processes for valence and arousal. Proc Natl Acad Sci USA 2004;101(9):3310–15.
31. Kilpatrick LA, Kutch JJ, Tillisch K, Naliboff BD, Labus JS, Jiang Z, Farmer MA, Apkarian AV, Mackey S, Martucci KT, et al. Alterations in resting state oscillations and connectivity in sensory and motor networks in women with interstitial cystitis/painful bladder syndrome. J Urol 2014;192(3):947–55.
32. Landis JR, Williams DA, Lucia MS, Clauw DJ, Naliboff BD, Robinson NA, van Bokhoven A, Sutcliffe S, Schaeffer AJ, Rodriguez LV, et al. The MAPP research network: design, patient characterization and operations. BMC Urol 2014;14:58.
33. May A. Chronic pain may change the structure of the brain. Pain 2008;137(1):7–15.
34. McDonald RJ, White NM. A triple dissociation of memory systems: hippocampus, amygdala, and dorsal striatum. Behav Neurosci 1993;107(1):3–22.
35. McGaugh JL. Memory—a century of consolidation. Science 2000;287(5451):248–51.
36. McGaugh JL. The amygdala modulates the consolidation of memories of emotionally arousing experiences. Annu Rev Neurosci 2004;27:1–28.
37. McIntyre CK, McGaugh JL, Williams CL. Interacting brain systems modulate memory consolidation. Neurosci Biobehav Rev 2012;36(7):1750–62.
38. Melzack R, Wall PD. Textbook of pain. London, UK: Churchill Livingstone; 1999.
39. Milad MR, Quinn BT, Pitman RK, Orr SP, Fischl B, Rauch SL. Thickness of ventromedial prefrontal cortex in humans is correlated with extinction memory. Proc Natl Acad Sci USA 2005;102(30):10706–11.
40. Mordasini L, Weisstanner C, Rummel C, Thalmann GN, Verma RK, Wiest R, Kessler TM. Chronic pelvic pain syndrome in men is associated with reduction of relative gray matter volume in the anterior cingulate cortex compared to healthy controls. J Urol 2012;188(6):2233–7.
41. Mutso AA, Petre B, Huang L, Baliki MN, Torbey S, Herrmann KM, Schnitzer TJ, Apkarian AV. Reorganization of hippocampal functional connectivity with transition to chronic back pain. J Neurophysiol 2014;111(5):1065–76.
42. Palazzo E, Fu Y, Ji G, Maione S, Neugebauer V. Group III mGluR7 and mGluR8 in the amygdala differentially modulate nocifensive and affective pain behaviors. Neuropharmacology 2008;55(4):537–45.
43. Pukall CF, Strigo IA, Binik YM, Amsel R, Khalife S, Bushnell MC. Neural correlates of painful genital touch in women with vulvar vestibulitis syndrome. Pain 2005;115(1–2):118–27.
44. Rodriguez-Raecke R, Niemeier A, Ihle K, Ruether W, May A. Brain gray matter decrease in chronic pain is the consequence and not the cause of pain. J Neurosci 2009;29(44):13746–50.
45. Schmidt-Wilcke T, Leinisch E, Straube A, Kampfe N, Draganski B, Diener HC, Bogdahn U, May A. Gray matter decrease in patients with chronic tension type headache. Neurology 2005;65(9):1483–6.
46. Schweinhardt P, Kuchinad A, Pukall CF, Bushnell MC. Increased gray matter density in young women with chronic vulvar pain. Pain 2008;140(3):411–9.
47. Seeley WW, Crawford RK, Zhou J, Miller BL, Greicius MD. Neurodegenerative diseases target large-scale human brain networks. Neuron 2009;62(1):42–52.
48. Seminowicz DA, Labus JS, Bueller JA, Tillisch K, Naliboff BD, Bushnell MC, Mayer EA. Regional gray matter density changes in brains of patients with irritable bowel syndrome. Gastroenterology 2010;139(1):48–57.e42.
49. Seminowicz DA, Wideman TH, Naso L, Hatami-Khoroushahi Z, Fallatah S, Ware MA, Jarzem P, Bushnell MC, Shir Y, Ouellet JA, et al. Effective treatment of chronic low back pain in humans reverses abnormal brain anatomy and function. J Neurosci 2011;31(20):7540–50.
50. Sherry DF, Schacter DL. The evolution of multiple memory systems. Psychol Rev 1987;94(4):439–54.
51. Smallwood RF, Laird AR, Ramage AE, Parkinson AL, Lewis J, Clauw DJ, Williams DA, Schmidt-Wilcke T, Farrell MJ, Eickhoff SB, et al. Structural brain anomalies and chronic pain: a quantitative meta-analysis of gray matter volume. J Pain 2013;14(7):663–75.
52. Smith KB, Pukall CF, Tripp DA, Nickel JC. Sexual and relationship functioning in men with chronic prostatitis/chronic pelvic pain syndrome and their partners. Arch Sex Behav 2007;36(2):301–11.

53. Squire LR, Alvarez P. Retrograde amnesia and memory consolidation: a neurobiological perspective. Curr Opin Neurobiol 1995;5(2):169–77.
54. Sutcliffe S, Colditz GA, Goodman MS, Pakpahan R, Vetter J, Ness TJ, Andriole GL, Lai HH. Urological chronic pelvic pain syndrome symptom flares: characterisation of the full range of flares at two sites in the Multidisciplinary Approach to the Study of Chronic Pelvic Pain (MAPP) Research Network. BJU Int 2014;114(6):916–25.
55. Sutcliffe S, Colditz GA, Pakpahan R, Bradley CS, Goodman MS, Andriole GL, Lai HH. Changes in symptoms during urologic chronic pelvic pain syndrome symptom flares: findings from one site of the MAPP Research Network. Neurourol Urodyn 2015;34(2):188–95.
56. Sutton KS, Pukall CF, Chamberlain S. Pain, psychosocial, sexual, and psychophysical characteristics of women with primary vs. secondary provoked vestibulodynia. J Sex Med 2009;6(1):205–14.
57. Takashima A, Nieuwenhuis IL, Jensen O, Talamini LM, Rijpkema M, Fernandez G. Shift from hippocampal to neocortical centered retrieval network with consolidation. J Neurosci 2009;29(32):10087–93.
58. Tracey I, Mantyh PW. The cerebral signature for pain perception and its modulation. Neuron 2007;55(3):377–91.
59. Tu CH, Niddam DM, Chao HT, Chen LF, Chen YS, Wu YT, Yeh TC, Lirng JF, Hsieh JC. Brain Morphological changes associated with cyclic menstrual pain. Pain 2010;150(3):462–8.
60. Tu CH, Niddam DM, Yeh TC, Lirng JF, Cheng CM, Chou CC, Chao HT, Hsieh JC. Menstrual pain is associated with rapid structural alterations in the brain. Pain 2013;154(9):1718–24.
61. Vincent K, Warnaby C, Stagg CJ, Moore J, Kennedy S, Tracey I. Dysmenorrhoea is associated with central changes in otherwise healthy women. Pain 2011;152(9):1966–75.

CHAPTER 29

Functional and Structural Neural Abnormalities in Temporomandibular Disorders

Massieh Moayedi and Karen D. Davis

Temporomandibular disorders (TMDs) represent the most common orofacial chronic pain disorder [22], and are more prevalent in women [21]. These patients suffer from pain that is located in the temporomandibular (TM) region, sometimes associated with jaw movement. The source of pain in TMD has been attributed to the muscles of mastication, the TM joint, or both, and the chief complaint tends to be muscular in nature [35]. TMD can be classified as either posttraumatic (e.g., following a motor vehicle accident) or idiopathic, with no clear precipitating event or pathology for the pain [23].

TRIGEMINAL NERVE ABNORMALITIES IN IDIOPATHIC TMD

In some cases, TMD can be considered "idiopathic" because there is no obvious and identifiable pathology in the TM region. However, our recent diffusion-weighted imaging (DWI) findings revealed microstructural abnormalities along the trigeminal nerves of patients with idiopathic TMD [58]. Specifically, we found that there was decreased fractional anisotropy (FA; an index of white matter integrity), and increased mean diffusivity (MD) and radial diffusivity (RD)—two metrics of neuroinflammatory processes [8, 9]—along the trigeminal nerve. Although the underlying sources of these types of DWI findings are still under debate, they have been attributed to increased membrane permeability or decreased myelin insulation [10]. Therefore, one possibility is that the pain in so-called idiopathic TMD begins at the level of the trigeminal nerves. Alternatively, trigeminal nerve abnormalities may arise secondarily as a result of abnormal motor function in line with the Pain Adaptation model (see below). It is, however, noteworthy that in contrast to our findings [58], Wilcox and colleagues [80] did not find any abnormalities along the trigeminal nerve (or in brain structure) in a cohort of subjects with TMD. The lack of findings in their study could be due to various factors, such as the characteristics of the cohort examined (diagnostic criteria are not provided for the TMD group) or the duration of pain of the cohort (for a full discussion, see [56]).

BRAIN MECHANISMS IMPLICATED IN TMD

Regardless of whether peripheral pathologies play a role in initiating pain in TMD, the CNS has been implicated in maintaining the pain [65]. This concept is supported by TMD symptomatology that has been attributed to central mechanisms such as widespread pain

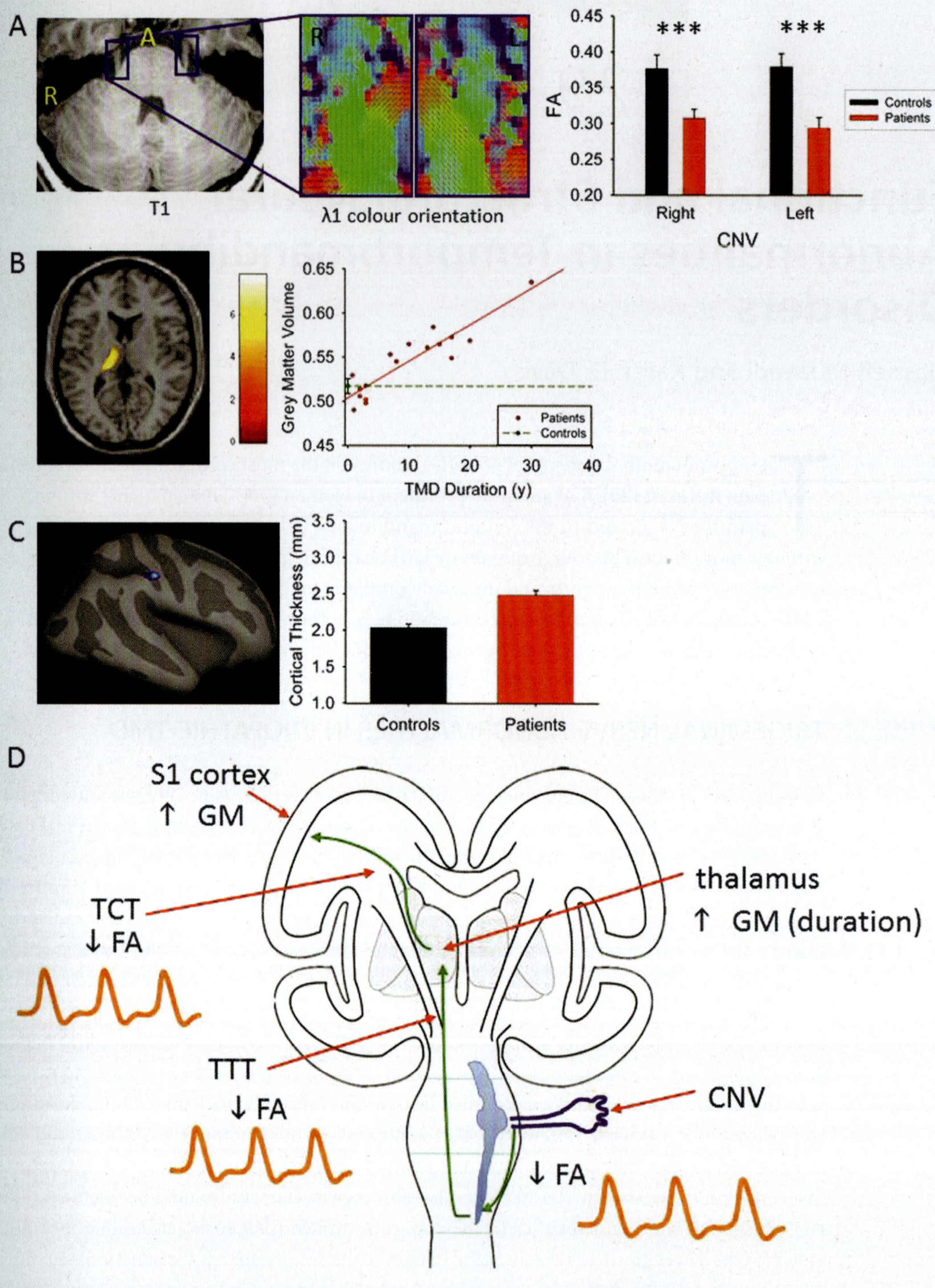

FIGURE 29-1 TMD patients have **(A)** lower fractional anisotropy (FA) along the trigeminal nerve (***$P < 0.005$), **(B)** progressively increased GM volume with TMD duration ($r = 0.91$, $P < 0.05$, corrected), and **(C)** thicker S1 cortex ($P < 0.05$, corrected). **D:** Proposed model of neural basis of sensory abnormalities in TMD. There is altered nociceptive activity (shown by *orange* action potentials) in the periphery and decreased FA in the trigeminal nerve (CNV), and along the trigeminothalamic tract (TTT) in the brainstem. These abnormalities may induce progressive increases in thalamic GM volume, reduced FA in the thalamocortical tract (TCT), and increased cortical thickness in the orofacial region of S1. (Modified from [58] with permission. Brain outline modified from the PHT500Y laboratory manual, University of Toronto.)

sensitivity [65], increased temporal summation of pain [52], and dysfunctional conditioned pain modulation (CPM) [42, 64]. Additionally, patients with TMD can exhibit cognitive [30–32] and motor dysfunction [72] possibly related to abnormalities in brain regions associated with these functions [69, 78]. Thus, TMD pain could be maintained via maladaptive brain plasticity [17, 81]. Additionally, this long-term aberrant nociceptive activity may lead to increased stress responses and deficits in learning and motivation, a process known as learned helplessness. This could also result in a reduced capacity for pain habituation/nociceptive adaptation, possibly related to diminished descending and top-down controls [11]. It is also possible that some individuals are more vulnerable to the development of TMD based on inherent personality-related factors that reduce the brain's capacity to modulate nociceptive activity.

Both functional and structural magnetic resonance imaging (fMRI, sMRI) have been used to examine the brain in chronic pain conditions [1, 20]. These methods can detect whether brain abnormalities are related to clinical findings or predisposing factors. The sMRI methods primarily used to evaluate brain grey matter are voxel-based morphometry and cortical thickness analysis, and white matter in the brain and cranial nerves can be evaluated using DWI.

There have been four studies investigating grey matter (GM) in TMD [29, 34, 57, 83]. Generally, these studies identified structural abnormalities in GM related to sensory, motor, and cognitive-modulatory functions. Of note, one of these studies did not reveal any abnormalities in brain GM in TMD [34], and follow-up studies of the same cohort did not find any structural differences in the primary somatosensory cortex (S1) [33] or along the trigeminal nerves [80]. Additionally, two studies have investigated white matter microstructure in patients with TMD [29, 58]. In contrast to the Wilcox et al. [80] study, our study [58] revealed widespread white matter abnormalities in white matter tracts related to sensory, motor, and cognitive-modulatory regions of the brain, and along the trigeminal nerve.

ABNORMALITIES ALONG SENSORY AND NOCICEPTIVE PATHWAYS IN TMD

Nociceptive information from the TM joint and the muscles of mastication is carried to the CNS via the trigeminal nerve. Nociceptive C and Aδ fibres project to second-order nociceptive-specific and wide dynamic-range neurons in the trigeminal brainstem sensory nuclear complex [67]. These cells ascend to various brainstem nuclei, and the thalamus via the trigeminothalamic tract, where they project to third-order neurons, which form thalamocortical tracts [67] (see Fig. 29-1D). Structural and functional abnormalities have been identified at several locations along the ascending nociceptive pathway of TMD patients.

As noted above, we have identified that there are structural abnormalities along the trigeminal nerve in a group of patients diagnosed with "idiopathic" TMD patients [58] (Fig. 29-1A). Further, these abnormalities were negatively correlated with TMD duration: patients who had only recently experienced TMD had trigeminal nerve FA values that were similar to those measured found in healthy controls, whereas patients with longer durations of TMD had lower FA values. These data suggest that the chronicity of TMD pain is related to changes in the microstructure of the trigeminal nerve. However, the factors that contribute to progressive microstructural nerve pathophysiology are not known. One possible source could be aberrant ongoing or ectopic activity along the nerve. This could arise from or induce neuroinflammation. Another possibility in line with the revised

Pain Adaptation model [38] is that prolonged alterations in motor activity in the orofacial region become pathological and a source of persistent nociceptive activity, which may alter trigeminal nerve microstructure.

In addition to peripheral pathophysiological processes, there may be central abnormalities. In support of this hypothesis, we found that thalamic GM volume positively correlated with TMD duration [57]. Similarly, Younger and colleagues [83] reported GM structural abnormalities in TMD related to pain characteristics. The concept that prolonged nociceptive input changes of chronic pain-driven gray matter changes comes from a study by Teutsch and colleagues [73], who reported increased S1 and midcingulate cortex (MCC) GM volume after 8 consecutive days of a 20-minute paradigm of acute nociceptive stimulation to the volar forearm. Subjects had thicker S1 and MCC. Additionally, we reported abnormalities along white matter tracts connecting the various levels of the ascending trigeminal nociceptive system—the trigeminothalamic tract, white matter coursing through the thalamus, thalamocortical tracts coursing through the somatomotor region of the internal capsule, and tracts adjacent to the somatosensory and motor cortices. For a summary schematic of proposed abnormalities along the main ascending sensory/nociceptive pathway, see Fig. 29-1D.

Abnormalities in central structures could reflect or contribute to abnormal functional responses in the brain. Evidence for this comes from an fMRI study that investigated nociceptive processing in patients with myofascial TMD with experimental pressure pain in the orofacial region [40]. The study did not investigate stimulus-evoked activity, but rather focused on functional connectivity of insular subregions, which are thought to have unique functions in nociceptive processing and pain modulation. During noxious stimulation, the TMD patients had greater functional connectivity (a measure of the correlation between brain regions, suggesting that they are working together) between cortical sensory areas and cognitive regions: the insula and the dorsomedial prefrontal cortex (dmPFC), including the rostral anterior cingulate cortex (ACC) and the medial frontal pole, compared with controls.

Taken together, the aforementioned findings suggest that there are functional and structural abnormalities along sensory and nociceptive pathways in TMD, and these abnormalities may be driven by prolonged pain.

ABNORMALITIES IN MOTOR REGIONS

The pain and motor systems interact at several levels within the nervous system. Several studies have identified GM and white matter abnormalities in regions associated with motor function in TMD patients [29, 57, 58, 83]. In some cases, the abnormalities were related to pain attributes. For example, we found that the thickness of the orofacial region of the primary motor cortex (M1) was negatively correlated with pain intensity in patients with TMD [57]. We also reported that patients with TMD had lower FA in motor pathways related to TMD pain intensity [58]. Furthermore, TMD patients had increased cortical activity in motor regions and sluggish cognitive task reaction times [78].

There are three mechanisms that may explain the observed abnormalities in the motor system (see Fig. 29-2): (1) nociceptive input dampens coordinated motor output to prevent further damage; (2) M1 modulates pain intensity; or (3) reduced movement to avoid pain may affect M1 thickness.

Previous studies have reported that nociceptive input inhibited M1 excitability [3], and that M1 stimulation modulated the perceived intensity of pain in chronic pain [27, 28, 49, 50]. Furthermore, a study by Boudreau and colleagues [13] reported that task

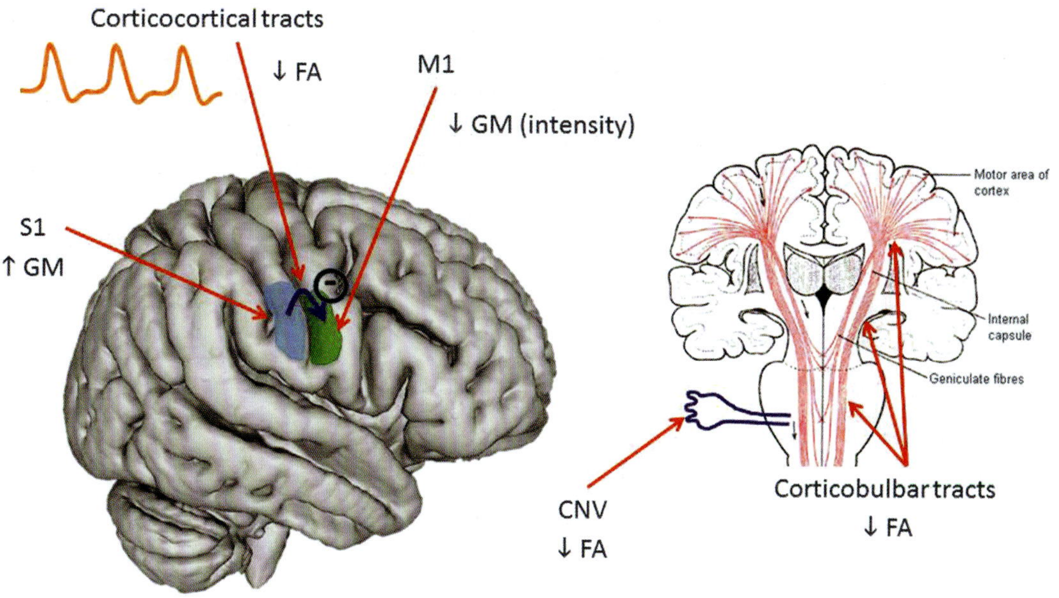

FIGURE 29-2 Proposed model for the neural basis of motor abnormalities in TMD. Left panel: Altered nociceptive input (shown by *orange* action potentials) inhibits motor cortex (M1) output in an intensity-dependent manner, and reduces fractional anisotropy (FA—a measure of white matter integrity) in corticocortical tracts connecting the primary somatosensory cortex and M1. Right panel: Decreased motor output causes disuse-related plasticity along corticofugal tracts (including corticobulbar tracts) and the motor portion of the trigeminal nerve (CNV).

training-related M1 plasticity was inhibited by noxious stimulation of the intraoral cavity. Additionally, several studies have reported abnormal stimulus-evoked fMRI activity in motor regions of chronic pain patients, although the implication of these abnormalities is not often discussed [1]. For instance, Kirveskari et al. [43] reported that patients with complex regional pain syndrome had weaker M1 reactivity with increased spontaneous pain ratings, and a negative correlation between pain intensity and M1 activation. Therefore, studies in experimental pain paradigms and in chronic pain patients have demonstrated that nociceptive activity modulates M1 function, and that M1 activity can modulate pain perception. Alternatively, the observed relationship between pain intensity and M1 thickness may be related to the possibility that patients with TMD make fewer jaw movements to avoid eliciting pain, although future studies are required to test this relationship. On the basis of the concepts of use-dependent plasticity [54] (or in this case disuse-dependent plasticity), this reduction in jaw activity may lead to atrophy of the orofacial region of the M1.

Finally, in a study of the relationship between helplessness in TMD patients and brain structure, we found that GM in motor regions, namely the supplementary motor area and the MCC, was related to helplessness in TMD, and that this relationship was mediated through (based on the Sobel test that suggests directionality) white matter tracts related to motor function, such as the corticofugal tracts (see Fig. 29-3). Therefore, it is possible that pain beliefs, such as helplessness, may alter brain structure, and further affect motor behaviours.

Therefore, TMD pain may alter motor function, which over time can become pathological, and a new source of pain. Additionally, prolonged pain can lead to changes in pain beliefs, further altering motor function in TMD.

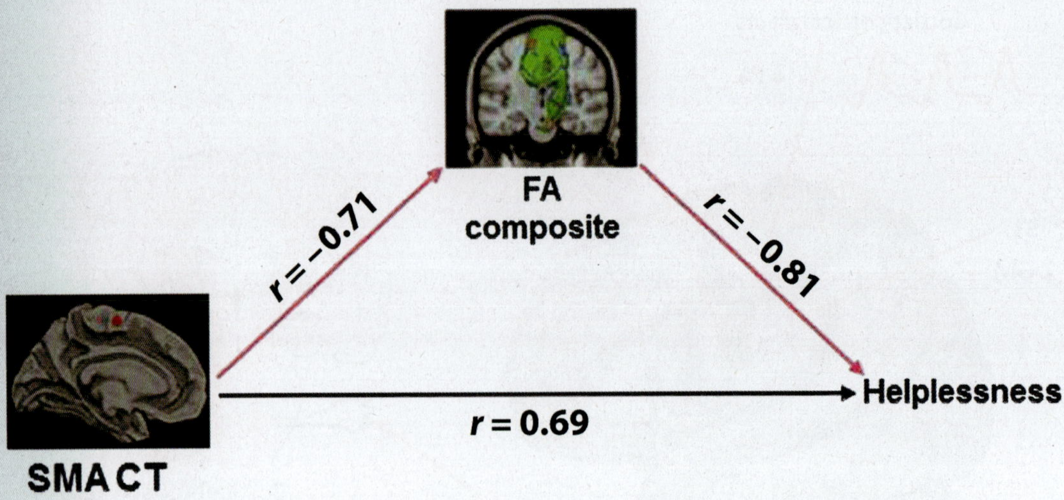

FIGURE 29-3 Brain structure and TMD pain helplessness. White matter along the corticospinal tract (CST) mediates the relationship between cortical thickness (CT) in the supplementary motor area (SMA) and pain helplessness. The correlation between SMA CT and helplessness (*black arrow*) was significantly mediated by the indirect pathway via the CST fractional anisotropy (FA) composite (*pink arrows*; Sobel statistic = 2.44, $P < 0.05$). The inverse mediation model was not significant (Sobel statistic = 0.7, $P = 0.48$), suggesting that the grey matter–helplessness relationship occurs by way of a descending circuit. *r*, Pearson correlation coefficient. (Reproduced with permission from [63].)

ABNORMALITIES IN COGNITIVE-MODULATORY BRAIN REGIONS

Structural brain abnormalities in cognitive-modulatory regions can provide a framework that could underlie the negative impact of chronic pain on cognitive abilities in TMD [30, 78]. An emerging concept is that the ventrolateral prefrontal cortex (vlPFC) is abnormal in TMD. Specifically, three studies found increased vlPFC GM [29, 57, 83], and one study found reduced white matter integrity adjacent to the vlPFC [58]. This region has been implicated in various aspects of pain, including anticipation [62] and modulation [77], as well as behavioural inhibition [2]. Thus, abnormalities in vlPFC may relate to hypervigilance in TMD [39, 70], which is related to increased pain anticipation.

We have also demonstrated that the frontal polar cortex is thicker in TMD compared with controls [57]. Additionally, probabilistic tractography revealed that the frontal polar cortices were more connected interhemispherically—the right and left frontal poles were more connected in TMD than in pain-free controls [58]. The frontal pole can be activated during spontaneous pain in patients with chronic pain [5]. Additionally, the frontal pole has also been implicated in complex executive cognitive functions such as learning behavioural routines [41, 45, 71], cognitive branching (the ability to put a pending task on hold to execute an ongoing one) [46], behavioural flexibility/adaptability [12], and *post hoc* monitoring or evaluating decisions based on feedback [74]. The concept of cognitive branching requires that working memory be a limited resource (there are only so many tasks that can be performed simultaneously). In this framework, tasks that are more behaviourally relevant (or salient) are prioritized [4, 44]. Specifically, the authors proposed that the frontal polar cortex functions to monitor salience (or value) of a given stimulus, so that behavioural outcomes can be selected accordingly. Given that pain is an inherently salient stimulus [19, 48], the presence of pain may engage the frontal pole. Further, a study

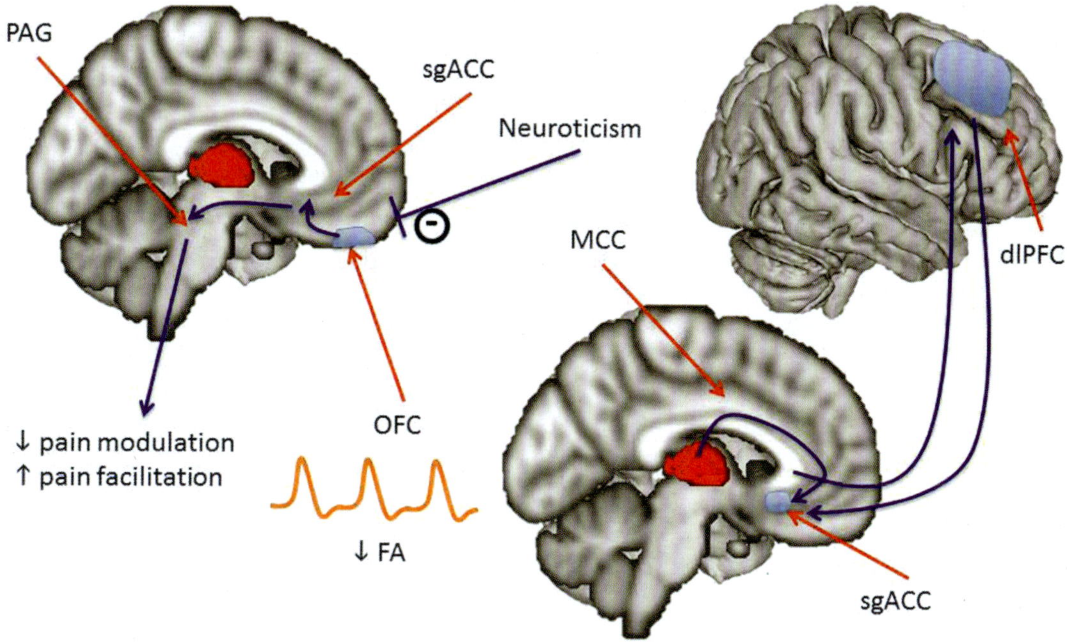

FIGURE 29-4 Proposed model for the neural basis of modulatory system abnormalities in TMD. The relationship of neuroticism and cortical thickness in the orbitofrontal cortex (OFC) alters the structure and antinociceptive function in pain-modulatory brain regions, including the subgenual anterior cingulate cortex (sgACC) and the periaqueductal grey (PAG). The dorsolateral prefrontal cortex (dlPFC) also has reduced white matter connectivity in patients with idiopathic TMD, which may be another substrate for dysfunctional pain modulation networks in TMD.

by Harman and Ruyak [37] reported that people with persistent low-level pain related to their work habits had cognitive deficits, indicative of an interference effect of pain. In the cases of acute pain, the frontal pole functions to direct behaviour to protect the subject. However, in chronic pain conditions, this region may be continuously engaged, and so to be able to perform a demanding cognitive task, would require the frontal pole to "put the pain on hold," allocating resources to the other, competing cognitive demand. Accordingly, Eccleston [24] showed that chronic pain patients could briefly be disengaged from pain during attentional switches. Further support for this hypothesis comes from studies that demonstrate that distraction can reduce pain perception [15, 55, 59]. These studies have demonstrated that distraction-based modulation of pain requires the recruitment of antinociceptive brain regions. However, these systems may not be effective in patients with TMD in two ways: there is evidence of dysfunctional antinociceptive systems [25, 42], and the cognitive branching model suggests that cognitive resources are limited [46]. Therefore, the cognitive load of chronic pain could impede the ability to engage in other tasks [47]. In support of this idea in TMD, we have shown that these patients have sluggish reaction times in cognitive interference tasks, but not for a simple sensorimotor task [78]. Therefore, in the context of use-dependent plasticity [54], frontal pole thickening and the increased white matter connectivity between the bilateral frontal poles may reflect the TMD cognitive load needed to be "put on hold" to address more immediate environmental demands.

Another brain imaging finding in TMD raises the issue of emotional regulation. Specifically, we found that unpleasantness is negatively correlated with GM in the orbitofrontal cortex (OFC) [57]. The OFC has been implicated in cognitive reappraisal and emotional regulation [61] related to interoception and somatovisceral stimuli, for directing our behaviour appropriately [7, 79]. The OFC is also thought to play a role in mental flexibility and adaptability (for a critical review, see [66]). Therefore, patients with TMD may have abnormal emotional regulation and reappraisal, which may lead to pain behaviours and exaggerated affective responses to pain.

Patients with TMD also had widespread white matter abnormalities in white matter tracts related to pain-modulatory brain regions. Specifically, patients had lower FA and increased MD and RD in white matter tracts coursing to the OFC and subgenual ACC (sgACC), the anterior corona radiata, which projects to the prefrontal cortex (PFC), and the external/extreme capsule adjacent to the right middle insula. The insula and MCC have been implicated in pain perception, negative emotion, and cognitive function [18, 68, 75]. The OFC and sgACC are thought to contribute to descending pain modulation [11]. Furthermore, patients with TMD had abnormal connectivity to the dorsolateral PFC, a region implicated in pain modulation [51], selecting information about the sensory environment (attention, self-monitoring, personality, working memory) and decision-making [6, 60] (see Fig. 29-4). Patients with TMD have widespread acute pain hypersensitivity [25, 52, 53], abnormal CPM [14, 42, 64], while having sluggish reaction times to a cognitive task [78]. These findings indicate that patients with TMD have dysfunctional descending modulation, likely related to abnormal structure and function of pain-modulatory brain regions.

PERSONALITY FACTORS AND TMD

Some individual factors can predispose persons to developing chronic pains, such as TMD. A prospective study by Fillingim and colleagues [26] reported that certain psychological traits could, to some extent, predict TMD onset, including neuroticism. We found that in patients with TMD, there is a positive correlation between neuroticism and cortical thickness in the left ventromedial PFC (part of the OFC) [57], an area that normally shows a negative correlation between GM and neuroticism [82]. Neuroticism has been defined as a stable personality trait associated with heightened sensitivity and/or processing of negative affective stimuli [76]. Therefore, it is not surprising that patients with high neuroticism scores have lower pain threshold and pain tolerance, and are more distressed by pain in experimental settings and chronic pain [36]. The mechanism by which inherent personality-related factors reduce the brain's capacity to effectively modulate nociceptive input and pain perception remains unclear. Crucially, high neuroticism is not common to all chronic pain patients, and not all highly neurotic persons suffer from chronic pain [16]. Therefore, neuroticism may only partially contribute to the development and severity of chronic pain. We propose that the relationship between neuroticism and abnormal GM in the OFC of TMD patients may contribute to the development of TMD (see Fig. 29-4). It is also possible that chronic pain may have modified the relationship between neuroticism and OFC thickness. However, the lack of correlation of TMD duration and neuroticism scores in our TMD sample does not support this hypothesis.

CONCLUSION

In sum, TMD is a complex chronic pain disorder associated with abnormalities in the sensory, motor, and cognitive-modulatory domains. These abnormalities are associated with functional and structural brain abnormalities in the brain. Neuroimaging techniques can help us understand the underlying brain mechanisms of TMD, and help us identify novel therapeutic targets. Here, we have reviewed evidence that suggests that both pre-existing structural abnormalities can predispose persons to developing TMD and that TMD pain can also initiate, maintain, and exacerbate functional and structural brain abnormalities.

REFERENCES

1. Apkarian AV, Bushnell MC, Treede RD, Zubieta J. Human brain mechanisms of pain perception and regulation in health and disease. Eur J Pain 2005;9:463–84.
2. Aron AR, Fletcher PC, Bullmore ET, Sahakian BJ, Robbins TW. Stop-signal inhibition disrupted by damage to right inferior frontal gyrus in humans. Nat Neurosci 2003;6:115–7.
3. Avivi-Arber L, Lee JC, Sessle BJ. Chapter 9—face sensorimotor cortex neuroplasticity associated with intraoral alterations. Prog Brain Res 2011;188:135–50.
4. Badre D, D'Esposito M. Is the rostro-caudal axis of the frontal lobe hierarchical? Nat Rev Neurosci 2009; 10:659–69.
5. Baliki MN, Chialvo DR, Geha PY, Levy RM, Harden RN, Parrish TB, Apkarian AV. Chronic pain and the emotional brain: specific brain activity associated with spontaneous fluctuations of intensity of chronic back pain. J Neurosci 2006;26:12165–73.
6. Barbas H. Anatomic basis of cognitive-emotional interactions in the primate prefrontal cortex. Neurosci Biobehav Rev 1995;19:499–510.
7. Barrett LF, Mesquita B, Ochsner KN, Gross JJ. The experience of emotion. Ann Rev Psychol 2007;58:373–403.
8. Basser PJ, Pierpaoli C. Microstructural and physiological features of tissues elucidated by quantitative-diffusion-tensor MRI. J Magn Reson B 1996;111:209–19.
9. Beaulieu C. The basis of anisotropic water diffusion in the nervous system—a technical review. NMR Biomed 2002;15:435–55.
10. Beaulieu C. The biological basis of diffusion. In: Johansen-Berg H, Behrens TEJ, editors. Diffusion MRI. London, UK: Elsevier; 2009. pp. 105–26.
11. Bingel U, Tracey I. Imaging CNS modulation of pain in humans. Physiology 2008;23:371–80.
12. Boorman ED, Behrens TE, Woolrich MW, Rushworth MF. How green is the grass on the other side? Frontopolar cortex and the evidence in favor of alternative courses of action. Neuron 2009;62:733–43.
13. Boudreau S, Romaniello A, Wang K, Svensson P, Sessle BJ, Arendt-Nielsen L. The effects of intra-oral pain on motor cortex neuroplasticity associated with short-term novel tongue-protrusion training in humans. Pain 2007;132:169–78.
14. Bragdon EE, Light KC, Costello NL, Sigurdsson A, Bunting S, Bhalang K, Maixner W. Group differences in pain modulation: pain free women compared to pain free men and to women with TMD. Pain 2002; 96:227–37.
15. Buhle J, Wager TD. Performance-dependent inhibition of pain by an executive working memory task. Pain 2010;149:19–26.
16. Costa PT, McCrae RR, Zonderman AB, Barbano HE, Lebowitz B, Larson DM. Cross-sectional studies of personality in a national sample: 2. Stability in neuroticism, extraversion, and openness. Psych Aging 1986;1:144–9.
17. Davis KD. Neuroimaging of pain: what does it tell us? Curr Opin Support Palliat Care 2011;5:116–21.
18. Davis KD, Moayedi M. Central mechanisms of pain revealed through functional and structural MRI. J Neuroimmune Pharmacol 2013;8:518–34.
19. Downar J, Mikulis DJ, Davis KD. Neural correlates of the prolonged salience of painful stimulation. NeuroImage 2003;20:1540–51.
20. Duerden EG, Albanese MC. Localization of pain-related brain activation: a meta-analysis of neuroimaging data. Hum Brain Mapp 2011;34:109–49.
21. Dworkin SF, Huggins KH, LeResche L, Von Korff M, Howard J, Truelove E, Sommers E. Epidemiology of signs and symptoms in temporomandibular disorders: clinical signs in cases and controls. J Am Dent Assoc 1990;120:273–81.
22. Dworkin SF, Leresche L. Research diagnostic criteria for temporomandibular disorders: review, criteria, examinations and specifications, critique. J Craniomandib Disord 1992;6:301–55.
23. Dworkin SF, Massoth DL. Temporomandibular disorders and chronic pain: disease or illness? J Prosthet Dent 1994;72:29–38.
24. Eccleston C. Chronic pain and attention: a cognitive approach. Br J Clin Psychol 1994;33(Pt 4):535–47.

25. Fernandez-de-las-Penas C, Galan-del-Rio F, Fernandez-Carnero J, Pesquera J, Arendt-Nielsen L, Svensson P. Bilateral widespread mechanical pain sensitivity in women with myofascial temporomandibular disorder: evidence of impairment in central nociceptive processing. J Pain 2009;10:1170–8.
26. Fillingim RB, Ohrbach R, Greenspan JD, Knott C, Dubner R, Bair E, Baraian C, Slade GD, Maixner W. Potential psychosocial risk factors for chronic TMD: descriptive data and empirically identified domains from the OPPERA case-control study. J Pain 2011;12:T46–60.
27. Fregni F, Freedman S, Pascual-Leone A. Recent advances in the treatment of chronic pain with non-invasive brain stimulation techniques. Lancet Neurol 2007;6:188–91.
28. Garcia-Larrea L, Maarrawi J, Peyron R. Thalamocingulate mechanisms of precentral cortex stimulation for central pain. In: Vogt B, editor. Cingulate neurobiology and disease. Oxford, UK: Oxford University Press; 2009. pp. 438–49.
29. Gerstner G, Ichesco E, Quintero A, Schmidt-Wilcke T. Changes in regional gray matter and white matter volume in patients with myofascial-type temporomandibular disorders: a voxel-based morphometry study. J Orofac Pain 2011;25:99–106.
30. Goldberg MB, Mock D, Ichise M, Proulx G, Gordon A, Shandling M, Tsai S, Tenenbaum HC. Neuropsychologic deficits and clinical features of posttraumatic temporomandibular disorders. J Orofac Pain 1996;10:126–40.
31. Grossi ML, Goldberg MB, Locker D, Tenenbaum HC. Reduced neuropsychologic measures as predictors of treatment outcome in patients with temporomandibular disorders. J Orofac Pain 2001;15:329–39.
32. Grossi ML, Goldberg MB, Locker D, Tenenbaum HC. Irritable bowel syndrome patients versus responding and nonresponding temporomandibular disorder patients: a neuropsychologic profile comparative study. Int J Prosthodont 2008;21:201–9.
33. Gustin SM, Peck CC, Cheney LB, Macey PM, Murray GM, Henderson LA. Pain and plasticity: is chronic pain always associated with somatosensory cortex activity and reorganization? J Neurosci 2012;32:14874–84.
34. Gustin SM, Peck CC, Wilcox SL, Nash PG, Murray GM, Henderson LA. Different pain, different brain: thalamic anatomy in neuropathic and non-neuropathic chronic pain syndromes. J Neurosci 2011;31:5956–64.
35. Hapak L, Gordon A, Locker D, Shandling M, Mock D, Tenenbaum HC. Differentiation between musculoligamentous, dentoalveolar, and neurologically based craniofacial pain with a diagnostic questionnaire. J Orofac Pain 1994;8:357–68.
36. Harkins SW, Price DD, Braith J. Effects of ex-traversion and neuroticism on experimental pain, clinical pain, and illness behavior. Pain 1989;36:209–18.
37. Harman K, Ruyak P. Working through the pain: a controlled study of the impact of persistent pain on performing a computer task. Clin J Pain 2005;21:216–22.
38. Hodges PW, Tucker K. Moving differently in pain: a new theory to explain the adaptation to pain. Pain 2011;152:S90–8.
39. Hollins M, Harper D, Gallagher S, Owings EW, Lim PF, Miller V, Siddiqi MQ, Maixner W. Perceived intensity and unpleasantness of cutaneous and auditory stimuli: an evaluation of the generalized hypervigilance hypothesis. Pain 2009;141:215–21.
40. Ichesco E, Quintero A, Clauw DJ, Peltier S, Sundgren PM, Gerstner GE, Schmidt-Wilcke T. Altered functional connectivity between the insula and the cingulate cortex in patients with temporomandibular disorder: a pilot study. Headache 2012;52:441–54.
41. Jenkins IH, Brooks DJ, Nixon PD, Frackowiak RSJ, Passingham RE. Motor sequence learning: a study with positron emission tomography. J Neurosci 1994;14:3775–90.
42. King CD, Wong F, Currie T, Mauderli AP, Fillingim RB, Riley JL III. Deficiency in endogenous modulation of prolonged heat pain in patients with irritable bowel syndrome and temporomandibular disorder. Pain 2009;143:172–78.
43. Kirveskari E, Vartiainen NV, Gockel M, Forss N. Motor cortex dysfunction in complex regional pain syndrome. Clin Neurophysiol 2010;121:1085–92.
44. Koechlin E. Frontal pole function: what is specifically human? Trends Cogn Sci 2011;15:241; author reply 243.
45. Koechlin E, Corrado G, Pietrini P, Grafman J. Dissociating the role of the medial and lateral anterior prefrontal cortex in human planning. Proc Natl Acad Sci U S A 2000;97:7651–56.
46. Koechlin E, Hyafil A. Anterior prefrontal function and the limits of human decision-making. Science 2007;318:594–600.
47. Legrain V, Damme SV, Eccleston C, Davis KD, Seminowicz DA, Crombez G. A neurocognitive model of attention to pain: behavioral and neuroimaging evidence. Pain 2009;144:230–2.
48. Legrain V, Iannetti GD, Plaghki L, Mouraux A. The pain matrix reloaded: a salience detection system for the body. Prog Neurobiol 2011;93:111–24.

49. Leo RJ, Latif T. Repetitive transcranial magnetic stimulation (rTMS) in experimentally induced and chronic neuropathic pain: a review. J Pain 2007;8:453–9.
50. Lima MC, Fregni F. Motor cortex stimulation for chronic pain: systematic review and meta-analysis of the literature. Neurology 2008;70:2329–37.
51. Lorenz J, Minoshima S, Casey KL. Keeping pain out of mind: the role of the dorsolateral prefrontal cortex in pain modulation. Brain 2003;126:1079–91.
52. Maixner W, Fillingim R, Booker D, Sigurdsson A. Sensitivity of patients with painful temporomandibular disorders to experimentally evoked pain. Pain 1995;63:341–51.
53. Maixner W, Fillingim R, Sigurdsson A, Kincaid S, Silva S. Sensitivity of patients with painful temporomandibular disorders to experimentally evoked pain: evidence for altered temporal summation of pain. Pain 1998;76:71–81.
54. May A. Experience-dependent structural plasticity in the adult human brain. Trends Cogn Sci 2011;15:475–82.
55. McCaul KD, Haugtvedt C. Attention, distraction, and cold-pressor pain. J Pers Soc Psychol 1982;43:154–62.
56. Moayedi M, Desouza D, Erpelding N. Making sense of gray matter abnormalities in chronic orofacial pain—synthesizing divergent findings. J Neurosci 2011;31:12396–7.
57. Moayedi M, Weissman-Fogel I, Crawley AP, Goldberg MB, Freeman BV, Tenenbaum HC, Davis KD. Contribution of chronic pain and neuroticism to abnormal forebrain gray matter in patients with temporomandibular disorder. NeuroImage 2011;55:277–86.
58. Moayedi M, Weissman-Fogel I, Salomons TV, Crawley AP, Goldberg MB, Freeman BV, Tenenbaum HC, Davis KD. White matter brain and trigeminal nerve abnormalities in temporomandibular disorder. Pain 2012;153:1467–77.
59. Petrovic P, Ingvar M. Imaging cognitive modulation of pain processing. Pain 2002;95:1–5.
60. Pochon JB, Levy R, Poline JB, Crozier S, LehÇricy S, Pillon B, Deweer B, Le Bihan D, Dubois B. The role of dorsolateral prefrontal cortex in the preparation of forthcoming actions: an fMRI study. Cereb Cortex 2001;11:260–6.
61. Ray RD, Ochsner KN, Cooper JC, Robertson ER, Gabrieli JD, Gross JJ. Individual differences in trait rumination and the neural systems supporting cognitive reappraisal. Cogn Affect Behav Neurosci 2005;5:156–68.
62. Salomons TV, Johnstone T, Backonja M, Shackman AJ, Davidson RJ. Individual differences in the effects of perceived controllability on pain perception: critical role of the prefrontal cortex. J Cogn Neurosci 2007;19:993–1004.
63. Salomons TV, Moayedi M, Weissman-Fogel I, Goldberg MB, Freeman BV, Tenenbaum HC, Davis KD. Perceived helplessness is associated with individual differences in the central motor output system. Eur J Neurosci 2012;35:1481–7.
64. Sarlani E, Greenspan JD. Evidence for generalized hyperalgesia in temporomandibular disorders patients. Pain 2003;102:221–6.
65. Sarlani E, Greenspan JD. Why look in the brain for answers to temporomandibular disorder pain? Cells Tissues Organs 2005;180:69–75.
66. Schoenbaum G, Roesch MR, Stalnaker TA, Takahashi YK. A new perspective on the role of the orbitofrontal cortex in adaptive behaviour. Nat Rev Neurosci 2009;10:885–92.
67. Sessle BJ. Acute and chronic craniofacial pain: brainstem mechanisms of nociceptive transmission and neuroplasticity and their clinical correlates. Crit Rev Oral Biol Med 2000;11:57–91.
68. Shackman AJ, Salomons TV, Slagter HA, Fox AS, Winter JJ, Davidson RJ. The integration of negative affect, pain and cognitive control in the cingulate cortex. Nat Rev Neurosci 2011;12:154–67.
69. Shibukawa Y, Ishikawa T, Kato Y, Shintani M, Zhang ZK, Jiang T, Tazaki M, Shimono M, Kumai T, Suzuki T, et al. Cortical dysfunction in patients with temporomandibular disorders. J Oral Biosci 2009;51:65–71.
70. Slade GD, Diatchenko L, Bhalang K, Sigurdsson A, Fillingim RB, Belfer I, Max MB, Goldman D, Maixner W. Influence of psychological factors on risk of temporomandibular disorders. J Dent Res 2007;86:1120–5.
71. Strange BA, Henson RN, Friston KJ, Dolan RJ. Anterior prefrontal cortex mediates rule learning in humans. Cereb Cortex 2001;11:1040–6.
72. Svensson P. What can human experimental pain models teach us about clinical TMD? Arch Oral Biol 2007;52:391–4.
73. Teutsch S, Herken W, Bingel U, Schoell E, May A. Changes in brain gray matter due to repetitive painful stimulation. NeuroImage 2008;42:845–9.
74. Tsujimoto S, Genovesio A, Wise SP. Evaluating self-generated decision in the frontal polar cortex of monkeys. Nat Neurosci 2010;13:120–6.
75. Vogt BA. Pain and emotion interactions in subregions of the cingulate gyrus. Nat Rev Neurosci 2005;6:533–44.

76. Wade JB, Dougherty LM, Hart RP, Rafii A, Price DD. A canonical correlation analysis of the influence of neuroticism and extraversion on chronic pain, suffering, and pain behavior. Pain 1992;51:67–73.
77. Wager TD, Scott DJ, Zubieta JK. Placebo effects on human μ-opioid activity during pain. Proc Natl Acad Sci USA 2007;104:11056–61.
78. Weissman-Fogel I, Moayedi M, Tenenbaum HC, Goldberg MB, Freeman BV, Davis KD. Abnormal cortical activity in patients with temporomandibular disorder evoked by cognitive and emotional tasks. Pain 2011; 152:384–96.
79. Wiech K, Seymour B, Kalisch R, Stephan KE, Koltzenburg M, Driver J, Dolan RJ. Modulation of pain processing in hyperalgesia by cognitive demand. NeuroImage 2005;27:59–69.
80. Wilcox SL, Gustin SM, Eykman EN, Fowler G, Peck CC, Murray GM, Henderson LA. Trigeminal nerve anatomy in neuropathic and non-neuropathic orofacial pain patients. J Pain 2013;14(8):865–72.
81. Woolf CJ, Salter MW. Neuronal plasticity: increasing the gain in pain. Science 2000;288:1765–9.
82. Wright CI, Williams D, Feczko E, Barrett LF, Dickerson BC, Schwartz CE, Wedig MM. Neuroanatomical correlates of extraversion and neuroticism. Cereb Cortex 2006;16:1809–19.
83. Younger JW, Shen YF, Goddard G, Mackey SC. Chronic myofascial temporomandibular pain is associated with neural abnormalities in the trigeminal and limbic systems. Pain 2010;149:222–8.

CHAPTER 30

Brain Activity and Reorganization in Complex Regional Pain Syndrome

Martin Lotze and Flavia Di Pietro

INTRODUCTION TO CRPS AND REASONS FOR NEUROIMAGING RESEARCH IN CRPS

Complex regional pain syndrome (CRPS) is a disorder characterized not only by persistent pain and disability but also by dysfunction in several body systems. What causes CRPS is unknown. The most common precipitating event for CRPS is minor trauma (i.e., fracture) to the upper extremity, particularly the wrist [6, 44]. Movement disorders are common, ranging from a decrease in active movement through to fixed dystonic positions. While CRPS is typically subgrouped into CRPS-I and CRPS-II—depending, respectively, on the absence or presence of peripheral nerve injury [29] —the signs and symptoms in both subgroups of CRPS converge over time, and a peripheral cause of the ongoing disorder becomes increasingly difficult to assign. As the disorder develops, neither CRPS-I nor CRPS-II can be explained by the initial trauma [3].

In recent decades, chronic CRPS has become recognized as a disease of the central nervous system [15, 40]. This is partly due to the generally poor response to CRPS treatments [34], which have largely been targeted towards the painful limb. There are also many examples of perceptual phenomena in CRPS, which implicate the brain, and suggest top-down influences of the brain on the body in this disorder. CRPS patients exhibit poor performance in two-point discrimination tasks [37], perceive their affected limb to be bigger than it actually is [30, 33], and report distortions in their mental image of the affected limb [20].

Neuroimaging studies in CRPS have all led to the widely accepted notion that chronic CRPS reflects a case of maladaptive neuroplasticity [3, 9, 22, 29]. There is currently much investigation into the role of the brain in CRPS, and the studies have yielded evidence of cortical reorganization in motor and sensory systems. Although the primary somatosensory (S1) and primary motor (M1) cortices are the focus here, it is worth noting that functional changes have also been noted in the secondary somatosensory cortex [16, 37] and in the premotor and supplementary motor area [23]. Early results from connectivity analyses in CRPS patients point to differences in functional connectivity (FC), specifically in the default brain network (cingulate cortex, dorsomedial prefrontal cortex, precuneus) and the thalamus, and increased connectivity within M1 and S1 and the intraparietal sulcus (IPS) [2]. Independent voxel-based morphometry (VBM) studies of the cortex have reported conflicting results from small samples.

Overall, there is a paucity of large studies on these rare patients; this offers some explanation for the inconsistencies in the neuroimaging results in this clinical group. In this chapter, we will discuss some of the CRPS and neuroimaging evidence for functional reorganization in cortical areas (namely S1 and M1), FC changes, and morphological changes. We will also discuss CRPS interventions in relation to neuroimaging findings.

FINDINGS OF REORGANIZATION IN THE PRIMARY SOMATOSENSORY CORTEX (S1)

The strength of the S1 response with stimulation of the CRPS-affected limb has been investigated with electroencephalography (EEG) and magnetoencephalography (MEG). Taken together, the studies yield varied results, and it seems there is no difference when comparing limbs between patients, or between patients and healthy controls, in the S1 activation strength after peripheral stimulation [7]. Interestingly, however, when the MEG studies alone are considered (all involving tactile stimulation to the digits), there is an increase in the S1 activation in response to stimulation of the CRPS-affected hand compared with the healthy hand [16, 28, 43].

Regarding the latency of the observed S1 response after peripheral stimulation, the results are again inconclusive. It seems that there is no difference in latency across the studies between limbs in CRPS patients, or between CRPS patients and controls [16, 28, 38, 42, 43]. Again, however, the use of different technologies and paradigms may well explain this lack of consensus.

A key mechanism thought to underlie some of the clinical features of CRPS is cortical disinhibition. However, in their investigation into CRPS with dystonia, van Rijn et al. [42] found no differences in spatiotemporal interaction between CRPS patients and healthy controls—taken to suggest against S1 disinhibition. Lenz et al. [18], however, found evidence of bilateral cortical disinhibition in CRPS patients compared with healthy controls; this may be important given the consistency in bilateral results across different tests of motor cortex function, which is discussed below.

As well as investigations into the strength and latency of S1 activation, groups have studied the spatial representation of the CRPS-affected limb in S1 by mapping the distance between areas of S1 activation that result from stimulation of distinct peripheral sites on the limb. Studies have demonstrated that CRPS is associated with a decrease in the size of the S1 area serving the affected limb [16, 26, 38, 43]. This is thought to be maladaptive—groups have also documented the association of cortical changes with pain intensity and the area and strength of mechanical hyperalgesia [26, 27] and lower spatial acuity in the affected limb [23, 37]. Furthermore, changes in S1 representation have been found to reverse with sensorimotor retraining [26, 37].

Changes in S1 as a key feature of CRPS have often been described [3, 29]. Interestingly, however, a recent systematic review demonstrated that although there is indeed a consistent result between limbs in CRPS patients—such that the affected limb is smaller in its representation—critically, there is limited evidence regarding comparison with controls [7]. Furthermore, the review highlighted that there have been no published functional magnetic resonance imaging (fMRI) studies to date to answer the question of S1 spatial representation in CRPS, and that there are issues regarding methodological risk of bias in the extant studies, namely due to lack of blinding in neuroimaging analysis [7]. Given that therapies for CRPS have stemmed from the notion of S1 functional reorganization, further work—namely using fMRI and comparing patients with healthy controls—is needed to clarify this issue.

FINDINGS OF REORGANIZATION IN THE PRIMARY MOTOR CORTEX (M1)

Motor impairments arise as CRPS progresses (i.e., after the acute inflammatory stage), and therefore central nervous system dysfunction is implicated [29, 44]. Although it is highly unlikely that motor dysfunction arises from a single brain structure, the primary motor cortex has become a source of investigation in CRPS patients. Primarily, M1 representation of the CRPS-affected limb has been investigated with fMRI (e.g., imaging the size or strength of the cortical response to a movement task or imagined movement task), MEG (e.g., evaluating the 20 Hz cortical rhythm), and transcranial magnetic stimulation (TMS; e.g., measuring cortical excitability or mapping the spatial representation of the limb). In contrast to what has become general consensus on the shrinkage in the size of the affected limb representation in S1, however, no definitive conclusions can be drawn regarding differences in spatial representation in M1. Furthermore, it is difficult to confirm differences between sides in CRPS patients, or between CRPS patients and controls, in many of the other outcomes measured using the different technologies.

What appears to be consistent across studies of M1 function is the presence of bilateral changes. In an fMRI investigation, Maihöfner et al. [26] found bilaterally increased activation in M1 with finger-tapping of the CRPS-affected hand compared with that of the healthy hand and that of healthy controls. Using MEG to record cortical rhythms resulting from digit stimulation, Juottonen et al. [16] found a significant difference in the 20 Hz rhythm (specifically, a shorter rebound duration) in patients compared with controls, but not between sides in patients. Finally, evidence of bilateral M1 changes has come from TMS studies. Using paired-pulse stimulation paradigms, Schwenkreis et al. [39] and Eisenberg et al. [8] demonstrated a bilaterally higher amplitude ratio in CRPS patients than in controls. Similar to the results above, again the differences existed only between patients and healthy controls, and not between sides in patients. These results have all been taken to indicate disinhibition, and are thought to underlie the movement abnormalities—for instance, the lack of fine motor control—often seen in CRPS patients [32]. Bilateral changes in brain function have also been proposed as a possible explanation for the spread of motor signs across the body midline, which has been noted clinically in some CRPS patients.

ABNORMALITIES IN OTHER CEREBRAL AREAS

Pleger and colleagues [37] described that reduced two-point discrimination performance in CRPS patients was associated with reduced S1 and S2 BOLD-effect magnitude with electrical stimulation of the index finger. Only S1 activation contralateral to stimulation of the affected index finger correlated positively with the mean sustained pain levels in the group. There was a weaker association between the extent of impaired motor performance and BOLD changes after index finger stimulation. The authors suggested that tactile hyposensitivity might be a consequence of central reorganization associated with chronic pain, rather than a consequence of immobilization. It might also be interesting to investigate neurobiologic correlates of impaired spatial tactile training in these patients reported before [24].

Since the work of Maihöfner and colleagues [25], on the association between parietal activation and allodynia in CRPS patients, there has been a focus on this area as well. CRPS patients exhibit a neglect-like syndrome and body perception disturbance; such clinical symptoms are comparable to those of patients with left-sided neglect after right parietal lesions. However, patients showing a neglect after right inferior parietal lesions have no insight to their symptoms, whereas CRPS patients usually have such an insight [20]. Interestingly, CRPS patients with signs of dystonia showed reduced inferior parietal activation during motor imagery of the affected hand, together with reduced premotor and posterior insula activation [12]. The posterior parietal lobe also showed a decreased magnetoencephalographic response to tactile stimulation of the affected hand in these patients compared with healthy controls [43]. By using double-coil TMS in healthy participants, a functional interaction of the right parietal lobe (around the IPS) with the left motor cortex, during motor imagery of the right hand, has been demonstrated [17]. It is possible that this interaction is altered in patients with CRPS who have problems with conjuring a vivid image of the affected limb. Consequently, therapeutic approaches in CRPS patients have also focused on the parietal lobe.

Another interesting direction for imaging research in these patients might be an altered representation and effectiveness of pain suppression. Freund and colleagues [10] found bilateral decreased periaqueductal grey and anterior cingulate cortex (ACC) activation during index finger electrical stimulation of both hand sides in 10 CRPS patients, in comparison with 15 healthy controls, during a pain suppression task. This was interpreted as decreased effectiveness of the descending opioid pathway in these patients.

STUDIES INVESTIGATING ALTERED FUNCTIONAL CONNECTIVITY IN CRPS PATIENTS

Changes to the representation of the affected limb in M1 and S1 and altered intracortical inhibition might well be associated with altered connectivity between cortical or subcortical regions. Bolwerk and colleagues [2] calculated FC during rest in a group of 12 patients with CRPS and 12 age- and gender-matched healthy controls. They selected regions from the default-mode network (DMN), which has been shown to be predominantly active during rest [13]. It has been suggested that the resting brain might be affected by chronic pain, given that the disinhibition in cortical areas could be associated with changes to the DMN. Bolwerk and colleagues investigated FC in areas previously reported to show alterations in CRPS patients, for instance S1 and S2, M1, and the IPS. They found reductions in functional DMN connectivity in patients and increased FC between S1, M1, and IPS in patients. Furthermore, there was a trend for correlation between alterations in FC and the intensity of neuropathic pain. It is beyond the scope of this chapter; however, it is important to note that FC studies have been conducted on paediatric populations [21]. There are distinct differences in the clinical picture and progression of CRPS in a paediatric population and we refer the reader to the relevant literature in that field [41].

MORPHOLOGICAL CHANGES

With respect to changes in grey and white matter volume, the results seem to be inconsistent between studies. Geha and colleagues [11] published the first comparison for grey matter density in a sample of 26 patients and 28 healthy controls. They found a decrease in the right ventromedial PFC (VMPFC) grey matter density in comparison with healthy controls. VMFPC-grey matter volume was negatively associated with pain duration. The same side of the brain was affected regardless of the side of the body that was affected by CRPS.

A methodologically different approach was used by Pleger and colleagues [36] 6 years later, using VBM to investigate differences in grey matter in a group of 20 patients and 20 age- and gender-matched healthy controls. They found an increase in grey matter volume in M1 and the dorsomedial PFC (DMPFC) contralateral to the affected hand. In this study, a decrease of white matter in the internal capsule correlated inversely with increased grey matter in the motor cortex. A third group reported contradictory results again [1]: the CRPS group showed decreased grey matter volume in several regions processing the affective dimensions of pain, including the dorsal insula, the left orbitofrontal cortex, and the cingulate cortex. Increased grey matter volume in CRPS patients was seen in the bilateral dorsal putamen and right hypothalamus. Pain duration was associated with decreased grey matter in the left dorsolateral PFC (DLPFC). Pain intensity was positively correlated with volume in the left posterior hippocampus and left amygdala, and negatively correlated with that in the bilateral DLPFC. Although these three studies demonstrated contradictory results, they used different methods. Future studies should recruit larger samples and apply consistent methodology if we are to draw conclusions on structural changes in CRPS. It is also important to note that the pathophysiology of grey matter changes in the brain is still not understood [5].

LONGITUDINAL STUDIES AND INTERVENTION STUDIES

Normalization of the seemingly decreased hand representation size with effective treatment for CRPS has been shown using MEG [27]. For the therapeutic application of spinal cord stimulation (SCS), which shows selective efficacy on pain intensity for the initial phase after implantation, a similar effect on the hand representation in S1 has been demonstrated [35].

Noninvasive therapies have stemmed from the findings of differences in excitability and spatial representation in CRPS patients for S1 and M1. It is feasible that the altered intracortical inhibition found in these patients might well be remedied by repetitive TMS (rTMS) or transcranial direct current stimulation (TDCS). Interestingly, rTMS applied to increase cortical excitability (5–20 Hz) was more effective when applied over M1 than rTMS with a lower frequency (1 Hz) [19].

A behavioural training approach has been developed to address altered body representation and problems associated with execution of movement, without inducing pain. This therapy is called graded motor imagery (GMI) training, and it comprises a three-step program: a left/right limb judgement task, followed by imagined movements, and then mirror therapy [31]. We were interested in the cerebral effect of GMI in a CRPS patient who experienced a positive effect from this intervention. We used fMRI to investigate the brain's response to fist clenching, imagined clenching, and mental rotation, with a highly controlled task paradigm prior to and following 2 weeks of therapy in a CRPS patient, and a healthy age-matched control. In addition, we recorded pain scores and used fMRI to test again 3 months after the cessation of therapy. Pain intensity after therapy was reduced by more than 6 points on a 10-point scale, showed a linear reduction over time, and remained approximately 4 points lower than baseline at the 6-month follow-up point. Areas that have been associated with the emotional processing of pain, such as the ACC and anterior insula, showed constant activation over time, whereas S1 and S2 activation decreased in association with the actual pain ratings. IPS activation also decreased, especially during the mental rotation training [45].

The usage of NMDA-receptor blockers, alone or together with morphine, has in both cases been reported as effective treatment for CRPS [4]. The neurophysiological background

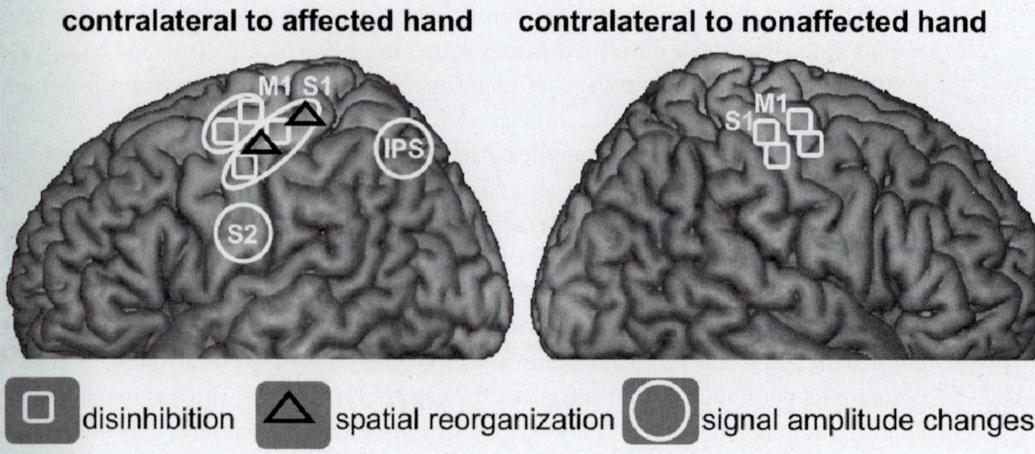

FIGURE 30-1 Examples of the findings obtained with different methods (fMRI, MEG, TMS, somatosensory evoked potential [SEP]) when comparing patients with CRPS with healthy controls. Patients show increased bilateral M1 and S1 disinhibition (*white square*), and some evidence of altered activation magnitude/signal amplitude in S1 and S2 after tactile stimulation of the affected side (*white circle*). In addition, a decrease has been reported over the parietal lobe (IPS, intraparietal sulcus) during motor imagery tasks. Only S1, representing the affected hand, shows a consistent decrease in the size of the representation of the affected hand (*black triangle*).

of this effect is possibly explained by ongoing Hebbian mechanisms—which might also be relevant for the development of chronic pain. Continuous stimulation, or repetitive signalling, increases the firing rate of the neurons; therefore, blocking the neural transmitters that mediate such learning processes might be effective to avoid the cortical reorganization associated with chronic pain. Since the NMDA receptor is essentially involved in cortical reorganization during repetitive training, such reorganization can be avoided by blocking this receptor. In a double-blinded placebo-controlled study, an NMDA blocker was combined with morphine and physiotherapy in a group of subacute CRPS patients [14]. Only the NMDA group experienced a reduction in pain, associated with a reduction in fMRI-activation magnitude for S1 and S2 contralateral to the affected hand when the hand was performing a clenching task. Although it has been proposed that the NMDA-receptor blocker might be most effective in combination with morphine during the period of time when pain is becoming chronic, it is possible that the effect observed might also be associated with decreased dependence on morphine when using the combination of pharmacological therapies.

CONCLUSION

Our knowledge of the brain's role in the pathophysiology of CRPS has been informed by several neuroimaging technologies, using vastly different paradigms. While many results are inconclusive, the findings of cortical reorganization in the primary somatosensory and primary motor cortices are the most consistent (see Fig. 30-1). A decrease in the size of the S1 representation of the CRPS-affected limb, together with bilateral M1 changes, seem the most viable targets for future research into the cerebral effects of treatments for this disorder. Furthermore, altered sensorimotor integration and alteration in parietal lobe function might well be associated with phenomena such as neglect, poor performance in motor imagery, and altered body perception. It might be fruitful to focus on interactions of these areas using connectivity analyses during activation and rest.

ACKNOWLEDGEMENT

This investigation was supported by a grant of the BMBF (01DR12044). FDP was supported by an Australian Postgraduate Award (APA) PhD scholarship.

REFERENCES

1. Barad MJ, Ueno T, Younger J, Chatterjee N, Mackey S. Complex regional pain syndrome is associated with structural abnormalities in pain-related regions of the human brain. J Pain 2014;15(2):197–203.
2. Bolwerk A, Seifert F, Maihöfner C. Altered resting-state functional connectivity in complex regional pain syndrome. J Pain 2013;14(10):1107–15.e8.
3. Bruehl SP. An update on the pathophysiology of complex regional pain syndrome. Anesthesiology 2010;113(3):713–25.
4. Cossins L, Okell RW, Cameron H, Simpson B, Poole HM, Goebel A. Treatment of complex regional pain syndrome in adults: a systematic review of randomized controlled trials published from June 2000 to February 2012. Eur J Pain 2013;17(2):158–73.
5. Davis KD, Moayedi M. Central mechanisms of pain revealed through functional and structural MRI. J Neuroimmune Pharmacol 2013;8(3):518–34.
6. de Mos M, de Bruijn AGJ, Huygen FJPM, Dieleman JP, Stricker BHC, Sturkenboom MCJM. The incidence of complex regional pain syndrome: a population-based study. Pain 2007;129(1–2):12–20.
7. Di Pietro F, McAuley JH, Parkitny L, Lotze M, Wand BM, Moseley GL, Stanton TR. Primary somatosensory cortex function in complex regional pain syndrome: a systematic review and meta-analysis. J Pain 2013; 14(10):1001–18.
8. Eisenberg E, Chistyakov AV, Yudashkin M, Kaplan B, Hafner H, Feinsod M. Evidence for cortical hyperexcitability of the affected limb representation area in CRPS: a psychophysical and transcranial magnetic stimulation study. Pain 2005;113(1–2):99–105.
9. Flor H, Diers M. Sensorimotor training and cortical reorganization. NeuroRehabilitation 2009;25(1):19–27.
10. Freund W, Faust S, Birklein F, Gaser C, Wunderlich AP, Muller M, Billich C, Juchems MS, Schmitz BL, et al. Substantial and reversible brain gray matter reduction but no acute brain lesions in ultramarathon runners: experience from the TransEurope-FootRace Project. BMC Med 2012;10:170.
11. Geha PY, Baliki MN, Harden RN, Bauer WR, Parrish TB, Apkarian AV. The brain in chronic CRPS pain: abnormal gray-white matter interactions in emotional and autonomic regions. Neuron 2008;60(4):570–81.
12. Gieteling EW, van Rijn MA, de Jong BM, Hoogduin JM, Renken R, van Hilten JJ, Leenders KL. Cerebral activation during motor imagery in complex regional pain syndrome type 1 with dystonia. Pain 2008;134(3):302–9.
13. Greicius MD, Krasnow B, Reiss AL, Menon V. Functional connectivity in the resting brain: a network analysis of the default mode hypothesis. Proc Natl Acad Sci USA 2003;100(1):253–8.
14. Gustin SM, Schwarz A, Birbaumer N, Sines N, Schmidt AC, Veit R, Larbig W, Flor H, Lotze M. NMDA-receptor antagonist and morphine decrease CRPS-pain and cerebral pain representation. Pain 2010;151(1):69–76.
15. Jänig W, Baron R. Complex regional pain syndrome is a disease of the central nervous system. Clin Auton Res 2002;12(3):150–64.
16. Juottonen K, Gockel M, Silen T, Hurri H, Hari R, Forss N. Altered central sensorimotor processing in patients with complex regional pain syndrome. Pain 2002;98(3):315–23.
17. Lebon F, Lotze M, Stinear CM, Byblow WD. Task-dependent interaction between parietal and contralateral primary motor cortex during explicit versus implicit motor imagery. PLoS One 2012;7(5):e37850.
18. Lenz M, Hoffken O, Stude P, Lissek S, Schwenkreis P, Reinersmann A, Frettloh J, Richter H, Tegenthoff M, Maier C. Bilateral somatosensory cortex disinhibition in complex regional pain syndrome type I. Neurology 2011;77(11):1096–101.
19. Leung A, Donohue M, Xu R, Lee R, Lefaucheur JP, Khedr EM, Saitoh Y, Andre-Obadia N, Rollnik J, Wallace M, et al. rTMS for suppressing neuropathic pain: a meta-analysis. J Pain 2009;10(12):1205–16.
20. Lewis JS, Kersten P, McCabe CS, McPherson KM, Blake DR. Body perception disturbance: a contribution to pain in complex regional pain syndrome (CRPS). Pain 2007;133(1–3):111–9.
21. Linnman C, Becerra L, Lebel A, Berde C, Grant PE, Borsook D. Transient and persistent pain induced connectivity alterations in pediatric complex regional pain syndrome. PLoS One 2013;8(3):e57205.
22. Lotze M, Moseley GL. Role of distorted body image in pain. Curr Rheumatol Rep 2007;9(6):488–96.

23. Maihöfner C, Baron R, DeCol R, Binder A, Birklein F, Deuschl G, Handwerker HO, Schattschneider J. The motor system shows adaptive changes in complex regional pain syndrome. Brain 2007;130(Pt 10):2671–87.
24. Maihöfner C, Decol R. Decreased perceptual learning ability in complex regional pain syndrome. Eur J Pain 2007;11(8):903–9.
25. Maihöfner C, Handwerker HO, Birklein F. Functional imaging of allodynia in complex regional pain syndrome. Neurology 2006;66(5):711–7.
26. Maihöfner C, Handwerker HO, Neundorfer B, Birklein F. Patterns of cortical reorganization in complex regional pain syndrome. Neurology 2003;61(12):1707–15.
27. Maihöfner C, Handwerker HO, Neundorfer B, Birklein F. Cortical reorganization during recovery from complex regional pain syndrome. Neurology 2004;63(4):693–701.
28. Maihöfner C, Neundorfer B, Stefan H, Handwerker HO. Cortical processing of brush-evoked allodynia. Neuroreport 2003;14(6):785–9.
29. Marinus J, Moseley GL, Birklein F, Baron R, Maihöfner C, Kingery WS, van Hilten JJ. Clinical features and pathophysiology of complex regional pain syndrome. Lancet Neurol 2011;10(7):637–48.
30. Moseley GL. Distorted body image in complex regional pain syndrome. Neurology 2005;65(5):773.
31. Moseley GL, Butler DS, Beames TB, Giles TJ. The graded motor imagery handbook. Adelaide, Australia: Noigroup Publications; 2012.
32. Moseley GL, Flor H. Targeting cortical representations in the treatment of chronic pain: a review. Neurorehabil Neural Repair 2012;26(6):646–52.
33. Moseley GL, Parsons TJ, Spence C. Visual distortion of a limb modulates the pain and swelling evoked by movement. Curr Biol 2008;18(22):R1047–8.
34. O'Connell NE, Wand BM, McAuley J, Marston L, Moseley GL. Interventions for treating pain and disability in adults with complex regional pain syndrome. Cochrane Database Syst Rev 2013;4:CD009416.
35. Pahapill PA, Zhang W. Restoration of altered somatosensory cortical representation with spinal cord stimulation therapy in a patient with complex regional pain syndrome: a magnetoencephalography case study. Neuromodulation 2014;17(1):22–7.
36. Pleger B, Draganski B, Schwenkreis P, Lenz M, Nicolas V, Maier C, Tegenthoff M. Complex regional pain syndrome type I affects brain structure in prefrontal and motor cortex. PLoS One 2014;9(1):e85372.
37. Pleger B, Ragert P, Schwenkreis P, Forster AF, Wilimzig C, Dinse H, Nicolas V, Maier C, Tegenthoff M. Patterns of cortical reorganization parallel impaired tactile discrimination and pain intensity in complex regional pain syndrome. NeuroImage 2006;32(2):503–10.
38. Pleger B, Tegenthoff M, Schwenkreis P, Janssen F, Ragert P, Dinse HR, Volker B, Zenz M, Maier C. Mean sustained pain levels are linked to hemispherical side-to-side differences of primary somatosensory cortex in the complex regional pain syndrome I. Exp Brain Res 2004;155(1):115–9.
39. Schwenkreis P, Janssen F, Rommel O, Pleger B, Volker B, Hosbach I, Dertwinkel R, Maier C, Tegenthoff M. Bilateral motor cortex disinhibition in complex regional pain syndrome (CRPS) type I of the hand. Neurology 2003;61(4):515–9.
40. Schwenkreis P, Maier C, Tegenthoff M. Functional imaging of central nervous system involvement in complex regional pain syndrome. Am J Neuroradiol 2009;30(7):1279–84.
41. Stanton-Hicks M. Plasticity of complex regional pain syndrome (CRPS) in children. Pain Med 2010;11(8): 1216–23.
42. van Rijn MA, van Hilten JJ, van Dijk JG. Spatiotemporal integration of sensory stimuli in complex regional pain syndrome and dystonia. J Neural Transm 2009;116(5):559–65.
43. Vartiainen NV, Kirveskari E, Forss N. Central processing of tactile and nociceptive stimuli in complex regional pain syndrome. Clin Neurophysiol 2008;119(10):2380–8.
44. Veldman PH, Reynen HM, Arntz IE, Goris RJA. Signs and symptoms of reflex sympathetic dystrophy: prospective study of 829 patients. Lancet 1993;342(8878):1012–6.
45. Walz AD, Usichenko T, Moseley GL, Lotze M. Graded motor imagery and the impact on pain processing in a case of CRPS. Clin J Pain 2013;29(3):276–9.

CHAPTER 31

Acupuncture, Pain, and Brain Imaging

Randy L. Gollub and Jian Kong

Acupuncture has been used since the beginning of human history [16, 47]. Acupuncture, as defined on the website of the National Center for Complementary and Alternative Medicine, refers to a family of procedures involving the stimulation of specific points on the body using a variety of techniques (http://nccam.nih.gov/health/acupuncture?nav=gsa). Despite its wide application in Eastern countries for thousands of years, lack of evidence for a therapeutic effect that is greater than a placebo treatment has slowed acceptance in Western countries.

Intriguingly, as more and more clinical trial approaches are applied to the study of acupuncture, what is perhaps most surprising is the relatively robust efficacy of genuine acupuncture treatments as well as sham acupuncture treatments to improve clinical outcomes over waitlist controls. In part, these findings reflect the complexity of identifying the "active ingredients" of acupuncture so as to enable the design of an appropriate sham condition [54]. However, increasing realization of the ability of acupuncture treatment to harness the self-healing mechanisms of the human mind and body is focusing efforts on directly investigating that phenomenon.

Since this evidence suggests that acupuncture treatment and placebo effects may work in part by activating self-healing mechanisms, it is not surprising that studies find the two share common pathways. Using pain as an example, studies show that both endogenous opioids and cholecystokinin are involved in acupuncture analgesia [7, 36] and placebo analgesia [1, 31]. Under the umbrella term of "self-healing," the distinction between the two could be blurred too far. A more useful construct holds that acupuncture, which is based on the stimulation of acupuncture points in the human body, should be regarded as having both "bottom-up" modulatory effects as well as "top-down" modulatory effects based on previous learning, expectation, therapeutic alliance, and other factors common to all placebo treatments. Brain imaging has the potential to illuminate these contributory mechanisms.

CHALLENGES AND LIMITATIONS OF CLINICAL TRIALS FOR ESTABLISHING TRUE EFFICACY OF ACUPUNCTURE TREATMENT

Randomized clinical trials (RCTs) are regarded as the gold standard method to determine therapeutic efficacy of a treatment. However, the ability of this method of investigation to yield meaningful information about whether and how acupuncture treatment relieves chronic pain works is fraught with problems, some specific to acupuncture and others that are more general limitations. To date, based on a search of PubMed (with acupuncture and chronic pain as key words), more than 250 clinical trials have been successfully performed with mixed results. In these trials, it is not uncommon for sham or placebo acupuncture to induce positive therapeutic effects similar in frequency and magnitude to those of verum (genuine) acupuncture. While individual patient outcomes vary widely, both verum and sham groups usually demonstrate superiority and clinical benefits compared with wait list control groups [2, 6, 15, 30, 33, 37] or even conventional treatment.

For instance, in a clinical trial on acupuncture treatment of chronic low back pain (cLBP), Cherkin and colleagues [4] investigated the treatment effects of four modes of treatment: individualized acupuncture, standardized acupuncture, simulated acupuncture, and usual care. They found that after 8 weeks of treatment, mean improvement on pain-related dysfunction for the individualized, standardized, and simulated acupuncture groups was similar, but all treatment modes had better outcomes than usual care.

In response to the contradictory results in the published clinical trials, a consortium of investigators pooled their data from multiple studies to estimate the effect size of acupuncture treatment to reduce chronic pain. In a recently published meta-analysis, Vickers and colleagues [50] used individual subject data from 29 high-quality RCTs (17,922 patients in total) to estimate the efficacy of acupuncture treatment on four chronic pain conditions: back and neck pain, osteoarthritis, chronic headache, and shoulder pain. They found acupuncture treatment superior to both sham and no acupuncture control for each of the four pain conditions. The results also indicated that the specific effect of acupuncture treatment over sham is relatively small, implying nonspecific effects are important contributors to acupuncture therapeutic effects.

To explore the relationship between the specific and nonspecific effects, we performed a crossover study in which the same subjects received verum acupuncture, sham acupuncture, placebo pills, and a rest control condition [27]. We used the change in their subjective pain ratings in response to calibrated heat pain stimuli as the primary outcome measure. We found that individuals' response to verum acupuncture and sham acupuncture was significantly positively correlated, further supporting the important contribution of nonspecific effects in acupuncture treatment.

Choice of outcome measurement is a crucial component of evaluating treatment effects in RCT investigations of acupuncture as well as any other treatment. For studies of chronic pain, most primary outcome measures are change scores of subjective assessments such as pain intensity and bothersomeness. Although these outcomes are easy to acquire, there are significant potential limitations.

First, subjective measurements can be easily biased by the context of the research [23]. It is well known that the action of deciding on a particular value to assign on a rating instrument is a complicated cognitive procedure [29]. Previous experience, context of treatment, expectancy, and the provider/patient relationship [12] can all significantly influence the final rating given by a patient [49] with or even without involvement of conscious thought [13]. For example, in a within-subject, repeated measures, crossover nonpain study where an objective measure of treatment outcome was available, the authors [53] randomly assigned 46 patients with asthma to active treatment with an albuterol inhaler, a placebo inhaler, sham acupuncture, or no intervention. At each visit, spirometry was performed repeatedly over a period of 2 hours. Maximum forced expiratory volume in 1 second (FEV(1)) was measured, and patients' self-reported improvement in breathing ratings were recorded. The results show that albuterol, but not the other treatments, results in a 20% increase in FEV(1). However, patients' reports of improvement after the intervention do not differ significantly for the albuterol inhaler, placebo inhaler, or sham acupuncture.

Further, since alternative medicine is not yet widely accepted in Western society, there may be a selection bias among those who choose to participate in clinical trials for acupuncture treatment to have high expectations for a positive outcome. Although it will not influence the resulting validity of RCTs, the nonspecific, self-healing effect in this particular population tends to be high [32]. This may partly explain the mixed results observed in the literature describing acupuncture treatment effects for clinical pain.

A second critical limitation to the use of subjective outcome measures is that they cannot elucidate the causal mechanism/pathways. This is of particular importance when one of the goals of the study is to distinguish between the contributions of potential multifactorial mechanisms that contribute to final outcome. Clearly, advances in acupuncture analgesia, specifically, and pain research, more generally, require more objective primary outcome measures, especially in alternative and integrative research where the nonspecific effects appear to play such an important role.

As an illuminating example, in a study of healthy subjects combining fMRI and an expectancy manipulation model using a two-by-two design, we found that although the analgesia effect as indicated by subjective pain rating decrease evoked by verum and sham acupuncture treatment is similar, the brain networks involved in mediating acupuncture and placebo analgesia to experimental pain stimuli are different [21, 22]. In a recent study with additional objective outcomes, Napadow and colleagues [42] used an event-related fMRI design coupled with autonomic monitoring and found that differential brain response to real and sham acupuncture stimuli in healthy adults is related to differential autonomic outflows that may have resulted from heterogeneity in evoked sensations. Moreover, objective physiological outcomes have also been explored in studies of acupuncture for chronic pain patients, and will be presented below.

THE ROLE OF BRAIN IMAGING IN ACUPUNCTURE RESEARCH USING EXPERIMENTAL PAIN AS A MODEL

Pain is a subjective experience; thus, there is no doubt that the brain plays an important role in mediating the experience. Nevertheless, if we agree that sensation originates in the activity of the brain, then it is possible to use indicators of brain function (e.g., specific changes in regional brain activity and network connectivity) as potential biomarkers. We must be cautious when we do this, since brain activity change, as measured by imaging tools, is not equal to subjective experience. In particular, we still do not know how conscious subjective experience is produced. Thus, all findings using imaging are indirect. Causal relation between what we measure and subjective experience remains to be proven. Even with this caveat, there is reasonable evidence that brain imaging will yield valuable insights into the underlying neural processes that constitute the experience of acute pain, its modulation, as well as the transitions into and out of chronic pain.

The current status of brain imaging techniques and their use in studies of acute and chronic pain are detailed in previous chapters. Here, we briefly summarize the points that are salient for description of the results of brain imaging studies of acupuncture analgesia. Many studies show that fMRI signal increases in a complex brain network including, but not limited to, insula, dorsal anterior cingulate cortex (ACC), thalamus, and primary and secondary sensory cortices when healthy subjects experience pain compared with when they experience no pain, or experience relatively lower-intensity pain [24, 48, 51]. These regions are often referred to as the "pain matrix" in the literature, and are investigated as potential imaging biomarkers for pain. In a recent study, Wager and colleagues [51] report a pattern of fMRI activity across brain regions that can distinguish heat pain from a warm stimulus, physical pain from mental pain, and the analgesia effect of the potent opioid analgesic drug remifentanil.

Acupuncture, because it is a somatically invasive treatment, also evokes a widespread response in the brain as recorded by fMRI. Actually, on the basis of traditional Chinese acupuncture theory, it is crucial for acupuncture to produce a unique type of somatosensation, referred to as *deqi*, for acupuncture to be effective. *Deqi* includes sensations such as soreness, aching, and dull pain [18]. Thus, it is not surprising that acupuncture needle stimulation evokes brain activity changes in a widespread network with reports of both fMRI signal increases and decreases [9–11, 19, 25, 45]. We note that this network is highly overlapping with the patterns of activation and deactivation when subjects experience heat pain [24]. For instance, in a test–retest reliability study in which we repeat identical acupuncture needle manipulation paradigms across six different imaging sessions [19], we find the most reliable activation/deactivation during electroacupuncture stimulation, irrespective of which acupuncture points are stimulated, are in insula (activation), operculum (activation), and medial orbital prefrontal cortex (deactivation). Meta-analytic techniques [3, 9], similarly, find that acupuncture needle stimulation produces consistent fMRI signal increases in insula, thalamus, ACC, and primary and secondary somatosensory cortices, as well as fMRI decreases in the medial prefrontal cortex, caudate, amygdala, and posterior cingulate cortex.

Thus, the challenge for imaging studies of acupuncture treatment effects on acute pain in healthy subjects as well as in patients with chronic pain disorders is to disambiguate fMRI signal changes that are due to the acupuncture treatment per se from those due to the experience of the experimental pain stimuli and most crucially from those due to the interaction that is the locus of treatment effect.

THE ROLE OF BRAIN IMAGING IN ACUPUNCTURE RESEARCH IN CHRONIC PAIN

It is now generally accepted that patients with chronic pain disorders have associated functional and anatomical changes in their brains. As an example, in a previous study, we have found enhanced resting functional connectivity in the pain descending control network in fibromyalgia patients [14]. Fibromyalgia patients also demonstrate enhanced connectivity between the insula and default mode network (DMN), which is associated with their subjective pain severity at the time of the scan [41]. Another study, conducted by Harris and colleagues [8], compares both short- and long-term effects of verum acupuncture and sham acupuncture treatment on *in vivo* μ-opioid receptor binding availability in patients with fibromyalgia. They find that different μ-opioid receptor binding processes may mediate clinically relevant analgesia effects for verum acupuncture and sham acupuncture although there is no significant difference in clinical outcome measurement between the two groups. As another example, using arterial spin labeling, our group finds [52] that exacerbation of clinical pain severity in cLBP patients is positively associated with statistically significant increases in regional cerebral blood flow in a widespread network of brain regions that are frequently noted in pain imaging studies, including the bilateral primary and secondary somatosensory cortices, and unilaterally in the right insula. In addition, we [35] also find that compared with healthy controls, cLBP patients demonstrate stronger DMN connectivity to the pregenual ACC, and right insula, with a strong association between DMN/insula connectivity and clinical pain intensity, corroborating the findings of Napadow et al. in fibromyalgia patients. In a more recent study on nonspecific LBP patients [26], we find a pattern of dynamic changes in the character of resting-state functional connectivity in the primary somatosensory cortex (S1) in cLBP patients, that is, S1 functional connectivity decreases when the patients experience low-intensity LBP compared with matched healthy controls, and functional connectivity at S1 increases when cLBP patients experience high-intensity LBP compared with the low-intensity condition. In addition, we also find increased cortical thickness in bilateral S1 somatotopically associated with the lower back in cLBP patients compared with healthy controls. In another study [12], we also find overlapping functional connectivity and brain structure changes also in fibromyalgia patients in rostral ACC (rACC), a key region in descending pain control system. Our results provide evidence of structural plasticity colocalized with areas exhibiting functional connectivity changes in chronic pain patients.

Studies also show that effective treatment can actually reverse the functional and anatomical changes in the brains of chronic pain patients. Seminowicz and colleagues [46] find that cLBP is associated with decreased cortical thickness and abnormal activity during attention-demanding tasks in the dorsolateral prefrontal cortex. Most intriguingly, after successful treatment, both cortical thickness and functional connectivity of the dorsolateral prefrontal cortex are normalized. In another study, investigators [44] also find that acupuncture (5-week treatment) reverses maladaptive brain plasticity (hyperactivation and overlapping/blurred representation of adjacent fingers within S1) in addition to reducing pain/paresthesia and the median nerve sensory latencies that characterize carpal tunnel syndrome patients. A recent study also shows that acupuncture reduces DMN/insula resting connectivity, in addition to pain levels, in fibromyalgia patients [40]. These results imply that brain imaging has the potential to be used as a biomarker for chronic pain treatment.

Brain response to acupuncture is also different for chronic patients. For instance, in a 2 × 2 ANOVA analysis, carpal tunnel syndrome patients responded to verum acupuncture with greater activation in the hypothalamus and deactivation in the amygdala compared with healthy adults, controlling for the nonspecific effects of sham acupuncture [39].

Whether and how acupuncture treatment might regulate/correct the functional and structural dysfunction of the brain associated with chronic pain disorders remains a mystery. Generally, acupuncture relieves pain by releasing endogenous opioids and activating the descending pain inhibitory control system [7]. Dysfunction of this descending pain inhibitory control network is one of the underlying mechanisms of chronic pain [14, 28]; thus, we hypothesize that acupuncture may relieve pain by correcting the dysfunction of the descending pain inhibitory control network. For instance, using the periaqueductal grey (PAG), a key region in descending pain inhibitory control network [28, 34], as a seed, we investigated differences in functional connectivity between subjects receiving verum and sham acupuncture with different expectancy levels [55]. We find that, compared with sham acupuncture stimulation, genuine electroacupuncture stimulation significantly enhances functional connectivity between the PAG and left posterior cingulate cortex and precuneus, and reduces functional connectivity between the PAG and right anterior insula.

In addition, studies have suggested that acupuncture can significantly modulate other empirically defined brain networks such as the DMN. For instance, Dhond and colleagues report that verum, but not sham, acupuncture can increase DMN connectivity with ACC, PAG, and amygdala—brain regions associated with pain perception and modulation [5]. Together, these results suggest that the changes in functional connectivity evoked by acupuncture needle stimulation may provide new information for our understanding of the mechanisms underlying verum and sham acupuncture analgesia.

SUMMARY AND FUTURE DIRECTIONS

Clinical trials suggest that verum acupuncture can significantly relieve the disease burden in chronic pain patients with evidence that nonspecific effects provide a significant contribution to the therapeutic benefits. Both acupuncture and placebo treatment (ritual effects) are very complicated phenomena, and we have a long way to go before we can harness and combine the two to obtain the best clinical outcome. Brain imaging may play a crucial role in this process. To reach this goal, several key questions need to be answered.

1. What is the association between brain functional/structural changes and subjective clinical symptom changes?
2. What is the relationship between brain response to acupuncture needle stimulation, neural correlates of deqi sensation [38], and clinical outcome?
3. Do different modalities of acupuncture (for instance, manual acupuncture vs. electroacupuncture [25]) work through the same mechanism? And if an individual responds to one mode of acupuncture (e.g., manual acupuncture), will he or she also respond to another mode of acupuncture (e.g., electroacupuncture) [17]?
4. What is the relationship between the specific and nonspecific effects of a particular treatment, and their underlying brain mechanism(s)?
5. Can we use brain imaging tools such as resting-state fMRI to predict an individual's response to acupuncture and placebo response, so that we can move individualized medicine one step forward [20]?
6. Are acupuncture mechanisms for pain relief similar to those of other subjective sensations, such as itch [43]?

REFERENCES

1. Benedetti F, Arduino C, Amanzio M. Somatotopic activation of opioid systems by target-directed expectations of analgesia. J Neurosci 1999;19(9):3639–48.
2. Brinkhaus B, Witt CM, Jena S, Linde K, Streng A, Wagenpfeil S, Irnich D, Walther H, Melchart D, Willich SN. Acupuncture in patients with chronic low back pain: a randomized controlled trial. Arch Intern Med 2006;166(4):450–7.
3. Chae Y, Chang DS, Lee SH, Jung WM, Lee IS, Jackson S, Kong J, Lee H, Park HJ, Lee H, et al. Inserting needles into the body: a meta-analysis of brain activity associated with acupuncture needle stimulation. J Pain 2013;14(3):215–22.
4. Cherkin DC, Sherman KJ, Avins AL, Erro JH, Ichikawa L, Barlow WE, Delaney K, Hawkes R, Hamilton L, Pressman A, et al. A randomized trial comparing acupuncture, simulated acupuncture, and usual care for chronic low back pain. Arch Intern Med 2009;169(9):858–66.
5. Dhond RP, Yeh C, Park K, Kettner N, Napadow V. Acupuncture modulates resting state connectivity in default and sensorimotor brain networks. Pain 2008;136(3):407–18.
6. Haake M, Muller HH, Schade-Brittinger C, Basler HD, Schafer H, Maier C, Endres HG, Trampisch HJ, Molsberger A. German Acupuncture Trials (GERAC) for chronic low back pain: randomized, multicenter, blinded, parallel-group trial with 3 groups. Arch Intern Med 2007;167(17):1892–8.
7. Han JS. Acupuncture: neuropeptide release produced by electrical stimulation of different frequencies. Trends Neurosci. 2003;26:17–22.
8. Harris RE, Zubieta JK, Scott DJ, Napadow V, Gracely RH, Clauw DJ. Traditional Chinese acupuncture and placebo (sham) acupuncture are differentiated by their effects on μ-opioid receptors (MORs). NeuroImage 2009;47(3):1077–85.

9. Huang W, Pach D, Napadow V, Park K, Long X, Neumann J, Maeda Y, Nierhaus T, Liang F, Witt CM. Characterizing acupuncture stimuli using brain imaging with fMRI—a systematic review and meta-analysis of the literature. PLoS One. 2012. 7(4):e32960.
10. Hui KK, Liu J, Makris N, Gollub RL, Chen AJ, Moore CI, Kennedy DN, Rosen BR, Kwong KK. Acupuncture modulates the limbic system and subcortical gray structures of the human brain: evidence from fMRI studies in normal subjects. Hum Brain Mapp 2000;9:13–25.
11. Hui KK, Liu J, Marina O, Napadow V, Haselgrove C, Kwong KK, Kennedy DN, Makris N. The integrated response of the human cerebro-cerebellar and limbic systems to acupuncture stimulation at ST 36 as evidenced by fMRI. NeuroImage 2005;27(3):479–96.
12. Jensen K, Srinivasan P, Spaeth R, Tan Y, Kosek E, Petzke F, Carville S, Fransson P, Marcus H, Williams SC, et al. Overlapping structural and functional brain changes in patients with long-term exposure to fibromyalgia. Arthritis Rheum 2013;65(12):3293–303.
13. Jensen KB, Kaptchuk TJ, Kirsch I, Raicek J, Lindstrom KM, Berna C, Gollub RL, Ingvar M, Kong J. Nonconscious activation of placebo and nocebo pain responses. Proc Natl Acad Sci USA 2012;109(39):15959–64.
14. Jensen KB, Kosek E, Petzke F, Carville S, Fransson P, Marcus H, Williams SC, Choy E, Giesecke T, Mainguy Y, et al. Evidence of dysfunctional pain inhibition in fibromyalgia reflected in rACC during provoked pain. Pain 2009;144(1–2):95–100.
15. Kaptchuk TJ. Acupuncture: theory, efficacy, and practice. Ann Intern Med 2002;136(5):374–83.
16. Kaptchuk TJ. Placebo studies and ritual theory: a comparative analysis of Navajo, acupuncture and biomedical healing. Philos Trans R Soc Lond B Biol Sci 2011;366(1572):1849–58.
17. Kong J, Fufa DT, Gerber AJ, Rosman IS, Vangel MG, Gracely RH, Gollub RL. Psychophysical outcomes from a randomized pilot study of manual, electro, and sham acupuncture treatment on experimentally induced thermal pain. J Pain 2005;6(1):55–64.
18. Kong J, Gollub R, Huang T, Polich G, Napadow V, Hui K, Vangel M, Rosen B, Kaptchup K. Acupuncture de qi, from qualitative history to quantitative measurement. J Altern Complement Med 2007;13(10):1059–70.
19. Kong J, Gollub RL, Webb JM, Kong JT, Vangel MG, Kwong K. Test-retest study of fMRI signal change evoked by electroacupuncture stimulation. NeuroImage. 2007;34(3):1171–81.
20. Kong J, Jensen K, Loiotile R, Cheetham A, Wey HY, Tan Y, Rosen B, Smoller JW, Kaptchuk TJ, Gollub RL. Functional connectivity of frontoparietal network predicts cognitive modulation of pain. Pain 2013;154(3): 459–67.
21. Kong J, Kaptachuk TJ, Polich G, Kirsch I, Vangel M, Zyloney C, Rosen B, Gollub RL. Expectancy and treatment interactions: a dissociation between acupuncture analgesia and expectancy evoked placebo analgesia. NeuroImage 2009;45:940–9.
22. Kong J, Kaptchuk TJ, Polich G, Kirsch I, Vangel M, Zyloney C, Rosen B, Gollub RL. An fMRI study on the interaction and dissociation between expectation of pain relief and acupuncture treatment. NeuroImage 2009;47(3):1066–76.
23. Kong J, Kaptchuk TJ, Polich G, Kirsch I, Gollub RL. Placebo analgesia: findings from brain imaging studies and emerging hypotheses. Rev Neurosci 2007;18(3–4):173–90.
24. Kong J, Loggia ML, Zyloney C, Tu P, Laviolette P, Gollub RL. Exploring the brain in pain: activations, deactivations and their relation. Pain 9 2010;148:257–67.
25. Kong J, Ma L, Gollub RL, Wei J, Yang X, Li D, Weng X, Jia F, Wang C, Li F, et al. A pilot study of functional magnetic resonance imaging of the brain during manual and electroacupuncture stimulation of acupuncture point (LI-4 Hegu) in normal subjects reveals differential brain activation between methods. J Altern Complement Med 2002;8(4):411–9.
26. Kong J, Spaeth R, Wey HY, Cheetham A, Cook AH, Jensen K, Tan Y, Liu H, Wang D, Loggia ML, et al. S1 is associated with chronic low back pain: a functional and structural MRI study. Mol Pain 2013:21;9(1):43.
27. Kong J, Spaeth R, Cook A, Kirsch I, Claggett B, Vangel M, Gollub RL, Smoller JW, Kaptchuk TJ. Are all placebo effects equal? Placebo pills, sham acupuncture, cue conditioning and their association. PLoS One 2013;8(7):e67485. doi:67410.61371/journal.pone.0067485.
28. Kong J, Tu PC, Zyloney C, Su TP. Intrinsic functional connectivity of the periaqueductal gray, a resting fMRI study. Behav Brain Res 2010;211(2):215–9.
29. Kong J, White NS, Kwong KK, Vangel MG, Rosman IS, Gracely RH, Gollub RL. Using fMRI to dissociate sensory encoding from cognitive evaluation of heat pain intensity. Hum Brain Mapp 2006;27(8):715–21.
30. Leibing E, Leonhardt U, Koster G, Goerlitz A, Rosenfeldt JA, Hilgers R, Ramadori G. Acupuncture treatment of chronic low-back pain—a randomized, blinded, placebo-controlled trial with 9-month follow-up. Pain 2002;96:189–96.
31. Levine JD, Gordon NC, Fields HL. The mechanism of placebo analgesia. Lancet 1978;2(8091):654–7.

32. Linde K, Niemann K, Meissner K. Are sham acupuncture interventions more effective than (other) placebos? A re-analysis of data from the Cochrane review on placebo effects. Forsch Komplementmed 2010;17(5): 259–64.
33. Linde K, Streng A, Jurgens S, Hoppe A, Brinkhaus B, Witt C, Wagenpfeil S, Pfaffenrath V, Hammes MG, Weidenhammer W, et al. Acupuncture for patients with migraine: a randomized controlled trial. JAMA 2005;293(17):2118–25.
34. Linnman C, Beucke JC, Jensen KB, Gollub RL, Kong J. Sex similarities and differences in pain-related periaqueductal gray connectivity. Pain 2012;153(2):444–54.
35. Loggia ML, Kim J, Gollub RL, Vangel MG, Kirsch I, Kong J, Wasan AD, Napadow V. Default mode network connectivity encodes clinical pain: an arterial spin labeling study. Pain 2013;154:24–33.
36. Mayer DJ, Prince DD, Rafii A. Antagonism of acupuncture analgesia in man by the narcotic antagonist naloxone. Brain Res 1977;121:368–72.
37. Melchart D, Streng A, Hoppe A, Brinkhaus B, Witt C, Wagenpfeil S, Pfaffenrath V, Hammes M, Hummelsberger J, Irnich D, et al. Acupuncture in patients with tension-type headache: randomised controlled trial. BMJ 13 2005;331(7513):376–82.
38. Napadow V, Dhond RP, Kim J, LaCount L, Vangel M, Harris RE, Kettner N, Park K. Brain encoding of acupuncture sensation—coupling on-line rating with fMRI. NeuroImage 2009;47(3):1055–65. doi:10.1016/j.neuroimage.2009.05.079.
39. Napadow V, Kettner N, Liu J, Li M, Kwong KK, Vangel M, Makris N, Audette J, Hui KKS. Hypothalamus and amygdala response to acupuncture stimuli in carpal tunnel syndrome. Pain 2007;130(3):254–66.
40. Napadow V, Kim J, Clauw DJ, Harris RE. Decreased intrinsic brain connectivity is associated with reduced clinical pain in fibromyalgia. Arthritis Rheum 2012;64(7): 2398–403.
41. Napadow V, LaCount L, Park K, As-Sanie S, Clauw DJ, Harris RE. Intrinsic brain connectivity in fibromyalgia is associated with chronic pain intensity. Arthritis Rheum 2010;62(8):2545–55.
42. Napadow V, Lee J, Kim J, Cina S, Maeda Y, Barbieri R, Harris RE, Kettner N, Park K. Brain correlates of phasic autonomic response to acupuncture stimulation: an event-related fMRI study. Hum Brain Mapp 2012;34(10):2592–606. doi:10.1002/hbm.22091.
43. Napadow V, Li A, Loggia ML, Kim J, Schalock PC, Lerner E, Tran TN, Ring J, Rosen BR, et al. The brain circuitry mediating antipruritic effects of acupuncture. Cerebral Cortex 2014;24(4)873–82.
44. Napadow V, Liu J, Li M, Kettner N, Ryan A, Kwong KK, Hui KKS, Audette J. Somatosensory cortical plasticity in carpal tunnel syndrome treated by acupuncture. Hum Brain Mapp 2007;28(3):159–71.
45. Napadow V, Makris N, Liu J, Kettner NW, Kwong KK, Hui KK. Effects of electroacupuncture versus manual acupuncture on the human brain as measured by fMRI. Hum Brain Mapp 2005;24(3):193–205.
46. Seminowicz DA, Wideman TH, Naso L, Hatami-Khoroushahi Z, Fallatah S, Ware MA, Jarzem P, Bushnell MC, Shir Y, Ouellet JA, et al. Effective treatment of chronic low back pain in humans reverses abnormal brain anatomy and function. J Neurosci 2011;31(20):7540–50.
47. Shapiro AK, Shapiro E. The powerful placebo: from ancient priest to modern physician. Baltimore, MD: The Johns Hopkins University Press; 1997.
48. Tracey I, Mantyh PW. The cerebral signature for pain perception and its modulation. Neuron 2007;55(3): 377–91.
49. Tracey I. Getting the pain you expect: mechanisms of placebo, nocebo and reappraisal effects in humans. Nat Med 2010;16(11):1277–83.
50. Vickers AJ, Cronin AM, Maschino AC, Lewith G, MacPherson H, Foster NE, Sherman KJ, Witt CM, Linde K, Cramer H. Acupuncture for chronic pain: individual patient data meta-analysis. Arch Intern Med 2012:1–10.
51. Wager TD, Atlas LY, Lindquist MA, Roy M, Woo CW, Kross E. An fMRI-based neurologic signature of physical pain. N Engl J Med 2013;368(15):1388–97.
52. Wasan AD, Loggia ML, Chen LQ, Napadow V, Kong J, Gollub RL. Neural correlates of chronic low back pain measured by arterial spin labeling. Anesthesiology 2011;115(2):364–74.
53. Wechsler ME, Kelley JM, Boyd IO, Dutile S, Marigowda G, Kirsch I, Israel E, Kaptchuk TJ. Active albuterol or placebo, sham acupuncture, or no intervention in asthma. N Engl J Med 2011;365(2):119–26.
54. Zhu D, Gao Y, Chang J, Kong J. Placebo acupuncture devices: considerations for acupuncture research. Evid Bas Compl Alternative Med 2013;2013:628907.
55. Zyloney CE, Jensen K, Polich G, Loiotile RE, Cheetham A, LaViolette PS, Tu P, Kaptchuk TJ, Gollub RL, Kong J. Imaging the functional connectivity of the Periaqueductal Gray during genuine and sham electroacupuncture treatment. Mol Pain 2010;6:80.

CHAPTER 32

Controversies in the Mechanism of Central Pain

J. H. Chien, J. H. Kim, J. J. Cheng, C. C. Liu, J. D. Greenspan, and F. A. Lenz

Lesions of the central nervous system (CNS) can produce human central pain syndromes and in animal models of those syndromes. Chronic pain syndromes associated with CNS injury in humans were first described by Dejerine and Roussy. They found that stroke-induced pain resulted from thalamic lesions, and coined the term "thalamic pain syndrome" ([21] c.f. [4]). Modern imaging has confirmed that central pain can arise from thalamic lesions and from multiple types and locations of lesions in the spinal cord (spinal cord injury [SCI]), brainstem, subcortical white matter, and cerebral cortex [3, 12, 32, 39, 59]. If central pain is caused by strokes of the brain, then these conditions are known as central poststroke pain (CPSP) syndromes.

Most studies of mechanisms of central pain in primates have been carried out in humans. In patients with CPSP and SCI central pain, loss of pain and/or thermal sensations is a uniform characteristic [3, 9, 11, 29, 59]. This pattern of sensory loss is associated with transection of the spinal cord, resulting in chronic pain localized below the level of the transection in SCI central pain, or after a stroke, resulting in chronic pain on the side of the body opposite the stroke in CPSP. The diagnosis of central pain is based on evidence of a CNS injury, evidence of pain and temperature sensory loss, and the exclusion of other mechanisms of pain. The clinical features and sensory testing in patients with central pain have advanced our understanding of the mechanism of this syndrome.

CLINICAL FEATURES OF SCI CENTRAL PAIN

Pain at or above the lesion level is often thought to be related, at least in part, to nociceptive input from somatic injuries associated with a traumatic spinal injury. Below-lesion pain, however, is more likely to be attributable to the neurological consequences of SCI. This may represent either the supraspinal consequences of denervation or a focus of hyperexcitability in the spinal cord, both consistent with a central pain syndrome [18].

Tasker and colleagues [58] reported clinical features and types of pain in 127 patients with SCI central pain [18]. The spontaneous pain was characterized as steady (95% of patients), intermittent (often shooting, 31%), and evoked (allodynia, hyperpathia, or hyperesthesia, 45%). Steady pain was described as thermal (burning in 75% and cold in 4%) or dysesthetic (tingling in 28%), and mechanical (aching in 13%, pressure in 18%, and rhythmic in 9%). A steady, burning, dysesthetic component was the most common in a study of 102 SCI patients [26].

Allodynia occurred in 47% of patients in Tasker's [57, 58] series, but only in areas of preserved sensation. Taking complete and incomplete SCI lesions together, it occurred in 21% as a band at the upper level of the sensory loss, as a diffuse sensation in 29%, and as a patchy sensation in 50%. In another series, allodynia was reported in dermatomes at the lesion level in 8 out of 20 patients with central pain resulting from SCI, below the lesion level in one patient and diffusely, including the face, in another patient [27].

SCI patients with central pain may also have an elevated heat pain threshold above the lesion level; and this threshold may be returned to normal or near normal following a pain-relieving dorsal root entry zone (DREZ) lesion [20]. This suggests that an intact afferent innervation sustains a pain-generating focus in the intact spinal or supraspinal structures. In a related study of SCI patients, Defrin and colleagues [20] found that both the threshold and the quality of pain produced by heat or cold were dependent upon the integrity of innocuous thermal sensations, a finding that highlights the interaction between nociceptive and non-nociceptive pathways in the CNS.

Patients with SCI central pain have a loss of spinothalamic tract (STT)-mediated thermal sensation, pain sensation, or both on quantitative sensory testing (QST) ([3, 28], see also [24]). This loss of sensation does not identify those patients with SCI central pain from among all patients with SCI [28]. Therefore, this pattern of sensory loss is a necessary but not sufficient condition for the development of SCI central pain. The pattern of sensory loss suggests that the STT must be damaged in patients with SCI central pain, an observation that is consistent with the incidence of central pain following anterolateral cordotomy [40].

SCI patients with central pain more frequently have hypersensitivity to mechanical and cold stimulation in dermatomes corresponding to the lesion level, compared with those without central pain [28]. The intensity of brush-evoked pain at the lesion level was correlated with spontaneous pain below the level of the injury. These findings suggest that activity at the lesion level mediates SCI central pain, and are consistent with the finding that sensory thresholds were returned to normal or near normal following a pain-relieving DREZ lesion in these patients [20]. These findings are also consistent with a model in which below injury level spontaneous pain results from brainstem, thalamic, and cortical neurons, which normally receive input in somatic sensory pathways (see below).

CLINICAL FEATURES OF CPSP

The clinical features of patients with SCI central pain are congruent with those of patients with CPSP. CPSP can arise from lesions of many different etiologies above the spinal–medullary junction, but is most commonly the result of a stroke [57]. Both CPSP and SCI central pain have sensory loss for thermal or pain modalities, in addition to spontaneous and evoked pain. Burning and aching are commonly endorsed qualitative pain descriptors [29, 39]. The pain may be increased in cold ambient temperatures even though cold allodynia is absent. Patients will often identify the temporal–spatial characteristics of the pain as diffuse, poorly localized, and constant. Clinical studies show that loss of thermal sensation, pain sensation, or both is necessary for the development of central pain [7, 12, 39, 53].

A descriptive report of 73 patients with CPSP found that the onset of pain is often delayed, consistent with the previous studies [57]. Pain in CPSP is commonly characterized as steady (usually burning 64.4%), dysesthetic (31.6%), intermittent (16.4%), and with allodynia or hyperalgesia (64.9%). The distribution of intermittent pain is similar to that of spontaneous pain overall, and to that of sensory loss. The onset of central pain was delayed between 1 and 4 weeks in 47–63%, and greater than 4 weeks in approximately 20% [1, 8, 57]. Distribution of pain was not related to features of the lesion, including size, side, or location of the lesion; similarly, neither quality nor severity of the pain was related to the degree of sensory loss, age, or sex of the patient.

There are three series of CPSP patients in which QST was carried out and descriptors of pain qualities were determined. In the most recent series, the patient's ongoing pain was described by most patients using temperature or mechanical descriptors [29], consistent with prior studies [9, 59]. Patients had average pain ratings of between 2.5 and 7.5 (visual analogue score, VAS).

QST can be used to identify both allodynia (pain evoked by a stimulus that is never normally painful) and hyperalgesia (increased pain evoked by a stimulus that is normally painful). Hypoesthesia and hypoalgesia are decreased sensations evoked by nonpainful and painful stimuli, respectively. Studies of QST in individual patients with CPSP documented tactile hypoesthesia in 27–52% of the patients tested [9, 29, 59] cf [11]). Tactile allodynia or hyperalgesia was found in 9–59%; the wide difference in incidence may be due to differences in the QST protocol [9, 59].

These studies reported a large proportion of CPSP patients with cool hypoesthesia (63–85%), although 0–23% showed cold allodynia [9, 29, 59]. All studies reported a large proportion of patients with warm hypoesthesia (85–100%), but no clear abnormal cases of heat allodynia (0% to borderline in 7%). A study correlating sensory loss with hypersensitivity found that tactile and cold hypoesthesia were significantly correlated with preservation in tactile and cold modalities, respectively [29]. As in the case of SCI central pain, cold and tactile hypoesthesia and allodynia were common but not necessary features among patients with CPSP. The development of these features of CPSP may be restricted to the anatomy of lesions involving different structures in the brain.

THE THALAMIC REGION OF Vc AND ITS IMPORTANCE IN PAIN PROCESSING

The thalamus has long been suggested to be the structure that acts as a generator for central pain by disinhibition [21]. Spontaneous thalamic neuronal activity is often categorized as either bursting activity (spike bursts, bursting mode) or tonic firing (tonic mode) [54]. Many studies have suggested that increased spike-bursting occurs in the thalamus of patients with chronic pain [35, 42, 51] and acute pain [38, 43].

Several lines of evidence demonstrate that the ventral caudal nucleus of the human sensory thalamus (Vc), the human analogue of the monkey ventral posterior (VP) nucleus [32], is important in human pain-signalling pathways. Studies of patients at autopsy following lesions of the STT show the densest STT termination in the Vc region, including posterior and inferior subnuclei of Vc, suprageniculate, and posterior subnuclei [10, 45, 46, 61]. In monkeys, STT terminations are found in the VMpo nucleus, which appears, by immunohistochemistry and physiology, to have a human analogue [6, 17]. In addition, neurons in Vc and VMpo respond to painful and thermal stimuli [37], while stimulation of this area leads to thermal and painful sensations [48], and lesions of this area diminish pain and thermal sensations [36]. These findings firmly establish Vc and VMpo as structures subserving thermal and pain sensations.

THE DISINHIBITION HYPOTHESIS: ANATOMY OF LESIONS RESULTING IN CPSP

In a study of patients with pure somatic sensory stroke (n = 21), the small vessel strokes were confined to the posterior lateral thalamus and probably involved the principal somatic sensory nucleus of the thalamus (Vc, ventral caudal). All involved either tactile or thermal/pain sensations or both, and nine were located in the VP lateral thalamus, which probably included the principal somatic sensory nucleus, Vc [32, 52]. Therefore, lesions of the pain and temperature somatic sensory pathway in the posterior thalamus are strongly associated with CPSP.

In another study, QST was carried out in four patients with CPSP and small lesions in the region of thalamic nucleus Vc, as shown in Fig. 32-1. These results were used as a test of the hypothesis that thalamic lesions leading to central pain and loss of cold sensitivity must include the region posterior to Vc, including VMpo (posterior part of the ventral medial nucleus); VMpo is indicated in Fig. 32-1 by the light grey shape marked with an asterisk. Most of the atlas maps shown in this figure do not include VMpo, because it is outside the borders of the lesion [6].

All four patients had lesions within the posterior half of Vc; in two patients, the thalamic lesion was limited to ventral Vc (patients 3 and 8). In the other two, the lesions were located in dorsal Vc and extended posterior to Vc proper into the Vcpor and pulvinar oral nuclei, that receive STT input (patients 13 and 18) [2, 45, 46]. In none of these lesions was there any involvement of VMpo. These patients demonstrate that involvement of Vc in lesions in a thalamic stroke is sufficient to cause CPSP or the central dysesthesia syndrome. VMpo need not be involved.

All four patients had alterations of cold pain sensation, while three patients had altered cool sensation (subjects 8, 13, and 18). The other patient (number 3) had the smallest lesion, which was limited to Vc. Heat pain perception was not impaired in any of the four lesions, but was impaired with a larger lesion of Vc [47]. Tactile perception was always impaired on the involved side. Therefore, lesions of Vc not involving regions posterior to Vc such as ventral medial posterior (VMpo [15]) are sufficient to impair cold sensibility and to produce CPSP.

The recent version of the disinhibition hypothesis proposes that central pain results from a lesion involving a cold-signalling pathway that projects to the insula through VMpo [16]. In patients with CPSP, the authors proposed that a lesion of this pathway disinhibits a medial STT pain-signalling pathway projecting to the anterior cingulate cortex (ACC) via the medial dorsal nucleus [14, 16]. According to this hypothesis, lesions of VMpo lead to cold hypoesthesia, and to the disinhibition of the ACC, which results in the burning pain of CPSP. Therefore, the location of thalamic and cortical strokes in CPSP provides a critical test of this hypothesis.

Prior studies have used computerized tomography to localize lesions in thalamus in patients with central pain (n = 12). In four cases, the lesions involved the thalamus, but all cases involved other structures in addition to the thalamus [1]. In a similar study of 27 patients with CPSP, 9 out of 27 had thalamic lesions, 2 of which were limited to the thalamus, and the rest could not be further specified [39]. In a more recent study, which used MRI scans, most patients (49/70) had lesions that included the "ventral posterior nucleus" (corresponding to Vc) [12]. As described above, MRI- and atlas-based methods have demonstrated thalamic small vessel strokes leading to CPSP that did not involve VMpo [36, 47], contrary to the disinhibition hypothesis.

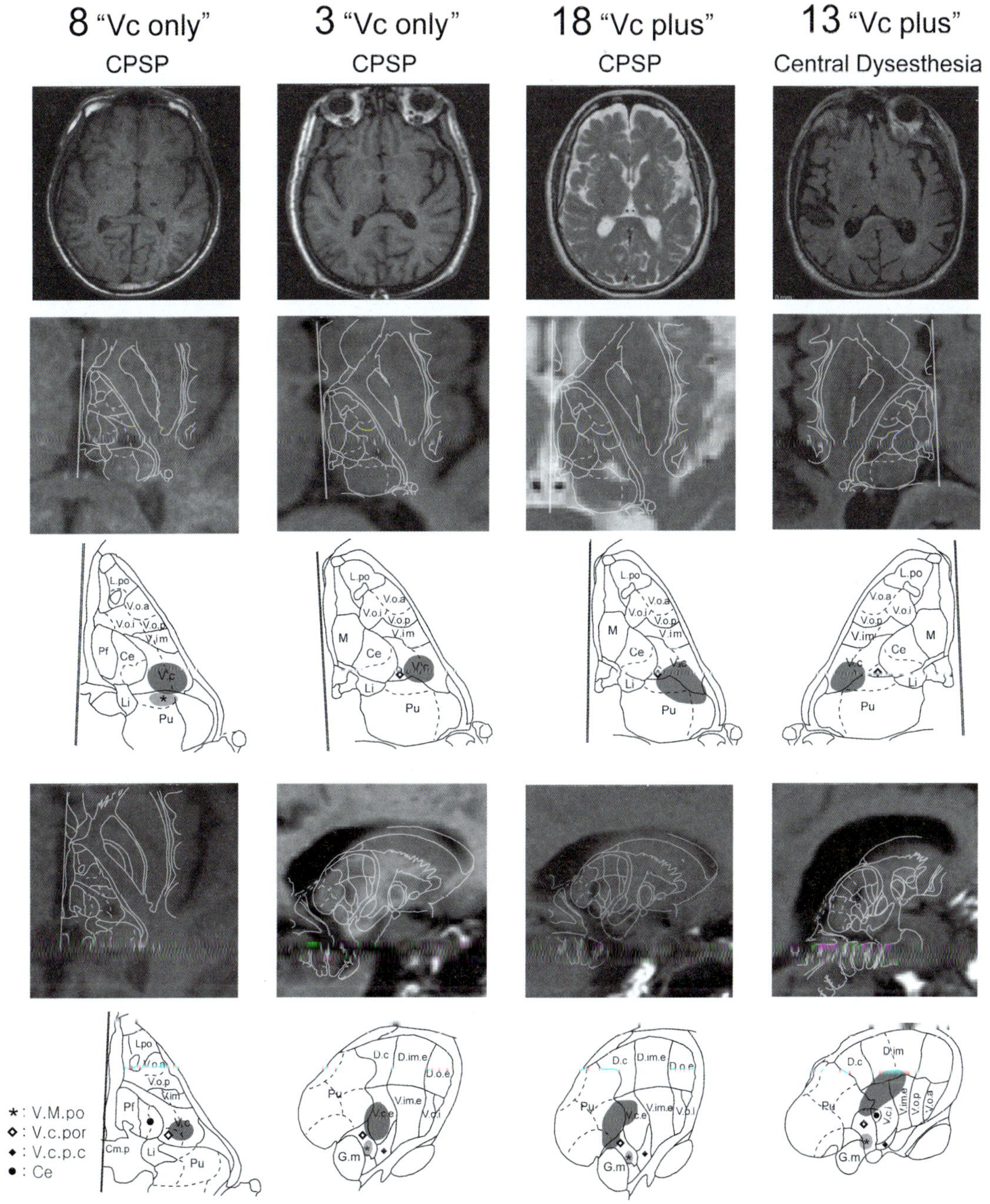

FIGURE 32-1 Locations of the thalamic lesions. Images taken through the centre of these lesions in the axial and sagittal planes are shown through thalamus and basal ganglia in rows 1, 2, and 4. Images in rows 2 and 4 are overlaid with outlines of the atlas maps of these structures as described above. Rows 3 and 5 show the area of the lesion relative to the outline of nuclei as estimated from the Schaltenbrand atlas for patients 3, 13, and 18. In patient 8, the axial section in row 4 is above the axial section above that in rows 1 and 2.

Other lines of evidence help to evaluate this hypothesis. Approximately 50% of patients with CPSP do not have pain described by temperature, and less than 30% have cold allodynia [29]. Cold allodynia was not associated with impaired cold sensibility, but was associated with preserved cold sensibility [29], although cool hypoesthesia was frequently present. Therefore, diminution of cold sensations is not necessary for the development of CPSP, as predicted by the disinhibition hypothesis.

In the cases of CPSP with cold allodynia, the disinhibition hypothesis suggests that ACC should be activated in response to cold stimuli. There are a number of imaging studies that do not support this suggestion. A subject with cold allodynia (patient 3) was studied with a single-subject PET protocol during the response to immersion of either hand in a 20°C water bath. The scan during stimulation of the affected hand was characterized by intense activation of contralateral sensorimotor cortex and no significant activation of ACC.

Activations are shown in Fig. 32-2 for the stimulation of the affected (A) and unaffected hands (U), as labelled. Stimulation of the allodynic hand produced strong activation of the sensorimotor cortex around the contralateral central sulcus (red arrowheads, left row, and bottom of middle row). There is no evidence of activation of the ACC, which is seen in the most dorsal nine MRI cuts. Among the more posterior structures, there was activation of the S2/inferior parietal lobule region contralaterally with S2 indicated by a dark blue circle (top right row) and by a light blue circle below the intraparietal sulcus (top middle row). Finally, there was increased blood flow in the contralateral insula/retroinsula and decreased blood flow in the ipsilateral insula/retroinsula (orange circle, right row—second image down). With stimulation of the unaffected hand, there was a similar pattern of activation involving contralateral sensorimotor cortex, inferior frontal gyrus, bilateral prefrontal cortex, inferior parietal lobule/secondary somatosensory cortex (S2), and insula/retroinsula and decreased blood flow in the ipsilateral insula/retroinsula.

These results demonstrate that in patient 3, immersion of the affected hand in 20°C water produced hyperalgesia and significantly increased activation in the contralateral cortex, compared with stimulation of the other hand. The largest PET study of CPSP-induced cold allodynia involved patients with a lateral medullary stroke (Wallenberg syndrome) [49] (see also [13, 33]). The allodynic test stimulus was a cold/mechanical cutaneous stimulus, which produced an activation similar to that with the water bath, described above. Therefore, the evidence from existing imaging studies demonstrates that cold allodynia is associated with activation of sensorimotor cortex, but not ACC.

Patients with SCI central pain uniformly had loss of pain or temperature sensation or both [3, 24, 28]. However, the degree of sensory loss for thermal or pain modalities is not a predictor of the presence of central pain among the population of patients with SCI [24, 28]. Therefore, the loss of STT function is a necessary but not sufficient condition for the development of central pain in patients with SCI. Abnormal hypersensitivity to tactile and thermal stimuli is more common in SCI patients with central pain than in those without. The intensity of tactile allodynia at the border of sensory loss is a significant predictor of the intensity of spontaneous pain in the levels below the lesion. SCI central pain patients show normalization of some changes in sensibility following successful DREZ lesions. This result suggests that intact afferent innervation sustains a pain-generating activity above the level of injury or in supraspinal structures. In addition, both the threshold and the quality of thermal pain were strongly dependent upon the integrity of innocuous thermal sensations [20], as in the study of CPSP described above [29].

The results of morphologic imaging suggest that lesions of Vc proper are more likely to lead to CPSP than are lesions of VMpo. Clinical and QST results are more consistent with spared, rather than impaired, sensory pathways contributing to hypersensitivity and spontaneous central pain. Functional imaging studies show that cold allodynia is more likely to be associated with activation of sensorimotor cortex rather than ACC. These results are consistent with a model in which central pain is due to disinhibition of the low-threshold pathway from dorsal columns to Vc thalamus to the sensorimotor cortex. In both CPSP and SCI central pain, a brain structure acts as a generator for signals that are responsible for the

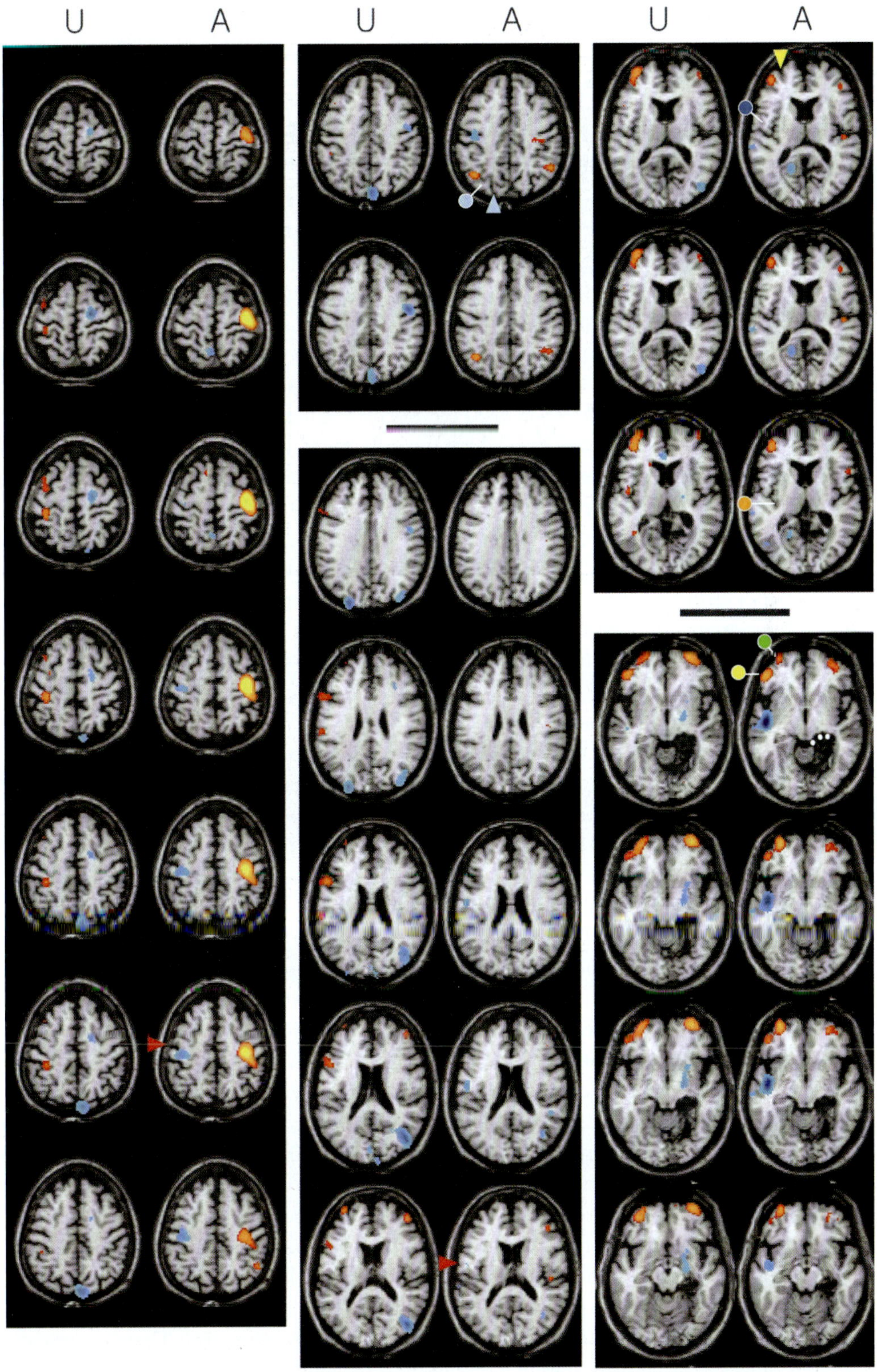

FIGURE 32-2 Blood flow consequences of 20°C water bath stimulation of the affected and unaffected hands in a patient with CPSP (patient 3)**.** PET blood flow data are displayed in colour on the structural MRI images as appropriate. The coloured areas on the scan indicate *t*-scores, red–yellow for increases, and blue for decreases in blood flow with respect to resting conditions. Coloured symbols indicate sulci (*arrowhead*) and gyri (*circles*) (see text).

symptoms of central pain. Characteristic changes in thalamic activity or functional mode may act as a generator of symptoms in central pain syndromes.

IS THALAMIC FUNCTIONAL MODE ALTERED IN CHRONIC PAIN STATES?

Spontaneous thalamic neuronal activity is often categorized as either bursting activity (spike bursts, bursting mode) or tonic firing (tonic mode) [54]. Many studies have suggested that increased spike-bursting occurs in the thalamus of patients with chronic pain [35, 42, 51] and acute pain [38, 43].

Spike-bursting activity refers to a particular pattern of interspike intervals (ISIs) between action potentials, such that a spike burst begins after a relatively long ISI (60 ms), and begins with a short ISI (typically <6 ms) [42]. Thereafter, the ISIs progressively lengthen, so that the cell's firing decelerates throughout the spike burst, from ISIs of less than 6 ms to an ISI of greater than 16 ms. Between bursts, cells fire in single spikes at a frequency of 10–20 Hz.

In patients with spinal transection, the highest rate of bursting occurs in cells that do not have peripheral receptive fields and that are located in the representation of the anaesthetic part of the body. These cells also have the lowest firing rates in the interval between bursts (principal event rate) [42]. The low firing rates suggest that these cells have decreased tonic excitatory drive and are hyperpolarized, perhaps due to loss of excitatory input from the STT [5, 23, 25]. Therefore, the available evidence suggests that affected thalamic cells in patients with spinal transection are dominated by spike-bursting consistent with membrane hyperpolarization [34, 55].

Spike-bursting activity is maximal in the region posterior and inferior to the core nucleus of Vc (Table 4 in [42]). Stimulation in this area evokes the sensation of pain more frequently than does stimulation in the core of Vc [22, 30, 31, 44, 48]. Thus, increased spike-bursting activity may be correlated with some aspects of the abnormal sensations (e.g., dysesthesia or chronic spontaneous pain) that patients with SCI central pain experience. In patients with spinal transection, the painful area and the area of sensory loss overlap [42, 50]. Here, the bursting activity might be related to sensory loss rather than to pain.

These findings about spike-bursting activity in spinal patients have been called into question by a study in patients with chronic pain [50]. It has been reported that the number of bursting cells per trajectory in patients with movement disorders (controls) is not different from that in patients with chronic pain. However, there are significant differences between the two studies [63] in terms of patient population (SCI vs. mixed chronic pain), location of cells studied (Vc vs. anterior and posterior to Vc), and analysis methods (incidence of bursting cells vs. bursting parameters). Clearly, the increase in bursting activity demonstrated in the earlier study is more applicable to the region of the principal somatic sensory nucleus of patients with central pain from spinal transection [60].

Further support for increased spike bursts occurring in patients with spinal cord transection is found in thalamic recordings from monkeys with thoracic anterolateral cordotomies [3]. Some of these animals showed increased responsiveness to electrocutaneous stimuli, and thus this may represent a model of central pain [55]. The most pronounced changes in firing pattern were found in thalamic multireceptive cells that respond to both cutaneous brushing and compressive stimuli with activity that is not graded into the noxious range. In comparison with normal controls, multireceptive cells in the monkeys with cordotomies showed significant increases in the number of bursts occurring spontaneously or in response to brushing or compressive stimuli. The changes in bursting behaviour were widespread, occurring in the thalamic representation of upper and lower extremities, both ipsilateral and contralateral to the cordotomy.

In addition to an increase in spike-bursting activity in chronic pain states, there also appears to be a relationship between spike-burst firing and acute pain. The cellular response in Vc to painful and nonpainful mechanical and thermal stimuli is characterized by spike bursts, which are preceded by periods of inhibition [38]. The cold response cells seem to exhibit this nonlinear response more readily than cells responding to other modalities.

Spike bursts are also found in the thalamic representation of the monkey upper extremity and in the thalamic representation of the arm and leg ipsilateral to the cordotomy. Pain is not typically experienced in these parts of the body in patients with thoracic spinal cord transection or cordotomy [42, 57]. Spike bursts are increased in frequency during slow wave sleep in all mammals studied, including humans [19, 41]. However, such bursting could cause pain if stimulation in the vicinity of the bursting cell produced the sensation of pain. This finding has been reported in two recent studies of sensations evoked by stimulation of the region of Vc in patients with chronic pain secondary to neural injury [41].

Thus, there is evidence from both human and nonhuman primate studies for a relationship between chronic pain states and an altered thalamic neuronal firing pattern [42, 62]. It appears that there is an increase in spike-burst firing in chronic pain conditions although spike-bursting is found in parts of VP thalamus representing parts of the body where patients with SCI experience spontaneous and evoked pain. This activity would result in increased activation of the primary somatic sensory cortex [36, 49, 56]. The exact physiological relationships that link the pattern of thalamic firing to the human perception of chronic pain have yet to be elucidated.

ACKNOWLEDGEMENT

This work was supported by the National Institutes of Health—National Institute of Neurological Disorders and Stroke (NS38493 to FAL) and the Johns Hopkins Neurosurgical Pain Research Institute.

CONFLICT OF INTEREST

None of the authors have conflicts of interest related to this work, which is in accordance with the statement of ethical standards for manuscripts submitted to *Journal of Neuroscience*.

REFERENCES

1. Andersen P, Vestergaard K, Ingeman-Nielsen M, Jensen TS. Incidence of post-stroke central pain. Pain 1995;61:187–93.
2. Apkarian AV, Hodge CJ. Primate spinothalamic pathways, III: thalamic terminations of the dorsolateral and ventral spinothalamic pathways. J Comp Neurol 1989;288:493–511.
3. Beric A, Dimitrijevic MR, Lindblom U. Central dysesthesia syndrome in spinal cord injury patients. Pain 1988;34:109–16.
4. Biemond A. The conduction of pain above the level of the thalamus opticus. AMA Arch Neurol Psychiatry 1956;75:231–44.

5. Blomqvist A, Ericson AC, Craig AD, Broman J. Evidence for glutamate as a neurotransmitter in spinothalamic tract terminals in the posterior region of owl monkeys. Exp Brain Res 1996;108:33–44.
6. Blomqvist A, Zhang ET, Craig AD. Cytoarchitectonic and immunohistochemical characterization of a specific pain and temperature relay, the posterior portion of the ventral medial nucleus, in the human thalamus. Brain 2000;123(Pt 3):601–19.
7. Bogousslavsky J, Regli F, Uske A. Thalamic infarcts: clinical syndromes, etiology and prognosis. Neurology 1988;38:837–48.
8. Boivie J, Leijon G. Clinical findings in patients with central poststroke pain. In: Casey KL, editor. Pain and central nervous system disease. New York, NY: Raven Press; 1991. pp. 65–75.
9. Boivie J, Leijon G, Johansson I. Central post-stroke pain—a study of the mechanisms through analyses of the sensory abnormalities. Pain 1989;37:173–85.
10. Bowsher D. Termination of the central pain pathway in man: the conscious appreciation of pain. Brain 1957;80:606–20.
11. Bowsher D. Central pain: clinical and physiological characteristics. J Neurol Neurosurg Psychiatry 1996;61:62–9.
12. Bowsher D, Leijon G, Thuomas KA. Central poststroke pain: correlation of MRI with clinical pain characteristics and sensory abnormalities. Neurology 1998;51:1352–8.
13. Cesaro P, Mann MW, Moretti JL, Defer G, Roualdes B, Nguyen JP, Degos JD. Central pain and thalamic hyperactivity: a single photon emission computerized tomographic study. Pain 1991;47:329–36.
14. Craig AD. The functional anatomy of lamina I and its role in post-stroke central pain. In: Sandkühler J, Bromm B, Gebhart GF, editors. Nervous system plasticity and chronic pain. Amsterdam, the Netherlands: Elsevier; 2000. pp. 137–51.
15. Craig AD, Blomqvist A. Is there a specific lamina I spinothalamocortical pathway for pain and temperature sensations in primates? J Pain 2002;3:95–101.
16. Craig AD, Reiman EM, Evans A, Bushnell MC. Functional imaging of an illusion of pain. Nature 1996;384:258–60.
17. Craig AD, Zhang ET. Retrograde analyses of spinothalamic projections in the macaque monkey: input to posterolateral thalamus. J Comp Neurol 2006;499:953–964.
18. Davidoff G, Roth E. Clinical characteristics of central (dysesthetic) pain syndrome in spinal cord injury patients. In: Casey KL, editor. Pain and central nervous system diseases: the central pain syndromes. New York, NY: Raven Press; 1991. pp. 77–83.
19. Davis KD, Kiss ZHT, Tasker RR, Dostrovsky JO. Thalamic stimulation-evoked sensations in chronic pain patients and nonpain (movement disorder) patients. J Neurophysiol 1996;75:1026–37.
20. Defrin R, Ohry A, Blumen N, Urca G. Sensory determinants of thermal pain. Brain 2002;125:501–10.
21. Dejerine J, Roussy G. La syndrome thalamique. Rev Neurol 1906;14:521–32.
22. Dostrovsky JO, Wells FEB, Tasker RR. Pain evoked by stimulation in human thalamus. In: Sjigenaga Y, editor. International symposium on processing nociceptive information. Amsterdam, the Netherlands: Elsevier; 1991. pp. 115–120.
23. Dougherty PM, Li YJ, Lenz FA, Rowland L, Mittman S. Evidence that excitatory amino acids mediate afferent input to the primate somatosensory thalamus. Brain Res 1996;278:267–73.
24. Eide PK. Pathophysiological mechanisms of central neuropathic pain after spinal cord injury. Spinal Cord 1998;36:601–12.
25. Ericson AC, Blomqvist A, Craig AD, Ottersen OP, Broman J. Enrichment of glutamate-like immunoreactivity in spinothalamic tract terminals in the nucleus submedius of cat. Soc Neurosci Abstr 1993;18:832.
26. Fenollosa P, Pallares J, Cervera J, Pelegrin F, Inigo V, Giner M, Forner V. Chronic pain in the spinal cord injured: statistical approach and pharmacological treatment. Paraplegia 1993;31:722–9.
27. Finnerup NB, Johannesen IL, Bach FW, Jensen TS. Sensory function above lesion level in spinal cord injury patients with and without pain. Somatosens Mot Res 2003;20:71–6.
28. Finnerup NB, Johannesen IL, Fuglsang-Frederiksen A, Bach FW, Jensen TS. Sensory function in spinal cord injury patients with and without central pain. Brain 2003;126:57–70.
29. Greenspan JD, Ohara S, Sarlani E, Lenz FA. Allodynia in patients with post-stroke central pain (CPSP) studied by statistical quantitative sensory testing within individuals. Pain 2004;109:357–66.
30. Halliday AM, Logue V. Painful sensations evoked by electrical stimulation in the thalamus. In: Somjen GG, editor. Neurophysiology studied in man. Amsterdam, the Netherlands: Excerpta Medica; 1972. pp. 221–30.
31. Hassler R, Reichert T. Klinische und anatomische Befunde bei stereotaktischen Schmerzoperationen im Thalamus. Arch Psychiat Nerverkr 1959;200:93–122.
32. Hirai T, Jones EG. A new parcellation of the human thalamus on the basis of histochemical staining. Brain Res Rev 1989;14:1–34.

33. Hirato M, Watanabe K, Takahashi A, Hayase N, Horikoshi S, Shibasaki T, Ohye C. Pathophysiology of central (thalamic) pain: combined change of sensory thalamus with cerebral cortex around central sulcus. Stereotact Funct Neurosurg 1994;62:300–3.
34. Jahnsen H, Llinas R. Electrophysiological properties of guinea-pig thalamic neurones: an in vitro study. J Physiol 1984;349:205–26.
35. Jeanmonod D, Magnin M, Morel A. A thalamic concept of neurogenic pain. In: Gebhart GF, Hammond DL, Jensen TS, editors. Progress in pain research and management. Proceedings of the 7th World Congress on Pain, Vol. 2. Seattle, WA: IASP Press; 1994. pp. 767–787.
36. Kim JH, Greenspan JD, Coghill RC, Ohara S, Lenz FA. Lesions limited to the human thalamic principal somatosensory nucleus (ventral caudal) are associated with loss of cold sensations and central pain. J Neurosci 2007;27:4995–5004.
37. Lee J, Dougherty PM, Antezana D, Lenz FA. Responses of neurons in the region of human thalamic principal somatic sensory nucleus to mechanical and thermal stimuli graded into the painful range. J Comp Neurol 1999;410:541–55.
38. Lee JI, Ohara S, Dougherty PM, Lenz FA. Pain and temperature encoding in the human thalamic somatic sensory nucleus (ventral caudal): inhibition-related bursting evoked by somatic stimuli. J Neurophysiol 2005;94:1676–687.
39. Leijon G, Boivie J, Johansson I. Central post-stroke pain-neurological symptoms and pain characteristics. Pain 1989;36:13–25.
40. Lenz FA, Casey KL, Jones EG, Willis WD Jr. The human pain system: experimental and clinical perspectives. New York, NY: Cambridge University Press; 2010.
41. Lenz FA, Gracely RH, Baker FH, Richardson RT, Dougherty PM. Reorganization of sensory modalities evoked by microstimulation in region of the thalamic principal sensory nucleus in patients with pain due to nervous system injury. J Comp Neurol 1998;399:125–38.
42. Lenz FA, Kwan HC, Martin R, Tasker R, Richardson RT, Dostrovsky JO. Characteristics of somatotopic organization and spontaneous neuronal activity in the region of the thalamic principal sensory nucleus in patients with spinal cord transection. J Neurophysiol 1994;72:1570–87.
43. Lenz FA, Ohara S, Gracely RH, Dougherty PM, Patel SH. Pain encoding in the human forebrain: binary and analog exteroceptive channels. J Neurosci 2004;24:6540–4.
44. Lenz FA, Seike M, Richardson RT, Lin YC, Baker FH, Khoja I, Jaeger CJ, Gracely RH. Thermal and pain sensations evoked by microstimulation in the area of human ventrocaudal nucleus. J Neurophysiol 1993;70:200–12.
45. Mehler WR. The anatomy of the so-called "pain tract" in man: an analysis of the course and distribution of the ascending fibers of the fasciculus anterolateralis. In: French JD, Porter RW, editors. Basic research in paraplegia. Springfield, MA: Charles C. Thomas; 1962. pp. 26–55.
46. Mehler WR, Feferman ME, Nauta WHJ. Ascending axon degeneration following anterolateral cordotomy. An experimental study in the monkey. Brain 1960;83:718–50.
47. Montes C, Magnin M, Maarrawi J, Frot M, Convers P, Mauguiere F, Garcia-Larrea L. Thalamic thermo-algesic transmission: ventral posterior (VP) complex versus VMpo in the light of a thalamic infarct with central pain. Pain 2005;113:223–32.
48. Ohara S, Lenz FA. Medial lateral extent of thermal and pain sensations evoked by microstimulation in somatic sensory nuclei of human thalamus. J Neurophysiol 2003;90:2367–77.
49. Peyron R, Garcia-Larrea L, Gregoire MC, Convers P, Lavenne F, Veyre L, Froment JC, Mauguiere F, Michel D, Laurent B. Allodynia after lateral-medullary (Wallenberg) infart: a PET study. Brain 1998;121:345–56.
50. Radhakrishnan V, Tsoukatos J, Davis KD, Tasker RR, Lozano AM, Dostrovsky JO. A comparison of the burst activity of lateral thalamic neurons in chronic pain and non-pain patients. Pain 1999;80:567–75.
51. Rinaldi PC, Young RF, Albe-Fessard DG, Chodakiewitz J. Spontaneous neuronal hyperactivity in the medial and intralaminar thalamic nuclei in patients with deafferentation pain. J Neurosurg 1991;74:415–21.
52. Schaltenbrand G, Walker AE. Stereotaxy of the human brain. New York, NY: Thieme-Stratton; 1982.
53. Schmahmann JD, Leifer D. Parietal pseudothalamic pain syndrome: clinical features and anatomic correlates. Arch Neurol 1992;49:1032–7.
54. Steriade M, Jones EG, Llinas RR. Thalamic oscillations and signaling. New York, NY: Wiley, John & Sons; 1990.
55. Steriade M, Jones EG, McCormick DA. Thalamic, organization and chemical neuroanatomy. In: Thalamus, Vol. 1. Amsterdam, the Netherlands: Elsevier; 1997. pp. 269–338.
56. Swadlow HA, Gusev AG. The impact of 'bursting' thalamic impulses at a neocortical synapse. Nat Neurosci 2001;4:402–408.

57. Tasker RR. Central pain states. In: Loeser JD, editor. Bonica's management of pain. Philadelphia, PA: Lippincott Williams & Wilkins; 2002.
58. Tasker RR, DeCarvalho GT, Dolan EJ. Intractable pain of spinal cord origin: clinical features and implications for surgery. J Neurosurg 1992;77:373–8.
59. Vestergaard K, Nielsen J, Andersen G, Ingeman-Nielsen M, Arendt-Nielsen L, Jensen TS. Sensory abnormalities in consecutive unselected patients with central post-stroke pain. Pain 1995;61:177–86.
60. Vierck CJ, Greenspan JD, Ritz LA. Long-term changes in purposive and reflexive responses to nociceptive stimulation following anterolateral chordotomy. J Neurosci 1990;10:2077–95.
61. Walker AE. Central representation of pain. Res Publ Assoc Res Nerv Ment Dis 1943;23:63–85.
62. Weng HR, Lee J-I, Lenz FA, Vierck CJ, Rowland LH, Dougherty PM. Functional plasticity in primate somatosensory thalamus following chronic lesion of the ventral lateral spinal cord. Neuroscience 2000;101:393–401.
63. Weng HR, Lenz FA, Vierck C, Dougherty PM. Physiological changes in primate somatosensory thalamus induced by deafferentation are dependent on the spinal funiculi that are sectioned and time following injury. Neuroscience 2003;116:1149–60.

CHAPTER 33

Pharmacological fMRI

David Borsook, Tor D. Wager, and Irene Tracey

In the early days of fMRI, if a study incorporated an acutely or chronically administered drug either alone or in combination with a task (i.e., giving a painful stimulus), it was referred to as a pharmacological MRI (phMRI) study. Many paradigms now include a drug challenge as part of the overall design or manipulation, and so there is nothing particularly "special" about phMRI; yet the expression and term remains and will be employed here. Several recent reviews provide a comprehensive overview of the field and the potential application and benefit for analgesic drug discovery in the industrial setting [7, 8, 67, 69]. Although other technologies could be used alongside drug administration, it is true that the field is led by clinical fMRI but with more preclinical studies now occurring. The key feature of fMRI use is its ability to measure alterations and responsivity of neural circuits with respect to pharmacological manipulation. Neural circuits provide "a language of translation" between preclinical species and humans [8], and as such, phMRI studies allow for extrapolation of efficacy from preclinical models to humans more objectively. Before we explicitly discuss the use of phMRI for analgesic drug discovery, we shall discuss some more generic aspects of how phMRI informs our understanding of pain, pain mechanisms, and their modulation as well as analgesia.

BACKGROUND

Whether neuroimaging information is neurochemical, structural, or functional, a range of CNS disorders have undoubtedly benefited from an improved scientific understanding of the mechanistic changes that occur *in vivo* and over time as the condition develops or improves naturally or with treatment. This is particularly true for acute and chronic pain where dramatic strides in our understanding of underpinning mechanisms have occurred, as discussed extensively in other chapters. We must remember that "functional" imaging is a powerful tool for measuring how the brain is processing and modulating nociceptive inputs to produce pain perceptions and not, as is often stated, the "holy grail" and objective "surrogate" of pain ratings. Rather, it is a "behind the scenes" measure distinct from, but obviously related to, subjective descriptions and ratings of pain—a process that uses its own tools for assessment. Many factors contribute to pain ratings that, irrespective of the nociceptive input or even the presence of strong analgesics, mean divergences and more complex relationships can occur between what a patient reports and his or her measured regional brain activity [18]. This has tremendous value for drug discovery and can provide confidence that your compound has target engagement or is attenuating nociceptive processing *in vivo*, so long as the conditions discussed at the end of this chapter are borne in mind and met.

The fact that subjects might not show a statistical improvement in subjective rating when using any of our developed pain scales is not an exclusive reason to throw the drug out at this early stage of development (e.g., at Phase 2), and yet this has very likely happened. A recent study by Harris and colleagues [23] alongside the study by Bingel and colleagues [5, 6] illustrates this point well [55].

CNS MODIFICATION VERSUS ANALGESIA

Additional measures, for example, structural or neurochemical, provide clues as to the underlying mechanisms sustaining and exacerbating a chronic pain state (e.g., central sensitization, alterations in descending pain modulation, anxiety, catastrophizing, and depression). Further, neuroimaging has powerfully illustrated how the pain condition itself changes the brain and spinal cord (both directly via nociceptive inputs and sensitization and indirectly via changes in lifestyle, biomechanics, etc.). Undoubtedly, neuroimaging highlighted the impact of unmanaged chronic pain on the brain and raised the stakes regarding better treatment and management. To test the clinical relevance of any of these neuroimaging-based measures, one can treat the patient, say pharmacologically, and see how the measures change relative to gold-standard clinical/behavioural measures. This helps our understanding of neuroimaging-based measures from being purely correlative to more causal in their nature. However, given the differences in sensitivity of behavioural and neuroimaging measures alongside the complex relationship between brain processing of nociceptive inputs and subjective pain ratings, it is possible that a treatment can change structure, function, or neurochemistry in the absence of a significantly altered pain rating on a particular scale chosen. This possibility throws up an interesting question. If neuroimaging shows that a patient's brain is "normalized" post-treatment to that of an age-matched healthy control subject, but there is no pain relief, is that a good thing? This is discussed in a recent editorial [55]. Correcting aberrant mechanisms with or without concomitant pain relief is now measurable because of brain imaging, but it raises interesting questions for the community. What has certainly been shown, thankfully, is that even patients with years of chronic pain and measurable changes in chemistry and structure when treated for their pain successfully reverse these changes and have "normal" looking brains from a structural perspective [22, 47], highlighting the tremendous plasticity of the CNS and our ability to intervene still.

EARLY OR BASELINE PREDICTORS OF RESPONSE

The next challenge for neuroimaging is to deliver statistically robust information at an individual level, rather than group averaging neural responses, which has been the common approach to date for phMRI studies examining analgesic mechanisms [27, 33, 66, 68, 70]. Individualized measures allow identified mechanisms with their concomitant neuroimaging markers to be related to your patient and their particular set of symptoms, possibly even providing measures that predict treatment response. Studies are now being published that highlight how neuroimaging measures (functional, network, and neurochemical) at baseline and pretreatment can contribute towards predicting treatment response (both behavioural and neuroimaging responses) [23, 65]. These studies firmly support the notion that the personalized medicine and stratification goals we need to aid clinical trials and treat our patients more effectively might be better realized using neuroimaging alongside other measures, such as quantitative sensory testing, being tested. Further, these studies and others highlight how brain imaging can be used to distinguish drug from placebo effects in patients.

Much has been learnt about the CNS mechanisms relevant to acute and chronic pain from human neuroimaging studies, and there is an opportunity to reverse-translate this knowledge to aid refinement of our preclinical models. If done, the following may be realized: (1) new targets within the CNS to assay for drug-related analgesic effects and (2) brain regions to record from that reflect symptoms difficult to measure from preclinical behavioural assessments (e.g., ongoing or tonic pain). Hopefully, in the coming years, by concerted effort and creation of consortia to share data and knowledge, progress in this domain will occur. Meanwhile, a number of studies have been done with the specific aim of improving analgesic drug discovery, and they span the preclinical to Phase 3 spectrum.

PRECLINICAL phMRI

A number of analgesic drugs have been evaluated using phMRI in rats (for a review, see [29]) either using preclinical chronic pain models or examining the effects of the drug on whole-brain systems (e.g., gabapentin on spinal nerve ligation model [25], celecoxib in an osteoarthritis model [59], buprenorphine in healthy rats [4], ketamine in healthy rats [16], and remifentanil in healthy rats [35]). In short, the studies have asked where the drug acts in the brain and what brain systems relevant to chronic or acute pain the drugs modulate.

The use of preclinical models allows for better comparisons with humans and the likelihood that such data are relevant to the patients, as illustrated by recent examples showing similar brain changes and responses to drug or pain across species [3, 4]. Further advantages proferred by the use of preclinical models include, among others, help with dosing as well as identifying potential side effect profiles based upon circuitry affected (e.g., those circuits involved in nausea and vomiting [15] or sedation [36]).

CLINICAL phMRI FOR ANALGESIC DRUG DISCOVERY

Phase 1

The reality is that few drugs make it to Phase 1 testing in humans (approximately 1 in 10). Although most Phase 1 trials enrol healthy subjects, there is a move to have earlier involvement of patients. Imaging can provide a number of novel insights into Phase 1 evaluation of a novel compound, including (1) CNS penetration validation and guidance on drug dosing [57]; (2) identification of neural circuits targeted [58]; (3) assessment of the predictive qualities of Phase 1 versus Phase 2; (4) assessment of potential efficacy, based on neural circuitry of activation and its connectivity [58]; and (5) potential side effects based on changes in brain regions involved with sleepiness, addiction, and nausea/vomiting.

Phase 2

Involving small groups of patients in Phase 2–based imaging studies will define similar features to not only those listed for Phase 1, but potentially also the following: (1) new drug versus best in class or comparator and (2) responders versus nonresponders. For example, the psychiatric side effects now noted for the antimalarial mefloquine [46] may have been determined prior to its marketing if an imaging-based study was done early in its development. There is no doubt that the use of imaging in early clinical trials and drug evaluation for analgesia is increasing [7]. Of the 70 drugs used and reported on clinicaltrials.gov that involved an imaging component, 10 involved analgesics (including for rheumatoid arthritis, migraine, fibromyalgia, and osteoarthritis) [7].

Phase 3

At this time, there are very few Phase 3 studies that use imaging to aid drug development (Clinicaltrials.gov) [7]. At this stage of a drug's evaluation, imaging may provide insights into the temporal course of drug effects (functional and morphological), potential long-term negative effects (e.g., opioids [57, 74]), disease modification, placebo/responder versus nonresponder issues, as well as baseline stratification to predict treatment response.

It is evident from the above that neuroimaging is being slowly adopted into analgesic drug development in both translational and clinical trials. Remaining issues to be cognizant of include the following: (1) Integration of imaging into trials without confounding regulatory processes and including added risks to the trial. If this approach shows valid outcomes, due to the increased power of the study, this could lead to fewer patients to be exposed to new drugs, particularly in Phase 2 studies. (2) Applying good imaging practice in trials [49, 50] to ensure standards across the industry; imaging may evolve into the validation of surrogate end points.

To implement these measures, some additional considerations are required, as discussed below.

IMPLEMENTING NEUROIMAGING FOR ANALGESIC DRUG DISCOVERY

Better practices for using neuroimaging to identify targets for drug development and evaluation are evolving rapidly. Over the past several years, the neuroimaging field across the neuroscience space has begun to mature from early proof-of-concept work and methods development into larger scale efforts to use neuroimaging in translational science, including datasets with multiple sites, cohorts, and outcome domains [42, 44, 60, 73]. This maturation includes a growing recognition of four kinds of needs: (1) outcome specificity, (2) clinically significant effects, (3) replication, and (4) evaluation of diagnostic properties. These four needs and their relevance to analgesia and measuring analgesic effects in phMRI studies will be discussed briefly below.

Outcome Specificity

It has long been recognized that distinct types and aspects of pain are not highly correlated, necessitating the targeting of specific behavioural and functional outcomes of interest. For example, sensitivity to different pain assays is uncorrelated or sometimes negatively correlated across mouse strains [40, 41], and effects on pain versus cognitive performance under pain can be unrelated [11]. It is now increasingly recognized that brain patterns that predict one pain-related outcome are not necessarily the patterns that predict another pain-related outcome. For example, placebo effects on pain reports are, in some cases, uncorrelated with placebo effects on brain responses to acute noxious events [63]. In addition, the brain patterns related to different kinds of acute and chronic pain in different patient groups may be distinct [1]. Such specificity motivates the need to identify brain markers related to specific outcomes of interest, and the evaluation of their construct validity as measures of those outcomes.

It is also critical to identify specific brain targets, and this is an ongoing challenge in the field. A central problem in identifying brain predictors of specific outcomes is that the smallest unit of analysis in fMRI, the "voxel" (about 1/100,000 of the volume of the brain), integrates activity across hundreds of thousands to millions of neurons with distinct functional properties. Thus, there is a many-to-one mapping between psychological processes and activity in each voxel [48, 72], which complicates the use of voxel-wise activation as a marker for pain. For example, fMRI correlates of pain have been identified in the anterior cingulate and insula (among other regions). Although these regions are certainly important for pain, they are the most frequently activated regions in the brain across all types of tasks (including emotion, judgement and decision-making, and tasks requiring mental effort [72]). Thus, activity in the anterior cingulate as a whole is not *specific* to pain or any other function, and is therefore unlikely to be useful as a diagnostic marker.

An important trend in the neuroimaging literature is the use of "statistical learning" or "machine learning" algorithms to identify distributed patterns of fMRI activity within and across regions [26, 39], and this approach is increasingly being applied to pain [10, 13, 37, 56, 64]. This approach, also called "Multivoxel Pattern Analysis," identifies patterns designed to be maximally predictive of a specific outcome. The algorithms can also be constrained to produce *neuroscientifically interpretable* patterns that can be used in reverse translation. They are suited to diagnostic development and testing because they are designed to optimize the prediction of outcomes such as pain (e.g., be sensitive to pain) and differentiate pain from related conditions (e.g., be specific to pain).

Another, powerful idea is that patterns derived from machine learning can circumvent some of the limitations in spatial resolution of fMRI, because patterns can be sensitive to the local structure of functional columns and differential functional organization across microvascular beds [14, 32]. Pattern information about functional topography is often preserved at a mesoscopic level, and is detectable even when the voxels sampled are larger than the columns themselves [14, 30, 31, 54]. In addition, mesoscopic organization is often preserved across individuals, permitting accurate inferences about individuals based on normative group-level data [45, 51, 52, 64]. This means that distributed local patterns of activity can be sensitive to the differential distribution of different types of neurons across a brain region. Thus, whereas any one voxel in a region such as the anterior cingulate may not be highly diagnostic of pain [61, 72], a particular local pattern across voxels within the anterior cingulate may be diagnostic [64].

Recent studies have suggested that brain markers based on distributed patterns of activity within and across brain regions can be used to predict forms of acute pain [10, 13, 37, 56, 64], identify brain targets of analgesic drugs (e.g., remifentanil [64]), and identify placebo responders [24, 63]. Related measures based on brain connectivity may identify individuals that will develop chronic back pain [2]. These findings are promising in terms of the ability to identify markers useful for multiple aspects of treatment development. Brain markers for outcomes (e.g., acute pain) can be used in reverse translation to identify animal models with homologous brain features and develop new treatments. Markers for neural systems involved in drug action can be used to identify the brain components affected by treatments. Combined with a scientific understanding of the aspects and types of pain that these brain components reflect, these markers can be used to (a) generate novel hypotheses about combined treatments based on targeting complementary brain systems and (b) match individuals to appropriate treatments based on the match between the brain systems that show abnormal responses and those targeted by a candidate treatment.

Clinically Significant Effects

MRI and fMRI images are a complex source of information, consisting of measures on the order of 50,000–200,000 voxels or more, reflecting activity in coherent, but spatially distributed systems across the brain. Like other measures distributed across many variables such as genome-wide scans, MRI analyses may show many statistically significant differences that are not large enough to be *clinically* significant. This has emerged as an important issue in the literature, as there have been widespread criticisms that effect sizes for brain–behaviour correlations are often dramatically overestimated [34, 62, 71]. Though machine learning fMRI approaches based on local patterns do not address this issue, some machine learning approaches can provide unbiased estimates of effect size and establish that brain patterns are robust enough to be meaningfully useful for prediction and diagnosis. These approaches integrate brain information across regions (and potentially imaging modalities) to make a *single* prediction about a patient's status or level of pain. Such approaches suggest that brain information can provide very robust markers that track acute pain magnitude [64], and may provide useful diagnostic information about patient status in pain [56] and other types of psychopathology [9, 17, 20, 75].

Replication

Another important problem in the development of brain markers is that the search for effects across many brain voxels and modalities has resulted in high false-positive rates, and there is an increasing recognition of the need for replication of results across laboratories [28, 43]. This is true across multiple fields that deal with complex data, including both neuroimaging [12] and genetics [21], and in other fields as well [53]. A second, related problem is that what constitutes a replication in neuroimaging studies has been unclear. Regions that are often treated as units of analysis in publications—such as the amygdala or dorsal anterior cingulate—include hundreds or thousands of voxels, and it is insufficient for replication purposes to find "anterior cingulate activity" in two or more studies.

When used in specific ways, machine learning–based approaches can circumvent both problems. These approaches use part of the data to estimate a distributed pattern that serves as a provisional brain marker, and another part of the data to test the diagnostic accuracy of that specific pattern. In some cases, brain predictors of pain may be identified in a group of individuals that provide information diagnostic of pain in other individuals, even when collected at different sites. Because the pattern is fixed across training and testing, this strategy provides an exact replication test of the brain marker [64].

Thus, although results in most previous neuroimaging studies are not used prospectively to quantitatively test responses in new samples and individuals, machine learning-derived patterns have shown promise in this regard.

Evaluation of Diagnostic Properties

Dominant paradigms in neuroimaging data analysis have not focused on diagnostic properties, which may be captured in part by analysis of the sensitivity and specificity of a specific brain pattern for a specific class of outcomes. However, as neuroimaging is increasingly used in clinical studies, there is increasing focus on the diagnostic value of brain patterns for clinical conditions using such criteria [2, 9, 17, 20, 75] and treatment responses [19, 38].

Another important concept is that brain markers that can be applied across individuals can be easily tested for generalization across samples and sites, which is essential if neuroimaging markers are to be validated and used clinically. In addition, the generalization and specificity of such markers—with respect to types of pain, body sites, and pain versus related psychological states—can be tested on existing data, accelerating the development–test cycle for brain markers.

There are now several promising candidate markers emerging for pain. For acute nociception-driven pain, a distributed pattern of regions that matches well with prototypical "pain-processing" regions in humans and animals can accurately track the magnitude of pain [64]. If two conditions are moderately different in pain (e.g., 2 points on a 10-point visual analogue scale [VAS]), activity in this pattern, the "neurologic pain signature" (NPS), as it has been termed by Wager, can correctly predict which is more painful for an individual person with 90–100% accuracy. It has been successfully tested across different sites, and work examining the transfer across types of pain (e.g., heat, cold, mechanical, inflammatory) is ongoing. In addition, it was shown to have 90% or greater sensitivity and specificity to somatic pain in comparison with nonpainful warmth, pain anticipation, pain recall, and emotionally evocative images, and it responded to remifentanil administration with a time course predicted by pharmacokinetic models of remifentanil.

However, the NPS is likely to be sensitive to only certain aspects of pain. In initial tests, it was not affected by a placebo treatment. In addition, a brain pattern that was optimized to predict placebo effects relied on very different systems from the NPS, including frontal cortical activity during pain anticipation [63]. Finally, recent work has suggested that brain markers can predict the transition from acute to chronic back pain with moderate accuracy (80% in a holdout sample; [2]). However, like the placebo-predictive pattern, it relies on very different brain systems from the NPS: It is based on connectivity between the ventromedial prefrontal cortex and nucleus accumbens, neither of which responds strongly to increases in noxious stimulus intensity. Together, these preliminary results suggest that there may be distinct, predictive markers for acute pain driven by nociceptive input and psychological factors. The development of acute back pain, in addition, is accompanied by a shift in the correlates of pain away from "nociception-centred" pain systems and towards systems broadly associated with value, emotion, stress, and autonomic regulation.

These markers hold promise for both providing new explanations of pain and clinical translation, though they must continue to be tested for replicability across samples and specificity versus generalization across types of pain, types of patients, and other contextual factors.

CONCLUSION

From what is presented in this chapter and the literature discussed, it is evident that phMRI is a significant and growing component of neuroimaging-based studies. Such paradigms provide insight into the neural bases of analgesia and pain relief, in the context of pain-related drugs, as well as enable a translational agenda by aiding analgesic drug development within industry. It is our belief that phMRI will play an increasing role in both clinical decision-making and drug discovery in the years to come.

REFERENCES

1. Apkarian AV, Hashmi JA, Baliki MN. Pain and the brain: specificity and plasticity of the brain in clinical chronic pain. Pain 2011;152(3 Suppl):S49.
2. Baliki MN, Petre B, Torbey S, Herrmann KM, Huang L, Schnitzer TJ, Fields HL, Apkarian AV. Corticostriatal functional connectivity predicts transition to chronic back pain. Nat Neurosci 2012;15(8):1117–9.

3. Becerra L, Navratilova E, Porreca F, Borsook D. Analogous responses in the nucleus accumbens and cingulate cortex to pain onset (aversion) and offset (relief) in rats and humans. J Neurophysiol 2013;110(5):1221–6.
4. Becerra L, Upadhyay J, Chang PC, Bishop J, Anderson J, Baumgartner R, Schwarz AJ, Coimbra A, Wallin D, Nutile L, et al. Parallel buprenorphine phMRI responses in conscious rodents and healthy human subjects. J Pharmacol Exp Ther 2013;345(1):41–51.
5. Bingel U, Tracey I, Wiech K. Neuroimaging as a tool to investigate how cognitive factors influence analgesic drug outcomes. Neurosci Lett 2012;520(2):149–55.
6. Bingel U, Wanigasekera V, Wiech K, Ni Mhuircheartaigh R, Lee MC, Ploner M, Tracey I. The effect of treatment expectation on drug efficacy: imaging the analgesic benefit of the opioid remifentanil. Sci Transl Med 2011;3(70):70ra14.
7. Borsook D, Becerra L, Fava M. Use of functional imaging across clinical phases in CNS drug development. Transl Psychiatry 2013;3:e282.
8. Borsook D, Becerra L, Hargreaves R. A role for fMRI in optimizing CNS drug development. Nat Rev Drug Discov 2006;5(5):411–24.
9. Brodersen KH, Schofield TM, Leff AP, Ong CS, Lomakina EI, Buhmann JM, Stephan KE. Generative embedding for model-based classification of fMRI Data. PLoS Comput Biol 2011;7(6):e1002079.
10. Brodersen KH, Wiech K, Lomakina EI, Lin CS, Buhmann JM, Bingel U, Ploner M, Stephan KE, Tracey I. Decoding the perception of pain from fMRI using multivariate pattern analysis. NeuroImage 2012;63(3): 1162–70.
11. Buhle JT, Stevens BL, Friedman JJ, Wager TD. Distraction and placebo: two separate routes to pain control. Psychol Sci 2012;23(3):246–53.
12. Button KS, Ioannidis JP, Mokrysz C, Nosek BA, Flint J, Robinson ES, Munafo MR. Power failure: why small sample size undermines the reliability of neuroscience. Nat Rev Neurosci 2013;14(5):365–76.
13. Cecchi GA, Huang L, Hashmi JA, Baliki M, Centeno MaV, Rish I, Apkarian AV. Predictive dynamics of human pain perception. PLoS Comput Biol 2012;8(10):e1002719.
14. Chaimow D, Yacoub E, Ugurbil K, Shmuel A. Modeling and analysis of mechanisms underlying fMRI-based decoding of information conveyed in cortical columns. NeuroImage 2011;56(2):627–42.
15. Chin CL, Fox GB, Hradil VP, Osinski MA, McGaraughty SP, Skoubis PD, Cox BF, Luo Y. Pharmacological MRI in awake rats reveals neural activity in area postrema and nucleus tractus solitarius: relevance as a potential biomarker for detecting drug-induced emesis. NeuroImage 2006;33(4):1152–60.
16. Chin CL, Upadhyay J, Marek GJ, Baker SJ, Zhang M, Mezler M, Fox GB, Day M. Awake rat pharmacological magnetic resonance imaging as a translational pharmacodynamic biomarker: metabotropic glutamate 2/3 agonist modulation of ketamine-induced blood oxygenation level dependence signals. J Pharmacol Exp Ther 2011;336(3):709–15.
17. Cuingnet R, Gerardin E, Tessieras J, Auzias G, Lehericy S, Habert MO, Chupin M, Benali H, Colliot O, Alzheimer's Disease Neuroimaging I. Automatic classification of patients with Alzheimer's disease from structural MRI: a comparison of ten methods using the ADNI database. NeuroImage 2011;56(2):766–81.
18. Denk F, McMahon SB, Tracey I. Pain vulnerability: a neurobiological perspective. Nat Neurosci 2014;17(2):192–200.
19. Doehrmann O, Ghosh SS, Polli FE, Reynolds GO, Horn F, Keshavan A, Triantafyllou C, Saygin ZM, Whitfield-Gabrieli S, Hofmann SG. Predicting treatment response in social anxiety disorder from functional magnetic resonance imagingtreatment prediction in social anxiety disorder. JAMA Psychiatry 2013;70(1):87–97.
20. Du W, Calhoun VD, Li H, Ma S, Eichele T, Kiehl KA, Pearlson GD, Adali T. High classification accuracy for schizophrenia with rest and task FMRI data. Front Hum Neurosci 2012;6:145.
21. Duncan LE, Keller MC. A critical review of the first 10 years of candidate gene-by-environment interaction research in psychiatry. The Am J Psychiatry 2011;168(10):1041–9.
22. Gwilym SE, Filippini N, Douaud G, Carr AJ, Tracey I. Thalamic atrophy associated with painful osteoarthritis of the hip is reversible after arthroplasty: a longitudinal voxel-based morphometric study. Arthritis Rheum 2010;62(10):2930–40.
23. Harris RE, Napadow V, Huggins JP, Pauer L, Kim J, Hampson J, Sundgren PC, Foerster B, Petrou M, Schmidt-Wilcke T, et al. Pregabalin rectifies aberrant brain chemistry, connectivity, and functional response in chronic pain patients. Anesthesiology 2013;119(6):1453–64.
24. Hashmi JA, Baria AT, Baliki MN, Huang L, Schnitzer TJ, Apkarian AV. Brain networks predicting placebo analgesia in a clinical trial for chronic back pain. Pain 2012;153(12):2393–402.
25. Hooker BA, Tobon G, Baker SJ, Zhu C, Hesterman J, Schmidt K, Rajagovindan R, Chandran P, Joshi SK, Bannon AW, et al. Gabapentin-induced pharmacodynamic effects in the spinal nerve ligation model of neuropathic pain. Eur J Pain 2014;18(2):223–37.

26. Horikawa T, Tamaki M, Miyawaki Y, Kamitani Y. Neural decoding of visual imagery during sleep. Science 2013;340(6132):639–42.
27. Iannetti GD, Zambreanu L, Wise RG, Buchanan TJ, Huggins JP, Smart TS, Vennart W, Tracey I. Pharmacological modulation of pain-related brain activity during normal and central sensitization states in humans. Proc Natl Acad Sci USA 2005;102(50):18195–200.
28. Ioannidis JP. Why most published research findings are false. PLoS Med 2005;2(8):e124.
29. Jenkins BG. Pharmacologic magnetic resonance imaging (phMRI): imaging drug action in the brain. NeuroImage 2012;62(2):1072–85.
30. Kamitani Y, Sawahata Y. Spatial smoothing hurts localization but not information: pitfalls for brain mappers. NeuroImage 2010;49(3):1949–52.
31. Kamitani Y, Tong F. Decoding the visual and subjective contents of the human brain. Nat Neurosci 2005;8(5):679–85.
32. Kriegeskorte N, Cusack R, Bandettini P. How does an fMRI voxel sample the neuronal activity pattern: compact-kernel or complex spatiotemporal filter? NeuroImage 2010;49(3):1965–76.
33. Lee MC, Ploner M, Wiech K, Bingel U, Wanigasekera V, Brooks J, Menon DK, Tracey I. Amygdala activity contributes to the dissociative effect of cannabis on pain perception. Pain 2013;154(1):124–34.
34. Lieberman MD, Berkman ET, Wager TD. Correlations in social neuroscience aren't voodoo: commentary on Vul et al. (2009). Perspect Psychol Sci 2009;4(3):299–307.
35. Liu CH, Greve DN, Dai G, Marota JJ, Mandeville JB. Remifentanil administration reveals biphasic phMRI temporal responses in rat consistent with dynamic receptor regulation. NeuroImage 2007;34(3):1042–53.
36. Liu X, Pillay S, Li R, Vizuete JA, Pechman KR, Schmainda KM, Hudetz AG. Multiphasic modification of intrinsic functional connectivity of the rat brain during increasing levels of propofol. NeuroImage 2013;83:581–92.
37. Marquand A, Howard M, Brammer M, Chu C, Coen S, Mourao-Miranda J. Quantitative prediction of subjective pain intensity from whole-brain fMRI data using Gaussian processes. NeuroImage 2010;49(3):2178–89.
38. Miller JM, Schneck N, Siegle GJ, Chen Y, Ogden RT, Kikuchi T, Oquendo MA, Mann JJ, Parsey RV. fMRI response to negative words and SSRI treatment outcome in major depressive disorder: a preliminary study. Psychiatry Res 2013;214(3):296–305.
39. Mitchell TM, Shinkareva SV, Carlson A, Chang K-M, Malave VL, Mason RA, Just MA. Predicting human brain activity associated with the meanings of nouns. Science 2008;320(5880):1191–5.
40. Mogil JS, Wilson SG, Bon K, Eun Lee S, Chung K, Raber P, Pieper JO, Hain HS, Belknap JK, Hubert L. Heritability of nociception I: responses of 11 inbred mouse strains on 12 measures of nociception. Pain 1999;80(1):67–82.
41. Mogil JS, Wilson SG, Bon K, Eun Lee S, Chung K, Raber P, Pieper JO, Hain HS, Belknap JK, Hubert L. Heritability of nociception, II: types' of nociception revealed by genetic correlation analysis. Pain 1999;80(1):83–93.
42. Mueller SG, Weiner MW, Thal LJ, Petersen RC, Jack CR, Jagust W, Trojanowski JQ, Toga AW, Beckett L. Ways toward an early diagnosis in Alzheimer's disease: the Alzheimer's Disease Neuroimaging Initiative (ADNI). Alzheimers Dement 2005;1(1):55–66.
43. Pashler H, Wagenmakers EÄ. Editors' introduction to the special section on replicability in psychological science a crisis of confidence? Perspect Psychol Sci 2012;7(6):528-530.
44. Poldrack RA, Barch DM, Mitchell JP, Wager TD, Wagner AD, Devlin JT, Cumba C, Koyejo O, Milham MP. Toward open sharing of task-based fMRI data: the OpenfMRI project. Front Neuroinform 2013;7:12.
45. Rissman J, Greely HT, Wagner AD. Detecting individual memories through the neural decoding of memory states and past experience. Proc Natl Acad Sci USA 2010;107(21):9849–54.
46. Ritchie EC, Block J, Nevin RL. Psychiatric side effects of mefloquine: applications to forensic psychiatry. J Am Acad Psychiatry Law 2013;41(2):224–35.
47. Rodriguez-Raecke R, Niemeier A, Ihle K, Ruether W, May A. Brain gray matter decrease in chronic pain is the consequence and not the cause of pain. J Neurosci 2009;29(44):13746–50.
48. Sarter M, Berntson GG, Cacioppo JT. Brain imaging and cognitive neuroscience: toward strong inference in attributing function to structure. Am Psychol 1996;51(1):13.
49. Schwarz AJ, Becerra L, Upadhyay J, Anderson J, Baumgartner R, Coimbra A, Evelhoch J, Hargreaves R, Robertson B, Iyengar S, et al. A procedural framework for good imaging practice in pharmacological fMRI studies applied to drug development #1: processes and requirements. Drug Discov Today 2011;16(13–14):583-93.
50. Schwarz AJ, Becerra L, Upadhyay J, Anderson J, Baumgartner R, Coimbra A, Evelhoch J, Hargreaves R, Robertson B, Iyengar S, et al. A procedural framework for good imaging practice in pharmacological fMRI studies applied to drug development #2: protocol optimization and best practices. Drug Discov Today 2011;16(15–16):671–82.

51. Shinkareva SV, Malave VL, Just MA, Mitchell TM. Exploring commonalities across participants in the neural representation of objects. Hum Brain Mapp 2012;33(6):1375–83.
52. Shinkareva SV, Mason RA, Malave VL, Wang W, Mitchell TM, Just MA. Using fMRI brain activation to identify cognitive states associated with perception of tools and dwellings. PLoS One 2008;3(1):e1394.
53. Simmons JP, Nelson LD, Simonsohn U. False-positive psychology: undisclosed flexibility in data collection and analysis allows presenting anything as significant. Psychol Sci 2011;22(11):1359–66.
54. Swisher JD, Gatenby JC, Gore JC, Wolfe BA, Moon C-H, Kim S-G, Tong F. Multiscale pattern analysis of orientation-selective activity in the primary visual cortex. J Neurosci 2010;30(1):325–30.
55. Tracey I. "Seeing" how our drugs work brings translational added value. Anesthesiology 2013;119(6):1247–8.
56. Ung H, Brown JE, Johnson KA, Younger J, Hush J, Mackey S. Multivariate classification of structural MRI data detects chronic low back pain. Cereb Cortex 2014;24(4):1037–44.
57. Upadhyay J, Anderson J, Baumgartner R, Coimbra A, Schwarz AJ, Pendse G, Wallin D, Nutile L, Bishop J, George E, et al. Modulation of CNS pain circuitry by intravenous and sublingual doses of buprenorphine. NeuroImage 2012;59(4):3762–73.
58. Upadhyay J, Anderson J, Schwarz AJ, Coimbra A, Baumgartner R, Pendse G, George E, Nutile L, Wallin D, et al. Imaging drugs with and without clinical analgesic efficacy. Neuropsychopharmacology 2011;36(13): 2659–73.
59. Upadhyay J, Baker SJ, Rajagovindan R, Hart M, Chandran P, Hooker BA, Cassar S, Mikusa JP, Tovcimak A, Wald MJ, et al. Pharmacological modulation of brain activity in a preclinical model of osteoarthritis. NeuroImage 2013;64:341–55.
60. Van Essen DC, Smith SM, Barch DM, Behrens TEJ, Yacoub E, Ugurbil K. The WU-Minn Human Connectome Project: an overview. NeuroImage 2013;80(0):62–79.
61. van Snellenberg JX, Wager TD. Cognitive and motivational functions of the human prefrontal cortex. In: A Christensen, E Goldberg, D Bougakov, editors. Luria's legacy in the 21st century. Oxford, UK: Oxford University Press; 2009. pp. 30–61.
62. Vul E, Harris C, Winkielman P, Pashler H. Puzzlingly high correlations in fMRI studies of emotion, personality, and social cognition. Perspect Psychol Sci 2009;4(3):274–90.
63. Wager TD, Atlas LY, Leotti LA, Rilling JK. Predicting individual differences in placebo analgesia: contributions of brain activity during anticipation and pain experience. J Neurosci 2011;31(2):439–52.
64. Wager TD, Atlas LY, Lindquist MA, Roy M, Woo CW, Kross E. An fMRI-based neurologic signature of physical pain. N Engl J Med 2013;368(15):1388–97.
65. Wanigasekera V, Lee MC, Rogers R, Kong Y, Leknes S, Andersson J, Tracey I. Baseline reward circuitry activity and trait reward responsiveness predict expression of opioid analgesia in healthy subjects. Proc Natl Acad Sci USA 2012;109(43):17705–10.
66. Wise RG, Lujan BJ, Schweinhardt P, Peskett GD, Rogers R, Tracey I. The anxiolytic effects of midazolam during anticipation to pain revealed using fMRI. Magn Reson Imaging 2007;25(6):801–10.
67. Wise RG, Preston C. What is the value of human fMRI in CNS drug development? Drug Discov Today 2010;15(21–22):973–80.
68. Wise RG, Rogers R, Painter D, Bantick S, Ploghaus A, Williams P, Rapeport G, Tracey I. Combining fMRI with a pharmacokinetic model to determine which brain areas activated by painful stimulation are specifically modulated by remifentanil. NeuroImage 2002;16(4):999–1014.
69. Wise RG, Tracey I. The role of fMRI in drug discovery. J Magn Reson Imaging 2006;23(6):862-876.
70. Wise RG, Williams P, Tracey I. Using fMRI to quantify the time dependence of remifentanil analgesia in the human brain. Neuropsychopharmacology 2004;29(3):626–35.
71. Yarkoni T. Big correlations in little studies: Inflated fMRI correlations reflect low statistical power—commentary on Vul et al. (2009). Perspect Psychol Sci 2009;4(3):294–8.
72. Yarkoni T, Poldrack RA, Nichols TE, Van Essen DC, Wager TD. Large-scale automated synthesis of human functional neuroimaging data. Nat Methods 2011;8(8):665–70.
73. Yarkoni T, Poldrack RA, Van Essen DC, Wager TD. Cognitive neuroscience 2.0: building a cumulative science of human brain function. Trends Cogn Sci 2010;14(11):489–96.
74. Younger JW, Chu LF, D'Arcy NT, Trott KE, Jastrzab LE, Mackey SC. Prescription opioid analgesics rapidly change the human brain. Pain 2011;152(8):1803–10.
75. Zeng L-L, Shen H, Liu L, Wang L, Li B, Fang P, Zhou Z, Li Y, Hu D. Identifying major depression using whole-brain functional connectivity: a multivariate pattern analysis. Brain 2012;135(5):1498–507.

SECTION 7

Future Directions

CHAPTER 34

Neuroethical Issues in Brain Imaging of Pain

Karen D. Davis

Advances in neuroimaging have spearheaded efforts to identify brain biomarkers of pain. This has raised great debate regarding neuroethical issues associated with pain biomarkers. This chapter reviews the key concepts and important factors pertaining to the development and neuroethics of brain imaging-based pain biomarkers. Important questions to be addressed regarding imaging-based biomarkers of pain are (Fig. 34-1):

1. Do we need them?
2. How good are they?
3. How would they be used?
4. Who sets guidelines?
5. Social and legal responsibility of neuroscientists and clinicians?

PAIN AND NOCICEPTION

Pain has been defined by the International Association for the Study of Pain as "an unpleasant sensory and emotional experience associated with actual or potential tissue damage, or described in terms of such damage . . . Pain is always subjective" (http://www.iasp-pain.org/Education/Content.aspx?ItemNumber=1698#Pain) [17]. As such, pain is a subjective experience and only known definitively by self-report [4]. Self-reports provide a reasonable assessment of the pain experience and are considered the gold standard. However, the presence of influential people can alter an individual's self-report of pain. Furthermore, self-reports are challenging in children, patients with dementia, and noncommunicative populations [27]. Thus, there are instances in which self-report cannot be obtained or does not accurately represent the true pain being experienced; as a result, proxies for pain are needed to guide treatment [15].

Historically, a major thrust in pain research has been to understand brain mechanisms underlying pain through the study of nociception. As noted above, pain is a subjective experience. In contrast, nociception simply refers to "The neural process of encoding noxious stimuli" (http://www.iasp-pain.org/Education/Content.aspx?ItemNumber=1698#Nociception) [17]. Therefore, nociception can reflect pain but, clearly, is not equivalent to pain. For example, there can be nociception but no pain, as exemplified by a general anaesthetic state in which nociceptive neurons may continue to respond to a noxious stimulus. Furthermore, there can be pain without usual nociceptive activity (e.g., poststroke pain, phantom pain). Nonetheless, measures of nociception are used by some as an objective biomarker of pain.

Imaging Biomarkers of Pain

Need?
- ❑ complementary to self-report

Validity?
- ❑ specificity
- ❑ sensitivity

Usage?
- ❑ acute pains, chronic pains
- ❑ diagnostics, prognostics, treatment planning

Guidelines and monitoring?
- ❑ medical associations, government, insurers, scientists, clinicians, scientific/medical societies

Social and legal responsibility?
- ❑ clinicians, scientist

FIGURE 34-1 Broad neuroethical questions for consideration in developing imaging-based biomarkers of pain.

THE NEED FOR BRAIN BIOMARKERS OF PAIN

The shortcoming of pain self-reports noted above has led some to develop an objective biomarker surrogate for pain. Much of this endeavour has been fuelled by patient groups who report challenges in receiving adequate medical treatment and insurance coverage for functional chronic pain disorders and thus are seeking an objective test to validate their pain experience. However, the use of an imaging-based brain biomarker for pain diagnostics is laden with neuroethical concerns (see below). Nonetheless, if brain biomarkers of pain were to be established, they could have utility for prognostics (i.e., prediction) and triage (i.e., personalized treatment based on efficacy) (Fig. 34-2). These latter two applications represent significant clinical value to streamline patient care (i.e., personalized medicine) based on knowledge of a patient's brain functional circuitry. Although it may seem that using brain imaging biomarkers for prognostics and treatment planning is less prone to ethical concerns than diagnostic applications, ethical issues for these usages clearly are important because of the potential for mistreatment.

PROS AND CONS OF BRAIN BIOMARKERS OF PAIN

The potential value of brain biomarkers of pain is significant [7] (Fig. 34-3 and see below): First, they would provide evidence for pain and suffering that may not be obtainable in some vulnerable populations that have no or limited ability to communicate accurately their personal feelings. This objective data would also validate a communicative patient's self-report of pain, thereby facilitating his or her access to treatment and insurance coverage. Second, brain imaging data could provide guidance for a more streamlined, personalized approach to treatment in an individual that could improve treatment efficacy and reduce potential side effects.

There are also significant arguments against the use of brain biomarkers of pain [7] because their shortcomings represent barriers to the humane treatment of real pain (Fig. 34-3). Fundamentally, a brain biomarker test could devalue the self-report of pain, essentially diminishing the patient's personal experience of pain. Factors of sensitivity and

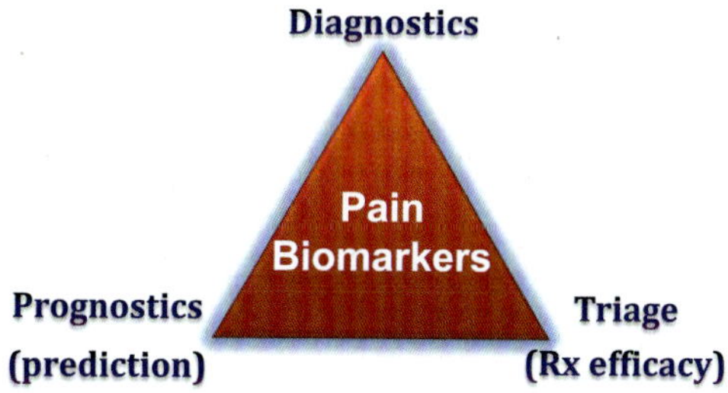

FIGURE 34-2 Three applications of pain biomarkers.

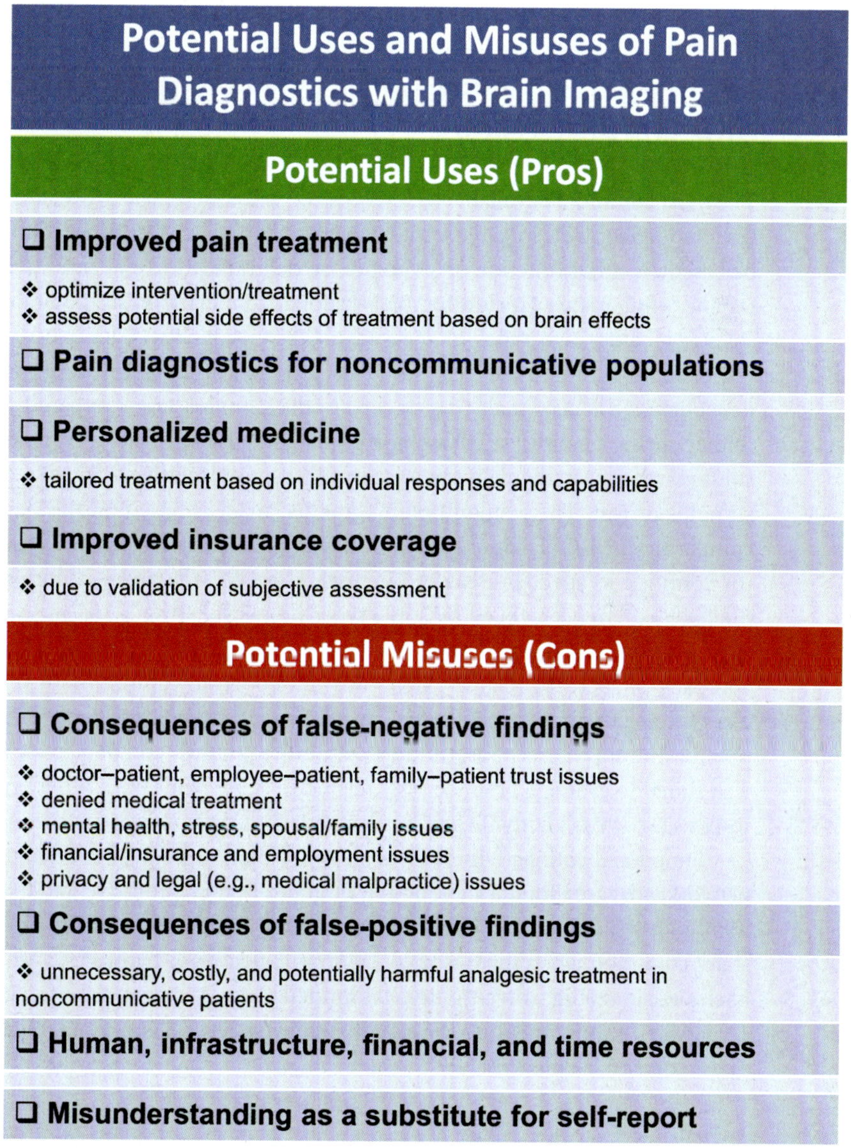

FIGURE 34-3 Potential advantages and negative consequences of using imaging-based biomarkers to the diagnosis of pain. (Reproduced with permission from Davis et al. [7].)

specificity are discussed below and speak to the enormous challenges in developing valid biomarkers, particularly for different types of chronic pains. One of the most important ethical issues of any biomarker used for clinical purposes is the false-negative problem. All medical tests have some level of false-negative outcomes. In the case of pain, a false biomarker test can also contradict a patient's own self-report of pain. This conflict could then have serious consequences in terms of denied treatment, access to insurance, as well as employment and quality-of-life issues, including stresses for the patient and his or her family. Conversely, a false-positive outcome in a noncommunicative patient could result in unnecessary, costly, and potential dangerous treatment. Finally, there are ethical issues pertaining to the privacy of brain imaging information, and financial and human resources that are needed to administer MRI-based testing represent a barrier to financially disadvantaged patients.

BRAIN IMAGING APPROACHES TO EVALUATE ACUTE AND CHRONIC PAINS

The most commonly available technology for brain imaging is MRI, and so brain biomarkers intended for widespread use will likely be MRI-based. Defining a brain biomarker could be based on either function or structure. Structural MRI can be used to measure grey matter and white matter (including inter-regional connectivity) in the brain. Functional MRI (fMRI) includes two types of measures: Conventionally, fMRI is used to determine the response to a stimulus or task based on a statistical comparison of blood oxygen level–dependent (BOLD) signals time-locked to the stimulus/task compared with a control level (either during a control stimulus/task or just a resting baseline). A typical pain fMRI protocol involves repeatedly delivering a painful stimulus interleaved with a control nonpainful stimulus or rest. The resultant pain stimulus "map" is based on the statistical outcome of comparing the BOLD signal during the pain and nonpain states in all voxels of the brain (or confined to specific areas of interest). However, the onset, duration, and intensity of the pain experience evoked by some types of painful stimuli and in some individuals can vary and may not occur exactly during the duration of the stimulus. For this reason, the approach of "percept-related fMRI" was developed to capture brain responses that more closely reflect pain experience (i.e., a pain map) rather than simply the application of a painful stimulus (i.e., a pain stimulus map) [6]. Stimulus- and percept-related fMRI are thus well suited to evaluate brain activity related to acute pains or to other types of evoked pain responses such as allodynia and hyperalgesia, but cannot evaluate chronic (ongoing) pain.

Functional connectivity (FC) is an application of fMRI that evaluates brain areas and networks that are thought to be acting as a unit. Brain regions are said to have FC if they exhibit highly synchronized low-frequency BOLD activity (<0.01 Hz) [6] during a "resting-state" condition when there is no overt stimulus or task. Thus, FC is well suited for studies of chronic, ongoing pain although it is limited to assessing very low-frequency synchronous activity and cannot measure the activity within specific regions or at higher (arguably more physiological) frequencies.

VALIDITY OF BIOMARKERS

Brain imaging has been used to study pain for over 20 years. However, the vast amount of data accumulated provides insight into the "average" pain response as detected across a group of studies. However, the concept of a brain biomarker for pain requires that a pain response be detectable in an individual person. The validity of a brain biomarker for pain thus critically depends on factors that impact its sensitivity and specificity. This requires examining the following key issues [7] (Fig. 34-4):

Operational Definition of the Biomarker

A biomarker of any kind must be defined on the basis of a set of strict criteria. For a pain-evoked fMRI paradigm, an "activation" would need to be established on the basis of a statistical decision as to whether a particular combination of brain areas has increased BOLD

Defining a Putative Pain "Biomarker"

❑ Imaging technique

❖ fMRI: BOLD (evoked, resting-state connectivity), perfusion (rCBF)
❖ PET: rCBF (water), glucose metabolism, receptor binding

❑ Activation features

❖ presence or absence of an evoked response
❖ magnitude of response
❖ sign (i.e., increase or decrease from baseline)
❖ anatomical location
❖ size and spatial extent
❖ connectivity with other brain areas
❖ behavioural correlation (e.g., pain intensity)

❑ Imaging parameters

❖ MRI field strength (e.g., 1.5 T, 3 T)
❖ pulse sequence (e.g., echoplanar, spiral)
❖ acquisition parameters (spatial and temporal resolution, etc.)

❑ Protocol design

❖ stimulus modality (heat, mechanical, electrical, laser, etc.)
❖ stimulus intensity (fixed stimulus, fixed evoked pain intensity)
❖ control condition (no stimulus, nonpainful (e.g., thermal, mechanical))
❖ duration and number of trials (block vs. single trial design)

❑ Preprocessing and statistical criteria

❖ hemodynamic response (stimulus-related vs. percept-related)
❖ spatial (Gaussian) and temporal filters
❖ height and extent (cluster) threshold
❖ correction for multiple comparisons
❖ whole brain versus region of interest analysis
❖ fixed effects versus random effects analysis

❑ Physiological issues

❖ brain areas are nonspecific and multiresponsive (fear, attention, salience, emotion, pain, etc.)
❖ overlap of pain and non-pain-responsive neurons for touch, etc. (i.e., no brain area contains only pain-responsive neurons)
❖ BOLD, rCBF ceiling effects

FIGURE 34-4 Technical and physiological factors impacting the definition of a universal brain-imaging pain biomarker. (Reproduced with permission from Davis et al. [7].)

signal compared with a particular control stimulus. The choice of statistical threshold is important since thresholds that are too liberal lead to false positives (i.e., type I errors) and thresholds that are too stringent produce false negatives (i.e., type II errors).

The fMRI criteria that could be considered to make such decisions include the magnitude, sign (i.e., activation, deactivation), location, and spatial extent of the responses, as well as connectivity patterns and correlations with measures of pain (for a review, see [3]). Likely, a variety of these criteria will need to be combined, and recent complex approaches including connectivity analyses and machine learning have shown some success in predicting acute [28] and chronic pain [1].

To establish a pain biomarker that could be applied to diagnostics, the normal range of brain responses, both in terms of magnitude and location, to a given type of painful stimulus must be understood. However, pain is a complex multidimensional subjective experience, characterized across many domains (intensity, unpleasantness, quality), and evokes a variety of feelings (emotions, anxiety, fear, etc.) and responses (motor, sympathetic, etc.). Furthermore, there are different types of pain experiences associated with different sources of pain (somatic, deep, visceral, heat, cold, mechanical, etc.). Some examples of the tremendous intersubject variability in pain experiences manifest in a range of (1) pain thresholds, suprathreshold responses, adaptation, and habituation [2, 8, 10, 12, 18, 29]; (2) prioritization between pain and cognitive challenges [9, 26]; (3) effects of mind-wandering [19]; (4) cognitive–behavioural modification of pain [25]; and (5) context. Furthermore, recent imaging studies have demonstrated vast intersubject variability in brain structure and function [23]. In light of the brain and behaviour variability across the healthy population, establishing a "normal pain biomarker" represents a significant challenge.

Technical, Statistical, and Design Factors

There are many technical factors that contribute to the reproducibility, specificity, and sensitivity of any fMRI result (Fig. 34-4). For example, the specific MRI scanner (field strength, gradients, pulse sequence, etc.), parameters of acquisition (pulse sequence, slice thickness, voxel size, TR and TE [times to relaxation and excitation], etc.), and preprocessing (spatial and temporal filters, normalization, etc.) all impact the signal-to-noise ratio and hence the detectability of an evoked response. The detectability of a BOLD response also critically depends on the statistical approach (whole brain vs. region of interest analyses, fixed vs. random effects, stimulus- vs. percept-related, etc.) and thresholds (magnitude of response, number of voxels, multiple comparisons corrections, etc.) that are chosen. As noted above, the criteria used to define a biomarker could influence a variety of metrics, including the magnitude, extent, and location of activations and deactivations and their connectivity and correlation with a behavioural measure. Finally, the design of the MRI protocol must be planned carefully, including the choice of stimulus modality (mechanical, heat, cold, ischemic, chemical, or resting state), duration, and its intensity (fixed or based on individually set to evoke a level of pain), as well as the control condition. These design attributes will dictate how findings can be interpreted, including whether the outcome pertains to a specific or general type of pain.

Neurophysiological Factors

Neurophysiological factors must be carefully considered in both the experimental design of fMRI protocols and the interpretation of the results.

First, it must be recognized that BOLD fMRI is only an indirect hemodynamic measure of neuronal activity. Although many types of neuronal responses can be approximated by the assumed hemodynamic response, this is not always the case. For example, the intensity and temporal pattern of many types of pains, particular chronic pains, can vary from the applied noxious stimulus. This is the case for repeated stimuli in which a variety of time-varying pain qualities are evoked, and there may be within-stimulus adaptation, between stimuli habituation, or prolonged pain after the stimulus [11, 12, 20, 21]. Therefore, the approach of percept-related fMRI (as described above) should be a consideration if one wishes to develop a pain biomarker rather than a nociception biomarker.

Second, the resolution of fMRI is quite coarse relative to the density of neurons in the brain. For example, there are hundreds of thousands of neurons that would reside within the volume of a typical fMRI voxel of 2 mm × 2 mm × 2 mm [24]. Therefore, the location of an fMRI response cannot precisely match the location of a particular cluster of nociceptive neurons.

Third, although spatial resolution in and of itself is not problematic for sensory, motor, and some cognitive functions that are subserved by dedicated areas of the brain, there are no such dedicated "pain spots" in the brain. Rather, the overall pain experience is thought to arise from a complex interaction amongst many brain regions, including those within an ascending "sensing" system, and a descending top-down "modulation and coping" system [13]. All nociceptive neurons are interspersed with (and outnumbered by) non-nociceptive sensory, motor, and/or cognitive neurons. Therefore, the choice of a control or baseline condition is crucial for pain fMRI studies (for discussion, see [5]). Furthermore, the multidimensional nature of pain engages many types of non-nociceptive neurons such as those responsible for salience detection, attention, emotion, fear, stress, anxiety, and motor responses. This raises the important possible confound of reverse inference errors in interpretation of fMRI results (for details, see [16]).

Fourth, normal variations in brain physiology and structure based on age, sex, and other group factors need to be considered.

New Developments

New sophisticated MRI approaches using multivariate pattern analysis and machine learning algorithms, and graph theory are being developed to identify widespread brain patterns of pain-evoked responses and connectivity that may be indicative and/or predictive of acute and chronic pains and treatment effects [1, 14, 16, 22, 28]. The sensitivity and specificity of these new approaches are promising but debatable given the validity issues described above, and so further work is needed to establish their applicability at the level of the individual subject. These MRI-based biomarkers could be strengthened by corroboratory evidence from more direct measure of neuronal activity such as magnetoencephalography.

MOVING FORWARD

Brain imaging biomarkers may be of clinical and basic science utility, but there are enormous scientific and ethical issues to be addressed, some generic and others specific to the intended use of the biomarker (diagnostics, prognostics, treatment decisions, etc.). In moving forward with the development of this and other imaging-based biomarkers, a broader discussion needs to consider issues of guidelines and monitoring. There are many stakeholders, including medical associations, government bodies, insurers, scientists, and medical and scientific societies, but it is not clear who will take social and legal responsibility for ensuring the validity of the biomarker and its ensured proper usage. Certainly, there are direction and lessons to be learned from other fields. For example, the pain imaging community can learn from the scientific, medical, legal, and ethical considerations and discussions pertaining to genetic testing. Therefore, future efforts to develop a brain-based biomarker for pain need to be coordinated across laboratories, disciplines, and with input from all interested stakeholders.

REFERENCES

1. Apkarian AV, Baliki MN, Farmer MA. Predicting transition to chronic pain. Curr Opin Neurol 2013;26:360–7.
2. Coghill RC, McHaffie JG, Yen YF. Neural correlates of interindividual differences in the subjective experience of pain. Proc Natl Acad Sci USA 2003;100:8538–42.
3. Davis KD. Recent advances and future prospects in neuroimaging of acute and chronic pain. Future Neurol 2006;1:203–13.
4. Davis KD. Is chronic pain a disease? Evaluating pain and nociception through self-report and neuroimaging. J Pain 2013;14:332–3.
5. Davis KD. Neurophysiological and anatomical considerations in functional imaging of pain. Pain 2003;105:1–3.
6. Davis KD, Moayedi M. Central mechanisms of pain revealed through functional and structural MRI. J Neuroimmune Pharmacol 2013;8:518–34.
7. Davis KD, Racine E, Collett B. Neuroethical issues related to the use of brain imaging: can we and should we use brain imaging as a biomarker to diagnose chronic pain? Pain 2012;153(8):1555–9.
8. Emerson NM, Zeidan F, Lobanov OV, Hadsel MS, Martucci KT, Quevedo AS, Starr CJ, Nahman-Averbuch H, Weissman-Fogel I, Granovsky Y, et al. Pain sensitivity is inversely related to regional grey matter density in the brain. Pain 2014;155:566–73.
9. Erpelding N, Davis KD. Neural underpinnings of behavioural strategies that prioritize either cognitive task performance or pain. Pain 2013;154:2060–71.
10. Erpelding N, Moayedi M, Davis KD. Cortical thickness correlates of pain and temperature sensitivity. Pain 2012;153:1602–9.
11. Hashmi JA, Davis KD. Effect of static and dynamic heat pain stimulus profiles on the temporal dynamics and interdependence of pain qualities, intensity, and affect. J Neurophysiol 2008;100:1706–15.
12. Hashmi JA, Davis KD. Women experience greater heat pain adaptation and habituation than men. Pain 2009;145:350–7.
13. Hashmi JA, Davis KD. Deconstructing sex differences in pain sensitivity. Pain 2014;155:10–13.
14. Hashmi JA, Kong J, Spaeth R, Khan S, Kaptchuk TJ, Gollub RL. Functional network architecture predicts psychologically mediated analgesia related to treatment in chronic knee pain patients. J Neurosci 2014;34:3924–36.
15. Herr K, Coyne PJ, McCaffery M, Manworren R, Merkel S. Pain assessment in the patient unable to self-report: position statement with clinical practice recommendations. Pain Manag Nurs 2011;12:230–50.
16. Iannetti GD, Salomons TV, Moayedi M, Mouraux A, Davis KD. Beyond metaphor: contrasting mechanisms of social and physical pain. Trends Cogn Sci 2013;17:371–8.
17. IASP Task Force on Taxonomy. Classification of chronic pain. Descriptions of chronic pain syndromes and definitions of pain terms. Seattle, WA: IASP Press; 1994.
18. Kim HS, Neubert JK, Miguel AS, Xu K, Krishnaraju RK, Iadarola MJ, Goldman D, Dionne RA. Genetic influence on variability in human acute experimental pain sensitivity associated with gender, ethnicity and psychological temperament. Pain 2004;109:488–96.
19. Kucyi A, Salomons TV, Davis KD. Mind wandering away from pain dynamically engages antinociceptive and default mode brain networks. Proc Natl Acad Sci USA 2013;110:18692–7.
20. Kwan CL, Diamant NE, Mikula K, Davis KD. Characteristics of rectal perception are altered in irritable bowel syndrome. Pain 2005;113:160–71.
21. Kwan CL, Diamant NE, Pope G, Mikula K, Mikulis DJ, Davis KD. Abnormal forebrain activity in functional bowel disorder patients with chronic pain. Neurology 2005;65:1268–77.
22. Liang M, Mouraux A, Hu L, Iannetti GD. Primary sensory cortices contain distinguishable spatial patterns of activity for each sense. Nat Commun 2013;4:1979.

23. Mueller S, Wang D, Fox MD, Yeo BT, Sepulcre J, Sabuncu MR, Shafee R, Lu J, Liu H. Individual variability in functional connectivity architecture of the human brain. Neuron 2013;77:586–95.
24. Pakkenberg B, Gundersen HJ. Neocortical neuron number in humans: effect of sex and age. J Comp Neurol 1997;384:312–20.
25. Salomons TV, Moayedi M, Erpelding N, Davis KD. A brief cognitive-behavioural intervention for pain reduces secondary hyperalgesia. Pain 2014;155(8):1446–52.
26. Seminowicz DA, Mikulis DJ, Davis KD. Cognitive modulation of pain-related brain responses depends on behavioral strategy. Pain 2004;112:48–58.
27. Stinson JN, Kavanagh T, Yamada J, Gill N, Stevens B. Systematic review of the psychometric properties, interpretability and feasibility of self-report pain intensity measures for use in clinical trials in children and adolescents. Pain 2006;125:143–57.
28. Wager TD, Atlas LY, Lindquist MA, Roy M, Woo CW, Kross E. An fMRI-based neurologic signature of physical pain. N Engl J Med 2013;368:1388–97.
29. Wang G, Erpelding N, Davis KD. Sex differences in connectivity of the subgenual ACC. Pain 2014;155:755–63.

CHAPTER 35

Neuroimaging Current Developments and Future Uses

Todd Parrish

Technological developments are very hard to predict. Most science fiction stories depict flying cars, teleportation, and sophisticated medical practices. Those predictions have yet to come to fruition. For example, it still takes the same 5½ hours to fly from New York to Los Angeles as it did in the 1960s, toast still takes 2 minutes to make, and space exploration is still limited. On the bright side, computing technology has grown by leaps and bounds. Most of us have more computing power in our phones than what was used to calculate the first images of functional magnetic resonance imaging (MRI) in the early 1990s. Computing power has revolutionized the medical field, especially the noninvasive field of MRI. The fantasy medical practices shown in science fiction are closer than the ideas of transportation or world economics depicted in these movies. This chapter highlights recent technological developments in MR data acquisition, reconstruction, and analysis that has brought us closer to the future that science fiction predicts. Finally, some predictions about the near future of neuroimaging and how that system may look are made.

BREAKTHROUGHS IN PRACTICE TODAY

The field of MRI has focused on increasing the static magnetic field to increase the overall signal to noise and contrast of the acquired images. This has led to more than a couple of dozen 7 T whole-body systems and a handful of 9.4 T magnets (mostly head only) and now a 10.5-T whole-body system just delivered to the Center for Magnetic Resonance Research at the University of Minnesota. Some of the current issues with manufacturing high-field magnets are the extreme cost and the dependence on liquid helium. Recently, the manufacturer of the 7 T whole-body magnets indicated they have stopped taking orders and will not deliver any more magnets because they are losing millions of dollars each time they make one. Worldwide there is a shortage of liquid helium, which is driving up the costs of operating MRI systems. Steps need to be taken to demonstrate a need for these high magnetic fields, and alternatives to liquid helium need to be implemented. One option is reliquification systems that recycle the helium and compress it back into the liquid form. Another solution is the development of high-temperature superconducting materials (77 K) that require only liquid nitrogen, which is more abundant. This has been an active area of research for many years, but has yet to deliver.

With the development of higher field magnets come challenges of exciting protons and receiving their signal. This is because the higher magnet fields cause protons to resonate at higher frequencies. The high frequencies have difficulty penetrating the body, thus leaving signal voids in the centre of the object. The solutions to these challenges developed at 7 T have trickled down to greatly improve the quality of the electronics used to transmit and receive on lower field systems (3 and 1.5 T). The result is higher-quality data at 3 T without the issues of higher field. A breakthrough has recently taken place in the use of a large number of array elements in head coil designs. The head coil has evolved from a 2-channel system to an 8- or 12-channel system. Currently, vendors are offering 32- and 64-channel head coils with experimental coils going as large as 128. The gain in signal to noise (the true currency of imaging) is incredible, but does come at a price of nonuniformity of the signal distribution. The closer the brain is to the coil, the higher the signal to noise. Thus, there is a spatial gradient of signal to noise, which affects the detection of the weak neuroimaging signals. The spatial variation will lead to difficulties in thresholding maps of activation or connectivity. For example, thalamic connections will have weaker signals compared with their cortical endpoints, which may lead to varying spatial thresholds to visualize the connections. The large number of coils can be used for accelerating the acquisition of the image as the coils can be used for spatial encoding. The advantage is reduced signal distortion and signal voids in areas of high susceptibility. This is known as parallel imaging and can be used in the phase and slice encoding directions to get large acceleration factors at the expense of signal to noise.

The improvements in image acquisition have allowed the full sampling of diffusion space with high levels of diffusion weighting (*b*-values between 5000 and 15,000 $s \cdot mm^{-2}$). This has led the field away from the Gaussian diffusion assumption towards high-order models of diffusion. The benefits of the higher order models are improved representation of the voxel's white matter coherence and multiple fibre orientations as distribution functions instead of ellipsoids. The results from the models have created astonishing maps of white matter sheets in the brain. A great deal of work is underway to identify the best models of the diffusion data coupled with the optimal data acquisition to provide a robust method of mapping white matter. Finally, the addition of navigated echoes (low-resolution images used to correct motion) to structural, functional, and diffusion image acquisitions has reduced the effects of gross motion as well as physiologic motion. Researchers can now push the voxel size further by spending some of the gained signal to noise on improving the resolution of their data without the confound of blurring due to motion.

BREAKTHROUGHS ON THE CUSP

Just recently, a major breakthrough in image acquisition was developed, which excites a number of slice positions during a single RF pulse instead of just a single slice, called multiband excitation [1]. The acceleration factors for the multiband method range from 2 to 8 currently. When multiband imaging is used in conjunction with parallel imaging acceleration (a method that uses coil information to accelerate spatial encoding), it allows "whole-brain" BOLD data collection in 200–500 ms, depending on the thickness and resolution. Acquiring data at these rates allows one to capture physiologic noise instead of aliasing it into the low-frequency range. Coupled with the concept of multiecho data for T^*_2 mapping and motion rejection [3] and large channel array coils, resting-state data stand to have a tremendous improvement in quality and sensitivity. Furthermore, diffusion data acquisitions will benefit from the ability to better sample diffusion space to provide more data for the diffusion models without commensurately increasing imaging time. This is accomplished by collecting more directions and multiple diffusion weightings (*b*-values) to collect different diffusion shells with significantly reduced repetition times (TRs). Diffusion spectrum imaging acquisitions that took hours could now be reduced to reasonable clinical times of 15 minutes.

With such a flood of data, developments on the analysis side are also occurring. These include the implementation of graphics processing unit (GPU)-based image reconstruction computers to handle the massive amount of data per second coming out of the scanners. Collecting high-resolution datasets requires the ability to automatically sift through them for features or characteristics of disease or plasticity. In this situation, support vector machines and other classifiers have the ability to identify similarities and abnormalities based on training sets. With proper data collection, screening and categorization of subjects, and cooperation between research groups, it will be possible to identify pathologic conditions and at what stage a patient may be at the time of the scan. More importantly, if the imaging data are integrated into patient databases and electronic records, it will be possible to determine the optimal treatment method and timeline tailored to that individual's disease.

In an interesting application of classifiers and data acquisition, a new method of acquiring and reconstructing MR data, called MR Fingerprinting, has been developed [5]. In this case, a set of largely undersampled data are acquired rapidly with a variety of MR contrasts by various sequence types and parameters. Using high-resolution dictionaries, the acquired data are reconstructed to form synthetic models of the subject's brain with whatever contrast one desires. MR Fingerprinting does not require protocoling, previous knowledge of the patient's condition, or long acquisition times. The time of normal clinical examination can be reduced from 40 minutes to less than a minute. Although these scans currently do not have functional information, one can easily imagine that this type of dictionary approach could be applied to connectivity measures in normal and impaired brains to aid in diagnosis and treatment. Combining all of the current hardware advancements and data acquisition strategies has led to the development of MR-encephalography [4]. The hope is that it would combine the temporal resolution of EEG and the spatial resolution of MRI to detect brain activity. It may be possible to take this concept one step further by adding spectroscopic information (measurement of the chemical metabolites in the brain) to the mix. Knowing the alterations in metabolites during rest or when synchronized with a task may provide even more insight on how the brain functions and where it breaks down in the face of disease.

PREDICTIONS FOR FUTURE MR NEUROIMAGING METHODS

Developments in hardware will lead the way to creating smaller imaging systems—not quite the handheld imaging devices promised in science fiction, but something that can easily be used in the general practitioner's office or kiosk-like imaging centres. Key developments will be creating magnetic fields with room temperature–superconducting devices, high-performance magnetic field gradients used to spatially encode the object, and head-only dedicated systems. A possibility is to combine MR Fingerprinting and rapid imaging methods with a pulsed field MR system. In this case, during brief and varying pulses of the magnetic field, different contrasts would be collected. Synthetic images would be reconstructed similarly to the MR Fingerprinting method. The advantages would be immense as one would not need a large static magnetic field, which is dangerous, expensive to operate, and difficult to move. The field generated would be brief and localized so as not to require large amounts of shielding. The system would have the advantages of high magnetic field data collection without the risk of the magnetic field existing for long periods of time. If one were interested in only projections (similar to x-rays) of the object, it would be possible to collect the data without the use of magnetic field gradients, making the implementation easier but the interpretation of the data more difficult. This could be overcome by collecting the data while rotating the device around the object (hand sweeping as in sci-fi) or having the object rotate during multiple acquisitions.

Such advancements in the hardware would allow for the use of MR as a screening tool and brain checkups. The checkup might consist of the rapid resting-state examination where the data are compared with known databases of disease and normal development. Parents would have peace of mind knowing that their children were developing at the correct pace. Utilizing the chemical specificity that MRI/MRS possesses, it would be possible to target imaging data at specific proteins (Chemical Exchange Saturation Transfer [2]) for their concentration or presence to assess biochemical systems. Current off-resonance saturation techniques of magnetization transfer and chemical exchange saturation transfer are capable of isolating specific proteins or molecules to provide concentration information at high spatial resolution. This information would provide metabolic clues about development and aging, as well as the genesis of disease conditions very early to facilitate the proper treatment.

A complex ethical issue will have to be dealt with as MRI technology develops. The issue is related to understanding people's thoughts and intentions through neuroimaging. Current research allows investigators to determine what word or object the participant is thinking about during the imaging session. The dictionary for these studies is currently limited to a few dozen elements; however, the methods are in place to allow the vocabulary to expand exponentially. The "mind reading" techniques are being applied to participants while they sleep and dream. The aim is to provide a movie of the dream state. One could imagine how the use of these methods would allow investigators to know what happened at a crime scene, getting detailed information about a terrorist plot, or having the ability to communicate with a patient who is "locked-in." However, with this ability comes the possibility for abuse (e.g., cheating spouses, employer interviews, scholarships, or grant awards). The advancement of brain imaging and neuroscience will lead to a better understanding of the brain itself; however, there could be serious consequences related to the use of this information. Because of the breadth of fields that these developments could impact, it is critical that researchers are cognizant of the ethical ramifications of their work.

THE IMAGING MACHINE OF THE FUTURE

Like few other body parts, the size and shape of the head and hence the brain are mostly the same across populations. This is not true for anatomy of the chest and abdomen, where there is a wide variety of circumference. Therefore, the concept of a head-only neuroimaging system makes sense. One could envision a high-tech version of the 1950s hairdryer that populated all the beauty salons.

The device would lower down over the head and have a viewing panel at eye level. The system would have at its core a pulsed magnetic field system to generate the main magnetic field as well as the gradient magnetic field for spatial encoding. It would be lightweight and utilize room temperature superconductors for power efficiency. The head coil would be made of a large number of coil arrays to facilitate rapid imaging with high signal to noise. The system may collect data using a sparse/undersampled reconstruction method similar to MR Fingerprinting for diagnostic and structural means. It would switch to a more traditional mode for obtaining resting-state and task-based data to gather information about the connectivity and functioning of the brain. Other modes could assess the metabolic levels, vascular compliance and reactivity (high blood pressure or atherosclerosis), blood–brain barrier integrity, and eye movements.

All data would be included in the individual's medical record, which would have evolved into an application similar to Google Earth for the individual brain, capable of displaying the temporal changes over the lifetime of the individual. All data will be analyzed automatically to generate a report that is uploaded to the physician, psychologist, psychiatrist, and parents, if applicable. If analyzed correctly, other features such as heart rate and blood pressure could be assessed. As a result, MR Neuroimaging will replace the standard blood pressure measure and give a complete picture of the anatomical and functional health of an individual.

REFERENCES

1. Feinberg DA, Moeller S, Smith SM, Auerbach E, Ramanna S, Gunther M, Glasser MF, Miller KL, Ugurbil K, Yacoub E. Multiplexed echo planar imaging for sub-second whole brain fMRI and fast diffusion imaging. PloS One 2010;5(12):e15710.
2. Kogan F, Hariharan H, Reddy R. Chemical Exchange Saturation Transfer (CEST) Imaging: description of technique and potential clinical applications. Curr Radiol Rep 2013;1(2):102–14.
3. Kundu P, Inati SJ, Evans JW, Luh WM, Bandettini PA. Differentiating BOLD and non-BOLD signals in fMRI time series using multi-echo EPI. NeuroImage 2012;60(3):1759–70.
4. Lee HL, Zahneisen B, Hugger T, LeVan P, Hennig J. Tracking dynamic resting-state networks at higher frequencies using MR-encephalography. NeuroImage 2013;65:216–22.
5. Ma D, Gulani V, Seiberlich N, Liu K, Sunshine JL, Duerk JL, Griswold MA. Magnetic resonance fingerprinting. Nature 2013;495(7440):187–92.

INDEX

Note: Page numbers followed by "*f*" and "*t*" denote figures and tables, respectively.

D

Q

R

S